# Nutrition Assessment

## Clinical and Research Applications

# Nutrition Assessment

## Clinical and Research Applications

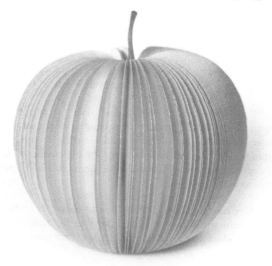

**Nancy Munoz, DCN, MHA, RDN, FAND**

Assistant Chief, Food and Nutrition Service
VA Southern Nevada Healthcare System
North Las Vegas, Nevada
Lecturer
University of Massachusetts, Amherst

**Melissa Bernstein, PhD, RD, LD, FAND**

Assistant Professor
Chicago Medical School
North Chicago, Illinois

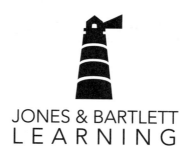

JONES & BARTLETT
LEARNING

*World Headquarters*
Jones & Bartlett Learning
5 Wall Street
Burlington, MA 01803
978-443-5000
info@jblearning.com
www.jblearning.com

Jones & Bartlett Learning books and products are available through most bookstores and online booksellers. To contact Jones & Bartlett Learning directly, call 800-832-0034, fax 978-443-8000, or visit our website, www.jblearning.com.

Substantial discounts on bulk quantities of Jones & Bartlett Learning publications are available to corporations, professional associations, and other qualified organizations. For details and specific discount information, contact the special sales department at Jones & Bartlett Learning via the above contact information or send an email to specialsales@jblearning.com.

13787-3

**Production Credits**
VP, Product Management: David D. Cella
Director of Product Management: Cathy L. Esperti
Product Manager: Sean Fabery
Product Specialist: Taylor Maurice
Director of Vendor Management: Amy Rose
Vendor Manager: Juna Abrams
Director of Marketing: Andrea DeFronzo
VP, Manufacturing and Inventory Control: Therese Connell
Composition: SourceHOV LLC
Project Management: SourceHOV LLC

Cover Design: Kristin E. Parker
Director of Rights & Media: Joanna Gallant
Rights & Media Specialist: Merideth Tumasz
Media Development Editor: Shannon Sheehan
Cover Image, Title Page: © Robert Bray/Getty Images
Part Opener, Chapter Opener Image: © SunnyChinchilla/Shutterstock
Printing and Binding: Edwards Brothers Malloy
Cover Printing: Edwards Brothers Malloy

**Library of Congress Cataloging-in-Publication Data**

Names: Munoz, Nancy, editor. | Bernstein, Melissa, editor.
Title: Nutrition assessment : clinical and research applications / [edited by] Nancy Munoz and Melissa Bernstein.
Other titles: Nutrition assessment (Munoz)
Description: Burlington, MA : Jones & Barlett Learning, [2019] | Includes bibliographical references and index.
Identifiers: LCCN 2017045352 | ISBN 9781284127669 (paperback : alk. paper)
Subjects: | MESH: Nutrition Assessment | Biomedical Research
Classification: LCC R853.C55 | NLM QU 146.1 | DDC 610.72/4–dc23 LC record available at https://lccn.loc.gov/2017045352

6048

Printed in the United States of America
23 22 21 20 19    10 9 8 7 6 5 4 3 2

*To Pedro, Peter, and Samantha Munoz:*

*You three are my "North, my South, my East, and West,*
*My working week and my Sunday rest;*
*My noon, my midnight, my talk, my song;*
*My everything!"*
*(Based on a poem by W.H. Auden)*

**–Nancy Munoz**

---

*To my family—with all my love.*

**–Melissa Bernstein**

# Brief Contents

# Contents

# Foreword

Nutrition is a topic of growing interest for individuals, health science students and professionals, researchers, healthcare think tanks, international health organizations, and government agencies. It is the basis of well-being from before birth to the end of life. Over the course of a life span, good nutrition equips the body to grow and develop to its full potential. Good nutrition serves as the foundation for effective learning at school and as preparation for a productive adulthood. It is essential for a robust immune system to ward off infections and diseases throughout the life cycle. Good nutrition builds and maintains the body on bedrock, while poor nutrition builds and attempts to maintain the body on shifting sands.

Improving the nutrition status of individuals is one of the most cost-effective investments for improving health outcomes and reducing healthcare costs, yet research on measuring the contributions of nutrition in terms of the aforementioned outcomes and costs is limited. Quantifying the population's needs for nutrition will require high-quality, evidence-based research and a data revolution in order to fill the gaps and prioritize the most effective actions to improve outcomes and reduce costs. It will require researchers to focus on two broad concepts. First, they will need to quantify what really counts as a measure of current and improving nutrition status, recognizing that some outcomes are readily visible and others are not clearly apparent. Second, they will need to identify what we are counting as metrics of improved nutrition status that lack sufficient sensitivity to measure changes.

As health sciences students, you have the opportunity to participate in health- and nutrition-related research to quantify the nutrition needs of populations and to develop measurement tools to demonstrate the valuable role that nutrition plays. As emerging leaders in the health sciences, you have the additional responsibility to communicate the role of nutrition as measured by high-quality research, with the findings of this research used to identify priority areas, set target goals, and establish actions for change.

Some nutrition programs will be more successful than others in improving healthcare outcomes and/or reducing healthcare costs. The less effective program outcomes give the trained professional an opportunity to use critical thinking skills to examine the root cause of disappointing outcomes and to develop stronger, more robust nutrition programs. It is through accurate assessment and evidence-based research that we can develop validated tools to differentiate definitive versus tentative relationships between nutrition and healthcare outcomes.

As a national or international nutrition advocate, you can use your academic training to shape not only your career but also the future health status of individuals living in the developed and developing world. Using *Nutrition Assessment: Clinical and Research Applications* as your guide, commit to developing and supporting the research-based innovations that are needed to meet the joint challenges of improving the lives of current and future generations.

*Mary Litchford, PhD, RDN, LDN*
*President, CASE Software & Books*

# Preface

Welcome to *Nutrition Assessment: Clinical and Research Applications*!

Almost half of all Americans have one or more preventable chronic diseases. Many chronic illnesses such as cardiovascular disease, hypertension, type 2 diabetes, some cancers, and poor bone health are related to poor eating habits and low levels of physical activity. In the United States, more than two-thirds of adults and approximately one-third of children and youth are overweight or obese, which is itself an underlying risk factor for chronic poor health. Nutrition scientists conduct research to elucidate how preventing and treating malnutrition, and considering both under- and over-nutrition, can promote better health outcomes for patients, clients, and communities.

This text is written for students in nutrition and health sciences programs and those involved in nutrition-related exploration. It is especially designed to meet the needs of nutrition researchers and students enrolled in masters and PhD courses in Nutrition and Dietetics, Public Health, Interprofessional Studies, and Population Health Science and Wellness programs. As such, it covers topics applicable and relevant to nutrition and health practitioners and those with advanced degrees, with a broad background in public health and advanced training in public health nutrition research. Complex topics are broken down into major key components to promote student understanding and build their practical knowledge base.

## ▶ The Goal of this Text

Evaluating the nutrition status of different segments of the population helps in measuring the prevalence of nutritional disorders and also in planning counteractive strategies. Our goal in writing this text was to provide nutrition and public health researchers and students with the knowledge and skills to identify nutrition problems and to develop research questions and study hypotheses. This text provides insights into planning community, clinical, and individual applications of nutrition prevention and treatments,

as well as provides fundamentals for critically evaluating published scientific research. We have written this text with the presumption that an understanding of government programs and a familiarity with the demographic profile of the U.S. population are necessary in order to appreciate nutrition in public health today.

The focus of this text is to help students select and use appropriate anthropometric, biochemical, clinical, dietary, functional, and socioeconomic assessment techniques to identify and prioritize the nutritional problems and needs of populations and communities. The contributors outline intervention strategies to guide students through the process of improving nutritional problems in target populations while also using critical thinking skills in evaluating the available literature.

## ▶ The Organization of this Text

This text is divided into six sections. The first section serves as an introduction, which provides historical perspective, as well as an overview of scientific and nutritional research. The next four sections address the different components of nutritional assessment: dietary, anthropometric, biochemical, and clinical. The final section concludes with an exploration of public health topics such as population wellness, coaching, nutrition interventions, and international research. Each chapter is enhanced with an array of learning feature.

## ▶ Features and Benefits

*Nutrition Assessment: Clinical and Research Applications* incorporates robust pedagogical features. These are deployed consistently across chapters, ensuring a uniform learning experience for the student and the reader.

Each chapter begins with a brief *Chapter Outline* and a series of *Learning Objectives*; together, these define expectations for each chapter. In that same vein, each section within each chapter begins with a *Preview* statement, which is, in turn, mirrored by a summarizing *Recap* statement at the end of the section.

Within the chapters, there are three recurring boxed features:

- *Viewpoint* is written from the perspective of a nutrition professional and highlights how the chapter content impacts his or her work. This feature is designed to be conversational and is meant to spur a discussion around the topic as it appears in practice.
- *Highlight* presents interesting topics pulled from current research in the nutritional sciences.
- A *Case Study* appears toward the end of each chapter and illustrates how topics discussed in the text can be applied in practice.

Each chapter concludes with a *Learning Portfolio*, which contains the following:

- Key Terms
- Study Questions
- Discussion Questions

- Activities
- Online Resources

## ▶ The Complete Learning Package

*Nutrition Assessment: Clinical and Research Applications* provides instructors with a full suite of resources, including:

- Test Bank, containing more than 500 questions
- Slides in PowerPoint format, featuring more than 300 slides
- Image Bank, collecting photographs and illustrations that appear in the text
- Instructor's Manual, including a number of educational tools:
  - Chapter Outlines
  - Answers to in-text Study Questions
  - Answers to in-text Case Studies

*Nancy Munoz*                    *Melissa Bernstein*

# The Pedagogy

*Nutrition Assessment: Clinical and Research Applications* incorporates an array of pedagogical features in order to facilitate active engagement.

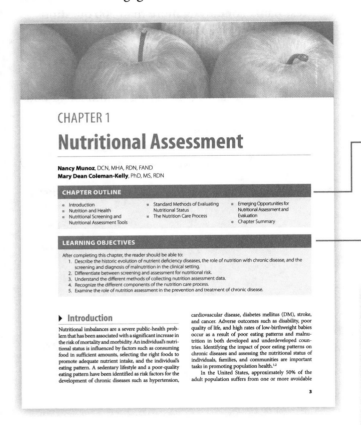

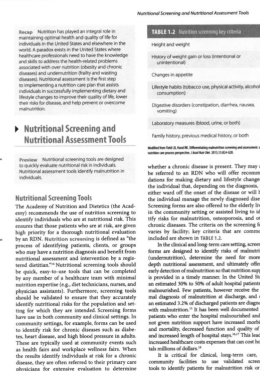

The **Chapter Outline** at the beginning of each chapter gives students a preview of topics that will be covered.

**Learning Objectives** focus students on the key concepts of each chapter and the material that they will learn.

Each section begins with a **Preview** statement, giving the reader a sense of what content to expect.

**Key Terms** are in boldface type the first time they are mentioned, with definitions appearing in the end-of-text Glossary.

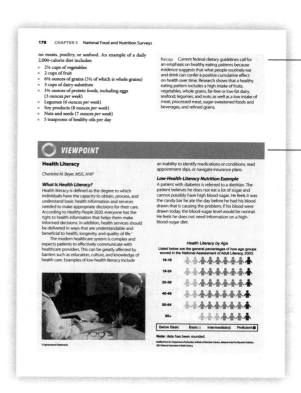

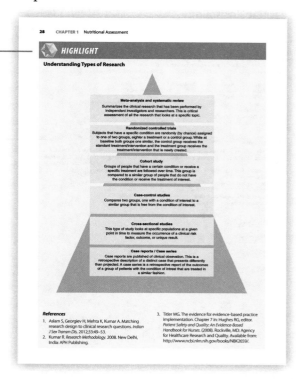

**Recap** boxes summarize each section.

Each **Viewpoint** feature is written by a nutrition professional and notes how the chapter content impacts his or her work.

**Highlight** presents topics of interest from current research literature.

At least one **Case Study** appears toward the end of each chapter and illustrates how topics discussed in the text might appear in practice.

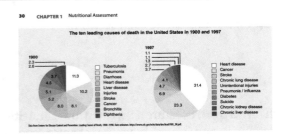

The ten leading causes of death in the United States in 1900 and 1997

## Learning Portfolio

### Key Terms

Anthropometry
Body mass index (BMI)
Bureau of Labor Statistics Consumer expenditure
survey data
Epidemiology
Food and Agriculture Organization of the United
Nations (FAO)
Healthy People 2020 (HP 2020)
Interprofessional
Nutrition assessment
Nutrition Care Process (NCP)

Nutrition Care Process Terminology (NCPT)
Nutrition Care Process and Model (NCPM)
Nutrition diagnosis
Nutrition-focused physical exam (NFPE)
Nutrition intervention
Nutrition screening
PES statement
Scurvy
Subjective global assessment (SGA)
Tumors

### Study Questions

1. The key difference between a nutrition-screening form and a nutrition-assessment form is:
   a. Screening forms provide a diagnosis for malnutrition
   b. Screening forms determine risk for malnutrition
   c. Screening forms diagnose chronic disease
   d. Screening forms determine risk for weight gain

2. The Academy of Nutrition and Dietetics recommends using the _____ screening form to assess risk for malnutrition in the adults in the clinical setting.
   a. MUST
   b. SNAQ
   c. Mini SNAQ
   d. Mini MUST

Each chapter concludes with a **Learning Portfolio**, which is an array of student-centered resources and activities.

The Learning Portfolio collects a comprehensive list of **Key Terms** specific to the chapter.

**Study Questions** provide multiple-choice and true/false questions, testing the reader's knowledge of information covered in the chapter. These can be used for self-assessment or as homework assignments; answers are included in the Instructor's Manual.

---

30. The most reliable indicator of poor nutritional status is:
    a. Weight loss
    b. Low albumin concentrations
    c. Low dietary intake of nutrients
    d. Poor handgrip strength

### Discussion Questions

1. How does the obesity rate affect the incidence of chronic disease in the United States?
2. Describe the shift from infectious disease to chronic disease that affects public health.

3. Nutrition screens allow individuals who are at risk of suboptimal nutritional status to be identified. List and describe the most commonly used screening tools. What are the benefits and drawbacks of each screening tool?

### Activities

1. Develop a marketing campaign targeting a specific segment of the community you live or study in that introduces population-based intervention strategies to reduce obesity and impact overall health.
2. Type 2 diabetes is widespread in all obese groups and now even in preteen children. Develop an education tool to teach young children the health risks associated with diabetes.

3. Select a chronic condition that is prevalent in the American population. Work with three to four classmates to develop "the top 10 must know topics" by the average person in efforts to prevent or manage the disease. Develop a wiki page to communicate the information. Use videos and graphics on the page to deliver the message.

### Online Resources

**Food and Agriculture Organization (FAO) of the United Nations**

The FAO develops methods and standards for food and agriculture statistics, provides technical assistance services, and disseminates data for global monitoring. It is the world's largest database of food and agriculture statistics:
http://www.fao.org/statistics/en/.

**Bureau of Labor Statistics Consumer Expenditure Survey Data**

This database provides information on the buying habits of American consumers, including data on their expenditures, income, and consumer unit (families and single consumers) characteristics:
http://www.bls.gov/cex/.

**Anthropometric Measurement Videos**

This website provides technical videos on how to conduct anthropometric measures:
https://wwwn.cdc.gov/nchs/nhanes/nhanes3/anthropometricvideos.aspx.

**The State of Obesity: Adults in the United States**

This website provides interactive maps on adult obesity in the United States:
http://stateofobesity.org/adult-obesity/.

**Malnutrition Universal Screening Tool (MUST)**

This website provides the background for the MUST tool, online calculator, and videos.
http://www.bapen.org.uk/screening-and-must/must.

**Mini Nutritional Assessment Tool (MNA)**

This website provides an overview of the MNA tool and videos and provides access to the required forms:
http://www.mna-elderly.com/.

### References

1. Herder R, Demmig-Adams B. The power of a balanced diet and lifestyle in preventing cardiovascular disease. *Nutr Clin Care.* 2004;7:46-55.

2. Price S. Understanding the importance to health of a balanced diet. *Nurs Times.* 2005;2005;101:30.

**Discussion Questions** provide prompts for greater engagement with the content.

Suggested **Activities** provide additional interactive avenues for grappling with the chapter content.

**Online Resources** direct students to additional materials relevant to the content.

# About the Authors

**Nancy Munoz, DCN, MHA, RD, FAND** holds a doctorate in clinical nutrition from Rutgers State University of New Jersey (previously known as the University of Medicine and Dentistry of New Jersey), a master's degree in healthcare administration from the University of Maryland, and a bachelor's degree in food and nutrition from Marymount College in Tarrytown, New York. She is a registered dietitian nutritionist and a member, as well as a Fellow, of the Academy of Nutrition and Dietetics.

While guiding the practice of registered dietitian nutritionists in the care of older adults has defined Dr. Munoz's career, she has also been caring for veterans who have served our nation as the Assistant Chief for Nutrition and Food Services at the VA Southern Nevada Healthcare System since 2015. She is involved in the development, communication, and implementation of effective and efficient clinical nutrition protocols to guide compliance to assessment and foodservice standards.

Since 2009, Dr. Munoz has been a lecturer at the University of Massachusetts, Amherst campus for the Masters in Public Health program. Teaching the Nutritional Assessment course for this institution helped inspire the development of this text, as Dr. Munoz wanted a resource with a fresh approach to teaching students the different methods that can be applied to addressing nutrition questions in diverse research situations.

Dr. Munoz has contributed to and authored numerous textbook chapters and peer-reviewed journal articles on the topics of nutrition for older adults, pressure injuries, and clinical nutrition. She coauthored *Nutrition for the Older Adult*, also published by Jones & Bartlett Learning.

**Melissa Bernstein, PhD, RD, LD, FAND** is a registered dietitian nutritionist, licensed dietitian, and Fellow of the Academy of Nutrition and Dietetics. She received her doctoral degree from the Gerald J. and Dorothy R. Friedman School of Nutrition Science and Policy at Tufts University (Boston, Massachusetts). As an Assistant Professor in the Department of Nutrition at Chicago Medical School, Dr. Bernstein is innovative in creating engaging and challenging nutrition courses. Her interests include introductory nutrition, health and wellness, geriatric nutrition, physical activity, and nutritional biochemistry. In addition to co-authoring leading nutrition textbooks—including *Nutrition, Discovering Nutrition, Nutrition Across Life Stages,* and *Nutrition for the Older Adult*—Dr. Bernstein has reviewed and authored textbook chapters, position statements, and peer-reviewed journal articles on the topics of nutrition and nutrition for older adults. She is the co-author of the *Position of the Academy of Nutrition and Dietetics: Food and Nutrition for Older Adults: Promoting Health and Wellness*. She serves on review and advisory committees for the Academy's Evidence Analysis Library and as a reviewer for upcoming position statements.

# Acknowledgments

This book would not have been possible without the guidance, contributions, and support of so many people. We are grateful for the support of Robin Dahm, RDN, LDN, throughout the project. Her attention to detail and dedication to the success of this project were invaluable. We are fortunate to have Robin's expertise in creating the instructor resources that accompany this book.

We would also like to thank everyone at Jones & Bartlett Learning who helped make this text a reality. Starting with Sean Fabery, Product Manager, who guided the project from inception to completion; along with Taylor Maurice, Product Specialist; Juna Abrams, Vendor Manager; Indraneil Dey, Project Manager for SourceHOV; Merideth Tumasz, Rights & Media Specialist; Shannon Sheehan, Media Development Editor; and Andrea DeFronzo, Director of Marketing.

To all of the contributors who shared their knowledge and expertise in this manuscript, we could not have done the project without each and every one of you. Thank you to our colleagues for their guidance, support, and contributions to our academic growth. We also express thanks to our past, present, and future students, from whom we continually learn and who inspire projects such as this one.

Thanks also to the reviewers who contributed their feedback and knowledge to truly help make this a better text.

Finally, to our families, we are profoundly thankful for all of the love, support, reassurance, and patience that you give us.

# Contributors

## ▶ Chapters

**Mary Beth Arensberg, PhD, RDN, LDN, FAND**
Director of Health Policy and Programs
Abbott Nutrition
Columbus, Ohio
Chapter 12

**Melissa Bernstein, PhD, RD, LD, FAND**
Assistant Professor
Department of Nutrition
Chicago Medical School
North Chicago, Illinois
Chapter 2

**Ashley L. Bronston, MS, RDN, LD**
Independent Nutrition Consultant
Columbus, Ohio
Chapter 12

**Chimene Castor, EdD, RDN, LDN, FAND, CHES**
Assistant Professor
Department of Nutritional Sciences
Howard University
Washington, D.C.
Chapter 10

**Karen Chapman-Novakofski, PhD, RDN**
Professor
Department of Food Science & Human Nutrition
University of Illinois at Urbana-Champaign
Urbana, Illinois
Chapter 11

**Mary Dean Coleman-Kelly, PhD, MS, RDN**
Assistant Professor
Department of Nutritional Sciences
The Pennsylvania State University
University Park, Pennsylvania
Chapter 1

**Dwight L. Davidson, PhD, LMHC**
Health Faculty
West Chester University
West Chester, Pennsylvania
Chapter 7

**Patricia Davidson, DCN, RDN, CDE, LDN, FAND**
Assistant Professor
Department of Nutrition
West Chester University
West Chester, Pennsylvania
Chapter 7

**Johanna T. Dwyer, DSc, RD**
Professor of Medicine (Nutrition) and Community
    Health
Tufts University Medical School
Professor
Tufts University Friedman School of Nutrition
    Science and Policy
Senior Scientist
Jean Mayer USDA Human Nutrition Research Center
    on Aging at Tufts University
Boston, Massachusetts
Senior Nutrition Scientist
Office of Dietary Supplements
National Institutes of Health
Bethesda, Maryland
Chapter 12

**Elizabeth Eilender, MS, RD, CDN**
Adjunct Professor
BSN Program
Saint Peter's University
Jersey City, New Jersey
Chapter 5

**Phyllis J. Famularo, DCN, RD, CSG, LDN, FAND**
Senior Manager, Nutrition Services
Sodexo
Gaithersburg, Maryland
Chapter 9

**Ana María Hernández Rosa, MS, RDN, LD**
Outpatient Clinical Dietitian-Renal Dietitian
University Health System
San Antonio, Texas
Chapter 2

**Francisco José Rosales Herrera, MD, ScD**
Medical Director, Research and Development
Abbott Nutrition
Columbus, Ohio
Chapter 12

**Nava Livne, PhD, MS**
Chapter 4

**Nancy Munoz, DCN, MHA, RDN, FAND**
Lecturer
Masters in Public Health Program
University of Massachusetts Amherst
Amherst, Massachusetts
Assistant Chief, Nutrition and Food Service
VA Southern Nevada Healthcare System
North Las Vegas, Nevada
Chapters 1 and 8

**Oyonumo E. Ntekim, PhD, MD, MDSA**
Assistant Professor
Department of Nutritional Sciences
Howard University
Washington, D.C.
Chapter 10

**Jessica Pearl, MS, RD, CSSD, CSCS, CLT, CDN, FAND**
Registered Dietitian
JPearl Nutrition
New York, New York
Chapter 3

**Diane Rigassio Radler, PhD, RD**
Associate Professor
Department of Nutritional Sciences
Rutgers, The State University of New Jersey
Newark, New Jersey
Chapter 11

**Lona Sandon, PhD, MEd, RDN**
Program Director and Assistant Professor
Department of Clinical Nutrition
UT Southwestern Medical Center
Dallas, Texas
Chapter 6

**Crystal L. Wynn, PhD, MPH, RD**
Assistant Professor and Dietetic Internship Director
Department of Family and Consumer Sciences
Virginia State University
Petersburg, Virginia
Chapter 4

## ▶ Viewpoint Contributors

**Charlotte M. Beyer, MSIS, AHIP**
Instruction and Reference Librarian
Rosalind Franklin University of Medicine and Science
North Chicago, Illinois
Chapter 5 Viewpoint: "Health Literacy"

**Diane R. Bridges, PhD, MSN, RN, CCM**
Associate Dean of Interprofessional and Distance
    Education
Associate Professor
Chicago Medical School
Rosalind Franklin University of Medicine and Science
North Chicago, Illinois
Chapter 2 Viewpoint: "Interprofessional Healthcare
    Teams"
Chapter 4 Viewpoint: "Determinants of Health
    and Their Impact on Obesity"

**Robin B. Dahm, RDN, LDN**
Freelance Technical Editor
Moab, Utah
Chapter 7 Viewpoint: "BMI: The Weight Categories
    for Older Adults Are Different"
Chapter 10 Viewpoint: "Easy Targets: Marketing Junk
    Food to Children"

**Deidra Devereaux, MS, RDN**
Clinical Nutrition Manager
Department of Veterans Affairs
Las Vegas, Nevada
Chapter 11 Viewpoint: "Building Motivational
    Interviewing Skills"

**Randi S. Drasin, MS, RDN**
Registered Dietitian Nutritionist
Brandman Centers for Senior Care
Reseda, California
Chapter 6 Viewpoint: "Apps"
Chapter 12 Viewpoint: "Cultural Competency"

Lauren Grosskopf, MS
Senior Scientist, Research & Development
Kraft Heinz Company
Glenview, Illinois
Chapter 3 Viewpoint: "Product Development
  Process"

Linda S. Eck Mills, MBA, RDN, LDN, FADA
Owner
Dynamic Communication Services
Bernville, Pennsylvania
Chapter 3 Viewpoint: "Food Service Perspectives"

Robin S. Rood, MA, MEd, RD, LD
Owner
Rood Nutrition Counseling
South Russell, Ohio
Chapter 1 Viewpoint: "Health Initiatives"
Chapter 10 Viewpoint: "Nutrition Policies and
  Politics"
Chapter 11 Viewpoint: "Health and Nutrition Blogs"

Ari S. Rubinoff
Executive Chef
Cincinnati, Ohio
Chapter 8 Viewpoint: "Nutrition and a Professional
  Chef"

J. Scott Thomson, MS, MLIS, AHIP
Library Director
Rosalind Franklin University of Medicine
  and Science
North Chicago, Illinois
Chapter 9 Viewpoint: "Predatory Publishing"

# Reviewers

**Dorothy Chen-Maynard, PhD, RDN, FAND**
Program Director, Didactic Program in Dietetics
Department of Health Science and Human Ecology
California State University, San Bernardino
San Bernardino, California

**Diane L. Habash, PhD, MS, RDN, LD**
Clinical Associate Professor
College of Medicine
The Ohio State University
Columbus, Ohio

**Laura Horn, MEd, RD, LD**
Professor
Cincinnati State Technical and Community College
Cincinnati, Ohio

**Andrea M. Hutchins, PhD, RD, FAND**
Associate Professor
Department of Health Sciences
University of Colorado, Colorado Springs
Colorado Springs, Colorado

**Louise E. Schneider, DrPH, RD**
Associate Professor, Retired
Nutrition and Dietetics
Loma Linda University
Loma Linda, California

**Claudia Sealey-Potts, PhD, RD, LDN, FAND**
Associate Professor and Dietetic Internship Director
Department of Nutrition and Dietetics
University of North Florida
Jacksonville, Florida

**Jennifer Tomesko, DCN, RD, CNSC**
Assistant Professor
Department of Nutritional Sciences
Rutgers, The State University of New Jersey
Newark, New Jersey

We would also like to offer a special thanks to the 2016–2017 dietetic interns from the Virginia State University dietetic internship program in Petersburg, Virginia, for participating in the literature review included in Chapter 4:

- Anna Arnett
- Meredith Bowers
- Katelyn Cianelli
- Kiersten Llewellyn
- Kate Lalancette
- Mary Obielodan
- Amber Porter
- Kierra Wilkins

# SECTION 1
# Introduction

© Robert Bray / Getty Images

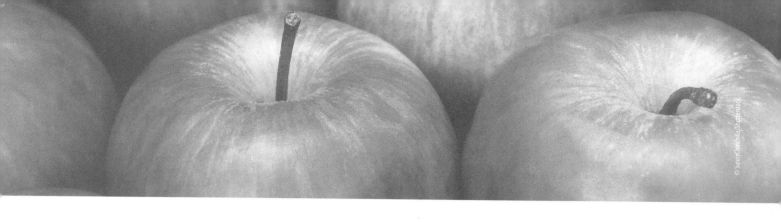

# CHAPTER 1

# Nutritional Assessment

**Nancy Munoz**, DCN, MHA, RDN, FAND
**Mary Dean Coleman-Kelly**, PhD, MS, RDN

## CHAPTER OUTLINE

- Introduction
- Nutrition and Health
- Nutritional Screening and Nutritional Assessment Tools
- Standard Methods of Evaluating Nutritional Status
- The Nutrition Care Process
- Emerging Opportunities for Nutritional Assessment and Evaluation
- Chapter Summary

## LEARNING OBJECTIVES

After completing this chapter, the reader should be able to:
1. Describe the historic evolution of nutrient deficiency diseases, the role of nutrition with chronic disease, and the screening and diagnosis of malnutrition in the clinical setting.
2. Differentiate between screening and assessment for nutritional risk.
3. Understand the different methods of collecting nutrition assessment data.
4. Recognize the different components of the nutrition care process.
5. Examine the role of nutrition assessment in the prevention and treatment of chronic disease.

## ▶ Introduction

Nutritional imbalances are a severe public-health problem that has been associated with a significant increase in the risk of mortality and morbidity. An individual's nutritional status is influenced by factors such as consuming food in sufficient amounts, selecting the right foods to promote adequate nutrient intake, and the individual's eating pattern. A sedentary lifestyle and a poor-quality eating pattern have been identified as risk factors for the development of chronic diseases such as hypertension, cardiovascular disease, diabetes mellitus (DM), stroke, and cancer. Adverse outcomes such as disability, poor quality of life, and high rates of low-birthweight babies occur as a result of poor eating patterns and malnutrition in both developed and underdeveloped countries. Identifying the impact of poor eating patterns on chronic diseases and assessing the nutritional status of individuals, families, and communities are important tasks in promoting population health.[1,2]

In the United States, approximately 50% of the adult population suffers from one or more avoidable

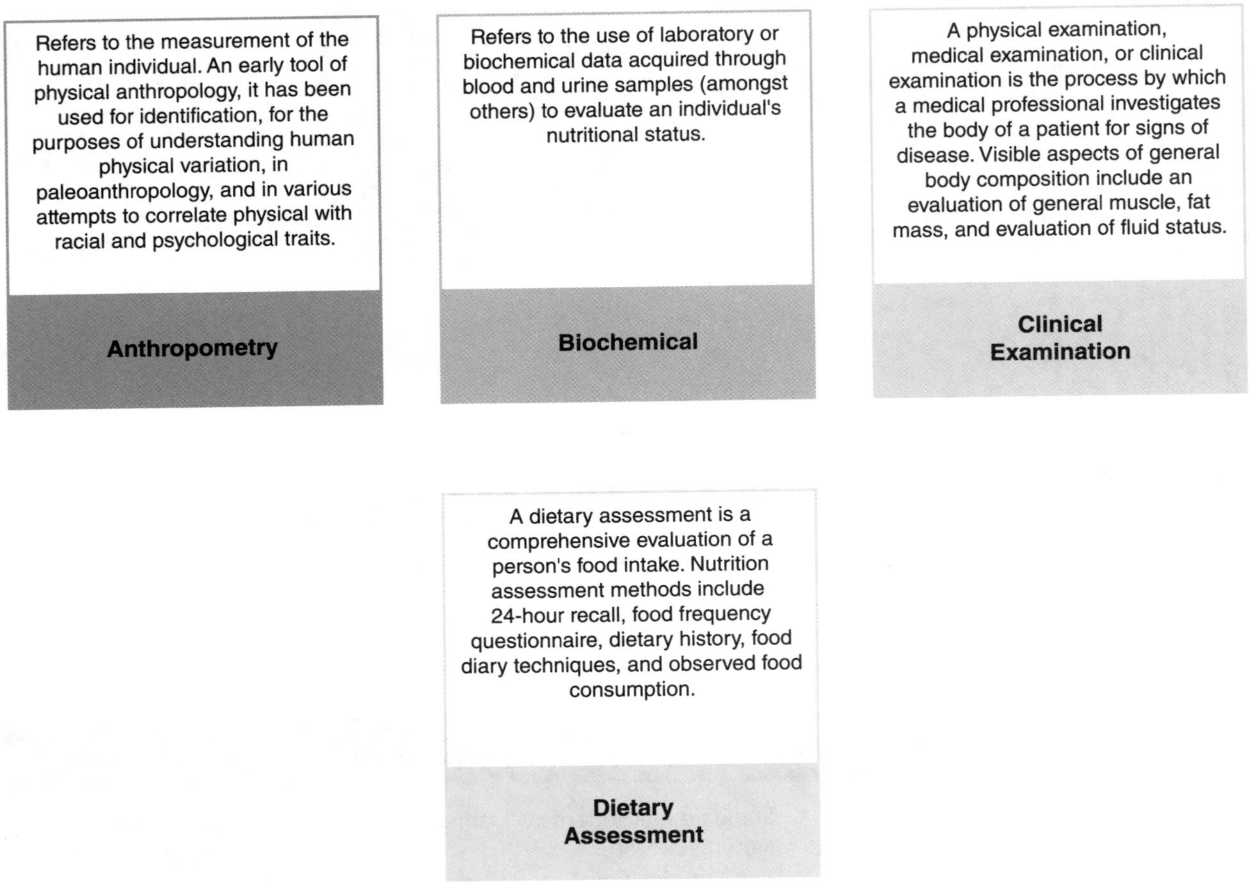

| | | |
|---|---|---|
| Refers to the measurement of the human individual. An early tool of physical anthropology, it has been used for identification, for the purposes of understanding human physical variation, in paleoanthropology, and in various attempts to correlate physical with racial and psychological traits. | Refers to the use of laboratory or biochemical data acquired through blood and urine samples (amongst others) to evaluate an individual's nutritional status. | A physical examination, medical examination, or clinical examination is the process by which a medical professional investigates the body of a patient for signs of disease. Visible aspects of general body composition include an evaluation of general muscle, fat mass, and evaluation of fluid status. |
| **Anthropometry** | **Biochemical** | **Clinical Examination** |

A dietary assessment is a comprehensive evaluation of a person's food intake. Nutrition assessment methods include 24-hour recall, food frequency questionnaire, dietary history, food diary techniques, and observed food consumption.

**Dietary Assessment**

**FIGURE 1.1** ABCDs of nutritional assessment

chronic disease. More than two-thirds of adults and approximately one-thirds of children and youth are overweight or obese. These extreme rates of overweight, obesity, and chronic disease have been a public-health concern for more than two decades and contribute not only to increased health risks but also to associated high medical costs.[3] In 2008, the medical costs connected with obesity were assessed at $147 billion. In 2012, the total estimated cost of diagnosed diabetes was $245 billion, including $176 billion in direct medical costs and $69 billion in decreased productivity.[4]

The evaluation of the nutrition status of different segments of the population helps in measuring the prevalence of nutritional disorders, and also to plan counteractive strategies (see **FIGURE 1.1**).

## ▶ Nutrition and Health

**Preview** Nutritional assessment is the first step to identify nutrition-related problems that arise from nutrient deficiency and lead to chronic disease or result in malnutrition.

## Nutrient Deficiency Diseases: A Historical Perspective

Good health and quality of life are desired by all individuals living in a society. Access to safe drinking water, nutritious food, and quality medical care are essential to the well-being of any person. Undernutrition and hunger are prevalent in underdeveloped as well as developed countries. An estimated 870 million adults and children worldwide have inadequate food intakes.[5] Chronic undernutrition leads to the onset of deficiency diseases, and physical signs of such diseases emerge when the intake of essential nutrients is inadequate and prolonged.

Keen observations by physicians in the early 1700s identified that in some instances the cause of human illness was related to the absence of certain foods; they proposed that those foods contained specific compounds whose absence led to the signs and symptoms of disease. One of the earliest known discoveries of the curative effects of foods with deficiency diseases was by Scottish physician James Lind in the mid-1700s. British sailors taking long voyages were developing **scurvy** and becoming severely ill or dying on the voyage. Observational research has progressed over time to the current

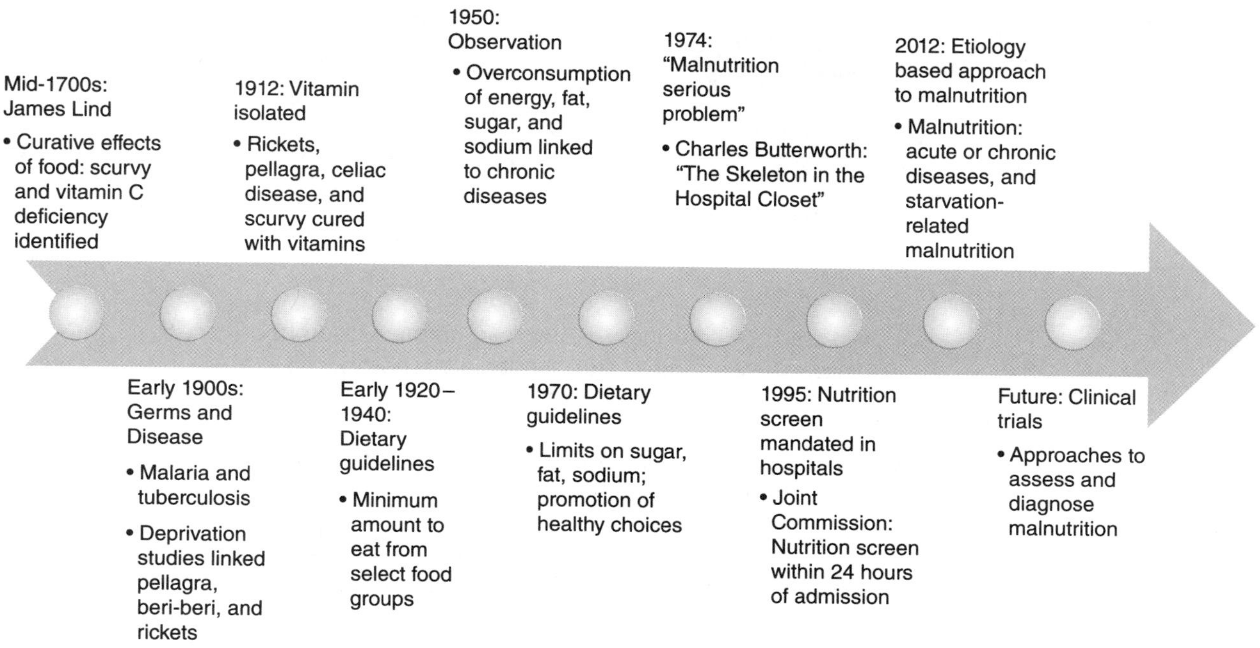

**FIGURE 1.2** Nutrition and health: A historical perspective

Data from Rosenfeld, L. (1997). "Vitamine—vitamin. The early years of discovery". *Clin Chem.* 43 (4): 680–5. Semba R. The Discovery of Vitamins. *Int J Vitamin Nutrition Research.* 2012;5:310-315. Funk C. The etiology of the deficiency diseases. Beri-beri, polynueritis in birds, epidemic dropsy, scurvy, experience scurvy in animals, infantile scurvy, ship beri-beri, pellagra. *J State Med.* 1912;20:341. Davis C, Saltos E. *Dietary Recommendations and How They Have Changed Over Time.* Ch. 2. America's Eating Habits: Changes and Consequences. http://purl.umn.edu/33604. Accessed January 24, 2017. Butterworth C. The Skeleton in the Hospital Closet. *Nutrition Today* 1974;March/April:436. Dougherty D, et al. Nutrition care given new importance in JCAHO standards. *Nutr Clin Pract.* 1995;10(1):26-31. White JV, Guenter P, Jensen G, et al. Consensus Statement: Academy of Nutrition and Dietetics and American Society for Parenteral and Enteral Nutrition: Characteristics Recommended for the Identification and Documentation of Adult Malnutrition (Undernutrition). *Journal of Parenteral and Enteral Nutrition.* 2012;36(3):275-283.

dietary guidelines. **FIGURE 1.2** shows a short historic timeline of nutrition and health.[6,7]

## Leading Causes of Death and Chronic Diseases

The interest in modifying diet to prevent chronic disease in Americans began when deficiency diseases and infectious diseases were eradicated. In addition, the implementation of government-mandated enrichment and fortification of food staples and the use of vaccinations to reduce deaths from infectious diseases also contributed to increased awareness of the American diet.[8]

**TABLE 1.1** ranks the 10 leading causes of death in the United States today. Four of the ten—heart disease, cancer, stroke, and diabetes mellitus[9]—are linked to diet and either can be prevented or have their onsets delayed by implementing healthy eating practices and making positive lifestyle choices.

Nutritionists today are challenged to find the optimal food pattern and nutrient profile that will optimize the quality of life and prevent chronic disease for their clients. Conducting nutritional assessment in the community setting is important when identifying early risks for chronic disease. Novel approaches such as evaluating the genetic profile of individuals to identify genetic determinates that lead to chronic disease

are being researched as a potential added "tool" that registered dietitian nutritionists (RDNs) can use along with traditional assessment measures. Understanding genomics in relationship to nutritional management of complex diseases is in its infancy, so routine genetic testing to provide dietary advice is not ready for practical application. The prospect for using nutritional genomics in the future, however, is exciting. It has the potential to offer RDNs and healthcare professionals the tools to create "genetically" personalized diet plans that are specific to any individual's genetic makeup.

## History of Diagnosing Malnutrition in the Clinical Setting

Identifying malnutrition and offering nutrition support to malnourished patients is relatively new in the clinical setting. In 1974, Dr. Charles Butterworth wrote a landmark paper, "The Skeleton in the Hospital Closet," in which he exposed malnutrition in the hospital as a serious problem.[10] In 1995, the Joint Commission (a US nonprofit healthcare accrediting organization), working with input from the American Society of Clinical Nutrition and the American Dietetic Association (now the Academy of Nutrition and Dietetics), created the standard requirement that hospitals provide a nutrition screening of each patient within 24 hours of admission.[11] Although this requirement offered a

**TABLE 1.1** Leading causes of death in the United States

| Rank | Disease | Contributing Risk Factors | Number of Deaths Annually |
|------|---------|---------------------------|---------------------------|
| 1 | Heart disease | Increasing age, family history, smoking, poor-quality diet, obesity, hypertension, increased cholesterol, stress, physical inactivity | 614,348 |
| 2 | Cancer | Increased age, smoking, excessive consumption of alcohol, excessive exposure to sun, obesity, family history, presence of some chronic conditions such as ulcerative colitis | 591,699 |
| 3 | Chronic lower-respiratory diseases | Exposure to tobacco smoke, chemicals, dust and burning fuel; advanced age and genetics | 147,101 |
| 4 | Accidents (unintentional injuries) | Motor-vehicle accidents most common; contributing factors include inexperience, teenage drivers, distractions | 136,053 |
| 5 | Stroke (cerebrovascular diseases) | Hypertension, tobacco use, diabetes, increased cholesterol, obesity, inactivity, coronary disease, excessive alcohol intake | 133,103 |
| 6 | Alzheimer's disease | Conditions that damage the heart and blood vessels such as diabetes, high cholesterol, and hypertension | 93,541 |
| 7 | Diabetes | Family history, dietary factors such as low vitamin D consumption, increased weight, obesity, inactivity, race, hypertension, increased cholesterol, polycystic ovarian syndrome, gestational diabetes, increased age | 76,488 |
| 8 | Influenza and pneumonia | Chronic disease, smoking, being immunocompromised | 55,227 |
| 9 | Nephritis, nephrotic syndrome, and nephrosis | Medical conditions that cause kidney injury such as diabetes, side effects of certain medications such as nonsteroidal anti-inflammatory drugs, infections such as HIV and malaria | 48,146 |
| 10 | Intentional self-harm (suicide) | Depression, previous self-harm | 42,773 |

Modified from Health United States. Table 19 (data are for 2014). 2015. www.cdc.gov. Accessed January 24, 2017.

framework for early identification of malnutrition, there has been considerable variance in the nutrition screening tools used and the procedures needed to follow and implement the rest of the nutrition care plan.[12] Many screening tools have used albumin as the primary indicator to identify malnutrition in patients. It is well documented, however, that albumin is a poor diagnostic indicator for malnutrition given the fact that it fluctuates in the presence of inflammation that could be induced by external factors such as trauma, surgery, or inflammatory diseases. The American Society for Parenteral and Enteral Nutrition (ASPEN) and the European Society for Clinical Nutrition and Metabolism has created an etiology-based approach to diagnose adult malnutrition in the clinical setting. This approach identifies malnutrition in the context of acute illness, chronic diseases, and starvation-related malnutrition.[13] This approach has been widely adopted by clinical dietitians across the United States. Clinical trials are currently underway to validate this approach to assessing and diagnosing malnutrition in the hospital setting.

**Recap** Nutrition has played an integral role in maintaining optimal health and quality of life for individuals in the United States and elsewhere in the world. A paradox exists in the United States where healthcare professionals need to have the knowledge and skills to address the health-related problems associated with over nutrition (obesity and chronic diseases) and undernutrition (frailty and wasting diseases). Nutritional assessment is the first step to implementing a nutrition care plan that assists individuals in successfully implementing dietary and lifestyle changes to improve their quality of life, lower their risks for disease, and help prevent or overcome malnutrition.

# ▶ Nutritional Screening and Nutritional Assessment Tools

**Preview** Nutritional screening tools are designed to quickly evaluate nutritional risk in individuals. Nutritional assessment tools identify malnutrition in individuals.

## Nutritional Screening Tools

The Academy of Nutrition and Dietetics (the Academy) recommends the use of nutrition screening to identify individuals who are at nutritional risk. This ensures that those patients who are at risk, are given high priority for a thorough nutritional evaluation by an RDN. **Nutrition screening** is defined as "the process of identifying patients, clients, or groups who may have a nutrition diagnosis and benefit from nutritional assessment and intervention by a registered dietitian."[14] Nutritional screening tools should be quick, easy-to-use tools that can be completed by any member of a healthcare team with minimal nutrition expertise (e.g., diet technicians, nurses, and physician assistants). Furthermore, screening tools should be validated to ensure that they accurately identify nutritional risks for the population and setting for which they are intended. Screening forms have use in both community and clinical settings. In community settings, for example, forms can be used to identify risk for chronic diseases such as diabetes, heart disease, and high blood pressure in adults. These are typically used at community events such as health fairs and workplace wellness fairs. When the results identify individuals at risk for a chronic disease, they are often referred to their primary care physicians for extensive evaluation to determine

| **TABLE 1.2** Nutrition screening key criteria |
|---|
| Height and weight |
| History of weight gain or loss (intentional or unintentional) |
| Changes in appetite |
| Lifestyle habits (tobacco use, physical activity, alcohol consumption) |
| Digestive disorders (constipation, diarrhea, nausea, vomiting) |
| Laboratory measures (blood, urine, or both) |
| Family history, previous medical history, or both |

Modified from Field LB, Hand RK. Differentiating malnutrition screening and assessment: a nutrition care process perspective. *J Acad Nutr Diet*. 2015;15:824-828.

whether a chronic disease is present. They may also be referred to an RDN who will offer recommendations for making dietary and lifestyle changes to the individual that, depending on the diagnosis, will either ward off the onset of the disease or will help the individual manage the newly diagnosed disease. Screening forms are also offered to the elderly living in the community setting or assisted living to identify risks for malnutrition, osteoporosis, and other chronic diseases. The criteria on the screening form varies by facility; key criteria that are commonly included are shown in **TABLE 1.2.**

In the clinical and long-term care setting, screening forms are designed to identify risks of malnutrition (undernutrition), determine the need for more-in-depth nutritional assessment, and ultimately offer an early detection of malnutrition so that nutrition support is provided in a timely manner. In the United States, an estimated 30% to 50% of adult hospital patients are malnourished. Few patients, however receive the formal diagnosis of malnutrition at discharge, and only an estimated 3.2% of discharged patients are diagnosed with malnutrition.[15] It has been well documented that patients who enter the hospital malnourished and are not given nutrition support have increased morbidity and mortality, decreased function and quality of life, and increased length of hospital stays.[16,17] This leads to increased healthcare costs expenses that can cost hospitals millions of dollars.[18]

It is critical for clinical, long-term care, and community facilities to use validated screening tools to identify patients for malnutrition risk or use validated screening tools to diagnose patients with malnutrition—and sometimes both. Using a validated screening tool ensures that (1) the individual who is identified at risk for malnutrition is indeed malnourished (high sensitivity), and (2) the individual who is not identified at risk for malnutrition is likely to be well nourished (high specificity).[14]

The Academy has identified several validated nutritional screening tools that have been researched for their ability to help identify malnutrition risk in individuals in community and clinical settings.[19] These tools largely use the same screening parameters to determine scores and risk levels. Commonly used risk-assessment parameters include recent weight loss, recent poor intake or appetite, and body mass index (BMI).[20] **TABLE 1.3** summarizes the most commonly used validated screening tools available and a description of their target populations when screening for malnutrition risk.

## Nutrition Assessment Tools

**Nutritional assessment** is defined by the Academy as "identifying and evaluating data needed to make decisions about a nutrition-related problem/diagnosis."[21] In essence, the difference between nutritional screening and nutritional assessment is that a screen identifies the "risk" for a nutrition problem or malnutrition, while the assessment "identifies the presence of or diagnosis" of a nutrition problem or malnutrition. Once identified, the practitioner creates an intervention to resolve the nutrition problem.[14] Validated nutritional assessment tools have been designed to allow RDNs and other healthcare professionals who are trained to use the tool to quickly and cost-effectively diagnose malnutrition in the acute care setting. The **subjective global assessment (SGA)** form initially started as a screening tool that has evolved as a validated diagnostic tool for malnutrition. When administrated

---

**TABLE 1.3** Commonly used nutrition screening tools

| Nutrition Screening Tool | Patient Population | Risk-Screening Parameters | Measures for Malnutrition Risk |
|---|---|---|---|
| Malnutrition screening tool | Acute-care hospitalized adults, oncology patients | ▪ Recent weight loss<br>▪ Recent poor intake | ▪ Score 0–1 for recent intake<br>▪ Score 0–4 for recent weight loss<br>▪ Total score: ≥2 = at risk for malnutrition |
| Mini Nutritional Assessment (MNA): Short Form | Subacute and ambulatory elderly patients | ▪ Recent intake<br>▪ Recent weight loss<br>▪ Mobility<br>▪ Recent acute disease or psychological stress<br>▪ Neuropsychological problems<br>▪ BMI | ▪ Score 0–3 for each parameter<br>▪ Total score: <11 = at risk for malnutrition |
| Malnutrition Universal Screening Tool (MUST) | Acute-care medical adults, medical surgical hospitalized adult patients | ▪ BMI<br>▪ Weight loss (%)<br>▪ Acute disease | ▪ Score 0–3 for each parameter<br>▪ Total score: >2 = high risk<br>1 = medium risk |
| Nutrition Risk Screening (NRS 2002) | Medical-surgical hospitalized, acute-care hospitalized patients | ▪ Recent weight loss (%)<br>▪ BMI<br>▪ Severity of disease<br>▪ Elderly (>70 years of age)<br>▪ Food intake or eating problems, skipping meals | ▪ Score 0–3 for each parameter<br>▪ Total score: >3 = start nutrition support |

Data from The Academy of Nutrition and Dietetics. *The Nutrition Care Manual.* https://www.nutritioncaremanual.org/. Accessed January 15, 2017.

by a trained professional, it is recognized as a validated method to diagnose malnutrition and predict postoperative complications, longer length of stay in postoperative patients and patients in the intensive care unit, readmission to the intensive care unit, and mortality.[22,23]

> **Recap** Nutritional screening tools are designed to quickly evaluate nutritional risk in individuals. Nutritional assessment tools are used to identify the presence of malnutrition in individuals. It is important that the RDN use validated screening and assessment tools to ensure that the results are correct for the population being evaluated.

## ▶ Standard Methods of Evaluating Nutritional Status

> **Preview** The use of nutrition assessment methods such as anthropometry, biochemical, and clinical dietary methods are essential tools to determine the health of individuals and groups.

Although the type of data collected to conduct nutritional assessments varies by clinical setting, the process and goal are the same. The evaluation of an individual or population nutritional status involves the interpretation of anthropometric, biochemical, clinical, and dietary data to define whether an individual or a group of individuals are well nourished or suffer from malnutrition. Malnutrition includes both overnutrition and undernutrition.

### Anthropometric Measures Method

**Anthropometry** is defined as the study of the measurement of the human body. It includes dimensions of bone, muscle, and adipose tissue. The area of anthropometry is a noninvasive process for determining body fat mass that incorporates several human body dimensions. Weight, standing height, horizontal length, skinfold thicknesses, limb lengths, wrist breadths, and head, chest, and waist circumferences are just a few examples of the different human body measurements that fall under anthropometric measures.[24]

Many indexes and ratios can be calculated from anthropometric measurements. One common indicator calculated from anthropometric measurements

**TABLE 1.4** Calculating body mass index

| BMI Formula | Weight (kilograms) ÷ height (meters²) |
| --- | --- |
| Interpretation | BMI values <18.5 = Underweight<br>BMI values 18.5–24.9 = Normal or desirable<br>BMI values 25.0–29.9 = Overweight<br>BMI values 30.0–34.9 = Obese (class I)<br>BMI values 35.0–39 = Obese (class II)<br>BMI values > 40.0 = Extreme obesity |

Data from National Institutes of Health. Clinical guidelines on the identification, evaluation, and treatment of overweight and obesity adults. 1988. Report no. 98-4083. https://www.ncbi.nlm.nih.gov/books/NBK2003/. Accessed December 3, 2016.

is the **body mass index (BMI)**. BMI is a measure of body fat utilizing height and weight for adult men and women. The National Academies of Science Engineering and Medicine (NASEM)—Health and Medicine Division, the Centers for Disease Control and Prevention (CDC), and many other organizations that conduct research on the health risks associated with excess weight and obesity use BMI as a measure.[25] **TABLE 1.4** shows the formula used to calculate BMI as well as the parameters used to interpret measures.

Anthropometry is a significant element in the nutrition assessment of individual children and adults, as well as segments of the population. Through the use of the National Health and Nutrition Examination Survey (NHANES), data collected through anthropometric measurements have been used to monitor growth and weight trends in the American population for more than 50 years.[26]

The anthropometric data for infants and children reveal general health status and dietary adequacy and are used to track trends in growth and development over time. The data collected have been used to produce national reference standards or growth charts.[27] Researchers from different health disciplines, for example, cardiovascular health, gerontology, nutrition, and occupational health, use anthropometric data to examine health status and healthcare utilization trends in U.S. adults.[24]

### Biochemical Measures Method

Variations in the quantity and composition of a person's diet are reflected in the concentration of chemical substances in tissue and body fluids and the appearance of different metabolites. The nutrition gamut ranges from an extreme of malnutrition because of deficiency, to optimal nutrition, to malnutrition because of overnutrition at the other end. Biochemical measures serve to identify nutritional status at any stage along the nutrition spectrum.

Although used commonly for identifying malnutrition, current literature is inconsistent for showing the validity of biochemical markers as determinants of individuals' nutritional status. The main consensus in the literature is that laboratory markers are not reliable as a stand-alone assessment.[28] The analysis of laboratory data can be difficult, and results are not always connected to clinical or nutrition findings. Biochemical results can be influenced by nonnutritional factors such as medications, hydration status, disease state, and stress.[28]

Not all content of body nutrients can be assessed by biochemical methods. Common deficiencies identified via biochemical or laboratory methods include[9]:

- Blood-forming nutrients such as iron, folacin, and vitamins $B_6$ and $B_{12}$
- Water-soluble vitamins such as thiamine, riboflavin, niacin, and vitamin C
- All of the fat-soluble vitamins (A, D, E, and K)
- Minerals such as iron, iodine, and trace elements; and
- Levels of blood lipids, including cholesterol, triglycerides, glucose, and enzymes linked to heart disease

The results of anthropometric, clinical, and dietary assessment methods can guide decisions concerning the need for biochemical or laboratory data.

## Clinical Method: History and Physical

A comprehensive look at an individual's or a group's nutrition assessment takes into account their history. A clinical history coupled with a physical examination is essential to identify signs and symptoms of malnutrition. A clinical history usually includes information such as medical diagnosis, recent hospital admissions, medications, changes in intake of food and fluids, food supply and preparation ability, and weight changes.

Once a history is obtained, a **nutrition-focused physical exam (NFPE)** should be conducted. An NFPE is a systematic way of evaluating an individual from head to toe, paying attention to his or her physical appearance and function to discover signs and symptoms related to malnutrition, nutrient deficiency, and toxicity.[29]

The presence of weight loss is an indicator of an individual's nutritional status.[30] In 2012, the Academy and the American Society for Parenteral and Enteral Nutrition put out a consensus statement defining malnutrition as the presence of two of the following symptoms: inadequate energy intake, weight loss, loss of muscle mass, loss of subcutaneous fat, localized or generalized accumulation of fluid, or decreased functional status as measured by handgrip strength.[12] Many of these characteristics are easily evaluated via an NFPE. See **TABLE 1.5** to review some of the signs and symptoms that can be identified as a result of conducting a systems-focused assessment.

## Dietary Methods

Dietary assessment methods are used to collect an individual's and group information on food supply and nutrients consumed. For groups of individuals (population groups), statistical databases such as the **Food and Agriculture Organization of the United Nations (FAO)** and the **Bureau of Labor Statistics Consumer expenditure survey data** provide information on food supply and purchasing habits. Actual food-intake data are obtained through the use of dietary surveys, food diaries, 24-hour recall, food-frequency questionnaires, food-habit questionnaires, or a combination of any of these methods. The NHANES is an example of a national survey program in the United States that has been designed to assess the health and nutritional status of adults and children.[26] This survey is unique in combining interviews and physical examinations.

A food diary requires that a participant report all food and fluids consumed for a specified period of time. A 24-hour recall involves listing all food and fluids consumed in the previous 24 hours. Foods and quantity consumed are recalled from memory with the assistance of a trained interviewer to facilitate the process. A food-frequency questionnaire is a structured listing of individual foods or groups of foods. For each food item or group, the participant must define the frequency in which the food is consumed in a specified time frame. This can be the number of times the food or group is consumed in a day, a week, or even a month. Diet histories are used to determine the usual intake of a specific individual. Food-habit questionnaires are used to collect either general information or specific details such as food perceptions and beliefs. Food likes and dislikes, food-preparation methods, and social surroundings related to meals are collected using this method. Combined dietary assessment methods can be pooled to improve accuracy and enable interpretation of the dietary data.[31]

Like all self-reported data, the complete accuracy of information obtained from dietary assessment methods such as surveys can be questioned. A study designed to evaluate the validity of the data reported by NHANES on caloric intake reported that in the 39 years of the history of the survey, data reported by the majority of participants were not physiologically reasonable.[32] These findings suggest that the ability to estimate population trends in caloric intake

**TABLE 1.5** Signs and symptoms of nutritional deficiency

| Body System | Sign or Symptom | Nutrient Deficiency |
| --- | --- | --- |
| General appearance | Wasting | Energy |
| Skin | Rash | Many vitamins, zinc, essential fatty acids |
| | Rash in sun-exposed area | Niacin (pellagra) |
| | Easy bruising | Vitamin C or K |
| Hair and nails | Thinning or loss of hair | Protein |
| | Premature whitening of hair | Selenium |
| | Spooning (upcurling) of nails | Iron |
| Eyes | Impaired night vision | Vitamin A |
| | Corneal keratomalacia (corneal drying and clouding) | Vitamin A |
| Mouth | Cheilosis and glossitis | Riboflavin, niacin, pyridoxine, iron |
| | Bleeding gums | Vitamin C, riboflavin |
| Extremities | Edema | Protein |
| Neurologic | Paresthesias or numbness in a stocking-glove distribution | Thiamin (beri beri) |
| | Tetany | Ca, Mg |
| | Cognitive and sensory deficits | Thiamin, niacin, pyridoxine, vitamin $B_{12}$ |
| Musculoskeletal | Wasting of muscle | Protein |
| | Bone deformities (e.g., bowlegs, knocked knees, curved spine) | Vitamin D, calcium |
| | Bone tenderness | Vitamin D |
| | Joint pain or swelling | Vitamin C |
| Gastrointestinal | Diarrhea | Protein, niacin, folate, vitamin $B_{12}$ |
| | Diarrhea and dysgeusia | Zinc |
| | Dysphagia or odynophagia (because of Plummer–Vinson syndrome) | Iron |
| Endocrine | Thyromegaly | Iodine |

to support the development of public policy relevant to diet and health relationships from the American nutrition surveillance system can be limited.[32]

**Recap** The use of the different nutrition assessment methods are valuable, simple, and practical tools used to describe nutrition problems in individuals as well as groups within the community.

# ▶ The Nutrition Care Process

**Preview** The Nutrition Care Process is a tool used by nutrition and dietetics professionals to improve the consistency and quality of individualized care for patients, clients, or groups.

## The Nutrition Care Process

The **Nutrition Care Process (NCP)** is a standardized model developed to assist the RDNs and dietetic technicians, registered (NDTR), in delivering high-quality nutrition care.[33] This process provides the framework for the RDN and NDTR to customize care, taking into account the individual's needs and values, while using the best scientific evidence at the time care decisions must be made. In 2003, the Academy endorsed the use of the NCP to afford nutrition specialists a strategy for critical thinking and decision making.

The NCP involves the use of unique yet interdependent—that is, distinct but interrelated—steps. This includes the completion of a nutrition assessment. Part of completing a nutrition assessment involves four steps. The first step is collecting and documenting information such as nutrition-related history, anthropometric measurements, laboratory data, clinical history, and NFPE findings. The second step is defining a nutrition diagnosis. This requires the RDN to evaluate the collected assessment information and name a specific problem that can be resolved through nutritional interventions. The third step requires the RDN to select nutrition interventions that will address the root of the nutrition diagnosis to resolve or control signs and symptoms. The last step of the NCP is monitoring and evaluation to determine whether the individual has achieved or is making progress toward the predetermined goal.[33]

## Nutrition Care Process and Model

The **Nutrition Care Process and Model (NCPM)** is a pictorial conception that shows the steps of the Nutrition Care Process as well as internal and external factors that influence application of the NCP (**FIGURE 1.3**).

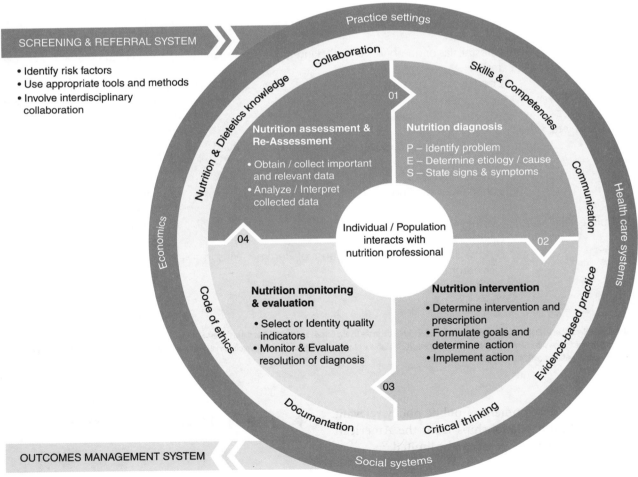

**FIGURE 1.3** The nutrition care process and model for nutrition and dietetics professionals

The relationship between the RDN and the individual or groups of individuals is at the center of the model, which defines the four steps of the NCP—nutrition assessment, diagnosis, intervention, and monitoring and evaluation. The NCP helps to identify external factors such as skill and ability of the RDN, application of evidence-based practice, application of the code of ethics, and knowledge of the RDN as some of the external factors influencing the process. This set of factors defines how individuals and groups of individuals receive nutrition information.

Other factors that impact the ability of individuals and groups to take advantage of the RDN services includes the healthcare system, socioeconomics, and the practice setting. The practice setting reveals rules and regulations that guide a practice and include the age and conditions qualifying for services and how the nutrition and dietetics professional apportions his or her time. The healthcare system defines the amount of time available for the nutrition and dietetics professional–patient interaction, the kind of services offered, and who provides the services. Social components reflect the health-related knowledge, values, and the time devoted to improving nutritional health of both individuals and groups. The economic aspect integrates resources assigned to nutrition care, including the value of a food and the nutrition professional's time expressed in the form of salary and reimbursement.[34]

The screening and referral process as well as outcomes management complete the components of the NCP. The NCPM offers a consistent structure and framework for nutrition and food professionals to use when providing nutrition care. The model is intended for use with individuals and groups of individuals of all ages with any healthcare condition and in all care settings.[13]

## Nutrition Care Process: Standardized Language

RDNs utilize **Nutrition Care Process Terminology (NCPT)** to describe all activities performed in the four steps of the NCP.[21] The NCPT is a controlled vocabulary used to depict the distinctive activities of nutrition and dietetics in completing the nutrition assessment, nutrition diagnosis, nutrition intervention, and nutrition monitoring and evaluation. It is intended to enable clear and reliable narratives of the services provided by RDNs.[35] Aside from facilitating communication, the NCPT enables researchers to define the types of nutrition problems observed in patient populations (nutrition diagnoses), the interventions to put in place, and the outcomes obtained.

The NCPT contains more than 1,000 terms and was developed with contributions from practitioners and researchers. Many of the terms have been matched for incorporation into the Systematized Nomenclature of Medicine—Clinical Terms and Logical Observation Identifiers Names and Codes. These are clinical terms in use worldwide for electronic health records. The NCPT's specific vocabulary allows for data gathering for nutrition research and documentation of quality measures.

The NCPT includes specific language for nutrition diagnosis. These statements help describe nutrition problems that the RDN can treat. The unique language developed to identify nutrition interventions helps outline actions intended to change a nutrition-related behavior, environmental condition, or aspect of health status for an individual or a group.[35] The NCPT also includes nomenclature to identify nutrition monitoring and evaluation parameters that can be used to determine changes in outcomes as they relate to nutrition diagnosis and intervention.

## Nutrition Care Process: Assessment

Nutrition assessment is a systematic method for obtaining, verifying, and interpreting data needed to identify nutrition-related problems, their causes, and their significances.[36] It is a continuous, nonlinear, and dynamic procedure that includes initial data gathering as well as recurrent reassessment and analysis of the individual's status compared to identified standards. Through the evaluation of the data collected for the nutrition assessment, the RDNs is able to determine whether a nutritionally diagnosable problem exists.[36]

The nutrition assessment terms are identified and grouped into five domains: food/nutrition-related history, anthropometric measurements, biochemical data, medical tests, and procedures.

A nutrition assessment commences after an individual is referred, as a consequence of an at-risk nutrition screen, or when an individual can benefit from nutrition care. Nutrition assessment allows the nutrition practitioner to determine if a nutrition diagnosis or problem exists. When that is the case, the RDN properly diagnoses the problem and generates a *problem, etiology, signs* or *symptoms* (PES) statement. This is step two of the NCP. In addition, RDNs create a plan to put in place interventions to resolve the nutrition diagnoses. In some instances, a plan of care identifies the need for further information or testing. If the initial completed assessment or reassessment shows that a nutrition problem is not present or that current problems cannot be improved by supplementary nutrition care, discharge from nutrition care services is appropriate.[21]

Data to complete a nutrition assessment of individuals is obtained from the person through interviews, observation, measurements, medical records, and information provided by the referring healthcare provider. For population groups, data from surveys, administrative data sets, and epidemiological or research studies are used to collect assessment information. The use of standardized language enables effective comparison of nutrition-assessment findings. When conducting the assessment, the RDN must determine which are the most appropriate data to collect, assess the need for additional data, select assessment tools and procedures that match the situation, and apply assessment tools in a reliable manner. The assessor must determine which data are relevant, important, and valid for inclusion in the nutrition assessment.[21]

## NCP: Nutrition Diagnosis

Defining a nutrition diagnosis is an important step between nutrition assessment and defining nutrition interventions. The purpose of a standardized nutrition diagnosis language is to designate nutrition problems reliably so that they are clear for all professionals. A **nutrition diagnosis** is used to identify and define a particular nutrition problem that can be solved or whose symptoms can be managed through nutrition interventions by a nutrition and food professional. A nutrition diagnosis (such as inadequate sodium intake) is different from a medical diagnosis (such as congestive heart failure). Unlike a nutrition diagnosis, a medical diagnosis defines a disease process or pathology such as congestive heart failure. It is not within the scope of nutrition and dietetics professionals to determine or assign medical diagnoses. The standardized language improves communication and documentation of nutrition care, and it offers a minimum data set and consistent data foundations for future research. The nutrition diagnosis falls into three domains: intake, clinical, and behavioral or environment. **TABLE 1.6** shows examples of nutrition diagnostic terminology that fall under each domain. A designation of "no nutrition diagnoses" can be used for individuals whose documented nutrition assessment indicate no nutritional problem requiring nutrition intervention and treatment.[21]

The outcome of the nutrition-diagnosis step of the NCP is the creation of a diagnosis statement, or **PES statement**, which has three elements: the problem (P), its etiology (E), and its signs and symptoms (S). The elements of the PES statement are joined by the phrases "related to" and "as evidenced by." The data collected and analyzed during the nutrition assessment

**TABLE 1.6** Nutrition diagnostic terminology

| Domain | Problem |
| --- | --- |
| Intake | Inadequate energy intake<br>Malnutrition |
| Clinical | Impaired nutrient utilization<br>Unintended weight loss |
| Behavioral/<br>Environmental | Not ready for diet or lifestyle change<br>Limited access to food or water |

Data from Academy of Nutrition and Dietetics. *Nutrition Terminology Reference Manual (eNCPT): Dietetics Language for Nutrition Care.* 2016. http://ncpt.webauthor.com/. Accessed December 8, 2016.

are used to generate the PES statement.[21] **FIGURE 1.4** shows how the standardized language is used to create a nutrition diagnosis and PES statement.

## NCP: Intervention

The third step of the NCP is determining the most appropriate intervention to resolve the nutrition problem. A **nutrition intervention** is the action taken by the nutrition and dietetics professional to correct or manage a nutrition problem. Its purpose is to target and resolve the diagnosis by eliminating signs and symptoms related to nutrition-related behaviors, environmental conditions, or conditions that affect nutrition and health. Nutrition interventions need to be individualized to meet the specific needs of each person.[21,36]

The NCP nutrition intervention has two distinct steps: planning and implementation. Planning involves selecting and prioritizing the nutrition diagnosis, collaborating with other caregivers, involving the patient and his or her representative, and reviewing evidence-based practice guidelines. With the patient at the center of the care, the FDN should work toward the expected outcome for the nutrition diagnosis, outline nutrition interventions, identify the frequency of the treatment, and identify the resources needed. The implementation step involves communicating and carrying out the care plan developed for the individual. Plan implementation involves monitoring the plan for acceptance (by the individual) and effectiveness. If the expected outcome for the individual is not being obtained, the interventions must be changed.[21,36]

Most often the nutrition intervention is designed to correct the etiology component of the PES statement.

**Patient Information**

Mrs. Smith is a 66-year-old female who was referred to your office by her primary care provider. The reason for the referral is outlined weight loss in the past 3 months.

Mrs. Smith's diagnosis includes diabetes, hypertension, and arthritis. Her height is 5'4". Her weight in the past three months: month 1 = 135 lbs, month 2= 127 lbs, month 3 = 122 lbs. Her usual body weight fluctuates between 137 and 134 lbs. Her current BMI = 20.9. This value is within the range for normal BMI.

Mrs. Smith's medical history is significant for diabetes and arthritis. During your interaction with the Mrs. Smith, you determine that overall her blood sugars are well controlled. She understands her medication regime and the importance of following her medication schedule. She reports that she has been "a bit out of sorts" since her husband died four months ago. Mr. Smith had been a world-renowned chef who had retired and turned his energy to shopping for and preparing every meal at home. Since his death, Mrs. Smith has not had the desire to shop for food or cook meals. This just does not seem important to her.

As the nutrition assessment is completed, you conclude that Mrs. Smith has poor intakes of calories and protein. Her intake is related to changes in her living situation following the death of her husband, who had supported her by preparing all meals. The poor intake has resulted in a 13-lb weight loss in three months.

Focusing on the poor intake as the key problem, the PES statement can be written as:

Inadequate protein-energy intake (NI-5.3) related to poor meal intake and loss of support for preparing meals as evidenced by a 13-lb weight loss in three months.

To address the weight loss, the PES statement can be written as:

Unintended weight loss (NC-3.2) related to poor meal intake and loss of support for preparing meals as evidenced by a 13-lb weight loss in 3 months.

**FIGURE 1.4** Using standardized language to create a PES statement

Data from Academy of Nutrition and Dietetics. *Nutrition Terminology Reference Manual (eNCPT): Dietetics Language for Nutrition Care.* 2016.http://ncpt.webauthor.com/. Accessed December 8, 2016.

Four domains are used when creating nutrition interventions: (1) food or nutrient delivery, (2) nutrition education, (3) nutrition counseling, and (4) coordination of care. The food or nutrient delivery domain encompasses provision of meals, snacks, and enteral and parenteral nutrition. Education and counseling tactics can help operationalize food and nutrient delivery efforts and guide individuals to make food choices that promote healthy eating patterns and optimize health. Nutrition education varies by care setting, desired outcome, and whether the person has a chronic or acute disease process. For instance, for home-dwelling individuals, food safety might be the focus of their nutrition education; therefore, counseling goes beyond understanding healthy eating patterns. It requires influencing and coaching individuals to foster lifestyle changes. Coordination of care is an **interprofessional** collaboration to identify the individual's needs and identify resources.[21,36]

## NCP: Monitoring and Evaluation

Nutrition monitoring and evaluation is the fourth step of the NCP. The purpose of this step is to measure the progress made by the individual in achieving the predetermined outcome. The individual's outcomes that are relevant to the nutrition diagnosis and interventions are monitored and measured. Data sources to aid in this step include self-monitoring information and material collected through records such as forms, spreadsheets, and computer programs. Information from anthropometric measurements, biochemical data, tests, and procedures also help to evaluate progress from current status to desired state. Data from pretests, questionnaires, surveys, and mail or telephone follow-up can also be used to measure the level of success of the plan of care.[21,36]

Outcomes associated with food and nutrient intake, nutrition-related physical signs and symptoms, and nutrition-related patient- and individual-centered outcomes are usually monitored by the nutrition and dietetics professional.[21,36]

The NCP's nutrition monitoring and evaluation step incorporates three unique and interconnected processes: monitoring process, measuring outcomes, and evaluating outcomes. Monitoring process involves ensuring that the client, patient, or individual understands and complies with the plan. This includes determining if the interventions were implemented as prescribed, providing evidence of how the plan is helping the patient to meet (or not meet) their goals, detecting other positive or negative outcomes, collecting information, identifying causes for absence of progress, and aggregating data that support the lack of progress as well as support conclusions with evidence. Measuring outcomes involves identifying markers that are relevant to the nutrition diagnosis or signs and symptoms, nutrition goals, medical diagnosis and outcomes, and quality-management goals. Evaluating outcomes requires that the nutrition care provider evaluate the change between the outcomes obtained to the individual's status at the beginning of the care process.[21,36]

> **Recap** The use of standardized indicators and criteria helps nutrition and dietetics professionals communicate using a common language understood inside and outside the profession. Data collected are used to promote continued development of the outcome data's validity and reliability.

## ▶ Emerging Opportunities for Nutritional Assessment and Evaluation

> **Preview** Micronutrient deficiencies are no longer the leading public-health priority in the United States. It is important to monitor individual and groups of individuals' diet and body weight as part of health-promotion and disease-prevention programs.

For more than a century, the role of nutrition in promoting health and preventing disease was over-shadowed by great achievements in medicine. In the same time frame, science and research increased our knowledge and understanding of micronutrient requirements and their role in supporting health. Changes in the food industry supporting the enrichment and fortification of food products have contributed to eradicating micronutrient deficiencies in some segments of the population. As a result, micronutrient deficiencies are no longer the highest public-health priority. Currently, a better understanding of the complex relationship between nutrition and health has placed the conduct of nutrition assessments as a key indicator in the surveillance of population health. Conducting population nutrition assessments provides data that help to continue advance healthcare practices.

## Healthy People 2020 Nutrition Objectives

One of the goals of the Healthy People 2020 initiative is to reduce the proportion of adults who are obese. The goal is to decrease this rate from a 2020 baseline of 33.9% to 30.5% by 2020. The 2011–2014 data reflecting rate of obesity per race are shown in Figure 1.4. These data show that the obesity rate for the white non-Hispanic or Latino rate is 34.4%. The obesity rate for African Americans is 47.9%. There is a 13.5 percentage-point difference between the groups with the best and worst obesity rates. This type of information is important for healthcare providers regardless of the practice setting. For the researcher interested in public health, this type of information is essential to demonstrate the need for additional research involving this segment of the population. **FIGURE 1.5** shows obesity disparities by race and ethnicity.

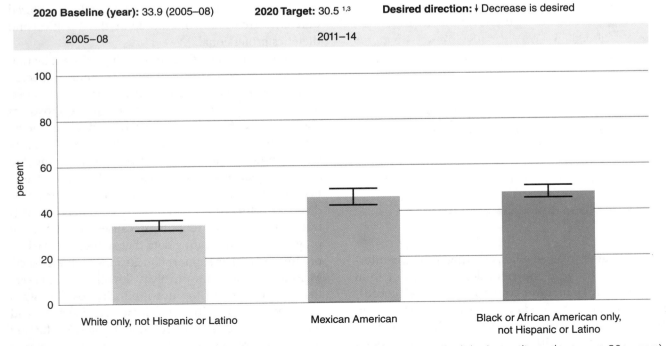

**2020 Baseline (year):** 33.9 (2005–08)      **2020 Target:** 30.5 [1,3]      **Desired direction:** ↓ Decrease is desired

2005–08                                          2011–14

**FIGURE 1.5** Disparities details by race and ethnicity for 2011–2014: Obesity among adults (age adjusted, percent, 20+ years)

## VIEWPOINT

### Health Initiatives

*Robin S. Rood, MA, MEd, RD, LD*

A health initiative is a strategy, action plan, or approach offered by an agency of the federal government, private business, or nonprofit organization to inform and direct people toward better health. In March 2010, the Affordable Care Act (ACA) was enacted into law, expanding access to health care to millions of people who had previously been unable to get health care because of preexisting conditions or simply because they could not afford it (**FIGURE A**).[1] One of the ACA's most popular features is that it allows children to remain on their parents' insurance until age 26 years.[2] In addition, preventive care services such as free flu shots, birth control, and annual physicals are more easily accessed.

In September 2010, First Lady Michelle Obama and National Football League (NFL) Commissioner Roger Goodell launched the "Let's Move" Campaign. Although the website is still available for public viewing, it is no longer being updated.[3] The "Play 60" campaign is now called the "Fuel Up to Play 60" and is an in-school nutrition and physical-activity program sponsored by the National Dairy Council, the NFL, and partners with the U.S. Department of Agriculture.[4] These programs encourage children, teens, and adults to engage in physical activity every day. The goal is to create a public and private partnership to combat childhood obesity.

The Presidential Active Lifestyle Award (PALA+) was created by the National Foundation on Fitness, Sports, and Nutrition to promote physical activity and good nutrition, and encourage Americans to meet the Physical Activity Guidelines and Dietary Guidelines for Americans. To win this award you can register at www.supertracker .usda.gov/PALAplus.aspx and log in to track foods and exercise for five weeks to earn a PALA+, or sign up at the

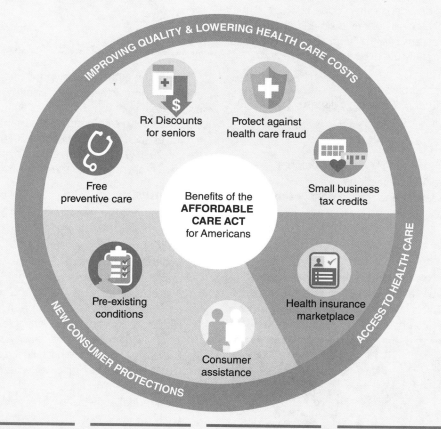

| Benefits for women | Your adult coverage | Strengthening Medicare | Holding insurance companies accountable |
|---|---|---|---|
| Providing insurance options, covering preventing service, and lowering costs. | Coverage available to children up to age 26 years. | Yearly wellness visit and many free preventing services for some seniors with Medicare. | Insures must justify any premium increase of 10% or more before the rate takes effect. |

**FIGURE A** Benefits of the Affordable Care Act

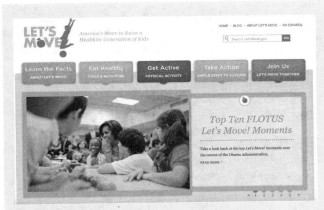

Reproduced from Let's Move! https://letsmove.obamawhitehouse.archives.gov.

National Fitness Foundation (www.fitness.foundation /pala), the only nonprofit officially chartered by Congress. Anyone who extends the challenge to weeks 6–8 will achieve a Presidential Active Lifestyle Premium Award.[5,6]

In December 2010, a health initiative called Healthy People 2020 was launched to assess the current health of Americans and offer health education programs targeted to their needs so that every population can live healthy lives.[7]

Now in its third decade, Healthy People 2020 is a science-based set of national objectives aimed at improving the health of all Americans. Healthy People 2020 reflects the need to address current issues in health care, including:

- Adolescent health
- Blood disorders and blood safety
- Dementias, including Alzheimer's disease
- Early and middle childhood
- Genomics
- Global health
- Health-related quality of life and well-being
- Healthcare-associated infections
- Lesbian, gay, bisexual, and transgender health
- Older adults
- Preparedness
- Sleep health
- Social determinants of health

The results of this ongoing collection of information can be found at www.healthypeople.gov. At this time, Healthy People 2030 is in development to project what areas of health are of concern to future generations.

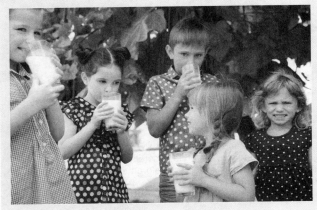

© Africa Studio/Shutterstock.

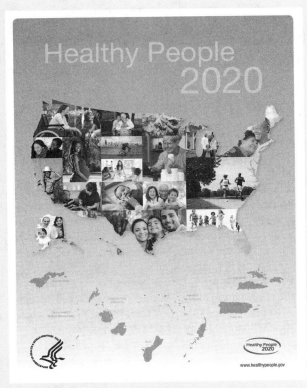

Reproduced from Healthy People 2020. U.S. Department of Health and Human Services. https://www.healthypeople.gov/.

A nation with a healthy population means a stronger and more productive society. Healthy minds and bodies also benefit economically from diet and physical exercise. Because health care costs have continued to increase, initiatives such as Healthy People 2020 and Healthy People 2030 will help keep costs down, create a healthier workforce, and stimulate the economy.

### References

1. HHS.gov. About the ACA [online]. (2017). Available at https://www.hhs.gov/healthcare/about-the-aca /index.html. Accessed July 10, 2017.
2. Healthcare.gov. Health Insurance Coverage for Children and Young Adults Under 26 [online]. (2017). Available at https://www.healthcare.gov/young-adults /children-under-26/. Accessed July 10, 2017.
3. Let's Move! [online]. (2017). Available at https://letsmove .obamawhitehouse.archives.gov/. Accessed July 10, 2017.
4. Fueluptoplay60.com. What Is Fuel Up to Play 60? [online]. (2017). Available at https://www.fueluptoplay60.com /funding/nutrition-equipment-grant.
5. Presidential Active Lifestyle Award (PALA+). [online]. (2017). Available at https://www.supertracker.usda .gov/PALAPlus.aspx. Accessed July 10, 2017.
6. President's Council on Fitness, Sports, and Nutrition. PALA+. [online]. (2017). Available at: https://www.hhs .gov/fitness/programs-and-awards/pala/. Accessed July 10, 2017.
7. Office of Disease Prevention and Health Promotion. Healthy People 2020. [online]. (2017). Available at: https://www.healthypeople.gov/. Accessed July 10, 2017.

**Healthy People 2020 (HP 2020)** is a set of goals and objectives with 10-year targets that are designed to guide national health-promotion and disease-prevention efforts to improve the health of all people in the United States. Released by the U.S. Department of Health and Human Services each decade, the Healthy People initiatives reflect the idea that setting objectives and providing science-based benchmarks to track and monitor progress can motivate and focus action. HP 2020 represents the fourth generation of this initiative, building on three decades of previous work.[38]

HP 2020 is a tool used for strategic management by the federal government, states, communities, and many other public- and private-sector partners. Its comprehensive set of objectives and targets is used to measure progress for health issues in specific populations as well as serve as a foundation for prevention and wellness activities across various sectors and within the federal government. It also serves as a model for measurement at the state and local levels. HP 2020 is committed to the vision of "a society in which all people live long, healthy lives." The initiative has four predominant goals:[38]

1. Help Americans have higher-quality and longer lives that are free of preventable diseases, disabilities, injuries, and premature death.
2. Help Americans achieve health equity, eliminate disparities, and improve the health of all groups.
3. Create social and physical environments that promote good health for all.
4. Promote quality of life, healthy development, and healthy behaviors across all life stages.

HP 2020 monitors approximately 1,200 objectives organized into 42 topic areas, each of which represents an important public-health area.[38] See **TABLE 1.7**.

The goal of the nutrition and health-status objective is to promote health and reduce chronic-disease risk through the consumption of healthful diets and achievement and maintenance of healthy body weights.[39]

The nutrition and weight status objectives for HP 2020 reflect strong science supporting the health benefits of eating a healthful diet and maintaining a healthy body weight. The objectives also emphasize that efforts to change diet and weight should address individual behaviors as well as the policies and environments that support these behaviors in settings such as schools, work sites, healthcare organizations, and communities.[39]

The goal of promoting healthy diets and healthy weight includes increasing household food security and eliminating hunger. A healthy diet includes a variety of nutrient-dense foods within and across the food groups, especially whole grains, fruits, vegetables, low-fat or fat-free milk or milk products, and lean meats and other protein sources. Individuals are also encouraged to limit the intake of saturated and *trans* fats, cholesterol, added sugars, sodium, and alcohol, as well as limit overall intake to meet caloric needs.[40]

Monitoring population diet and body weight is an important part of any health-promotion and disease-prevention program. Good nutrition is especially important to the growth and development of children. A healthy diet also helps Americans reduce their risks for many health conditions, including overweight and obesity, malnutrition, iron-deficiency anemia, heart disease, hypertension, dyslipidemia, type 2 diabetes, osteoporosis, oral disease, constipation, diverticular disease, and some forms of cancer.[22,39]

Diet reflects the variety of foods and beverages consumed over time in the home and in settings such as work sites, schools, and restaurants. Interventions that support the consumption of a healthier diet help ensure that individuals will have the knowledge and skills to make healthier choices.

Because weight is influenced by the balance between number of calories consumed versus calories expended, interventions put in place to improve weight should support changes in diet as well as physical activity. As new and innovative policies and environmental interventions to support diet and physical activity are implemented, it will be important to identify which are most effective. A better understanding of how to prevent unhealthy weight gain is also needed.[39] HP 2020 includes 22 objectives[21] as shown in **TABLE 1.8**.

## Diabetes Mellitus

Diabetes mellitus is perhaps one of the oldest disorders known to medicine. Clinical descriptions describing what we now call DM were portrayed 3,000 years ago by the ancient Egyptians.[41] See **FIGURE 1.6** for a quick history of DM.

Because DM is so widespread, it is now considered a 21st-century global emergency. An estimated 415 million adults worldwide live with DM. In addition, 318 million adults suffer from impaired glucose tolerance, thus increasing their risk for developing DM.[24] In the United States, 29.1 million people—9.3% of the American population—have diabetes, out of which only 21 million individuals have been diagnosed. During 2008–2009, an estimated 18,436 people younger than 20 years in the United States were newly diagnosed with type 1 diabetes annually, and 5,089

**TABLE 1.7** Healthy People 2020 topic areas

| Public-Health Area | | |
|---|---|---|
| **Access to Health Services** | **Genomics\*** | **Nutrition and Weight Status** |
| Adolescent health\* | Global health\* | Occupational safety and health |
| Arthritis, osteoporosis, and chronic back conditions Blood disorders and blood safety\* | Healthcare-associated infections\* Health communication and health information technology | Older adults\* Oral health |
| Cancer | Health-related quality of life and well-being\* | Physical activity |
| Chronic kidney disease | Hearing and other sensory or communication disorders | Preparedness\* |
| Dementias, including Alzheimer's disease\* | Heart disease and stroke | Public-health infrastructure |
| Diabetes | HIV | Respiratory diseases |
| Disability and health | Immunization and infectious diseases | Sexually transmitted diseases |
| Early and middle childhood\* | Injury and violence prevention | Sleep health\* |
| Educational and community-based programs | Lesbian, gay, bisexual, and transgender health\* | Social determinants of health\* |
| Environmental health | Maternal, infant, and child health | Substance abuse |
| Family planning | Medical product safety | Tobacco use |
| Food safety | Mental health and mental disorders | Vision |

\*These topics were not included in HP2010 and are new to HP2020.

Data from Centers for Disease Control and Prevention. *HP 2020*. https://www.cdc.gov/nchs/healthy_people/hp2020.htm. 2015. Accessed December 17, 2016.

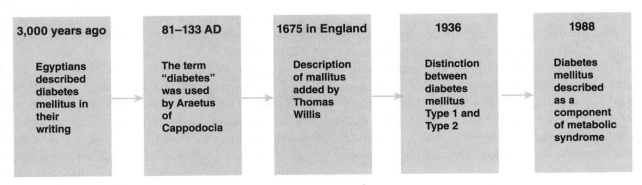

**FIGURE 1.6** History of diabetes mellitus

Data from Ahmed AM. History of diabetes mellitus. *Saudi Med J*. 2002. Apr;23(4):373-378.

**TABLE 1.8** HP 2020 nutrition and weight status objectives

| Area | Objectives |
| --- | --- |
| **Healthier Food Access** | Increase the number of states with nutrition standards for foods and beverages provided to preschool-aged children in childcare |
| | Increase the proportion of schools that offer nutritious foods and beverages outside of school meals |
| | ■ Increase the proportion of schools that do not sell or offer calorically sweetened beverages to students |
| | ■ Increase the proportion of school districts that require schools to make fruits or vegetables available whenever other food is offered or sold |
| | Increase the number of states that have state-level policies that incentivize food retail outlets to provide foods that are encouraged by the *Dietary Guidelines for Americans* |
| | Increase the proportion of Americans who have access to a food retail outlet that sells a variety of foods that are encouraged by the *Dietary Guidelines for Americans* |
| **Health Care and Work-Site Settings** | Increase the proportion of primary care physicians who regularly measure their patients' body mass index (BMI) |
| | ■ Increase the proportion of primary care physicians who regularly assess BMI in their adult patients |
| | ■ Increase the proportion of primary care physicians who regularly assess BMI for age and gender in their child or adolescent patients |
| | Increase the proportion of physician office visits that include counseling or education related to nutrition or weight |
| | ■ Increase the proportion of physician office visits made by patients with a diagnosis of cardiovascular disease, diabetes, or hyperlipidemia that include counseling or education related to diet or nutrition |
| | ■ Increase the proportion of physician office visits made by adult patients who are obese that include counseling or education related to weight reduction, nutrition, or physical activity |
| | ■ Increase the proportion of physician visits made by all child or adult patients that include counseling about nutrition or diet |
| | Increase the proportion of work sites that offer nutrition or weight-management classes or counseling |
| **Weight Status** | Increase the proportion of adults who are at a healthy weight |
| | Reduce the proportion of adults who are obese |
| | Reduce the proportion of children and adolescents who are considered obese |
| | ■ Reduce the proportion of children ages 2 to 5 years who are considered obese |
| | ■ Reduce the proportion of children ages 6 to 11 years who are considered obese |
| | ■ Reduce the proportion of adolescents ages 12 to 19 years who are considered obese |
| | ■ Reduce the proportion of children and adolescents ages 2 to 19 years who are considered obese |
| | Prevent inappropriate weight gain in youth and adults |
| | ■ Prevent inappropriate weight gain in children ages 2 to 5 years |
| | ■ Prevent inappropriate weight gain in children ages 6 to 11 years |
| | ■ Prevent inappropriate weight gain in adolescents ages 12 to 19 years |
| | ■ Prevent inappropriate weight gain in children and adolescents ages 2 to 19 years |
| | ■ Prevent inappropriate weight gain in adults ages 20 years and older |
| **Food Insecurity** | Eliminate the worst food insecurity among children |
| | Reduce household food insecurity and thus reduce hunger |

*(continues)*

| **TABLE 1.8** *(continued)* | |
| --- | --- |
| **Area** | **Objectives** |
| **Food and Nutrient Consumption** | Increase the contribution of fruits to the diets of the population age 2 years and older<br>▪ Increase the variety and contribution of vegetables to the diets of the population age 2 years and older<br>▪ Increase the contribution of total vegetables to the diets of the population age 2 years and older |
| | Increase the contribution of dark green vegetables, red and orange vegetables, and beans and peas to the diets of the population age 2 years and older |
| | Increase the contribution of whole grains to the diets of the population age 2 years and older |
| | Reduce consumption of calories from solid fats and added sugars in the population age 2 years and older<br>▪ Reduce consumption of calories from solid fats<br>▪ Reduce consumption of calories from added sugars<br>▪ Reduce consumption of calories from solid fats and added sugars |
| | Reduce consumption of saturated fat in the population age 2 years and older |
| | Reduce consumption of sodium in the population age 2 years and older |
| | Increase consumption of calcium in the population age 2 years and older |
| **Iron Deficiency** | Reduce iron deficiency among young children and females of childbearing age<br>▪ Reduce iron deficiency among children ages 1 to 2 years<br>▪ Reduce iron deficiency among children ages 3 to 4 years<br>▪ Reduce iron deficiency among females ages 12 to 49 years |
| | Reduce iron deficiency among pregnant females |

Data from US Department of Health and Human Services. (2015), *Heathy People 2020*. https://www.healthypeople.gov/. Accessed December 17, 2016.

people younger than 20 years were newly diagnosed with type 2 diabetes annually (see **FIGURE 1.7**).[42]

Diabetes was the seventh-leading cause of death in the United States in 2010 based on the 69,071 death certificates that listed diabetes as the underlying cause of death. Studies have found that only 35% to 40% of deceased people with diabetes had death certificates that listed diabetes; 10% to 15% had diabetes listed as the underlying cause of death. From 2003–2006, after adjusting for population age differences, death rates from all causes were 1.5 times higher among adults 18 years of age and older with diagnosed diabetes than among adults without diagnosed diabetes.[42]

## Managing DM

Diabetes can be treated and managed when someone adopts a healthy eating pattern, engages in regular physical activity, and takes prescribed medications to lower blood glucose levels. Another critical part of diabetes management is reducing cardiovascular disease risk factors such as high blood pressure, high lipid levels, and the use of tobacco. Patient education and self-care practices also are important aspects of

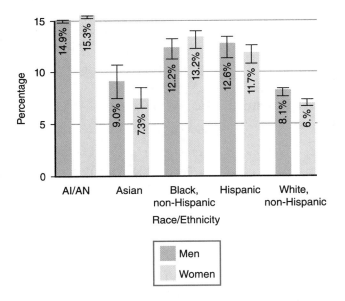

AI/AN = American Indian/Alaska Native.

Note: Error bars represent upper and lower bounds of the 95% confidence interval.

**FIGURE 1.7** New cases of DM in individuals younger than 20 years of age-2013–2015

Reproduced from Center for Disease Control and Prevention, *National Diabetes Statistics Report, 2014*. http://www.thefdha.org /pdf/diabetes.pdf.

disease management that help people with diabetes stay healthy. Nutritional assessment has been vital in identifying risks and diagnosing symptoms and comorbidities associated with DM.[42] Medical nutrition therapy is key to preventing DM, managing individuals who have been diagnosed with DM, and preventing—or at least reducing—the development of DM comorbidities.[43]

## Weight Management

From 2011–2014, 36.5% of adult Americans were considered obese. Overall, the prevalence of obesity among middle-aged adults ages 40 to 59 years (40.2%) and older adults ages 60 years and older (37.0%) was higher than among younger adults ages 20 to 39 years (32.3%). The prevalence of obesity among women (38.3%) was higher than among men (34.3%).[44] In 2015, the rate of obesity by state was higher in states such as Texas, Oklahoma, Missouri, and South Carolina. Obesity increases the risk for morbidity because of higher risks for; or the presence of hypertension, dyslipidemia, diabetes, coronary heart disease, stroke, gallbladder disease, osteoarthritis, sleep apnea and respiratory problems, and some cancers. Obesity is also related to increased risks of mortality. The biomedical, psychosocial, and economic effects of obesity have significant repercussions for the health and well-being of the US population.[45] **FIGURE 1.8** shows the rate of obesity and the rate of coronary heart disease by state for 2015.

The worldwide rate of obesity has more than doubled since 1980. In 2014, more than 1.9 billion adults ages 18 and older (39% of the world's population) were classified as overweight. Of these, more 600 million (13%) were deemed obese. Sadly, most of the world's population lives in countries where being overweight or obese kills more people than being underweight. In 2014, 41 million children over the age of five years fell into the category of overweight or obese. The silver lining in this epidemic is that obesity is preventable.[46]

The World Health Organization (WHO) defines overweight and obesity as "abnormal or excessive fat accumulation that presents a risk to health."[47] Different measuring indexes are used to capture weight measurements, depending on the age group. For children up to 5 years of age, the WHO's child growth standards introduced in April 2006 are recommended. For individuals 5 to 19 years of age, the WHO has developed growth reference data. The data are a reconstruction of the 1977 National Center for Health Statistics (NCHS) and WHO reference and uses the original NCHS data set supplemented with data from the WHO child growth standards sample for young children up to age 5 years. Body mass index is the most frequently used measure of overweight and obesity in adults. BMI is calculated by dividing an individual's weight in kilograms by the square of his or her height in meters (kg $\div$ m$^2$).[47] See **TABLE 1.9** for a list of BMI ranges and corresponding weight classifications.

The BMI provides the most useful population-level measure of overweight and obesity, as it is the same for both genders and for all ages of adults. It is important to note that one of the limitations of BMI measurement is that it may not correspond to the same body-fat percentage in different individuals.[47]

Globally, increased BMI is a risk factor for noncommunicable diseases such as cardiovascular disease, DM, musculoskeletal disorders (such as osteoarthritis), and cancer (particularly endometrial, breast, ovarian, prostate, liver, kidney, and colon). The risk for these noncommunicable illnesses rises for individuals with higher BMIs. Childhood obesity is linked with a higher chance of adult obesity, premature death, and adult disability. Aside from health risks in their future, obese children suffer from breathing problems and have higher risks for fractures, hypertension, cardiovascular disease, insulin resistance, and attendant psychological consequences.[46]

## What Is Being Done About the Obesity Epidemic?

In 2004, the World Health Organization implemented the "WHO Global Strategy on Diet, Physical Activity and Health" program, which outlines the steps needed to promote healthy diets and active lifestyles. This initiative challenges all stakeholders to get involved at global, regional, national, and local levels to improve diet and physical-activity patterns for all members of the population. The WHO has also put in place its "Global Action Plan for the Prevention and Control of Non-Communicable Diseases 2013–2020." Endorsed by heads of state and government in September 2011, this program seeks a 25% reduction in premature mortality from noncommunicable diseases by 2025. In 2016, the World Health Assembly requested a plan from the director general of the WHO's Commission on Ending Childhood Obesity to address the obesogenic environment and critical periods in the life course to tackle childhood obesity.[46] In the United States, HP 2020 addresses nutrition and weight status as one of its topic areas.

## Heart Disease

Every 42 seconds, someone somewhere in the United States has a heart attack. Every minute, an American

(A)

**2015**

Rate of coronary heart disease mortality among US adults (18+)

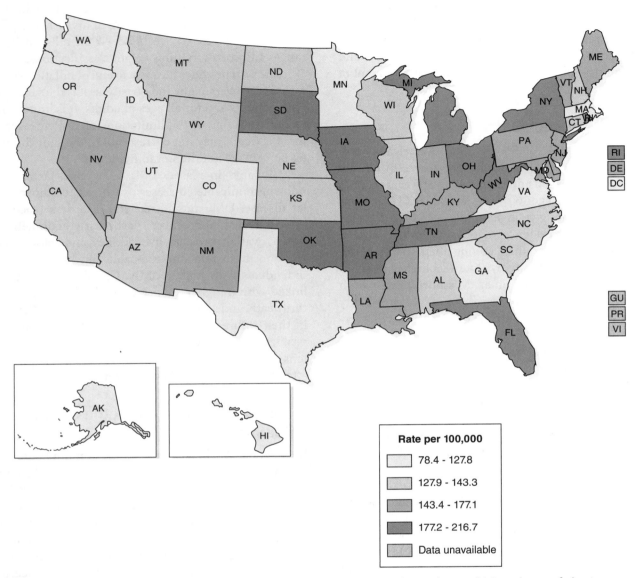

Rate per 100,000

- 78.4 - 127.8
- 127.9 - 143.3
- 143.4 - 177.1
- 177.2 - 216.7
- Data unavailable

**FIGURE 1.8** Coronary heart disease and obesity rate, 2015 (a) Rate of coronary heart disease (b) Prevalence of obesity

Data from CDC Data Trend Interactive Maps. https://www.cdc.gov/dhdsp/maps/dtm/index.html Accessed July 3, 2017. Map developed by Nancy Munoz using CDC interactive data tools

dies from a condition related to heart disease.[48] In fact, heart disease is the leading cause of death for both men and women. More than half of those who died from heart disease in 2009 were men. In the United States, one out of every four deaths results from heart disease, and approximately 610,000 Americans die from heart disease every year.[49] Heart disease includes several types of heart conditions such as coronary artery disease, heart attacks, and related conditions such as angina. The most common type of heart disease in the United States is coronary artery

disease, which affects the blood flow to the heart. In 2014, approximately 356,000 people died from coronary artery disease.[49]

Heart disease is the leading cause of death for people of most racial and ethnic groups in the United States, including African Americans, Hispanics, and whites. For Asian Americans or Pacific Islanders and American Indians or Alaska Natives, heart disease is second only to cancer.[50] The United States spends some $207 billion per year in caring for individuals with heart disease when healthcare services,

(B)

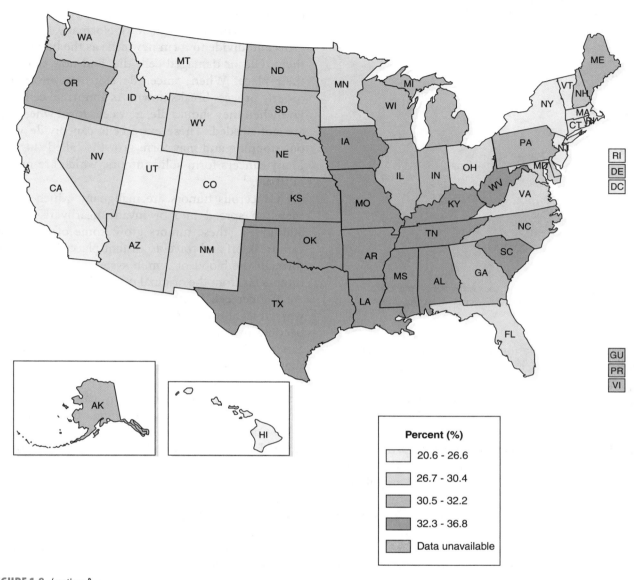

**2015**
Prevalence of obesity among US adults (20+)

**Percent (%)**
- 20.6 - 26.6
- 26.7 - 30.4
- 30.5 - 32.2
- 32.3 - 36.8
- Data unavailable

**FIGURE 1.8** *(continued)*

Data from CDC Data Trend Interactive Maps. https://www.cdc.gov/dhdsp/maps/dtm/index.html Accessed July 3, 2017. Map developed by Nancy Munoz using CDC interactive data tools.

medications, and loss of productive time are included in this amount.[49]

Additionally, heart disease is also the leading cause of death around the world. In 2012, 15.5 million people reportedly died from heart disease, accounting for 31% of all worldwide deaths. Of these deaths, 7.4 million died from coronary heart disease and 6.7 million died from strokes. More than three-quarters of the deaths related to heart disease occur in countries with low to middle incomes.[49]

Most cardiovascular diseases can be prevented when an individual focuses on behavioral factors such as the use of tobacco, being obese and over-weight, engaging in unhealthy eating patterns, having a physically inactive lifestyle, and consuming alcohol in higher-than-recommended amounts. Individuals with heart disease or who have a high risk for developing heart disease (by having one or more risk factors such as hypertension, diabetes, hyperlipidemia, or a preexisting diagnosis of the disease) need early detection and intervention as appropriate.[51] The WHO has identified both population-wide and individual low-resource interventions that, when used jointly, can help decrease the burden associated with

**TABLE 1.9** BMI classification

| Classification | BMI Range |
|---|---|
| Underweight | < 18.5 |
| Normal | 18.5–24.9 |
| Overweight | > 25.0 |
| Pre-obese | 25–29.9 |
| Obese | > 30.0 |
| Obese I | 30–34.9 |
| Obese II | 35–39.0 |
| Obese III | > 40 |

Data from World Health Organization. (2016). *Global Strategy on Diet, Physical Activity, and Health.* http://www.who.int/dietphysicalactivity/childhood_what/en/. Accessed August 18, 2017.

heart disease. Population-wide strategies that can be implemented to decrease heart disease include the implementation of comprehensive tobacco policies and the use of taxation to decrease the intake of foods that are considered high in sodium, fat, and sugar. Adjusting the environment by constructing walking and bicycling paths, helping people limit their consumption of alcohol, and providing heathy school meals to children are also examples of population strategies.[51]

At the individual level, systems must be in place to identify individuals with overall high total risk factors or single risk factors such as hypertension and hypercholesterolemia. Secondary prevention of heart disease in individuals with a diagnosis of the disease includes the use of medications such as aspirin, beta blockers, angiotensin-converting-enzyme inhibitors, and statins.[51]

Health benefits achieved by implementing these interventions are mostly independent. When smoking cessation is added to these strategies, 75% of recurrent vascular events are preventable.[51]

In 2013, WHO members agreed on global strategies to decrease the avoidable noncommunicable-disease burden. This includes reducing the global prevalence of hypertension by 25% and ensuring that at least 50% of eligible individuals would receive drug therapy and counseling to prevent heart attacks and strokes.[51]

In the United States, one HP 2020 goal is focused on improving the cardiovascular health of all Americans by 20% and reducing deaths from cardiovascular diseases and stroke by 20% by the year 2020.[52]

# Cancer

Cancer is the name given to a collection of related diseases. Some types of cancer can start in any of the trillion cells in the human body. Normally, these cells grow and divide to form new cells as the body needs them. Old or damaged cells die, and new cells take their place. When cancer develops, however, this orderly process breaks down. As abnormal cells survive when they should die, new cells form when they are not needed. These extra cells can divide without stopping and may form growths called **tumors**. Many cancers form solid tumors, which are masses of tissue.[53]

Cancerous tumors are malignant, which means they can spread into or invade nearby tissues. In addition, as these tumors grow, some of their cells can break off and travel to distant places in the body through the blood or lymph systems and form new tumors far from the original tumor.[53]

Cancer cells differ from normal cells in many ways that allow them to grow out of control and become invasive. One important difference is that cancer cells are less specialized than normal cells—that is, where normal cells mature into highly distinct cell types with specific functions, cancer cells do not. This is one reason why cancer cells continue to divide without stopping, unlike normal cells. Cancer cells are able to ignore signals that tell normal cells to stop dividing or that begin apoptosis (cell death), which the body uses to rid itself of unneeded cells.[36]

Each year in the United States, more than 1.5 million people are diagnosed with cancer—and more than 500,000 Americans die of cancer. By 2020, the number of new cancer cases is expected to increase to nearly 2 million a year.[54]

More than half of all cancer deaths could be prevented by healthy choices, screening, and vaccinations. Not smoking, drinking alcohol in moderation or not at all, getting enough sleep, eating a diet rich in fruits and vegetables and low in red meat, and getting enough physical activity have been shown to improve overall health and lower the risk of developing some cancers.[54]

Smoking causes approximately 90% of lung cancer deaths in men and almost 80% in women. Smoking also causes cancers of the larynx, mouth, throat, esophagus, bladder, kidney, pancreas, cervix, colon, and stomach, as well as a type of blood cancer called acute myeloid leukemia.[54]

The CDC supports comprehensive efforts at local, state, and national levels to prevent and control cancer for all Americans. To optimize public-health efficiency and effectiveness, the CDC recommends coordinating chronic-disease prevention efforts in four key domains:[54]

1. Epidemiology and surveillance to monitor trends and track progress
2. Environmental approaches to promote health and support healthy behaviors
3. Healthcare system interventions to improve the effective delivery and use of clinical and other high-value preventive services
4. Community programs linked to clinical services to improve and sustain the management of chronic conditions

These four domains help organize and focus the effective work done by the public-health community for many years. At the same time, they help concentrate efforts to strengthen programs and build expertise to address gaps in services. Finally, they help government agencies, state and local grantees, and diverse public and private partners find new ways to work together and support each other's efforts.[54]

Worldwide, cancer is among the leading cause of morbidity and mortality. In 2012, 14 million new cases and 8.2 million cancer-related deaths were reported. New cases of cancer are expected to grow by 70% over the next 20 years. The most-common cancer sites in men were lung, prostate, colon and rectum, stomach, and liver. In women, cancer is most commonly diagnosed in the breast, colon and rectum, lungs, cervix, and stomach. Approximately one-third of cancer-related deaths are associated with lifestyle behaviors such as increased BMI, minimal intake of fruit and vegetables, sedentary lifestyles, and habitual use of tobacco and alcohol.[55]

In excess of 60% of all new annual cases of cancer arise in Africa, Asia, and Central and South America. These regions account for 70% of the world's cancer deaths.[56]

In 2013, the WHO rolled out its Global Action Plan for the Prevention and Control of Non-Communicable Diseases 2013–2020. One aim of the plan includes reducing premature mortality from cancer by 25%.[55]

## Nutritional Epidemiology

**Epidemiology** concerns itself with the causes of diseases in populations and how diseases they develop and spread. The patient is the community, and individuals are viewed collectively. By definition, epidemiology is the scientific, systematic, and data-driven study of the distribution (frequency, pattern) and determinants (causes, risk factors) of health-related states and events (not just diseases) in specified populations (neighborhood, school, city, state, country, global). It is also the application of such study to controlling health problems.[57] Epidemiology is an essential element of public health, offering the basis for guiding practical and appropriate public-health interventions grounded in this science and in causal reasoning.[58]

Results obtained from epidemiologic studies are used to assess a community's health, make individual decisions, complete a clinical picture, and look for causes.[57] Public-health officials accountable for policy development, implementation, and evaluation use epidemiologic data as a factual framework for decision making. Many individuals may not recognize that they use epidemiologic evidence to make daily decisions affecting their health. When someone decides to quit smoking for example, or climbs the stairs rather than wait for an elevator, or eats a salad rather than a cheeseburger with fries for lunch, he or she may be influenced, consciously or unconsciously, by epidemiologists' assessment of risk.[57]

As epidemiologists research illness occurrence, they depend on healthcare providers to determine the correct diagnosis of each individual. On the other hand, epidemiologists offer providers an increased understanding of the clinical presentation and history of the condition being evaluated. A considerable number of epidemiologic studies are focused on finding causal elements that affect any individual's possibility of developing disease.[57]

Nutritional epidemiology is a moderately new field of medical research that looks at the association between nutrition and health. Diet and physical activity are difficult to measure accurately, which may partly explain why nutrition has received less attention than other risk factors for disease in epidemiology.[42]

The rigor of the research associated with nutritional epidemiology varies. Meta-analyses with questionable design and execution have helped to disperse contradictory messages about nutrition and health. One example of this is Flegal et al.,[59] who concluded that being overweight lessens the risk of all-cause mortality. Similarly, a contradicting meta-analysis reported that substituting saturated fat with polyunsaturated fats has no significant effect on cardiovascular risk.[59] These types of conclusion can be dangerous. Misleading or contradicting messages can prevent the public from adopting healthy lifestyles.[60]

Nutritional epidemiology requires design and analysis strategies that are unique to the field of food and nutrition. Appreciating the particulars of nutritional epidemiologic research demands a thorough understanding of nutritional science and its methodological background.[60]

## Measuring Nutrition Intake

Although the methods to collect information on nutrient intake have many limitations, numerous procedures have been created to determine nutrient intake from individuals and populations at large. Tools such as food-composition tables, food-frequency questionnaires, and

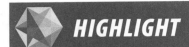

## HIGHLIGHT

### Understanding Types of Research

**Meta-analysis and systematic review**
Summarizes the clinical research that has been performed by independent investigators and researchers. This is critical assessment of all the research that looks at a specific topic.

**Randomized controlled trials**
Subjects that have a specific condition are randomly (by chance) assigned to one of two groups, eighter a treatment or a control group. While at baseline both groups one similar, the control group receives the standard treatment/intervention and the treatment group receives the treatment/intervention that is newly created.

**Cohort study**
Groups of people that have a certain condition or receive a specific treatment are followed over time. This group is compared to a similar group of people that do not have the condition or receive the treatment of interest.

**Case-control studies**
Compares two groups, one with a condition of interest to a similar group that is free from the condition of interest.

**Cross-sectional studies**
This type of study looks at specific populations at a given point in time to measure the occurrence of a clinical risk factor, outcome, or unique result.

**Case reports / Case series**
Case reports are published of clinical obsevation. This is a retrospective description of a distinct case that presents differently than projected. A case series is a retrospective report of the outcomes of a group of petients with the condition of intrest that are treated in a similar fashion.

### References

1. Aslam S, Georgiev H, Mehta K, Kumar A. Matching research design to clinical research questions. *Indian J Sex Transm Dis.* 2012;33:49–53.
2. Kumar R. *Research Methodology.* 2008. New Delhi, India: APH Publishing.
3. Titler MG. The evidence for evidence-based practice implementation. Chapter 7 in: Hughes RG, editor. *Patient Safety and Quality: An Evidence-Based Handbook for Nurses.* (2008). Rockville, MD: Agency for Healthcare Research and Quality. Available from: http://www.ncbi.nlm.nih.gov/books/NBK2659/.

biomarkers have shown good validity with the use of several criteria. The strengths unique to each method make it appropriate for use in particular applications.

The gold standard for determining nutrient information is the multiple-week diet record. With this tool, individuals document all items they consume over a period of several weeks. The method is different from other data-collection processes because an individual does not have to depend on his or her memory. The high contributor burden as well as the cost of maintaining diet records has reduced their use in large-scale epidemiologic studies. The capacity of these records to convey thorough diet data makes them valuable in validation studies for other dietary assessment techniques. Another drawback of diet records is that the procedure of logging data can alter an individual's diet, thus rendering the data nonrepresentative of actual and usual intake. On the other hand, projected intakes from diet records have shown high correlation with results from multiple 24-hour recalls.[61] In recurrent 24-hour recalls, a participant details all foods eaten in the preceding 24 hours or calendar day to a skilled interviewer in person or over the phone. This technique has been commonly used in dietary-intervention trials. It is also used in national surveys to discover trends in nutritional intake.[60]

## Nutritional Epidemiology in Illness Cause and Effect

One of the main reproaches stacked against nutritional epidemiology is that it depends heavily on observational data. This research method is believed to be secondary to experimental data in defining causation. When evidence from randomized controlled trials is not available, nutritional epidemiologists characteristically rely on prospective cohort studies, the strongest observational study design in terms of diminishing bias and deducing causality.[60]

**Recap**  The incidence of obesity is associated with increased risks for morbidity associated with the presence of hypertension, dyslipidemia, diabetes, coronary heart disease, stroke, gallbladder disease, osteoarthritis, sleep apnea, respiratory problems, and some cancers. Obesity has also been linked to increased risk of mortality. Nutritional epidemiology is a moderately new field of medical research that looks at the association between nutrition and health.

## ▶ **Chapter Summary**

Consuming healthy foods and living an active lifestyle are basic ways to promote health and well-being. Getting adequate nutrition is particularly important during periods of rapid growth and development. Following an unhealthy eating pattern during pregnancy, infancy, childhood, and adolescence can contribute to underdeveloped physical and mental abilities that have lifelong consequences. Prolonged nutrition deficiency, whether from excessive or inadequate intake, will promote or exacerbate a range of ailments and affect an individual's quality and length of life.

The use of nutrition screening allows for the identification of individuals who are at nutritional risk so that a full nutrition assessment can be completed. The Academy defines a nutrition assessment as "identifying and evaluating data needed to make decisions about a nutrition-related problem/diagnosis."[21] Nutrition-assessment techniques can be classified as one of four types: anthropometric, biochemical, clinical, or dietary.

The increased understanding of the role of nutrition in promoting health and well-being has made the evaluation of individuals, families, and communities key to monitoring public health.

 **CASE STUDY**

In the 21st century, the incidence of chronic disease has displaced the previous prevalence of nutrient deficiency as the primary area of public-health concern as population conditions. Leading causes of death have shifted from infectious diseases to chronic conditions. Approximately one-half of all American adults—117 million individuals—have one or more preventable chronic diseases, many of which are related to poor-quality eating patterns and physical inactivity.

Dr. Jones is a researcher who was just awarded a grant by the National Institute of Health (NIH) to measure the prevalence of diabetes in a selected sector of Camden, New Jersey.

### *Questions:*

1. As you go through the information in this chapter, determine which nutrition assessment methods you would incorporate in your procedure.
2. What drives your assessment-method selection?

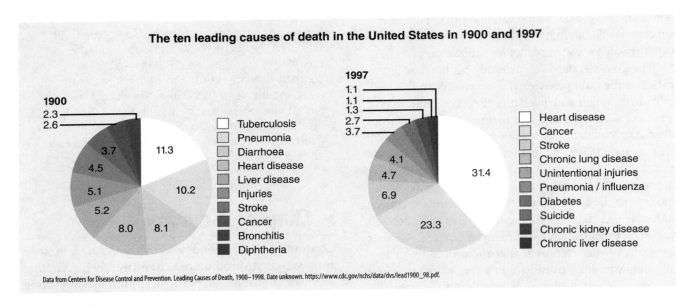

The ten leading causes of death in the United States in 1900 and 1997

Data from Centers for Disease Control and Prevention. Leading Causes of Death, 1900–1998. Date unknown. https://www.cdc.gov/nchs/data/dvs/lead1900_98.pdf.

# Learning Portfolio

## Key Terms

Anthropometry
Body mass index (BMI)
Bureau of Labor Statistics Consumer expenditure survey data
Epidemiology
Food and Agriculture Organization of the United Nations (FAO)
Healthy People 2020 (HP 2020)
Interprofessional
Nutrition assessment
Nutrition Care Process (NCP)

Nutrition Care Process Terminology (NCPT)
Nutrition Care Process and Model (NCPM)
Nutrition diagnosis
Nutrition-focused physical exam (NFPE)
Nutrition intervention
Nutrition screening
PES statement
Scurvy
Subjective global assessment (SGA)
Tumors

## Study Questions

1. The key difference between a nutrition-screening form and a nutrition-assessment form is:
   a. Screening forms provide a diagnosis for malnutrition
   b. Screening forms determine risk for malnutrition
   c. Screening forms diagnose chronic disease
   d. Screening forms determine risk for weight gain

2. The Academy of Nutrition and Dietetics recommends using the _____ screening form to assess risk for malnutrition in the adults in the clinical setting.
   a. MUST
   b. SNAQ
   c. Mini SNAQ
   d. Mini MUST

3. When writing PES statements, the section that includes the cause of the nutrition problem is the _____.
   a. Problem
   b. Etiology
   c. Signs and symptoms
   d. Intervention

4. Which of the following is *not* one of the four steps of the Nutrition Care Process?
   a. Screening and referral
   b. Nutrition assessment
   c. Nutrition intervention
   d. Nutrition diagnosis

5. The part of the Nutrition Care Process that involves data collection, reviewing the data for key factors, and comparing that data against nutrition care criteria is:
   a. Nutrition diagnosis
   b. Nutritional assessment
   c. Nutrition intervention
   d. Nutrition monitoring and evaluation

6. The HP 2020 Nutrition objectives:
   a. Are released by the Food and Drug Administration
   b. Are objectives to measure progress for health concerns in specific populations
   c. Has 10 prominent goals
   d. Provides strategic management for use only at the national level

7. Which of the following is *not* one of the four prominent nutrition goals for HP 2020?
   a. Eliminate all tobacco use by adults, teenagers, and children
   b. Attain high-quality longer lives free of preventable disease, disability, injury, and premature death
   c. Create social and physical environments that promote good health for all
   d. Achieve health equity, eliminate disparities, and improve the health of all groups

8. Which of the following is an objective that falls in the "weight status" category of the HP 2020 objectives?
   a. Reduce the proportion of adults who are at a healthy weight
   b. Reduce the number of women who are morbidly obese
   c. Increase the proportion of adults who are at a healthy weight
   d. Reduce the proportion of men who are underweight

9. Which of the following is *not* one of the objectives for the area of food and nutrient consumption for individuals age 2 years and older?
   a. Increase the consumption of fruits
   b. Increase the consumption of dairy
   c. Reduce the consumption of calories from solid fats
   d. Reduce the consumption of sodium

10. Diabetes is the _____ leading cause of death in the United States.
    a. First
    b. Second
    c. Seventh
    d. 10th

11. The most useful population-level measure of overweight and obesity in adults is:
    a. Ideal body weight
    b. Body mass index
    c. Body fat and lean mass percentages
    d. Growth charts

12. Which of the following is the leading cause of death for Americans?
    a. Diabetes mellitus
    b. Heart disease
    c. Stroke
    d. Osteoporosis

13. Half of all cancer deaths could be prevented by:
    a. Frequent primary care provider visits
    b. Sedentary lifestyle
    c. Polypharmacy
    d. Healthy eating practices and lifestyle choices

14. The strongest observational study design used in nutritional epidemiology is the:
    a. Meta-analysis
    b. Randomized placebo-controlled trial
    c. Prospective cohort
    d. Case control

15. Information included in the clinical history includes all of the following *except*:
    a. Medication
    b. Changes in food intake
    c. Medical diagnosis
    d. Laboratory tests

16. When should the nutrition-focused physical exam be conducted?
    a. After the lab values are in the medical record
    b. At the time of admission
    c. After the history is obtained
    d. Before any procedure is performed

17. According to the consensus statement by the Academy of Nutrition and Dietetics and ASPEN, malnutrition is diagnosed when the following two symptoms are present:
    a. Loss of muscle mass and loss of fluid
    b. Excessive energy intake and excessive subcutaneous fat
    c. Inadequate energy intake and weight loss
    d. Improved handgrip strength and fluid loss

18. Which of the following are two distinct steps in the intervention part of the Nutrition Care Process?
    a. Planning and implementation
    b. Communication and nutrient delivery
    c. Coordinating care and education
    d. Collecting and assessing data

19. Which of the following is a reason why micronutrient deficiency is not as prevalent in the United States today?
    a. Food staples were required by law to be enriched or fortified with important nutrients
    b. More people have access to antibiotics
    c. It is a farm-to-table philosophy
    d. Megadoses of nutrients are frequently used

20. The phrase "inadequate intake" is found in the _____ part of the nutrition diagnostic statement:
    a. Problem
    b. Signs and symptoms
    c. Etiology
    d. Assessment

21. Measuring weight, height, and body composition are examples of the data collection for the _____ method.
    a. Biochemical
    b. Anthropometric
    c. Clinical
    d. Dietary

22. Measuring blood nutrient concentrations, urinary metabolites, and blood lipid concentrations are examples of data collected in the _____ assessment method.
    a. Clinical
    b. Anthropometric
    c. Biochemical
    d. Dietary

23. The dietary data-collection method that uses a structured listing of individual foods or groups of foods that an individual consumes over a period of time is called a _____.
    a. 24-hour recall
    b. Food-frequency questionnaire
    c. Diet history
    d. Three-day food record

24. In the early 1700s, Dr. James Lind discovered an association between the consumption of citrus fruits and the prevention of which deficiency disease?
    a. Osteoporosis
    b. Rickets
    c. Pellegra
    d. Scurvy

25. During the so-called germ theory era, physicians believed that the cause of frequent illnesses in the general population were from _____.
    a. Infectious organisms
    b. Nutrient deficiencies
    c. Nutrient toxicity
    d. Nutrient excesses

26. _____ is the method used to find the causes of health outcomes and diseases in populations.
    a. Assessment
    b. Nutrition-focused physical exam
    c. Epidemiology
    d. Nutrition care process

27. Once micronutrient deficiency diseases were eradicated in the United States, health officials focused their attention on the dietary practices associated with chronic disease. These dietary practices include all of the following *except*:
    a. Excessive sugar intake
    b. Excessive fruit and vegetable intake
    c. Excessive saturated fat intake
    d. Excessive sodium intake

28. The part of the Nutrition Care Process that determines the extent to which intervention goals are met is:
    a. Assessment
    b. Intervention
    c. Diagnosis
    d. Monitoring and evaluation

29. The assessment tool that has been validated to accurately predict poor outcomes and longer length of hospital stay after surgery is the:
    a. Mininutritional assessment form
    b. Mini SNAQ
    c. Malnutrition Universal Screening Tool (MUST)
    d. Subjective global assessment

30. The most reliable indicator of poor nutritional status is:
    a. Weight loss
    b. Low albumin concentrations
    c. Low dietary intake of nutrients
    d. Poor handgrip strength

## Discussion Questions

1. How does the obesity rate affect the incidence of chronic disease in the United States?
2. Describe the shift from infectious disease to chronic disease that affects public health.
3. Nutrition screens allow individuals who are at risk of suboptimal nutritional status to be identified. List and describe the most commonly used screening tools. What are the benefits and drawbacks of each screening tool?

## Activities

1. Develop a marketing campaign targeting a specific segment of the community you live or study in that introduces population-based intervention strategies to reduce obesity and impact overall health.
2. Type 2 diabetes is widespread in all obese groups and now even in preteen children. Develop an education tool to teach young children the health risks associated with diabetes.
3. Select a chronic condition that is prevalent in the American population. Work with three to four classmates to develop "the top 10 must know topics" by the average person in efforts to prevent or manage the disease. Develop a wiki page to communicate the information. Use videos and graphics on the page to deliver the message.

## Online Resources

### Food and Agriculture Organization (FAO) of the United Nations

The FAO develops methods and standards for food and agriculture statistics, provides technical assistance services, and disseminates data for global monitoring. It is the world's largest database of food and agriculture statistics:
http://www.fao.org/statistics/en/.

### Bureau of Labor Statistics Consumer Expenditure Survey Data

This database provides information on the buying habits of American consumers, including data on their expenditures, income, and consumer unit (families and single consumers) characteristics:
http://www.bls.gov/cex/.

### Anthropometric Measurement Videos

This website provides technical videos on how to conduct anthropometric measures:
https://wwwn.cdc.gov/nchs/nhanes/nhanes3/anthropometricvideos.aspx.

### The State of Obesity: Adults in the United States

This website provides interactive maps on adult obesity in the United States:
http://stateofobesity.org/adult-obesity/.

### Malnutrition Universal Screening Tool (MUST)

This website provides the background for the MUST tool, online calculator, and videos.
http://www.bapen.org.uk/screening-and-must/must.

### Mini Nutritional Assessment Tool (MNA)

This website provides an overview of the MNA tool and videos and provides access to the required forms:
http://www.mna-elderly.com/.

## References

1. Herder R, Demmig-Adams B. The power of a balanced diet and lifestyle in preventing cardiovascular disease. *Nutr Clin Care.* 2004;7:46-55.

2. Price S. Understanding the importance to health of a balanced diet. *Nurs Times.* 2005;2005;101:30.

3. Centers for Disease Control and Prevention. What we eat in America. DHHS-USDA Dietary Survey Integration. 2015. https://www.cdc.gov/nchs/nhanes/wweia.htm. Accessed February 3, 2017.

4. Centers for Disease Control and Prevention. Adult obesity causes and consequences. 2016. https://www.cdc.gov/obesity/adult/causes.html. Accessed February 3, 2017.

5. Academy of Nutrition and Dietetics. Nutrition security in developing nations: sustainable food, water, and health. *J Acad Nutr Diet.* 2013;113:581-595.

6. Funk C. The etiology of the deficiency diseases. Beri-beri, polyneuritis in birds, epidemic dropsy, scurvy, experience scurvy in animals, infantile scurvy, ship beri-beri, pellagra. *J State Med.* 1912;20:341.

7. Semba R. The discovery of vitamins. *Int J Vit Nutr Res.* 2012;5:310-315.

8. Davis C, Saltos E. Dietary recommendations and how they have changed over time. Ch. 2 in *America's Eating Habits: Changes and Consequences.* 1999. http://purl.umn.edu/33604. Accessed January 24, 2017.

9. Centers for Disease Control and Prevention. Leading causes of death. 2016. https://www.cdc.gov/nchs/fastats/leading-causes-of-death.htm. Accessed January 22, 2017.

10. Butterworth C. The skeleton in the hospital closet. *Nutrition Today.* 1974 (March–April):436.

11. Dougherty D, Bankhead R, Kushner R, Mirtallo J, Winkler M. Nutrition care given new importance in JCAHO standards. *Nutr Clin Pract.* 1995;10(1):26-31.

12. White JV, Guenter P, Jensen G, et al. Consensus statement: Academy of Nutrition and Dietetics and American Society for Parenteral and Enteral Nutrition: characteristics recommended for the identification and documentation of adult malnutrition (undernutrition). *J Parenter Enteral Nutr.* 2012;36(3):275-283.

13. Lacey K, Pritchett E. Nutrition care process and model: ADA adopts road map to quality care and outcomes management. *J Am Diet Assoc.* 2003;103:1061-1071.

14. Field LB, Hand RK. Differentiating malnutrition screening and assessment: A nutrition care process perspective. *J Acad Nutr Diet.* 2015;15:824-828.

15. Donini LM, De Felice MR, Savina C, et al. Predicting the outcome of long-term care by clinical and functional indices: the role of nutritional status. *J Nutr Health Aging.* 2011;15:586-592.

16. Donini LM, Bernardini LD, De Felice MR, et al. Effect of nutritional status on clinical outcome in a population of geriatric rehabilitation patients. *Aging Clin Exp Res.* 2004;16:132-138.

17. National Alliance for Infusion Therapy, American Society for Parenteral and Enteral Nutrition Public Policy Committee and Board of Directors. Disease-related malnutrition and enteral nutrition therapy: a significant problem with a cost-effective solution. *Nutr Clin Pract.* 2010;25:548–554.

18. Jensen GL, Bistrian B, Roubenoff R, Heimburger DC. Malnutrition syndromes: a conundrum vs continuum. *J Parenter Enteral Nutr.* 2009;33:710-716.

19. Academy of Nutrition and Dietetics Evidence Analysis Library. Nutrition screening (NSCR) (2009–2010). 2010. http://www.andeal.org/topic.cfm?menu=3584. Accessed November 16, 2016.

20. Watterson C, Fraser A, Banks MI, et al. Evidence based practice guidelines for the nutritional management of malnutrition in adult patients across the continuum of care. *Nutr Diet.* 2009;66 (suppl):S1-S34.

21. Academy of Nutrition and Dietetics. International Dietetics and Nutrition Terminology (IDNT) 2008; Reference Manual. ISBN-13: 978-0880914451.

22. Detsky A, Smalley P, Change J. Is this patient malnourished? *JAMA.* 1994;271:54-58.

23. Lew C, Yandell R, Fraser RJ, Chua AP, Chong MF, Miller M. Association between malnutrition and clinical outcomes in the intensive care unit: a systematic review. *J Parenter Enteral Nutr.* 2016;41(5):744-758.

24. Centers for Disease Control and Prevention. *National Health Nutrition Examination Surveys (NHANES).* 2013. http://www.cdc.gov/nchs/data/nhanes/nhanes_13_14/2013_Anthropometry.pdf. Accessed December 3, 2016.

25. National Institutes of Health. *Clinical Guidelines on the Identification, Evaluation, and Treatment of Overweight and Obesity Adults.* 1998; Report no. 98-4083. https://www.ncbi.nlm.nih.gov/books/NBK2003/. Accessed December 3, 2016.

26. National Center for Health Statistics. *National Health and Nutrition Examination Survey.* 2016; https://www.cdc.gov/nchs/nhanes/. Accessed December 16, 2016.

27. National Center for Health Statistics. *Growth Charts.* 2010. https://www.cdc.gov/growthcharts/. Accessed December 3, 2016.

28. Bharadwaj S, Ginoya S, Tandon P, et al. Malnutrition: laboratory markers vs nutritional assessment. *Gastroenterol Rep.* 2016; 4(4):272-280.

29. Lichford M. Putting the nutrition-focused physical assessment into practice in long-term care. *Ann Longterm Care.* 2013;21(11):38-41.

30. Jensen GL Hsiao PY, Wheeler D. Adult nutrition assessment tutorial. *J Parenter Enteral Nutr.* 2012;36:267-274.

31. Frank-Stromborg M, Olsen SJ. *Instruments for Clinical Health-care Research.* 3rd ed. 2004. Sudbury, MA: Jones and Bartlett.

32. Archer E, Hand GA, Blair SN. *Validity of U.S. Nutritional Surveillance: National Health and Nutrition Examination Survey Caloric Energy Intake Data, 1971–2010.* Johannsen D, ed. PLoS ONE. 2013. 8(10):e76632.

33. Academy of Nutrition and Dietetics. NCP 101. 2016. http://www.eatrightpro.org/resources/practice/nutrition-care-process/ncp-101. Accessed December 4, 2016.

34. Bueche J, Charney P, Pavlinac J, Annalynn S, Thompson E, Meyers E. Nutrition care process and model part I: The 2008 update. *J Am Diet Assoc.* 2008; 108(7):1113-1117. https://www.ncbi.nlm.nih.gov/pubmed/18589014.

35. Bueche J, Charney P, Pavlinac J, Annalynn S, Thompson E, Meyers E. Nutrition care process and model part II: the 2008 update. *J Am Diet Assoc.* 2008;108(8):1113-1117. http://jandonline.org/article/S0002-8223(08)01203-0/references.

36. Academy of Nutrition and Dietetics. *Nutrition Terminology Reference Manual (eNCPT): Dietetics Language for Nutrition Care.* 2016. http://ncpt.webauthor.com/. Accessed December 8, 2016.

37. Healthy People 2020. Disparities details by race and ethnicity for 2011–14. 2017. https://www.healthypeople.gov/2020/data/disparities/detail/Chart/4968/3/2014. Accessed July 1, 2017.

38. Centers for Disease Control and Prevention. Healthy People 2020. 2015. https://www.cdc.gov/nchs/healthy_people/HP2020.htm. Accessed December 17, 2016.

39. US Department of Health and Human Services. Heathy People 2020. 2016. https://www.healthypeople.gov/. Accessed December 17, 2016.

40. US Department of Health and Human Services. *Dietary Guidelines for Americans.* 2005. Washington, DC: US Government Printing Office.

41. Ahmed AM. History of diabetes mellitus. *Saudi Med J.* 2002;23(4):373-379.

42. Centers for Disease Control and Prevention. *National Diabetes Statistics Report, 2014.* 2015. http://choosehealth.utah.gov

/documents/pdfs/factsheets/national-diabetes-report-web
.pdf. Accessed December 17, 2016.

43. American Diabetes Association. Nutrition recommendations and interventions for diabetes: a position statement of the American Diabetes Association. *Diabetes Care.* 2008;31(suppl 1):S61-S78.

44. Ogden CL, Carroll MD, Fryar CD, Flegal KM. Prevalence of obesity among adults and youth: United States, 2011–2014. NCHS Data brief, No. 219. 2015. https://www.cdc.gov/nchs /data/databriefs/db219.pdf. Accessed December 17, 2016.

45. US Department of Health and Human Services. *Managing Overweight and Obesity in Adults: Systematic Review from the Obesity Expert Panel—2013.* 2014. Washington, DC: National Heart, Lung, and Blood Institute. https://www.nhlbi.nih.gov /sites/www.nhlbi.nih.gov/files/obesity-evidence-review.pdf. Accessed December 17, 2016.

46. World Health Organization. Obesity and overweight. 2016. http://www.who.int/mediacentre/factsheets/fs311/en/. Accessed December 18, 2016.

47. World Health Organization. *Global Strategy on Diet.* 2016. http://www.who.int/dietphysicalactivity/childhood_what/en/. Accessed August 18, 2017.

48. Mozzafarian D, Benjamin EJ, Go AS, et al. Heart disease and stroke statistics—2015 update: a report from the American Heart Association. *Circulation.* 2015;131:e29–e322.

49. Mozzafarian D, Benjamin EJ, Go AS, et al. Heart disease and stroke statistics—2016 update: a report from the American Heart Association. *Circulation.* 2016; 133(4):e38-e360.

50. Heron M. Deaths: leading causes for 2008. *Natl Vital Stat Rep.* 2012; 60. https://www.cdc.gov/nchs/data/nvsr/nvsr60 /nvsr60_06.pdf. Accessed December 18, 2016.

51. World Health Organization. Cardiovascular diseases (CVDs). 2016. http://www.who.int/mediacentre/factsheets/fs317/en/. Accessed December 18, 2016.

52. American Heart Association and American Stroke Association. Heart disease and stroke statistics—at-a-glance. 2015. http://www.onebraveidea.com/submissions/ucm_470704.pdf. Accessed December 18, 2016.

53. National Cancer Institute. What is cancer? 2015. https:// www.cancer.gov/about-cancer/understanding/what-is-cancer. Accessed December 19, 2016.

54. Centers for Disease Control and Prevention. Preventing one of the nation's leading causes of death at a glance 2016. 2016. https://www.cdc.gov/chronicdisease/resources/publications /aag/dcpc.htm. Accessed December 19, 2016.

55. World Health Organization. Cancer. 2015. http://www.who.int /mediacentre/factsheets/fs297/en/. Accessed December 19, 2016.

56. International Agency for Research in Cancer. *World Cancer Report 2014.* 2015. http://publications.iarc.fr/Non-Series-Publications /World-Cancer-Reports/World-Cancer-Report-2014. Accessed December 19, 2016.

57. Centers for Disease Control and Prevention. What is epidemiology? 2016. https://www.cdc.gov/careerpaths /k12teacherroadmap/epidemiology.html. Accessed December 21, 2016.

58. Cates W. Epidemiology: applying principles to clinical practice. *Contemp Ob/Gyn.* 1982;20:147–161.

59. Chowdhury R, Warnakula S, Kunutsor S, et al. Association of dietary, circulating, and supplement fatty acids with coronary risk: a systematic review and meta-analysis. *Ann Intern Med.* 2014;160:398-406.

60. Satija A, Yu E, Willett WC, Hu FB. Understanding nutritional epidemiology and its role in policy. *Adv Nutr.* 2015;1(5):5-18.

61. Hebert JR, Hurley TG, Chiriboga DE, Barone J. A comparison of selected nutrient intakes derived from three diet assessment methods used in a low-fat maintenance trial. *Public Health Nutr.* 1998;1:207-214.

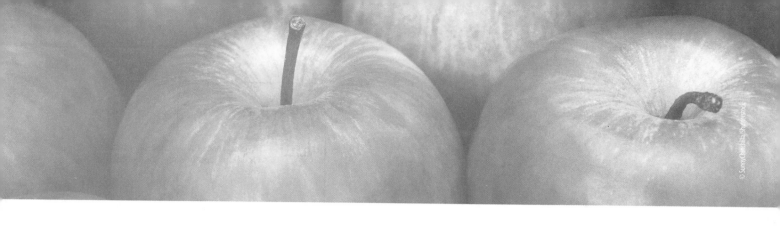

# CHAPTER 2
# Health Research Methods

**Melissa Bernstein**, PhD, RD, LD, FAND
**Ana María Hernández-Rosa**, MS, RDN, LD

## CHAPTER OUTLINE

- Introduction
- The Research Process
- Research Considerations
- Study Approaches
- Analyzing, Interpreting, and Communicating Research
- Why Publish?
- Chapter Summary

## LEARNING OBJECTIVES

After reading this chapter, the learner will be able to:

1. Discuss the professional relevance for establishing competency in reading and evaluating scientific literature.
2. Explain the key features of a research question and a study hypothesis.
3. List the importance of a clearly written literature review.
4. Describe study approaches commonly used in nutrition research, including the strengths and limitations.
5. Describe the tools used to critically evaluate scientific literature.
6. Describe the historical evolution of ethics in clinical research.
7. Identify the primary guidelines and key ethical considerations when conducting research with human subjects.
8. List key issues that may arise when conducting industry-sponsored research.
9. Define the differences between quantitative and qualitative research.
10. Identify the benefits of publishing findings to contribute to evidence-based practice.
11. Understand the use of information for assessing and evaluating nutrition research for relevancy, accuracy, reliability, relevance, and ethical practices.

## ▶ Introduction

Understanding the purpose and importance of **research**, as well as the process of conducting informative and ethical research by health professionals, serve as a fundamental basis for evidence-based nutrition care. Identifying a problem or a question is the origin of a study and leads an investigator to develop a research question and hypothesis. Research provides a systematic process for uncovering answers to questions and

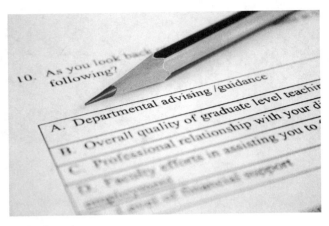

© alexskopje/Shutterstock.

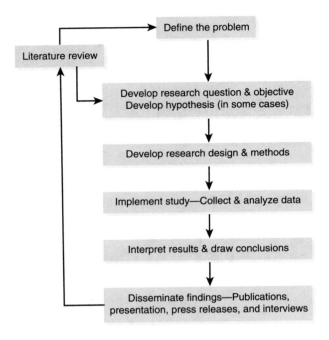

**FIGURE 2.1**  The scientific method.

expanding current knowledge that can be applied to clinical practice, education, and public health. Study methodology for sound research must be well defined and in a format that can be investigated. Choosing the right study design to answer the research question and test a hypothesis can make or break a study. In fact, study design determines the validity, reliability, strength of results, and conclusions. Errors in study design can lead to bias, confounding, weakened findings, and even lead to inaccuracies in results. It is thus essential to the research process that the study design be suitable for achieving the research purpose. The aim of this chapter is to introduce health professionals to scientific inquiry and the study designs common in nutrition research.

# ▶ The Research Process

> **Preview**   Reading and appraising scientific research is an essential skill for healthcare professionals and nutrition practitioners. Scientific research is the basis for evidence-based nutrition practice across the spectrum of professional responsibilities that run from individual clinical patient care to broader public-health policy and recommendations.

Understanding the scientific process and research are fundamental for nutrition professionals to practice evidence-based care, provide current and informed medical nutrition therapy, and establish expertise as a source of accurate, current, and reliable nutrition information. Learning about the process, methods, data analysis, results interpretation, and dissemination of scientific research will enable practitioners to better understand the foundations of clinical practice and reasoning, which are the basis for nutrition and

health recommendations and advancing the dietetics profession. The organized process of research is illustrated in **FIGURE 2.1**. Learning how to interpret medical research, healthcare literature, and research findings is an essential baseline skill for nutrition and healthcare professionals.

Research is an ongoing and dynamic process in which the results and findings from one study can stimulate new inquiry and perpetuate further investigation contributing to lifelong learning, professional advancement, and overcoming healthcare challenges. The opportunities to apply the knowledge gained from research are varied. Research findings, for example, can be used to improve patient care, establish or streamline food-delivery programs, educate consumers, and market dietary supplements. Going beyond what is currently "known" to dig deeper and further understand what is not known drives ongoing discovery. **Applied research** compels investors to further clinical reasoning, advance the knowledge base, and translate findings into practical applications for patient care and education.

The overall purpose of nutrition research is to solve nutrition-related problems and build a body of knowledge that supports and advances nutrition-related practices, whether for improved patient care, national nutrition guidance, or community-related food programs. **Evidence-based nutrition practice** is based on the body of knowledge built from scientific research and serves as the foundation for nutrition professionals regardless of the setting. Understanding nutrition research and the ability to critically interpret published scientific studies enables nutritionists to make appropriate and informed decisions about patient care and communicate as reliable food and nutrition professionals.

## The Research Question

The ambition to further knowledge, dig deeper, and explain more drives research further and advances nutrition practice. Research begins with a question. At its most basic level, identifying a problem, asking a question about how to solve the problem, and then searching for the answer is the foundation of research. Even if the **research question** is not fully constructed to spark an actual scientific research process, critical inquiry is what frequently drives a new research initiative. The form that a research study will take depends directly on the research question. Sometimes this question is based on personal interests, societal problems, or previous research. Whatever the inspiration for the topic or problem, the research question should be systematically planned, thoughtfully organized, and deliberately constructed.

A research question is designed to shed light on a problem and starts by asking about a relationship between two or more variables. The question may originate from a current gap in knowledge or result from conflicting findings in previous studies. A well-stated research question should be focused to describe the who, what, and how of the research project: Who will be assessed? What is the variable of interest that will be examined, or the intervention being implemented? How will the outcome be evaluated?[1] The research question should be clearly written, measurable, and straightforward. In scientific publications, the research question often will be clearly stated in the study introduction.

## The PICOT Format and FINER Criteria

A carefully constructed research question will serve as the foundation for the study hypothesis and therefore the study design. The research question should be evaluated for its clinical relevance and must be deemed answerable before proceeding with establishing a research agenda. A research question should be straightforward and include only one variable to be assessed.[2] Two commonly used tools for the development of a good research question are the PICOT format (which stands for, population, intervention, comparison group, outcome, and time) and the FINER criteria (which stands for feasible, interesting, novel, ethical, and relevant; see **TABLES 2.1** and **2.2**). The PICOT format is useful when developing a

### TABLE 2.1 The PICOT format

| P = Population (participants, patients) | What population will be examined? |
|---|---|
| I = Intervention (observations) | What is the intervention or exposure of interest? |
| C = Comparison group | Who will be the comparison group? |
| O = Outcome | What is the outcome being examined or measured? |
| T = Time | What is the time frame for assessment or follow-up? |

### TABLE 2.2 The FINER criteria

| F = Feasible | Is the study feasible? |
|---|---|
| I = Interesting | Is the study interesting? |
| N = Novel | Is the study novel? |
| E = Ethical | Is the study ethical? |
| R = Relevant | Is the study relevant? |

specific research question; it considers the population to be examined, the intervention to be studied, the comparison group, and the outcome of interest, and it may also include the study's time frame. Similarly, following the FINER criteria improves the creation of a good research question. A worthwhile study question is feasible, interesting, novel, ethical, and relevant to furthering current knowledge.

## Developing a Research Hypothesis

Moving forward with a research idea requires three initial steps[3]:

1. Stating a research question.
2. Identifying subjects and variables.
3. Stating a specific and measurable hypothesis that will define the study design and methods.

A study **hypothesis** can logically be developed from a well-written research question. A hypothesis is written following a review of available evidence and identification of variables of interest. Hypotheses are

*Alternate hypothesis*: In older adults, an 8-week community-based nutrition education program will significantly ($p < 0.05$) increase daily intake of fruits and vegetables as measured by a food-frequency questionnaire, compared with older adults who attend a weekly community meeting that does not include nutrition education.

*Null hypothesis*: In older adults, attending an 8-week community-based nutrition education program there will be no significant ($p < 0.05$) increase in daily intake of fruits and vegetables as measured by a food-frequency questionnaire, compared with older adults who attend a weekly community meeting that does not include nutrition education.

**FIGURE 2.2** Alternate and null hypothesis examples.

prediction statements about what the investigators expect to happen during the study. A hypothesis is designed to test the relationship between the dependent and independent variables—that is, whether an **independent variable** affects a **dependent variable**. The null hypothesis considers the possibility that the change could be the result of chance and therefore tests for the possibility that no difference results from the study (see **FIGURE 2.2**). Hypotheses must clearly define and specify relationships between two or more variables being investigated.[2] A hypothesis, whether written in as an **alternate hypothesis** or as **a null hypothesis**, should have the following attributes:[1]

- It should be measurable—that is, a hypothesis should be written in a form that can yield measurable results that can be analyzed and compared against the null hypothesis (stating that there will be no difference in primary outcome).
- It should specify the population being studied, including characteristics of the participant sample such as gender, age, and disease status.
- It should identify the time frame or the period over which the study will take place.
- It should specify the type of relationship being investigated or examined. When applicable, the hypothesis specifies the intervention type.
- It should clearly define the study variables, including comparison and outcome variables as well as any dependent variable(s).
- It should state the level of significance. When formally testing for statistical significance, the hypothesis should be stated as a null hypothesis.

- It should clearly identify the control group.
- It should clearly identify the study's setting.

Hypothesis-driven research is the foundation for studies in clinical nutrition.[1] A hypothesis will determine the design, methods, and statistical analysis for any study. Statistical inference is based on testing a null hypothesis—that there is no difference or effect.[2] The goal of most studies is therefore to "reject" the null hypothesis being tested to "accept" the alternate hypothesis. In other words, "there is" a statistically significant difference resulting from the effects of the independent variable on the dependent variable.

## Conducting a Literature Review

When faced with a research question, the first step is to determine if someone else has already found an answer to the question. A thorough and extensive **literature review** and systematic search is the basis to advance knowledge. A review of the literature may turn up hundreds of thousands of studies that need to be reviewed and summarized. Studies need to be collected, assessed, analyzed, and synthesized using prestated, standardized, rigorous, and transparent methods to lead to evidence-based conclusions. Performing a critical review of previously published work provides the foundation for which a research question and study hypothesis can be based and a new research project developed. Going back to the FINER criteria, for example, a comprehensive review of the existing scientific literature enables the investigators to begin to determine if their project is feasible, interesting, novel, ethical, and relevant. Performing a literature review provides a basis for what is already known about the topic of interest.

When beginning a literature review, the first task after establishing a topic is to complete a comprehensive search for relevant articles to include. During this process, a reference librarian can be a valuable source of assistance in choosing search criteria, search terms, and keywords; determining subject hearings; and providing tutorials on various search engines and other database-navigation techniques. When choosing articles, remember that the literature review will need to establish a clear line of argument to justify why the study should be conducted.[4] Once the relevant studies have been identified and critically read, those that will be included in the literature review are selected. To help organize research to aid in comparing and contrasting multiple studies, a summary of studies table maybe helpful (**TABLE 2.3**).

The introductions to most articles in scientific journals serve as opportunities for authors to review

**TABLE 2.3** Summary of studies table

| Author | Study Purpose/ objective or hypothesis | Subjects / Participants | Study Length or Duration | Study Design and Key Methods | Key Outcome Variables | Significant Findings | Study Strengths and Limitations | Strength of Evidence |
|---|---|---|---|---|---|---|---|---|
| **Study 1** | | | | | | | | |
| **Study 2** | | | | | | | | |
| **Study 3** | | | | | | | | |

the literature and provide readers with essential background, as well as state what is currently known about the topic and establish the basis for the research question and study hypothesis. The primary purpose of the literature review is to clearly define and describe what is already known about the topic of interest and identify the gaps in current knowledge, in attempt to justify why additional research is warranted. The literature review also provides an opportunity to critically analyze existing studies and then compare the methods and results from multiple studies with consideration of the individual study's strengths and limitations. The literature review should be written as a summary of all the studies synthesized and not simply as a list of individual study summaries one after the next. This is a challenging part of scientific writing and takes significant thought and analysis. An informative literature review is a synthesis of carefully selected and relevant studies that have been critically analyzed and compared and contrasted for their common themes and findings. A literature review should also offer insight into differences between studies and conflicting findings to establish a gap in knowledge that needs further investigation. Guidelines for writing a literature review are listed in **FIGURE 2.3**.

## Understanding and Evaluating Scientific Evidence

To stay current on new nutrition research is challenging. With approximately 2.5 million new scientific publications each year,[5] and more than 35,460 entries that include the key term *nutrition* on Medline in 2016,[6] this task can be quite overwhelming, especially if you don't have the skills, experience, or training in

how to read and review scientific literature. In July 2017, a Google search for the term *nutrition* brought up 158,000,000 results in just 2 seconds—with 387,168 articles in PubMed alone. Unfortunately, professionals know they cannot simply believe everything they read, even if a source appears reputable. To maintain the highest level of professionalism, be

1. Start with a clear introduction that explains how the review is organized and the purpose of the proposed research.
2. Use headings to organize the literature review in a logical manner that will guide the reader.
3. Start each paragraph with a strong topic sentence that clearly states the main idea of the paragraph. Use active voice rather than passive tense.
4. Use transitional words and phrases to connect ideas between sentences and paragraphs so that narrative flows logically and smoothly.
5. Acknowledge and be respectful of results and opinions of other research—even those that do not agree with your thesis. It is okay to indicate when results are conflicting or inconclusive and why you think so. Use a professional tone in doing so.
6. Use quotations when necessary, but do so sparingly. A literature review should be primarily your own synthesis of the research.
7. Write in an academic style.
8. Consistently reference the literature in your discussion.
9. Reference sources and be careful not to plagiarize.
10. Write a summary and conclusion at the end.

**FIGURE 2.3** Guidelines for writing a literature review.

reliable sources of nutrition information, and provide the most current and timely clinical nutrition patient care, nutritionists must be comfortable and confident in reading, reviewing, and interpreting published scientific literature. A critical appraisal of research should not be thought of as a "critique"—it is a systematic process used to identify the strengths and limitations of a research article in attempt to assess the validity and utility of the findings in professional or clinical settings.[7]

Critically reviewing scientific literature can be daunting. Ever since standardized evaluation tools became widely used, the process has become streamlined and objective. Interpreting literature, however, still requires that reviewers be knowledgeable about their subject areas. This assumes familiarity with the language, techniques, and methods used and allows for an understanding of as many aspects of a study as possible. When approaching a critical review of a scientific research article, there are important questions to ask before making assumptions about the study (**TABLE 2.4**).

Numerous tools and resources are available to guide investigators during critical review of scientific literature. The evidence analysis library (EAL) of the Academy of Nutrition and Dietetics (the Academy) has analysts who use a quality criteria checklist to objectively evaluate a study's design and methods. Additional tools are available to evaluate specific types of studies. The Consolidated Standards of Reporting Trials (CONSORT) 2010 Checklist (see Appendix A), for example, describes information to include when reporting a randomized trial. The CONSORT group is an independent panel of experts who developed a checklist with the goal of increasing the transparency of randomized controlled trials and to identify when there are deficiencies in a study design. Cochrane (www.cochrane.org) is a global network of researchers. The aim is to provide quality information to help those who want to make informed healthcare decisions by publishing independent systematic reviews and tools for assessing and evaluating studies.[8] A Swiss organization (www.strobe-statement.org) describes its online purpose as "*Strengthening the Reporting of Observational Studies in Epidemiology*" (STROBE). It offers a checklist of items that should be included in observational studies (see Appendix B). To improve the quality of reporting for systematic reviews, the *Preferred Reporting Items for Systematic Reviews and Meta-Analysis* (PRISMA) (www.prisma-statement .org) checklist is an evidence-based minimum set of items for reporting in systematic reviews and meta-analyses. It can also be used as a basis for reporting

| **TABLE 2.4** Questions to ask and answer when reviewing scientific literature |
| --- |
| 1. What is the source (journal) of the article? |
| 2. Was the publication peer reviewed? |
| 3. Who are the authors and what are their affiliations? |
| 4. What (or who) is the main subject of the study? |
| 5. What problem(s) were investigated? |
| 6. What is the purpose or rationale for the study? |
| 7. Who or what constituted the sample or population? |
| 8. What was the design of the study? |
| 9. What statistical analyses were used? |
| 10. What are the results? |
| 11. Are the results clear? |
| 12. Did the results answer the identified questions? |
| 13. Do the results seem valid? |
| 14. Are the interpretations (conclusions) of the results consistent with the study design and analysis? |
| 15. Are the results consistent with findings from similar studies? |
| 16. What do the results mean to medicine and health care, and you and your patients? |
| 17. Can the results be applied to your research or clinical practice? |

systematic reviews for other types of research, such as evaluations of interventions (see Appendix C).[9] Many of these checklists also have "extension" checklists that can be used for other study designs. STROBE version 4, for example, has STROBE checklists for cohort, case-control, and cross-sectional studies, and these are available for download from the organization's website.

**Recap**   Research begins with a question, identifies a problem, asks a question about how to solve the problem, and then searches for the answer. From a well-written research question, a hypothesis is written following a review of available evidence and the identification of variables of interest. Hypotheses are prediction statements about what investigators expect to happen during a study. An informative literature review is a synthesis of the relevant studies that have been carefully selected, critically analyzed, and then compared and contrasted for their common themes and findings. The review should provide insight into differences between studies and conflicting findings, to establish a gap in knowledge that needs further investigation. Numerous tools and resources are available to guide investigators in the critical-review process of scientific literature.

# ▶ Research Considerations

**Preview** This section discusses how research with human subjects became regulated. It also describes the most important ethical principles and challenges of working with human subjects.

Research is the pursuit of knowledge, often with the hope it will contribute to the betterment of society. Investigators have the responsibility to conduct studies and interventions in a way that maximizes the benefits and minimizes the harms for research participants. The possible benefits and burdens of science must be distributed evenly among all participants. Health professionals, including registered dietitians, must competently conduct research and be knowledgeable about federal regulations, rules, and laws that govern research practices as well as the guidelines and ethical standards set forth by professional organizations. While conducting research with human subjects, the protection of the rights and welfare of all persons must always be a priority.

## Ethical Considerations in Health Research

The cruel acts against and abuse of human subjects performed by Nazis during World War II (see the next section), as well as the Tuskegee study and the Willowbrook study, have negatively affected the public's trust in behavioral and biomedical research. The Tuskegee Study of Untreated Syphilis in the Negro Male (**FIGURE 2.4**) was designed by the Public Health Service

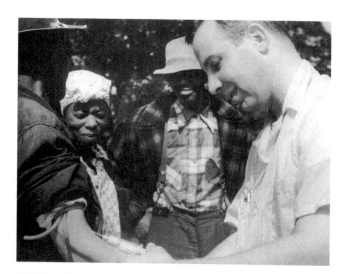

**FIGURE 2.4** Tuskegee syphilis study.

Reproduced from National Archives, Atlanta, GA (1932) Tuskegee Syphilis Study Pictures: Unidentified subject. https://upload. wikimedia.org/wikipedia/commons/3/3a/Tuskegee-syphilis-study_doctor-injecting-subject.jpg.

in 1932. The aim of this 40-year research study was to investigate the history of syphilis so that prevention and treatment programs could be developed for black men. The study had the following major ethical violations[10]:

1. The study initially involved 600 black men; 399 had syphilis and 201 did not. The study was conducted without telling these men whether or not they had syphilis and thus they could not give informed consent. None received proper treatment to cure their illnesses, even when penicillin became the drug of choice for treating syphilis in 1947.
2. Participants were never given proper treatment for their disease. Even after penicillin was discovered as an effective treatment for syphilis in 1947, researchers never offered treatment to the study's subjects.
3. An ad hoc advisory panel appointed by the assistant secretary for Health and Scientific Affairs concluded that the Tuskegee Study was "ethically unjustified." This means that the knowledge gained was sparse when compared with the risks the study posed for its subjects.

On the other hand, the Willowbrook experiments were performed with children who experienced intellectual disabilities.[11] These children received care in the Willowbrook State School in Staten Island, New York. They were intentionally exposed to hepatitis—mostly hepatitis A—with the goal of tracking the virus's development in the human body. The study continued for 14 years. The following issues made this study highly unethical:

1. The subjects in this **experiment** constituted a **vulnerable population**, which can be defined as a group of people who are relatively (or absolutely) incapable of protecting their own interests and who may be exposed to harm.
2. The interference with informed consent violated the subjects' rights.
3. The nontherapeutic nature of the experiment did not justify the deliberate infections and exposure to hepatitis.

These historic and high-profile research studies have raised appropriate concerns and questions.[12] For this reason, ethical considerations must always be put in place when planning a research study involving living subjects.

## Historical Context and the Nuremberg Code

The **Nuremberg Code** of 1947 was the most important document in the history of medical ethics and research, and it included principles that govern research with human subjects. The code includes informed-consent procedures and gives subjects the right to withdraw from a research study at any time without penalties. The code was enacted after the world learned of the atrocities and abuse committed by German scientists against human subjects during World War II. The experiments can be divided into three categories[13]:

1. *High-altitude experiments done by the German Experimental Institution for Aviation using a low-pressure chamber.* The objective was to determine the maximum altitude from which passengers of an aircraft could parachute to safety. Scientists also carried out freezing experiments to find an effective treatment for hypothermia. They carried out these experiments with prisoners who were also used to test different methods for turning seawater into drinking water.

2. *Testing and development of medications and therapies to treat illnesses of German military personnel.* Nazi scientists tested immunization compounds and sera for the prevention and treatment of contagious diseases such as malaria, typhus, tuberculosis, typhoid fever, yellow fever, and infectious hepatitis. Prisoners of concentration camps were also exposed to phosgene and mustard gas to test possible antidotes.

3. *Experiments to trace the genetic origins of various diseases.* Dr. Josef Mengele performed a wide variety of cruel and deadly experiments with Jewish and Roma twins, most of whom were minors.

## Nuremberg Code Regulations

The Nuremberg Code's regulations state the following:[14]

1. The voluntary consent of the human subject is essential. This means that the person involved should have legal capacity to give consent; should be so situated as to be able to exercise free power of choice, without the intervention of any element of force, fraud, deceit, duress, overreaching, or other ulterior form of constraint or coercion; and should have sufficient knowledge and comprehension of the elements of the subject matter involved as to enable him to make an understanding and enlightened decision. This latter element requires that before the acceptance of an affirmative decision by the experimental subject there should be made known to him the nature, duration, and purpose of the experiment; the method and means by which it is to be conducted; all inconveniences and hazards reasonable to be expected; and the effects upon his health or person which may possibly come from his participation in the experiment. The duty and responsibility for ascertaining the quality of the consent rests upon everyone who initiates, directs or engages in the experiment. It is a personal duty and responsibility that may not be delegated to another with impunity.

2. The experiment should be such as to yield fruitful results for the good of society, unprocurable by other methods or means of study, and not random and unnecessary in nature.

3. The experiment should be so designed and based on the results of animal experimentation and a knowledge of the natural history of the disease or other problem under study that the anticipated results will justify the performance of the experiment.

4. The experiment should be so conducted as to avoid all unnecessary physical and mental suffering and injury.

5. No experiment should be so conducted where there is an *a priori* reason to believe that death or disabling injury will occur—except, perhaps, in those experiments where the experimental physicians also serve as subjects.

6. The degree of risk to be taken should never exceed that determined by the humanitarian importance of the problem to be solved by the experiment.

7. Proper preparations should be made and adequate facilities provided to protect the experimental subject against even remote possibilities of injury, disability, or death.

8. The experiment should be conducted only by scientifically qualified persons. The highest degree of skill and care should be required through all stages of the experiment of those who conduct or engage in the experiment.

9. During the experiment the human subject should be at liberty to bring the experiment to an end if he has reached the physical or mental state where continuation of the experiment seems to the subject to be impossible.

10. During an experiment, the scientist in charge must be prepared to terminate the experiment at any stage, if there is probable cause to believe, in the exercise of the good faith, superior skill and careful judgment required of him that a continuation of the experiment is likely to result in injury, disability, or death to the experimental subject.

## The Declaration of Helsinki

The **Declaration of Helsinki of 1964** was developed by the World Medical Association (WMA).[15] Its purpose was to elaborate the ethical principles for medical research with human subjects that were previously presented in the Nuremberg Code. The most recent amendment of the declaration was done during the WMA General Assembly in Fortaleza, Brazil, in October 2013. In 2014, the WMA produced a celebratory publication to mark the 50th anniversary of the adoption of the Declaration of Helsinki. This document contains the general ethical principles and the terms related to possible risks, burdens, and benefits of research studies. It also mentions the groups and individuals considered particularly vulnerable. The declaration details the tasks of research ethic committees and explains the importance of safeguarding the privacy and confidentiality of research subjects' personal health information. The specific requirements of **informed consent** are also noted.

## The National Commission for the Protection of Human Subjects of Biomedical and Behavioral Research

The **National Commission for the Protection of Human Subjects of Biomedical and Behavioral Research** (1974–1978) was established through the **National Research Act of 1974**.[16] The commission is generally recognized as the first national bioethics commission. This commission developed the document known as the Belmont Report.

## Belmont Report: Principles (Beneficence, Autonomy, Justice)

The **Belmont Report of 1979** was published April 18, 1979, by the National Commission for Protection of Human Subjects of Biomedical and Behavioral Research.[17] The report is a statement of basic ethical principles and guidelines that should help resolve the ethical problems that surround the conduct of research with human subjects. The document is divided into three main sections. The first section establishes the difference between the objectives and methods used in research versus the ones in practice. The second section highlights the fundamental ethical principles that must guide research with human subjects, including respect for persons, beneficence, and justice.

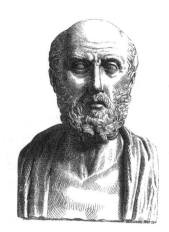

**FIGURE 2.5** Hippocrates.

Reproduced from 1881 Young Persons' Cyclopedia of Persons and Places.

The principle of **respect for persons** includes two moral requirements: the requirement to acknowledge autonomy and the requirement to protect those with diminished autonomy. Respect for persons requires that subjects be accepted to participate in research studies voluntarily and with adequate information and discussion before they consent to participate.

On the other hand, the concept of **beneficence** is widely used in the medical field and is based on the Hippocratic oath's ethical code (**FIGURE 2.5**), which requires that physicians treat their patients "according to their best judgment." The principle focuses on maximizing good results while minimizing harms.

With regard to **justice**, researchers must ensure they will provide all subjects with equitable and fair treatment and that each person can access the benefits of science. The recruitment of research participants needs to happen under critical observation and examination. This will help determine whether certain groups or social classes are being systematically chosen because of manipulability or accessibility, among other reasons, instead of being chosen for reasons that are closely related to the problem under study. When financial support for the research study comes from public funds, justice requires that the findings do not provide advantages only to those individuals who can afford to pay for new therapies and devices. Therefore, research should not disproportionately enroll participants from groups that would have barriers in receiving benefits from the applications of the research study.

The third section of the Belmont Report identifies and describes informed-consent procedures, risk-benefit analysis, recruitment of subjects, and justice in terms of bearing the possible benefits and burdens of a research intervention.

## Informed Consent

Informed consent is one of the most basic concepts of responsible biomedical and behavioral research. The purpose of an informed-consent document is to demonstrate the respect of subjects' autonomous determination to make informed, rational, and voluntary decisions to participate in research studies.[18] The informed-consent process must be done by protecting members of vulnerable populations from participation decisions that could be harmful or result in exploitation. Informed consent must meet the following requirements:

1. *Information.* First, the most relevant information and details about the research study must be disclosed to the participant in a way that can be readily comprehended. This information should summarize the purpose of the research and its procedures, timeline, and methods to protect the subject's privacy and confidentiality.
2. *Voluntariness.* The second requirement is that consent must be voluntary and that the subject was not pressured or coerced by the research staff to participate in the study.
3. *Comprehension.* The third requirement is that the consent is rational, meaning that participants understand the information that was discussed with them. This includes the possible risks and benefits of participation.

## Assessment of Risks and Benefits

The assessment of risks and benefits requires a display of relevant information, including other ways of obtaining the benefits sought from the research intervention. This evaluation therefore presents an opportunity to gather systematic and comprehensive details about the proposed study. The researcher must evaluate whether the study has been designed properly. From the review committee point of view, it is a way to determine if the risks to study participants are justified. This assessment will help the prospective participants decide whether to participate.

## Institutional Review Board

Under federal regulations, an **institutional review board (IRB)** is a group of experts who have been formally assigned to review and monitor biomedical research with human subjects. Any institution that receives federal funds must have an IRB. All research conducted by students, faculty, and staff must be reviewed.[19]

The IRB oversees the ethical and safety aspects of the research study.[20] The IRB must be composed of at least five members, one of whom must be a community member who does not have a scientific background and another who has no affiliation with the institution of the primary investigator. Members of the IRB assess the risks and benefits of the proposed study. The IRB is responsible for approving the study protocol, the informed-consent form, and all advertisements designed to recruit participants before their involvement. The study protocol must be reviewed annually.

## Types of Research and the IRB

Three main types of research are supposed to be evaluated by an IRB committee.[21] **Exempt research** refers to risk-free research. In this case, review is not required.[22] An example is when a study looks at the routine food-service practices in a hospital. If the research staff does not interact with the subjects, then review is not required. The second type is **minimal-risk research**. In this scenario, the risk of harm is no greater than the risk encountered in daily life or routine examinations. This type of research requires routine review by the IRB. The third type of research is a study that poses **greater than minimal risk**. This type of research may involve physical or psychological stress. In this case, a thorough review needs to be conducted by the IRB.

## Conflict of Interest

The term **conflict of interest** can be used in different ways. It can be defined as "a set of circumstances that creates a risk that professional judgment or actions regarding a primary interest will be unduly influenced by a secondary interest." A clearer definition of conflict of interest is "a conflict between the private interests and the official responsibilities of a person in a position of trust." A conflict of interest thus occurs when an individual must choose one set of interests against another.[23]

Health professionals and biomedical investigators collaborate with the pharmaceutical industry, medical device and biotechnology companies to conduct research and develop new treatments. This interdisciplinary relationship has produced important discoveries that benefit individuals and improve quality of care. However, this partnership has also created conflicts regarding financial gain of the pharmaceutical industry versus the values and goals of healthcare professionals. Therefore, physicians, healthcare institutions, and research centers must always put patients' safety and interests first. They should also oversee studies so that investigators carry out unbiased research.

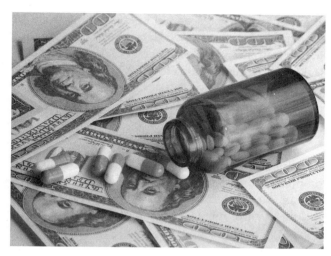

© lenetstan/Shutterstock.

The issues of conflict of interest arise when a member of a research team seeks financial gain or other benefits rather than focusing on the pursuit of knowledge, promotion of health, prevention of disease, or cure of disease.[24] Patients, participants in a research study, scholars, and the public should all have confidence that doctors and investigators will make ethical judgments. The primary interests of professionals conducting research with human subjects should include the promotion and protection of the integrity of research, the welfare of individuals enrolled in the study, and the quality of training and education of future public-health professionals.

Secondary interests are not limited to financial gain. Other examples of secondary interests include the desire for professional advancement; personal achievement; recognition within a field; and favors to colleagues, friends, or family members. Financial interests are more worrisome and common because the industry and for-profit companies mainly influence health professionals and researchers through their economic support. For a researcher, this financial gain should be subsidiary to sharing his or her findings in an unbiased way in scientific conferences, journals, and other peer-reviewed publications.

According to social science research findings, individuals can be influenced without even being conscious of it. Under certain conditions, there is always a risk of influencing an individual's professional judgment. This occurs more by secondary interest than by the primary interests previously mentioned.

## Conflict-of-Interest Policies

Policies must be in place to avoid conflict of interest. These policies must serve two interrelated purposes: (1) sustaining public trust in research, and (2) maintaining the integrity of professional judgment.[25] Conflict-of-interest policies attempt to decrease the influence of secondary interests through the following practices:

- Publishing findings in a timely manner
- Providing quality care
- Developing and updating professional practice guidelines
- Informing patients about advancements in treatment
- Encouraging other researchers and health professionals through teaching

As a rule of thumb, all policies should be clear, reasonable, and fair. Although a one-size-fits-all conflict-of-interest policy does not exist, at a minimum a basic policy should ask the following:[26]

- Who does the policy apply to?
- How should the disclosure be made?
- What are the enforcement procedures?
- What are the consequences of noncompliance?

## Industry-Sponsored Research

Although biases can come from diverse sources, recent emphasis has been focused on industry-sponsored research. Consider the historical context in which industry has been involved in scientific research. Before World War II, most food-related research was funded and conducted by food-industry researchers. In the years after World War II, the United States went through a period of rapid technological evolution and scientific development. This evolution also included the transformation of agriculture in terms of production and a steady increase in industry growth. The companies that experienced this steady growth were those involved in medical, pharmaceutical, chemical, and food production.

Currently, industry-funded research studies account for a large proportion of all nutrition and research related to food science.[27] Economic support from industry is inevitably a major component of the scientific environment, although it is just one component of an extremely complex system. Issues of conflict of interest and possible bias need to be approached with experience and skills to manage and correct these problems effectively. Furthermore, guidelines and recommendations should be in place.

## Guidelines for Industry-Sponsored Research

The International Life Sciences North America Working Group on Guiding Principles proposed eight conflict-of-interest guidelines. The guidelines presented in **FIGURE 2.6** appeal to industry funding and aim to safeguard the integrity and credibility of scientific findings, especially with respect to nutrition professionals, human health, and food science.

In conjunction with a strong peer-review system, open declarations of research sponsorship, and policies, these guidelines provide a framework for conducting industry-sponsored research that is beyond reproach.

## Bias

**Bias** is defined as any tendency that prevents unprejudiced consideration of a question. Bias can happen at any stage of the research process, starting from the design continuing through data analysis, and ending in publication. Examples of bias at each stage of a clinical trial are presented in **FIGURE 2.7**.

## Research and Protection for Vulnerable Populations

A vulnerable population is "the state of an individual or population being vulnerable to a particular disease or event."[28] The **factors** determining risks may include environmental, psychological, psychosocial,

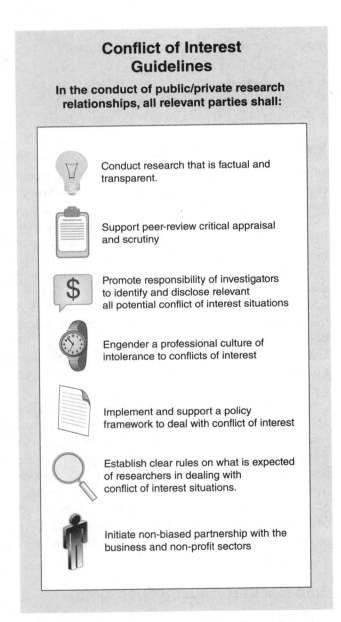

**FIGURE 2.6** Conflict-of-interest guidelines for public and private research affiliations.

Modified from Rowe et al. Funding food science and nutrition research: financial conflicts and scientific integrity. *Am J Clin Nutr* 2009;89:1285–91. http://ajcn.nutrition.org/content/89/5/1285.full.pdf+html. Accessed May 7, 2017.

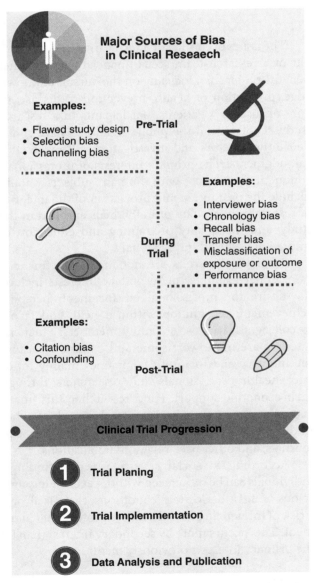

**FIGURE 2.7** Major sources of bias in clinical research and the stages of the trial affected.

Data from Pannucci C, Wilkins E. Identifying and avoiding bias in research. *Plast Reconstr Surg*. 2010 August; 126(2): 619–625. doi:10.1097/PRS.0b013e3181de24bc. https://www.researchgate.net/publication/45461983_Identifying_and_Avoiding_Bias_in_Research. Accessed August 6, 2017.

# HIGHLIGHT

## Confused about Nutrition? You Are Not Alone

We've all seen the flashy headlines, read the hyped-up blogs or glanced at the must-read social media posts about nutrition, diet, supplements, and health. They appear daily—multiple times—as shown in **FIGURE A**.

Nutrition and health professionals have long known that exaggerated science not only confuses the public but makes the job of credentialed nutritionists (RDNs) and committed scientists even harder.

Sensational news stories in newspapers, coupled with the premature dissemination of research findings, are "damaging" to the field of academic research on nutrition and have eroded the public's trust of nutrition science.[1] According to the report,

> "The detrimental impact of poor nutrition on the health and wellbeing of individuals, healthcare systems and the economy is substantial. Nutrition research has the potential to make a profound positive impact on human health in the UK and globally. The failure to adequately address nutrition research in an organized and structured way seriously undermines the ability to achieve best health at lowest cost."

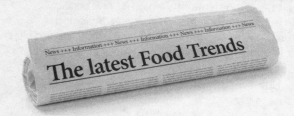

**FIGURE A** Headline example.

© Zerbor/Shutterstock.

Additionally, there has been, and rightfully so, much skepticism of industry sponsored research and the appointment of nutrition scientists to industry-backed committees and boards, leading to further discredit of research findings and increased suspicion of conflict of interest.[2] This further leads to discouraged and confused consumers, perpetuating the "quick fix" mentality.

Take the popularity of fad diets, for example. Whether scientist of celebrity endorsed, fad diets are a multi-billion dollar revolving door of short-lived, disappointing diets that usually lack substantial scientific support. **FIGURE B** shows a visual overview of some of the more well-known fad diets over the past 200 years.

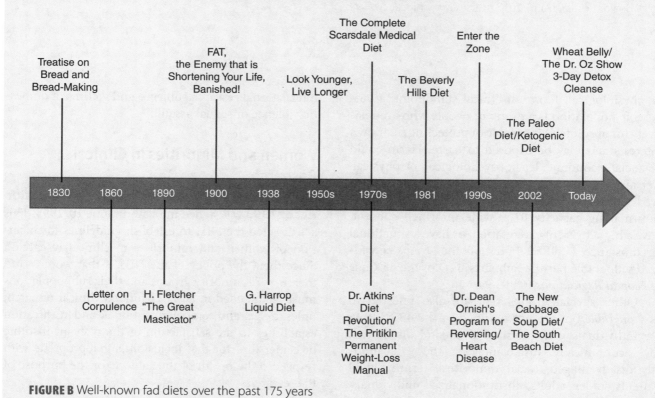

**FIGURE B** Well-known fad diets over the past 175 years

Nutrition research is extremely complex. It encompasses many different areas of study with important links to health and disease research, public health, environmental sustainability, and social and behavioral influences. The far-reaching and interconnected nature of nutrition makes it hard to filter out a single, simple, take-home, one line answer that many people are seeking.

Nutrition research is also exciting and always changing. Nutrition scientist are constantly discovering more and more about how the body works and how the food/ fuel we eat affects health. This means that in this area of study there is always more to learn, always something new to figure out. As nutritionists, scientists, and educators our job is a big one. We have to possess the tools to compare any headline to scientifically sound, evidence-based recommendations to determine the accuracy of the findings and communicate clearly to the public. The goal being, to empower informed consumers (**FIGURE C**). The hallmark of a healthy diet, however, is unfortunately not usually "sensational" or "headline worthy" The Academy of Nutrition and Dietetics (as well as lots of other credible nutrition and health experts) recommend getting all the nutrients your body needs by first attempting to eat a varied diet of "real," whole foods, meaning less-processed foods and a more plant-based diet, as the best strategy for living a healthful life and avoiding many chronic degenerative diseases. Plus regular exercise, of course.

### References

1. Medical Research Council. National Institute for Health Research July 2017 https://www.nihr.ac.uk/

### Be a Safe and Informed Consumer

o Let your health care professional advise you on sorting reliable information from questionable information.

o Contact the manufacturer for information about the product you intend to use.

o Be aware that some supplement ingredients, including nutrients and plant components, can be toxic. Also, some ingredients and products can be harmful when consumed in high amounts, when taken for a long time, or when used in combination with certain other drugs, substances, or foods.

o Do not self-diagnose any health condition. Work with health care professionals to determine how best to achieve optimal health.

o Do not substitute a dietary supplement for a prescription medicine or therapy, or for the variety of foods important to a healthful diet.

o Do not assume that the term "natural" in relation to a product ensures that the product is wholesome or safe.

o Be wary of hype and headlines. Sound health advice is generally based upon research over time, not a single study.

o Learn to spot false claims. If something sounds too good to be true, it probably is.

**FIGURE C** Be a safe and informed consumer

Reproduced from US Food and Drug Administration http://www.fda.gov/ForConsumers/ConsumerUpdates/ucm050803 .htm. Accessed August 1, 2017.

news-and-events/documents/Review%20of%20 Nutrition%20and%20Human%20Health_final.pdf accessed 8.1.17.

2. Nestle, M. Food Politics www.foodpolitics.com. accessed 8.1.17

or physiological. From an ethical standpoint, a vulnerable population is a group of people who are relatively (or absolutely) incapable of protecting their own interests and may be exposed to harm. Harm could be social, economic, legal, psychological, or physical. Certain groups and individuals may be considered vulnerable because: they do not have the decision-making capacity to provide informed consent, have a higher risk of exploitation, or have a situational circumstance. **FIGURE 2.8** presents the groups considered vulnerable per the Subparts B–D of the 45 *Code of Federal Regulations* (CFR) Part 46.

Other special groups that are also referred to as *vulnerable* but are not outlined in the 45 CFR 46 are individuals with physical or mental disabilities, the economically disadvantaged, the educationally disadvantaged, racial minorities, terminally ill patients, older adults, institutionalized individuals, international research subjects, and victims of domestic violence or sexual assault.[29]

## Women and Minorities in Clinical Research

The **National Institutes of Health Revitalization Act of 1993** was signed into law on June 10, 1993. This act directed the NIH to establish guidelines for inclusion of women and minorities in clinical research.[30] Since then, the policy of the NIH is that women and members of minority groups and their subpopulations must be included in all NIH-funded clinical research, unless a clear and compelling rationale and justification establishes to the satisfaction of the relevant institute or center director that inclusion is inappropriate with respect to the health of the subjects or the purpose of the research.

**1**   Pregnant women and neonates          **2**   Children                    **3**   Prisoners

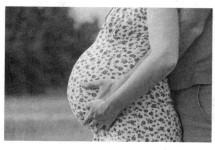 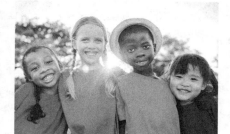 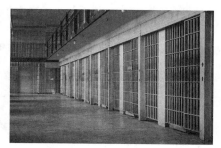

**FIGURE 2.8** Vulnerable populations.

© aragami12345s/Shutterstock; © Rawpixel.com/Shutterstock; © txking/Shutterstock.

## Theory Development

Principal investigators should assess the theoretical or scientific linkages between gender, race and ethnicity, and their topics of study.[31] Following this evaluation, the principal investigator and the applicant or research institution will address the policy in each application and study proposal, providing the required information on inclusion of women and minorities and their subpopulations in clinical research. They must also state any required justifications for exceptions to the established policy.

## Challenges and Barriers: Recruitment and Informed Consent

Challenges to recruiting efforts and obtaining informed consent are developing as demographics change and clinical trials become more inclusive. One major recruitment challenge and a significant barrier to communicate with potential research subjects is the prevalence of low **health literacy**, or how much individuals are able to obtain, process, and understand basic health information and services needed to make appropriate health decisions.[32]

### Prevalence of Low Health Literacy

The National Assessment for Adult Literacy has reported that low health literacy tends to be higher in immigrant individuals who spoke a language other than English before starting their formal school education.[30] Members of minority groups or adults living below the poverty level also have lower average health literacy. Low health literacy affects both research and the economy because the patient needs to read and understand important healthcare information. As previously mentioned, cultural and language barriers negatively affect effective communication with patients. According to the Agency for Healthcare Research and Quality, differences in health literacy level were consistently associated with increased hospitalizations, greater emergency-care use, lower use of mammography, lower receipt of influenza vaccine, less ability to demonstrate taking medications appropriately, less ability to interpret labels and health messages, and, among seniors, poorer overall health status and higher mortality. Health literacy level potentially mediates disparities.

In 2004, the National Academy of Medicine estimated that 90 million people in the United States had limited health literacy.[33] Both healthcare professionals

## HIGHLIGHT

### Morbid Obesity

Morbidly obese patients are usually excluded from clinical trials since a weight over 300 pounds is a common exclusion criterion. Oseltamivir (Tamiflu®) pharmacokinetics in Morbid Obesity (OPTIMO trial) was one of the first clinical trials that emphasized the importance of studying drug dosing for morbidly obese patients. The alarming rates of life-threatening complications and deaths from Influenza H1N1 affecting obese patients triggered investigators to examine the possible causes of the disparity.

Data from L. M. Thorne-Humphrey, K. B. Goralski, K. L. Slayter, T. F. Hatchette, B. L. Johnston, S. A. McNeil, (The 2009 OPTIMO Study Group); Oseltamivir pharmacokinetics in morbid obesity (OPTIMO trial). *J Antimicrob Chemother* 2011; 66 (9): 2083–2091. doi: 10.1093/jac/dkr257 Link to Full Text https://academic.oup.com/jac/article/66/9/2083/768948/Oseltamivir-pharmacokinetics-in-morbid-obesity

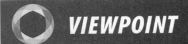

## VIEWPOINT

### Interprofessional Healthcare Teams

*Diane R. Bridges, PhD, MSN, RN, CCM*

*400,000. What do you think this number represents? The answer is…MEDICAL ERRORS!*

In 1999, the National Academy of Medicine (formerly called the Institutes of Medicine) report, "To Err is Human: Building a Safer Health System," charged that mistakes and unsafe practices in American hospitals kill at least 44,000 patients and perhaps as many as 98,000 Americans die in hospitals each year as a result of medical errors."[1]

In 2013, it was reported this figure may be as high as 400,000 deaths a year.[2] In this same year, hospital medical errors were listed as the third-leading cause of death in the U.S.[3] Additionally, medical errors cost the nation $1 trillion each year.[4]

To put this number in perspective: It is equivalent to two fully occupied 747 planes crashing every day!

We as a society would not tolerate this happening, so why do we tolerate medical errors?

Medical errors were noted to be one of the ten most common *sentinel events*. A sentinel event is a "patient safety event (not primarily related to the natural course of the patient's illness or underlying condition) that reaches a patient and results in either severe temporary harm, permanent harm or death."[5]

The 10 most-cited reasons sentinel events occur are due to a person or a lack of the following[6]:

1. Human factors
2. Communication (provider to provider and provider to patient)
3. Leadership
4. Assessment
5. Information management
6. Physical environment
7. Care planning

8. Continuum of care
9. Medication use
10. Operative care

### So what can we do to reduce medical errors?

The American Medical Association stated "With an aging population and surge for newly insured patients entering the system, we encourage other states to consider adopting this innovative approach to helping facilitate the work of highly functioning teams of medical professionals who can meet the growing demand for healthcare".[7,8] The answer to how we can reduce medical errors is to develop highly skilled and functional interprofessional healthcare teams that communicate, collaborate, and cooperate with each other and the patient families to provide the highest quality care.

An interprofessional team includes healthcare providers from different professional backgrounds who work together and alongside patients, carers, patient families, and communities to deliver the best quality care they can provide.[9,10] Based on their knowledge and skills, each team member assumes profession-specific roles.[8,11] Then as a team they combine resources, identify and analyze problems, and assume joint responsibility for the patient care plans they devleop.[8,11] It is through these deliberate acts of collaboration and communication with other healthcare professionals that highly functioning interprofessional teams are formed.[12] Outcomes of a collaborative interprofessional team approach have been shown to reduce adverse events, improve patient

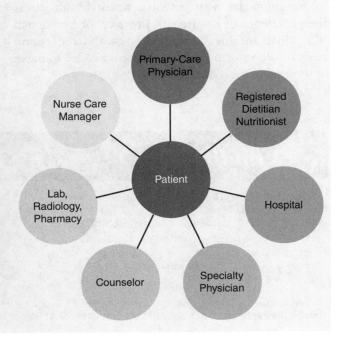

outcomes, as well as, improve patient and employee satisfaction.[13]

The team involves all healthcare providers including registered dietitian nutritionists (RDN's) as they are a vital member of the healthcare team. It is a known fact that the diets people eat, impact their health, development, morbidity and mortality.[14] Communication between RDNs and patients and RDNs and other healthcare providers are essential to providing the best care possible to patients. It is up to each individual healthcare provider to forge these relationships, become an active member of the healthcare team and work together on conducting research that will help demonstrate positive patient outcomes when interprofessional teamwork is practiced.

### References

1. Institute of Medicine; Committee on Quality of Health Care in America. *To err is human: Building a safer health system*. Washington D.C.: National Academies Press; 1999.
2. James J. A new, evidence-based estimate of patient harms associated with hospital care. *Journal of Patient Safety*. September2013; 9(3):122–128. doi: 10.1097/PTS.0b013e3182948a69.
3. Makary M, Daniel M. Medical error-The third leading cause of death in the US. *BMJ*. 2016; 353:i2138. doi: http://dx.doi.org/10.1136
4. Andel C, Davidow S, Hollander M, Moreno D. The economics of health care quality and medical errors. *J Health Care Finance*. Fall 2012; 39(1):39–50.
5. Joint Commission: Comprehensive Accreditation Manual for Hospitals. *Sentinel Events* (SE). Comprehensive Accreditation Manual for Hospitals. January 2016. Available at: https://www.jointcommission.org/assets/1/6/CAMH_24_SE_all_CURRENT.pdf. Accessed November 1, 2016.
6. Rodak S. 10 Most Identified Sentinel Event Root Causes. *Becker's Infection Control and Clinical Quality*. September 2013. Available at: http://www.beckershospitalreview.com/quality/10-most-identified-sentinel-event-root-causes.html. Accessed November 1, 2016.
7. American Medical Association. *AMA Passes Recommendations for Payment Models that Support New Approaches to Team-Based Health Care*. 2013. Available at: http://www.ama-assn.org/ama/pub/news/news/2014/2014-06-09-policy-to-define-team-based-medical-care.page. Accessed November 2, 2016.
8. Lumague M, Morgan A, Mak D, Hanna M, Kwong J, Cameron C, et al. Interprofessional education: the student perspective. *Journal of Interprofessional Care*. 2008; 20(3):246–253.
9. Counsell SR, Kennedy RD, Szwabo P, Wadsworth NS, Wohlgemuth C. Curriculum recommendations for resident training in Geriatrics Interdisciplinary Team Care. *Journal of the American Geriatrics Association*. 1999; 47(9):1145–1148.
10. Freeth D, Reeves S, Koppel I, Hammick M, Barr H. *Evaluating Interprofessional Education: A Self-Help Guide*. London: Higher education Academy Health Sciences and Practice Network; 2005.
11. Barker KK, Oandasan I. Interprofessional care review with medical residents: Lessons learned, tensions aired-A pilot study. *Journal of Interprofessional Care*. 2005; 19(3):207–214.
12. Barr H, Koppel I, Reeves S, Hammick M, Freeth, D. *Effective Interprofessional Education: Development, Delivery and Evaluation*. Oxford: Blackwell Publishing;2005.
13. Epstein N. Multidisciplinary in-hospital teams improve patient outcomes: A review. *Surg Neurol Int*. 2014; 5(Suppl 7): S295–S303. doi:10.4103/2152-7806.139612.
14. World Health Organization. Diet, nutrition and the prevention of chronic diseases. 2003. Available at: http://health.euroafrica.org/books/dietnutritionwho.pdf. Accessed November 7, 2016.

and patients play active roles in health literacy. The skills needed to achieve health literacy are summarized in **FIGURE 2.9**.

### Cultural Competency

**Cultural competence** refers to how well individuals understand the importance of social and cultural influence on their beliefs and behaviors. Cultural differences can interfere in the informed-consent process. Cultural competency (also referred to as *cultural sensitivity*) applies when working with diverse groups or special populations. **TABLE 2.5** presents a comparison of how culture impacts the informed-consent process in high-resource research sites versus low-resource research sites where individuals have been discriminated against.

### Strategies When Working with Diverse Populations
### Diverse Populations

A variety of strategies can be used when working with research subjects from diverse populations. The most important one is to learn about their history and cultural factors. As a researcher, it is important to focus on past events that may have caused misunderstandings or dissatisfaction with, or abuse from, biomedical research or healthcare providers.[34] Furthermore, an investigator who puts cultural competence into practice should review the literature and contact local

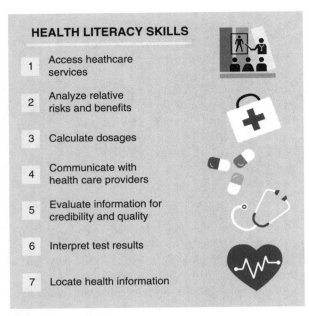

**FIGURE 2.9** Health literacy skills.

Reproduced from National Network of Libraries of Medicine. Health Literacy. Available at https://nnlm.gov/outreach/consumer/hlthlit.html. Accessed October 28, 2016 https://www.hhs.gov/ohrp/regulations-and-policy/regulations/45-cfr-46/index.html.

organizations or researchers in the setting where the research will be done. This will help the investigator have a better grasp of the community.

Another essential strategy is to achieve community engagement, especially in cases in which there is a difference in power between the investigator and the members of the community. This holds true particularly when the research project is sponsored by high-income countries and is implemented in low- to middle-income countries. It was for these reasons that community advisory boards (CABs) were created.[34] CABs help formalize partnerships between members of academia and individuals living in a community. These partnerships guide community-based participatory research (CBPR). The purpose of CBPR is to study chronic diseases, and it aims to reduce disparities in health outcomes.

According to the Office of Disease Prevention and Health Promotion, the term *disparities* is often interpreted to mean racial or ethnic disparities; however, there are many other dimensions of disparity across

**TABLE 2.5**   How culture may affect the informed-consent process

| Features Affecting Consent Forms and Consent Processes in High-Resource Culture Settings | Features Affecting Consent in Low-Resource or Tribal Settings or in Subpopulations Suffering from Discrimination |
| --- | --- |
| <ul><li>Written consent is stressed.</li><li>Contracts and contract law are firmly established.</li><li>"If it is not written, it didn't happen."</li></ul> | <ul><li>The population may be an "oral tradition" society.</li><li>The population may have had rights or property taken away by signing documents.</li><li>Members may wonder, "Why isn't my word good enough?"</li></ul> |
| <ul><li>Individual autonomy in decision making is emphasized.</li></ul> | <ul><li>Members may emphasize community and consultation with others: "community consent."<br>Example: Women may not be allowed to consent on their own; researchers may need agreement of a village or tribal chief to conduct the research with the population.</li></ul> |
| <ul><li>Allows specimens or tissues to be stored and used for future research, often without consent or knowledge.</li></ul> | <ul><li>Members may believe that body parts or specimens contain the essence of the person's being or power.</li><li>Members may suspect that the "other culture" is benefiting from research on their samples, and not the culture that donated the samples.</li></ul> |
| <ul><li>Population believes in science; explains concepts scientifically.</li></ul> | <ul><li>Members may hold different beliefs about of what causes disease.</li><li>Members may not be scientifically or medically literate.</li><li>Religious or cultural beliefs may be more important.</li></ul> |
| <ul><li>More-compartmentalized thinking: "You are separate from your community; your specimens are separate from you."</li></ul> | <ul><li>More-integrated thinking: "You are not separate from your community; your body parts represent a part of you."</li></ul> |

Data from Collaborative Institutional Training Initiative. Consent and Cultural Competence. Authors: Renee Holt and Gary L. Chadwick. Available at: https://www.citiprogram.org/members/index.cfm?pageID=125 Accessed on December 10, 2016.

the United States.[35] If a health outcome is seen to a greater or lesser extent between different populations, then a **health disparity** exists. Demographic factors such as race, ethnicity, gender, sexual identity, age, disability, socioeconomic status, and geographic location can all contribute to an individual's ability to achieve his or her well-being. It is important to recognize the impact that social determinants of health have on the lives of certain populations. Examples of social determinants of health include:

- The availability of resources to meet daily needs such as educational and job opportunities, living wages, or healthful foods
- Social norms and attitudes, such as discrimination
- Exposure to crime, violence, and social disorder such as the presence of trash
- Social support and social interactions
- Exposure to mass media and emerging technologies such as the Internet and cell phones
- Socioeconomic conditions such as concentrated poverty
- Quality schools
- Transportation options
- Public safety
- Residential segregation

The National Institutes of Health has established the National Institute on Minority Health and Health Disparities (NIMHD). NIMHD leads scientific research to improve minority health and eliminate health disparities. **TABLE 2.6** presents the framework developed by the NIMHD to encourage and support researchers working with minority populations and attempting to effectively address health disparities in their communities.

> **Recap** A thorough assessment of risks and benefits must be done before initiating any research project. The Nuremberg Code was the first effort to document important principles governing research with human subjects, and it was further elaborated through the Declaration of Helsinki. Subsequently, the Belmont Report established the basic ethical principles of beneficence, autonomy, and justice. When research is conducted with human subjects, the protection of all persons' rights and welfare must remain a priority. This is extremely important when recruiting and obtaining informed consent from individuals considered part of a vulnerable population. Certain groups and individuals may be considered vulnerable because they do not have the decision-making capacity to provide informed consent or they have a higher risk of exploitation.

# ▶ Study Approaches

> **Preview** Understanding different study approaches is essential when designing a research project. This section discusses the differences between the various study approaches and study designs and how they are used to conduct health and nutrition research.

The main purposes of research are to build knowledge and confirm previous scientific findings. A research study must be able to use the systematic scientific methodology to formulate a research question, design a study, collect data, and analyze the data to draw conclusions.[36] Research should employ thinking and action processes that are logical, understandable, confirmable, and useful to the clinical, professional, and consumer communities. Different types of approaches can be taken, depending on the specific aims of a research study. Note that naturalistic inquiry, experimental-type research, and mixed methods are equally important in building the knowledge base of human health and guidelines for professional practice.

The six general steps to integrate scientific principles are:

1. Define the problem
2. Determine the possible causes
3. Determine probable solutions
4. Select the best solution
5. Test the chosen solution
6. Evaluate

## Basic Research

**Basic research**, also known as "fundamental or pure" science, follows the scientific method and is focused on exploring unknown information.[37] In this type of research, all confounding variables must be controlled carefully. Therefore, most basic research studies are conducted in laboratory settings. The results of the experiments and contributions to the body of knowledge are not expected to be applied in practice immediately. Furthermore, basic research builds the foundation for the applied research studies that follow. Basic research questions are narrowly defined and are investigated with only one level of analysis: prove or disprove theory or confirm or not confirm previous research findings reported in literature.

Some examples of basic research studies in the field of nutrition and dietetics include food-science experiments comparing the effectiveness of innovative

**TABLE 2.6** National Institute on Minority Health and Health Disparities research framework

| **Health Disparity Populations: Race/Ethnicity, Low SES, Rural, Sexual/Gender Minority** <br> **Other Fundamental Characteristics: Sex/Gender, Disability, Geographic Region** | | | | |
|---|---|---|---|---|
| **Domains of Influence** | **Levels of Influence** | | | |
| | **Individual** | **Interpersonal** | **Community** | **Societal** |
| **Biological** | Biological vulnerability and mechanisms | Caregiver–child interaction <br> Family microbiome | Community illness exposure <br> Herd immunity | Sanitation <br> Immunization <br> Pathogen exposure |
| **Behavioral** | Health behaviors <br> Coping strategies | Family functioning <br> School, work functioning | Community functioning | Policies and laws |
| **Physical, Built Environment** | Personal environment | Household Environment <br> School, work Environment | Community environment <br> Community resources | Societal structure |
| **Sociocultural Environment** | Sociodemographics <br> Limited English <br> Cultural identity <br> Response to discrimination | Social networks <br> Family, peer norms <br> Interpersonal discrimination | Community norms <br> Local structural discrimination | Societal norms <br> Societal structural discrimination |
| **Healthcare System** | Insurance coverage <br> Health literacy <br> Treatment preferences | Patient–clinician relationship <br> Medical decision-making | Availability of health services <br> Safety net services | Quality of healthcare |
| **Health Outcomes** | **Individual Health** | **Family/ Organizational Health** | **Community Health** | **Population Health** |

*(Vertical label along left of domain rows: Lifecourse)*

Reproduced from NIMHD Research Framework. www.nimhd.nih.gov, https://www.nimhd.nih.gov/about/overview/research-framework.html. Accessed March 15, 2017.

food-preservation methods, in vitro chemoprevention experiments using bioactive food compounds, and in vivo metabolism and dietary intervention experiments on diabetes mellitus type 2 using animal models.

## Applied Research

Applied research has been defined as "inquiry using the application of scientific methodology with the purpose of generating empirical observations to solve critical problems in society."[37] Furthermore, applied research aims to modify existing concepts, information, and products. This type of research is used to inform public policy, contribute to applied behavioral analysis, and support operational decision making. The ultimate goal of applied research is to help improve the human condition by identifying gaps in knowledge and the best approaches for addressing contemporary issues. Applied research questions are generally open-ended because the study will be conducted in a setting that will be influenced by societal factors and several stakeholders. Members of a multidisciplinary team will have different perspectives about the problem under study.

Investigators have identified four main differences between applied research and basic research.

The two types of research differ in terms of purpose, context, validity, and methods. Implementing a research study in the home, community, academia, or a healthcare facility can be more challenging than conducting the research in a laboratory or a setting that the researcher can control.

Examples of applied research studies in the nutrition and dietetics field include the evaluation of interventions to maintain and improve the health and well-being of vulnerable populations, including nutrition education and food-assistance programs; conducting focus groups to identify barriers to achieving lifestyle changes; and examining the effects of nutrition policies in an enforced setting.

## Nutrition Research

The Academy of Nutrition and Dietetics states that nutrition research encompasses a wide range of activities within the field. These activities go from tracking patient outcomes, quality-improvement projects, and testing new interventions to surveying customer acceptance of menu items and conducting community-needs assessments.[38] The specific aims of these research activities are to improve patient care and the effectiveness of nutritional interventions. The findings from both basic and applied sciences can help improve nutrition practices in all work scenarios: food-service management, community nutrition, and clinical practice.

## Descriptive Studies

In a **descriptive study**, information is collected without changing the environment (i.e., no manipulation occurs).[39] In human research, a descriptive study can provide information about the naturally occurring health status, behavior, attitudes, or other characteristics of a group. Descriptive studies are also conducted to demonstrate associations or relationships between factors in society. Descriptive studies differ by time frame. A researcher might want to study a population at one point in time instead of following subjects for a extended period.

## Qualitative Research

**Qualitative research** focuses on behavior in natural settings. It studies small groups in a setting. Data gathered in qualitative research are non-numerical and presented in language and/or pictures. The conclusion of a qualitative research study is based on the interpretations drawn by a group of researchers. Some of the most common techniques used in qualitative research

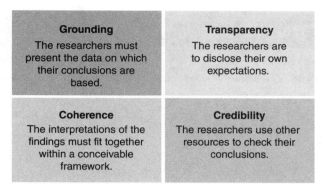

**FIGURE 2.10** Guidelines to evaluate the trustworthiness of qualitative research findings.

Data from Pistrang N, Barker C. Varieties of Qualitative Research: A Pragmatic Approach to Selecting Methods. In: *APA Handbook of Research Methods in Psychology: Vol 2*. Washington, DC. 2012; 4-16.

include observations, face-to-face or telephonic interviews, and surveys or questionnaires.

Qualitative research is evaluated based on trustworthiness. This type of research has no exact concept of validity and reliability. Therefore, members of academia have set forth guidelines to evaluate the trustworthiness of qualitative research findings. Those guidelines are presented in **FIGURE 2.10**.

## Quantitative Research

**Quantitative research** focuses on gathering numerical data and generalizing it across groups of people or to explain a phenomenon. Quantitative methods emphasize objective measurements and the statistical, mathematical, or numerical analysis of data collected through polls, questionnaires, and surveys; as well as manipulating preexisting statistical data using computational techniques.

Quantitative approaches focus on specific behaviors that can be easily quantified. For the data to be representative, large samples of the population are used.[40] Quantitative approaches must assign numerical values to responses, and conclusions are based on the results of statistical analysis. Four types of designs in quantitative research are described in **TABLE 2.7**.

Quantitative research designs are either descriptive or experimental. A descriptive study establishes associations between variables; an experimental study establishes causality.[41] Proving causality in nutrition research is extremely challenging. Criteria for causal inference and rationale are described in **TABLE 2.8** and provide a framework for determining causality in scientific research.

Good examples of quantitative approaches are nutrition surveys for dietary assessment. Data collected from quantitative surveys can help food and

**TABLE 2.7** Quantitative research designs

| Type of Design | Key Focus | Intervention | Common Study Designs |
|---|---|---|---|
| Descriptive | ■ Observational<br>■ Variables are not controlled | No | ■ Cross-sectional<br>■ Longitudinal<br>■ Observational<br>■ Secondary data analysis |
| Correlational | ■ Relationships among variables<br>■ Variables are not controlled | No | ■ Descriptive<br>■ Correlation<br>■ Predictive<br>■ Model testing |
| Quasi-Experimental | ■ Causality<br>■ Suboptimal variable control<br>■ Independent variable not manipulated | Yes | ■ Pre- and post-test designs<br>■ post-test only<br>■ Interrupted time-series designs |
| Experimental | ■ Tests causality with optimal variable control<br>■ Independent variable manipulated | Yes | ■ Classic experimental designs<br>■ Randomized designs<br>■ Crossover<br>■ Nested |

Modified from Center of Innovation in Research and Teaching. Understanding Research Design. https://cirt.gcu.edu/research/developmentresources/research_ready/researchreadyintroduction/research_design. Accessed May 7, 2017.

**TABLE 2.8** Hill's criteria for causal inference

| Criteria | Rationale |
|---|---|
| Strength of Association | Strong associations have a higher likelihood of being causal than do weak associations |
| Consistency | A causal association should be stable when tested with various study designs |
| Specificity | An exposure can only cause a single outcome |
| Temporality | The cause or exposure must come before the effect or outcome |
| Biologic Gradient | The ability to demonstrate a dose-response relationship. This quality may not always be present |
| Plausibility | Is there scientific justification for the relationship between cause and effect? |
| Coherence | Do the cause and effect make sense with what is known about the facts of the exposure and the disease? |
| Experimental Evidence | Do randomized controlled trials exist and support the cause and effect? |
| Analogy | Analogies provide insight into the causal pathways and add to the weight of the evidence |

Modified from Hill AB. The environment and disease: Association or causation? *Proc R Soc Med.* 1965;58:295-300. Adapted from Figure 3. Hill's criteria for causal inference. Bruemmer B, Harris J, Gleason P, et al. Publishing nutrition research: A review of epidemiologic method. *J Am Diet Assoc.* October 2009;109(10).

nutrition professionals inform policy.[42] The results of this quantitative approaches can suggest the following:

- The average consumption of foods and nutrients by socioeconomic and demographic groups
- The frequency of consumption of specific food groups or products
- The adequacy of diet for different populations

The strengths of using quantitative approaches include greater precision of measurement, the ability to make comparisons, and the ability to test causal hypotheses using experimental designs.

## Commonly Used Study Designs in Health and Nutrition Research

Primary research—also called *original research*—is a single study designed and conducted by researchers themselves as compared to secondary or tertiary research in which information is collected from primary (and secondary) sources. Review articles in which the authors review, organize, interpret, summarize, and draw conclusions from many primary research studies is considered a secondary study design. Systematic reviews are a rigorous form of tertiary research because data and information come from primary and secondary sources.

## Survey Research

The purpose of survey research is to describe and quantify characteristics of a chosen population based on a stated research objective. Survey research used to measure people at one point in time is considered a basic cross-sectional study design. Surveys that ask about one point of time in the past are considered retrospective. Longitudinal surveys are administered more than once over a longer study period. For example, the Nurses' Health Study, conducted by researchers at Harvard's School of Public Health and Brigham and Women's Hospital in Boston, is a cohort study that surveys more than 280,000 nurses ages 19 to 51 years annually about their health and wellness.[43] Surveys that are deliberate in their design are useful to establish baseline data about the prevalence of a disease or food intake, establish associations among variables, and provide insight into areas of future research, although causal relationships cannot be concluded from survey findings. If the sample represents the target population, then the results of a survey can usually be generalized to the population of interest, making survey research one of the most widely used methods in public-health nutrition for planning dietary services. Common concerns with survey research are the population (sample) selection and selection bias, which will limit the generalizability of the findings. Nutrition monitoring in the United States is frequently conducted by a combination of multiple surveys of various target populations.[44] The National Nutrition Monitoring and Related Research Program (NNMRRP) is a survey that is used to gain information about the diet and nutritional status of Americans, factors that affect diet and nutritional status, and how diet affects health. The National Health and Nutrition Examination Survey (NHANES) part of NNMRRP obtains 24-hour dietary recall information from a nationally representative sample of people of all ages living in the United States. A dietary behavior questionnaire that asks about food-related behaviors is also included.[45]

## Epidemiologic Study Designs

Epidemiologic study designs are *observational*, meaning the investigators only observe the natural relationships between risk factors and outcomes and ask participants questions.[4] Epidemiologic studies are common and valuable in nutrition and public-health research because they frequently look at risk factors such as exposure and the chance that an outcome such as a disease will occur. Epidemiologic research involves three key elements: (1) common terms, (2) a conceptual framework, and (3) concepts of causal association.[46]

Study designs can be grouped as observational, (which includes cross-sectional, case-control, or cohort) and experimental such as clinical trials that are distinguished by the intervention that accompanies the experimental design.[3] In **observational studies**, the investigator allows for natural occurrences, observes relationships between variables and outcomes, and does not intervene with study participants. Observational study design can include studies that are cross-sectional, case study, prospective, and retrospective cohort, depending on the time data are collected.[47] Observational studies can also be used to investigate exposure-outcome relationships.

## Cross-Sectional Studies

**Cross-sectional studies** are retrospective epidemiologic research ventures that collect information from a population of interest at one point in time, as opposed to cohort and case-control studies that collect data over a determined time period. The goal of cross-sectional studies is to investigate the associations between exposures and outcomes at one point in time and provide a "snapshot" of the population being studied. The cross-sectional study design includes surveys and laboratory experiments, and it may also sometimes be described as a "prevalence" study because it measures the prevalence of disease or exposure and thus is descriptive and useful for identifying associations. A cross-sectional study examines associations at only one point in time and does not examine a sequence of events; therefore, temporality cannot be established because both the exposure and the outcome are being assessed simultaneously, which prevents consequent determination of cause and effect. Other limitations of this study design are the possibility of selection and measurement bias. Random sampling of the population being investigated helps reduce potential biases. Cross-sectional studies are, however, less expensive than other study designs because they collect information at one point in time only. The NHANES is an example of a large-scale cross-sectional study design.

## Longitudinal Studies

When study participants are observed and data are assessed over a long period of time, the study is considered *longitudinal*, as compared to a cross-sectional study for which data are collected at just one point in time. A longitudinal study, for example, would follow the same group over 10 years. Prospective longitudinal studies look forward in time, and retrospective studies look backward in time. A **prospective study** will follow a group (cohort) of participants who do not have the disease or condition of interest forward through time, collecting data at defined intervals in time and focusing on potential causal factors (exposure) to determine whether the disease or other health outcome develops. Prospective studies have better control of variables and standardization in data collection because the study methods are planned variable occurrences. In comparison, retrospective studies examine data that have already occurred (such as past medical records) or ask study participants to remember exposures or outcomes. Retrospective studies are therefore usually less expensive than prospective studies but prone to recall bias. Prospective and retrospective study designs can be used to avoid ethical concerns in populations in which the risk of exposure is thought to be harmful—for example, alcohol and drug use and health outcomes—because the researchers observe free-living individuals. **FIGURE 2.11** contains details about each type of descriptive study. **TABLE 2.9** lists the strengths and limitations of observational study designs.

## Case-Control Studies

**Case-control studies** start with a group of participants (cases) with an outcome (such as a disease) and

**Cross-sectional study**
• There is a one-time interaction with the subjects.

**Longitudinal study**
• Subjects are followed over time.
• Data collection occurs at multiple time points.

**Observational study**
• The researcher does not interact with the subject.
• Observations are made within the subject's environment.

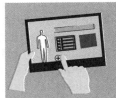

**Existing records**
• Data can be obtained from existing records without interacting with the subjects.
• Example: electronic health records.

**FIGURE 2.11** Types of descriptive studies.

Modified from The Office of Research Integrity. https://ori.hhs.gov/content/module-2-research-design. Accessed August 6, 2017.

investigate looking back (retrospectively) at possible exposures. Once a group of cases (people with a disease) are identified, matched controls (people without a disease) are located. **Controls** must be carefully chosen to make sure they had the same chance of exposure and are similar to the cases in all ways, except that they do not have the disease. Therefore, the two groups being compared are defined based on the presence or absence of the outcome, and the previous exposure of the cases (with the outcome or disease) are compared to the controls (those without the outcome or disease) in an attempt to identify what factors could have influenced the development of the outcome.

The researchers investigate common exposures with questionnaires and surveys. The aim is to determine the similarities and differences between the cases and controls in effort to identify past exposures or risk factors that could explain the odds of having the exposure among those with the outcome divided by the odds of having the exposure among those without the outcome.[4,46] An *odds ratio* can be used to estimate risk in cross-sectional and case control studies when the study is designed to investigate outcome rather than exposure.[48] In other words, researchers will take a group of people with a disease

**TABLE 2.9** Strengths and limitations of observational study designs

| Study Design | Strengths | Limitations |
|---|---|---|
| Cross-sectional: exposure and outcome measured at the same time. | Inexpensive<br>Timely<br>Individualized data<br>Ability to monitor for multiple confounders<br>Can assess multiple outcomes | No insight in to temporal sequence leading to evidence on causal factors<br>Not good for rare diseases or for diseases of short duration<br>Cannot provide answers to cause and effect |
| Case control: start with the outcome and look for exposures.<br>Also known as a *retrospective study*. | Inexpensive<br>Timely<br>Individualized data<br>Ability to monitor for multiple confounders<br>Can assess multiple outcomes<br>Good for rare diseases<br>Cases and controls can usually be easily identified based on outcome status | Cannot calculate prevalence<br>Can only assess one outcome<br>Poor selection of controls can introduce bias<br>May be difficult to identify enough cases<br>Possibility for recall bias<br>Cannot demonstrate temporality<br>Maybe challenging to target the past time period that represents plausible biologic period of exposure |
| Cohort (retrospective or prospective): prospective cohort study starts with exposure and looks for an outcome. | Temporality demonstrated<br>Individualized data<br>Ability to control for multiple confounders<br>Multiple exposures and outcomes can be assessed over time | Expensive<br>Time intensive<br>Not good for rare diseases because of the inefficiency of gathering information on participants who may not contract the disease<br>Maintain contact and follow up with many participants |

Modified from Thiese MS. Observational and interventional study design types; An overview. *Biochemia Medica* 2014;24(2):199-210. http://dx.doi.org/10.11613/BM.2014.022 and Bruemmer B, Jeffrey H, Gleason P, et al. Publishing nutrition research: A review of epidemiologic methods. J Am Diet Assoc. 2009;109(10).

and a group without the disease and then compare the exposure of interest in the cases to the controls. The benefits of case-control studies are that they are simple to perform, are usually less expensive, and are less time-consuming than many other study designs. Case-control studies are feasible for examining rates diseases and conditions. The limitations of this study design are the potential for *recall bias*: the cases and controls will remember things such as diet differently because of the presence of the disease and the findings are not generalizable to other groups. In addition, case-control studies can investigate only one disease at a time.

## Cohort Studies

**Cohort studies** begin with a group of individuals with common characteristics who are observed over time for exposure to risk factors such as diet. Then exposed and nonexposed individuals are compared based on an outcome of interest. This is in contrast with case-control studies, which begin with the disease. Cohort studies are designed to track individuals and their health information over time to observe the natural course of disease occurrence. In this design, risks and exposures are assessed as they occur during the study period. Retrospective cohort studies look back in time to examine exposures before the outcome occurs, whereas prospective studies move forward in time with an identified cohort (**FIGURE 2.12**). Prospective (prospective cohort and intervention) studies that follow study participants forward through time are best suited for suggesting causation.[47]

Cohort studies provide information about the **relative risk (RR)** of developing a disease based on the presence of an exposure. RR is an estimate used in prospective studies that compares the probability of an outcome in two groups, and expresses how much more or less likely it is for an exposed person to develop an outcome relative to a nonexposed person.

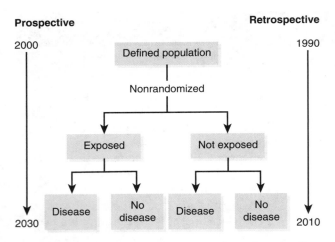

**FIGURE 2.12** Prospective and retrospective cohort studies.

Cohort studies are feasible for examining common diseases in which the exposure to risk factors leads to measurable outcomes in a relatively short time period after exposure. Other strengths of this study design are that they can provide information on the time-based sequence of events; for example, they allow for the measurement of exposures such as diet before disease occurs. Cohort studies are easier to conduct and less expensive than experimental studies but require extensive resources and monitoring, as well as following large numbers of people over long periods of time.

## Systematic Reviews

Review articles are an informative way to evaluate, summarize, and communicate a current body of knowledge. Reviews are a common form of secondary research useful in identifying inconsistencies in evidence and gaps in research; they they provide a basis for ongoing investigation. Systematic reviews are a high-level, clearly defined, and rigorous critical review process often initiated to answer a specific research question in a balanced and unbiased manner from multiple research papers. The Academy of Nutrition and Dietetics defines a systematic review as "a summary of scientific literature on a specific topic or question that uses explicit methods to conduct a comprehensive literature research and identify relevant studies, critically appraise the quality of each study, and summarize the body of literature or evidence to answer the question."[48] In a systematic review, the studies are collected, assessed, and critically evaluated following identified and established criteria. Each step is systematic and documented for transparency and reproducibility.

Systematic reviews take a long time to perform. The possibility exists that by the time a systemic review is published, more-recent research has emerged that supersedes the conclusion or recommendation from the systematic review. Despite limitations, systematic reviews play an important role in evidence-based practice by providing practitioners with a concise and authoritative understanding of a specific health issue. Nutritionists and other healthcare providers can use results from systematic reviews to drive their clinical practice without conducing the critical review of each article personally, leaving more time for thoughtful patient care.

**Meta-analysis** is a method of secondary research. This statistical technique is used frequently in systematic reviews to combine studies and add strength to the findings through greater statistical power. In a meta-analysis, results from many studies that are similar in study design are united into a single, larger pool of results and simultaneously analyzed in an attempt to determine an independent conclusion. Meta-analyses are useful as a foundation for public policy and when developing evidence-based practice recommendations.[2] Strengths of meta-analysis are its rigor and its objectivity as compared to research reviews because of its statistical analysis of data. The findings are more powerful than the included individual studies because the methods are precise, the inclusion criteria of multiple similar studies limit bias, and study methods are replicable. However, because data come from multiple different studies, measurements of variables and outcomes may differ.

The Academy of Nutrition and Dietetics evidence analysis review process is the source for evidence-based practice guidelines for nutrition patient care and diet therapy decision making. Evidence analysis is a complex process, so the EAL manual divides the analysis process into five defined steps for evaluating food and nutrition questions conducted by a team of subject-matter experts and trained research analysts.[49] See **FIGURE 2.13**.

The **Nutrition Care Process (NCP)** is a standardized model intended to guide RDNs in providing high-quality nutrition care.[50] The NCP (**FIGURE 2.14**) has four distinct and interrelated phases that give nutrition and dietetics practitioners a systematic structure to scientifically manage nutrition care and help patients meet health and nutrition goals. Using the NCP does not mean that all patients receive the same nutritional care; instead, it provides a framework for the RDN to take into account each patient's needs and values and use the best evidence available to make decisions to individualize care.[51] The Academy of Nutrition and Dietetics Health

Step 1. *Formulate the evidence analysis question*: Specify a focused question in a defined area of practice. Three key items are used to generate good-quality questions: an analytical framework to identify links between factors and outcomes, the PICOT format to write questions, and the Nutrition Care Process to serve as a framework.

Step 2. *Gather and classify the evidence*: This step involves developing a search plan to conduct a detailed literature search. The plan clearly defines the inclusion and exclusion criteria and identifies the key search terms and outcomes necessary to conduct a comprehensive search. The search plan and all literature searches results are documented and assessed for inclusion eligibility. Excluded articles are listed along with reason for exclusion.

Step 3. *Critically appraise each article (risk of bias)*: This step involves critically assessing each included article for methodological quality. Each study is evaluated based on appropriateness of study design and how well the study was conducted by using the Academy's risk-of-bias tool, called the *quality criteria checklist*.

Step 4. *Summarize the evidence*: This step involves achieving two major tasks. First, key data from the included articles are extracted by using the Academy's web-based data-extraction template. Second, evidence extracted from each study is distilled into a brief, coherent, and easy-to-read summary. The result of this phase is called the *evidence summary*.

Step 5. *Write and grade the conclusion statement*: This step includes developing a concise conclusion statement for the research question and assigning a grade to the conclusion statement. The grade reflects the overall strength and weakness of evidence in forming the conclusion statement. The grading scale used by the Academy: grade I = good or strong, II = fair, III = limited or weak, IV = expert opinion only, and V = not assignable.

**FIGURE 2.13** Steps in the evidence analysis systematic review process.

Reproduced from Academy of Nutrition and Dietetics EAL Systematic Review Process. https://www.andeal.org/eal-sr. Accessed July 8, 2017.

Informatics Infrastructure (ANDHII) enables RDNs to track nutrition care outcomes and advance their evidence-based nutrition practice research by offering secure online data collection.[52] The objective of ANDHII is that knowledge gained through the collection and analysis of nutrition information will add to the evidence basis for nutrition practice and translate into higher-quality patient care.

## Experimental Design Studies

During an experiment; a procedure, treatment, or intervention is tested and an outcome is observed. An experiment is therefore defined as "a test under controlled conditions that is made to demonstrate a known truth, to examine the validity of a hypothesis, or to determine the efficacy of something that has not been tried before."[53] Any true experiment should have three elements: (1) manipulation of an independent variable, (2) a control group, and (3) random assignment. These are defined in **TABLE 2.10**.

## Control/Experimental Groups

In an **experimental research design**, to help determine the cause and effect with the experimental group all factors are held constant except those that are manipulated by the researcher.[54] This will allow for the results of the control group and the experimental group to be compared. A control is used to prevent additional variables from influencing the outcome of the experiment. Therefore, the **control condition** represents the effect that exists in the absence of the experimental treatment. For the control condition to function appropriately, it must be as similar as possible to the treatment group—for example, placebo diet versus experimental diet. This means that the researcher must identify the variables that need to be controlled. Experimental designs also have a series of essential components that will be discussed further.

## Randomization

The first essential component of an experimental design is known as *randomization*. The word *random* in this context means that every individual in a particular population has an equal chance of being selected to participate. Moreover, **randomized assignment** refers to how the subjects are randomly placed into the control group or the experimental group. In a randomized clinical trial, treatments are randomly assigned to the subjects. The random assignment limits bias in how treatments are assigned to human subjects and helps establish the base for statistical tests and further analysis.

### Multilevel Randomized Design

An extension of the basic randomized design is known as a **multilevel randomized design**. This design has more than two levels of the independent variable; here

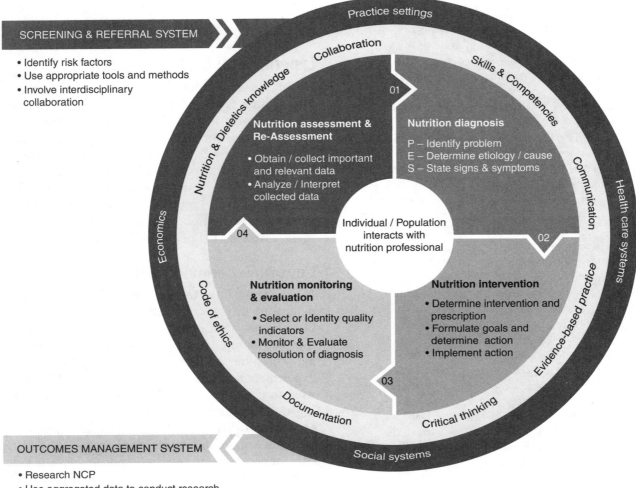

- *Nutrition assessment*: The RDN collects and documents information such as food or nutrition-related history; biochemical data, medical tests, and procedures; anthropometric measurements; nutrition-focused physical findings; and client history.
- *Diagnosis*: Data collected during the nutrition assessment guide the RDN in selection of the appropriate nutrition diagnosis (i.e., naming the specific problem).
- *Intervention*: The RDN then selects the nutrition intervention that will be directed to the root cause (or etiology) of the nutrition problem and aimed at alleviating the signs and symptoms of the diagnosis.
- *Monitoring and evaluation*: In the final step of the process, the RDN determines whether the patient or client has achieved or is progressing toward the planned goals.

**FIGURE 2.14** Nutrition care process.

Reproduced from Academy of Nutrition and Dietetics. Nutrition Terminology Reference Ma nual (eNCPT): *Dietetics Language for Nutrition Care*. 2016. http://ncpt.webauthor.com. Accessed December 8, 2016.

level refers to the number of variations of the independent variable. In clinical trials testing the efficacy of an experimental drug, for example, it would be advantageous to determine not only whether the drug produced an outcome different than the placebo treatment condition but also whether the different doses of the experimental drug produced different results. In this case, participants would be randomly assigned to different groups, depending on the quantity of experimental drug and control conditions.

| **TABLE 2.10** Essential criteria for good experiments | |
| --- | --- |
| **Criterion** | **Meaning** |
| Manipulation | Induce a change in the hypothesized cause to determine whether the hypothesized consequence occurs. |
| Control | Prevent other possible causal factors from intruding on and contaminating the experiment. |
| Random Assignment | Procedure used in experiments to create multiple study groups that include participants with similar characteristics so that the groups are equivalent at the beginning of the study. |

Reproduced from U.S. Department of Health and Human Services. The Office of Research Integrity. Module 2 Research Design Section 2. https://ori.hhs.gov/content/module-2-research-design-section-2.

| **TABLE 2.11** Mechanisms of the placebo effect | |
| --- | --- |
| **Mechanisms of the Placebo Effect** | |
| Psychological | ▪ Expectations<br>▪ Conditioning<br>▪ Learning<br>▪ Memory<br>▪ Motivation<br>▪ Somatic focus<br>▪ Reward<br>▪ Anxiety reduction<br>▪ Meaning |
| Neurobiological | ▪ Immune responses<br>▪ Hormonal responses<br>▪ Depression |

Reproduced from Finniss DG, Kaptchuk TJ, Miller F, Benedetti F. Placebo Effects: Biological, Clinical and Ethical Advances. *Lancet.* 2010;375(9715):686-695. doi:10.1016/S0140-6736 (09)61706-2. Accessed on 05/7/17.

### Placebo

Placebo groups are used to ensure that external validity is maintained. Placebo groups can help control the experiment. A **placebo** is a simulation of therapy that has no physiological effect.[55] Moreover, a **placebo effect** is "a way of describing, quantifying, and understanding everything that surrounds the placebo treatment."[55] This includes the interaction between the patient and his or her provider, the support given to this patient, and every factor in the healthcare environment that could have a potential influence on the outcomes of a subject participating in the research study.

It is evident that several placebo-effect mechanisms can affect both healthy individuals and patients with different medical conditions. Possible psychological and neurobiological mechanisms of the placebo effect are presented in **TABLE 2.11**.

## Double-Blind Studies

Randomized double-blind placebo studies are known as the "gold standard" in intervention-based research. A **double-blind study** is an experiment designed to test the effect of a treatment or substance by using groups of experimental and control subjects in which neither the subjects nor the investigators know which treatment is being administered to which group.[56]

In a double-blind test of a new drug, the substance may be identified to the investigators by a random number or code and never a name. The purpose of a double-blind study is to eliminate the risk of bias by the participants, which could affect outcomes. A double-blind study may be augmented by a crossover experiment in which experimental subjects unknowingly become control subjects—and vice versa—at some point in the study.

## Factorial Designs

A **factorial design** is a design that investigates the independent and interactive effect that two or more independent variables have on the dependent variable.[57] A *factor* is simply a categorical variable with two or more values, which are commonly referred to as *levels*. The types of information that can be obtained from a factorial design are main effects and interaction effects.

The advantages of factorial designs include the following.

▪ The effect of more than one factor can be tested. This means that more than one hypothesis can be tested.
▪ Control of a potentially confounding variable can be created by incorporating it into the design of the experiment.
▪ The researcher can test for interactive effects among the various factors.

For example, in a dietary-intervention study, subjects may differ in terms of the amount of a specific micronutrient they receive (one factor), whether the supplementation is taken orally or administered intramuscularly (second factor), and by their gender (third factor). If there are three doses of a supplement (A, B, and C), two different methods of administration (I and II), and two genders (male and female), there will be a total of 12 (3 × 2 × 2) groups of subjects for comparison of the outcome.

## Crossover Design

A **crossover design** describes a clinical trial in which groups of human subjects receive two or more interventions in a particular order.[58] For example, a two-by-two crossover design involves two groups of participants. One group receives drug A during the initial phase of the trial followed, by drug B during a later phase. The other group receives drug B during the initial phase, followed by drug A. During the trial, participants "crossed over" to the other drug. All participants receive drug A and drug B at some point during the trial, but in a different order, depending on the group to which they are assigned. The main purpose served by this design is to provide a basis for distinguishing treatment effects from period effects. A crossover design has the potential of confounding the influence of order, or what is known as **carryover effects**.[59] The existence of carryover effects must be ruled out for the crossover method to have validity.

Carryover effects refers to when the effect of the previous treatment carries over to influence the response of the next treatment. To decrease carryover effects or ensure that none are present, the carryover design often includes a rest period or washout between the administration of a different treatment. When evidence exists that a rest or washout period is able to eradicate any carryover effects, the design is efficient. This might happen in some biomedical and pharmaceutical studies.

## Counterbalancing

**Counterbalancing** is when a series of sequences is administered in such a way that it balances out order effects.[60] The most common issue when studying the between-subjects factor of counterbalancing is that more participants will be needed to have statistical power. This disadvantage of needing more participants however, is often offset by being able to discover more effects. There are two types of counterbalancing: complete counterbalancing and Latin square.[61] In **complete counterbalancing**, all possible orders of presentation are included in the experiment. This is easier with small numbers of experimental conditions. On the other hand, a **Latin square** is constructed for using the

counterbalancing technique to control for order effects without having all possible orders. This ensures that all possible orders are received by different subjects.

## Familiarization

In research, repeated exposure of subjects to certain tests or procedures can lead to **familiarization**, which is defined as becoming well acquainted with something.[62] A good example is the assessment of memory. Imagine a sample of older adults participating in a research study investigating the potential benefits of bioactive compounds found in blueberries in the prevention of memory loss. The repeated completion of the tests may at some point influence the subjects' performance and improve the results as the subjects become more experienced. The improvements in memory could be to the result of practice effects and not the dietary intervention itself. This happens mostly when collecting longitudinal data. Therefore, researchers must be aware of familiarization and retest effects, particularly regarding the problem under study.

## Translational Research

**Translational science** has been described as a spectrum that integrates each phase of research and can be thought of as "bench to bedside."[63] The process goes from the fundamentals of biology regarding health and disease to the potential interventions that could improve human health. Therefore, translation is the process of turning observations in the laboratory, clinic, and community into interventions that improve the health of individuals and the public—from diagnostics and therapeutics to medical procedures and behavioral changes. Translational science is the field of investigation focused on understanding the scientific and operational principles underlying each step of the translational process. **FIGURE 2.15** presents the relationship between the stages of translational research, with the patient at its core.

> **Recap**  An understanding of research terminology and essential criteria for reviewing and evaluating scientific studies is a highly effective way to expand your knowledge and skills and improve patient and client care. Common study designs in nutrition research include both qualitative and quantitative research methods such as large-scale population-wide surveys, systematic reviews, and meta-analysis as well as cohort studies, intervention and experimental designs, and translations research.

(A)

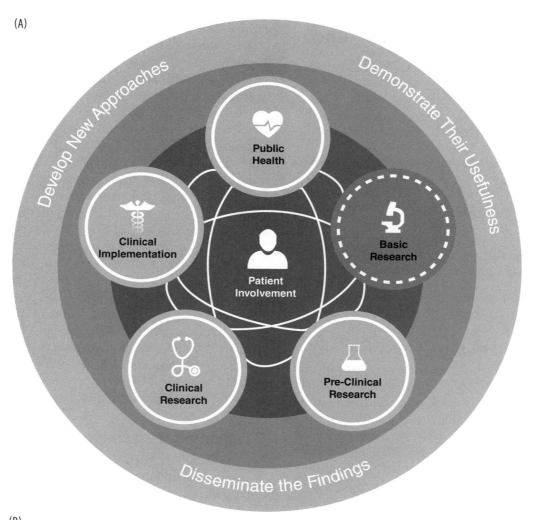

(B)

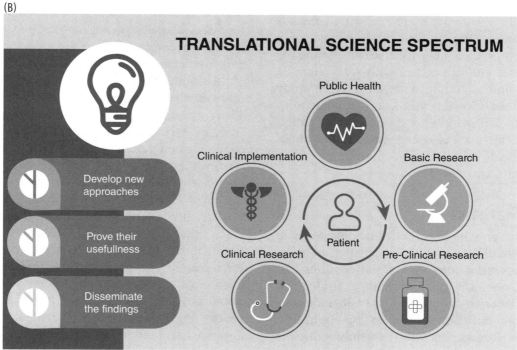

**FIGURE 2.15** The translational science spectrum (A) (B).

Reproduced from US Department of Health and Human Services, NIH. National Center for Advancing Translational Sciences Translational Science Spectrum. National Center for Advancing Translational Sciences Web Site. https://ncats.nih.gov/translation/spectrum. Accessed on Aug 6, 2017.

# ▶ Analyzing, Interpreting, and Communicating Research

**Preview**　Evaluating scientific research requires synthesizing many steps. The process begins with a topic of interest and the development of a research question. The next steps involve acquiring knowledge through the use of available technology, establishing evaluation criteria for selecting and assessing research, and then evaluating and integrating all of the needed information in a systematic, clear, and understandable way to answer the research question. The selection of appropriate statistical analysis of research data results in greater confidence in a study's results and conclusions.

## Informational Health Literacy

It goes without saying that there is a level of proficiency and skill to become an information-literate healthcare provider. In research, identifying a topic of interest and developing a research questionare necessary first steps. This is followed by acquiring the knowledge needed through the efficient use of current technologies such as search engines and online and electronic resources. Next, establishing evaluation criteria for selecting and assessing research, and then evaluating and integrating all of the needed information in a systematic, clear, and understandable way to answer the research question is no small task. All this must be done while also considering the highest level of ethical practice with study subjects and clearly understanding and interpreting study methods and statistical analysis. Informational health literacy enables providers to translate information about risk factors, diseases, and medical and nutritional treatments to effectively communicate with patients, clients, and consumers.

## Research Statistics

For healthcare practitioners, understanding research methodology and data analysis is a key part of informational literacy for interpreting and communicating nutrition research. At a minimum, analyzing and interpreting research data requires a basic understanting of common statistical techniques used in healthcare research. Researchers will frequently enlist the help of an expert scientific statistician during the planning, execution, and analysis of a study. Enlisting the guidance of research statistician is helpful to determine the appropriate statistical tests to test a

hypothesis. Determining correlation versus causation, for example and assisting in data analysis, interpreting results, and extrapolating findings. Selection of appropriate statistical tests and accurate data analysis results in greater confidence in the study's results and conclusions. To conclude that the results from a study are statistically significant, the appropriate statistical test needs to be chosen.[64] A statistically significant finding is an observed effect that is large enough so that it is unlikely to have occurred by chance.

Many statistical procedures are available, and selecting one depends on the study design and type of data being collected. Choosing the right statistical tests when designing a research project is an important task because it adds power to the findings and provides strong support for the study outcomes and conclusions. Using the appropriate methods for the study objectives to test the results of data collection, and then interpreting findings accurately, can be a significant challenge. Statistical tests that are commonly used in nutrition research are described in **TABLE 2.12**. **TABLE 2.13** contains a list of research purposes along with some common statistical procedures.[2]

## Communicating Findings

Once data have been analyzed and findings summarized, areas for future investigation are developed that perpetuate the scientific process for ongoing critical inquiry and research and ultimately drive the nutrition profession forward. Advances in patient care, food-service delivery, appropriate diet therapy, and nutrition recommendations are evolving, improving, and advancing with ongoing inquiry and research.

Accurate, timely, and effective communication of research findings bridges research to practice. There are many vehicles to communicate research findings. Effective dissemination of nutrition knowledge relies on varied methods, with the key aim of transmitting knowledge and practices to target audiences. Drummond and Murphy-Reyes discuss the three P's of disseminating nutrition research—posters, presentations, and publications—that will reach other like-minded scientists and researchers.[4] Social media has also become a common method for researchers to promote their findings and reach a wider consumer base. The use of blogs, organizational websites, podcasts, electronic journals, and newsletters as well as other personal social media apps are becoming more widely approved as acceptable means to reach and communicate with a larger population. This latter form of communicating nutrition findings aligns with emerging areas of innovative nutrition research. to generate approaches that

**TABLE 2.12** Descriptions of statistical tests commonly used in nutrition research

| | |
|---|---|
| Descriptive Statistics[a,b] | The four trends of the sample are mean, mode, median, and range. They are used to describe the sample and sometimes to demonstrate how the sample may represent a population—if that population's measures of central tendencies (descriptive statistics) are known. |
| *t*-tests[a] | Tests the difference between two groups' means; can be one-tailed or two-tailed; can be used with paired or unpaired samples. Sometimes called called a student's *t*-test. |
| Chi-square | Method used to analyze variables to find differences between groups. It is a nonparametric test calculated when analyzing nominal or ordinal data. |
| Analysis of variance (ANOVA)[a] | Tests the difference among the means of three or more groups for one or more variables. |
| Analysis of covariance (ANCOVA)[a] | A variant of ANOVA that allows adjusting for extraneous, additional, or undesired variables. |
| Multiple analysis of variance (MANOVA)[a] | A variant of ANOVA that allows for the study of multiple dependent variables. If MANOVA results are significant, ANOVA must be done for each variable. |
| Cochran's Q test[b] | Compares proportions among three or more matched groups. |
| Duncan Range test[a] | A test used after ANOVA to identify means that differ significantly from one another. |
| Kendall's rank correlation[a,b] | A test of the linear relationship between two ordinal or continuous variables. |
| Kruskal-Wallis test[b] | A nonparametric test for significance when using two independent samples. It is comparable to ANOVA, but for rank-ordered data. |
| Mann-Whitney test[b] | Sometimes called the Mann-Whitney U-test, it is the nonparametric equivalent of a *t*-test. Used with ordinal data for two groups. |
| Multiple regression analysis[a] | Any statistical method that evaluates the results of more than one independent variable on a single dependent variable. |
| Newman-Keuls test | Tests for significance in multiple *post hoc* comparisons. |
| Pearson's 2'η test[b] | A test of categorical data for goodness of fit or comparisons of observations. |
| Person's product movement test[a] | A test of the strength of the linear relationship between two interval or ratio (continuous) variables. |
| Regression analysis[a] | A method of predicting dependent variable variability by one or more independent variables. Most commonly used are simple linear regression and multiple linear regression. |
| Spearman's rho[b] | A test that demonstrates the degree of relationship between two ordinal variables that may not have normal distribution. |
| Tukey test[a] | A test to identify significantly different groups after ANOVA. |
| Wilcoxon Rank sum test[b] | A test of significance for two paired, ordinal data samples. |

**Key**
[a]Tests that can be used with continuous data
[b]Tests that can be used with ordinal data
Covariance = the measure of effect by two or more variables
Nonparametric = inferential statistics involving nominal-level or ordinal-level data to make inferences about the population
Parametric = inferential statistics involving interval or ratio data to make inferences about the population
Ordinal variable = the assignment of numbers to identify ordered relations among a variable with unspecified, unequal, or nonuniform intervals
Continuous variable = variables that can take on an infinite range of values on a continuum with equal variables

**TABLE 2.13**  Uses for common statistical procedures

| | |
|---|---|
| **To summarize data:** | Descriptive statistics |
| **To examine the frequency relationship of one variable to a theoretical distribution:** | Chi-squared test for goodness of fit |
| **To examine the frequency relationship of two variables to each other:** | Chi-squared test for association |
| **To examine the measured relationship between two variables:** | |
| ▪ For ordinal data: | Spearman's rho test |
| ▪ For continuous data: | Pearson's correlation coefficient |
| **To examine the measured relationship of multiple variables:** | Multiple regression test |
| **To examine the significance of difference between groups:** | |
| ▪ For one group: | *t*-test |
| ▪ For two independent groups: | |
| – Ordinal data: | Mann-Whitney test |
| – Continuous data: | Wilcoxon matched pairs test |
| ▪ For two related groups | |
| – Ordinal data: | Independent samples *t*-test |
| – Continuous data: | Paired samples *t*-test |
| ▪ For multiple independent groups: | |
| – One independent variable: | One-way ANOVA |
| – Multiple independent variables: | MANOVA |
| ▪ For multiple related groups: | Repeated measures ANOVA |

are based on the desire to produce actionable knowledge. This mode of transdisciplinary research uses approaches that tend to be more engaged, participatory, and holistic.[65] Regardless of the method used, when communicating scientific results, the message has to be audience appropriate and uphold the highest level of ethical standards while providing a clear, honest, and accurate report of the findings, along with a full disclosure of any and all potential conflicts of interest.

**Recap**  Analyzing and interpreting nutrition research can be a complicated task because of the complexity of diet. The far-reaching and interconnected nature of lifestyle behaviors, including nutrition, make it hard to predict outcomes and control for all possible variables. Enlisting the help of a trained statistician and developing a study with appropriate statistical tests are essential for accurately interpreting nutritional research findings.

# ▶ Why Publish?

**Preview**  This section encourages the graduate student or doctoral candidate to participate in research to advance the profession, and it summarizes the potential benefits for all—the individual, the academic institution, and the public.

## Research Potential, Productivity, and Merit

Have you ever heard the phrase "publish or perish"?[66] In the academic and scientific environment, it is critical to be an active researcher and to publish the findings of your work. The private sector, government institutions, and academia are continuously searching for candidates who have demonstrated research potential, productivity, and competence in their fields of study. Having a strong record of publications as an entry-level food and nutrition professional can be challenging, but it will make you a highly competitive candidate. In the research context, *merit* mainly means the quality and quantity of publications in important journals in a particular discipline. However, getting involved in interdisciplinary research teams forms a professional collaboration among scholars and peers from other fields of science. This can ultimately lead to a greater pool of employment and professional development opportunities. This could also influence the potential trajectory of your career path.

## Research to Influence Policy

In 2014, the Academy of Nutrition and Dietetics established the Council on Research. This council is responsible for coordinating the Academy's research efforts.[67] Subsequently, the Academy published the International and Scientific Affairs Strategic Plan to establish a new structure for research initiatives the Academy.[68] Research also forms the basis for the Academy's decisions, policies, and communications and guides the Academy in advocacy work with government, research, and philanthropic agencies.[68] This facilitates the establishment of partnerships and collaborations to advance the science of nutrition. **Advocacy research** attempts to influence the formal and informal policies established by policymakers and other stakeholders. Thus, it is important to collect good data and present findings in a compelling manner.[69]

## Disseminate Your Findings

Presenting findings at national and international conferences can help the student engage in conversations and obtain feedback from experts in the field. Preparing a poster, abstract, or presentation may be especially beneficial in helping the authors identify strengths and weaknesses in their own projects and analyze how limitations can be approached. This is part of a critical-thinking process that can contribute to the generation of new ideas and organizing arguments to defend the methodology of the study. Traveling to international conferences can be highly attractive and rewarding for students competing for scholarships, awards, and possible fellowships in other countries.

## Applied Practice

The ultimate goal of research in the nutrition and dietetics arena is to continue improving patient care by assessing and analyzing findings from various nutrition interventions.[70] With this goal in mind, the AND has developed its evidence analysis library (EAL) and the Dietetics Practice Based Research Network (DPBRN).[71] The EAL is an online tool that provides professionals with a summary of the best available research on different nutrition-related themes.[72] The DPBRN conducts, supports, promotes, and advocates for practice-based research that answers questions that are important to dietetics practice.[73] As you become more experienced you will start to develop a focus based on your personal research interests. Once you have chosen a particular area, you can to network with other professionals with similar interests and hopefully initiative collaborations between research centers, professional organizations, the industry, and the community. Other factors that can influence your focus area include state of the literature, importance of the topic to your discipline, the availability of potential mentors, and funding.

Research will not be possible without adequate financial support. Having scientific publications will increase your access to economic resources and funding opportunities. The Academy of Nutrition and Dietetics Foundation has a series of grants that support research projects conducted by members.[74] A list of websites to find grant opportunities can be found at the end of this chapter.

## Manuscript Submission

When you are in the process of getting your manuscript finished, it is important to start a log of potential journals as possible submission targets. **FIGURE 2.16**

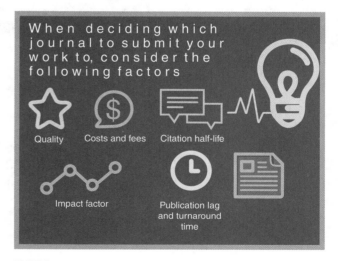

**FIGURE 2.16** How to decide to which journal to submit your work.

Data from Bartkowski JP, Deem CS., Ellison CG. Publishing in academic journal strategic advice for doctoral students and academic mentors. *Am Soc.* 2015; 46, 99–115.

presents the factors you should consider when making a final decision.

Your mentors can guide you in this process. Once the research team has identified which journal to submit the manuscript make sure to read the submission requirements carefully and format the document according to the author's guidelines.

## Benefits of Research Publications

As a graduate student or doctoral candidate, you may see the benefits of getting your work accepted and published. The immediate benefits as a master or doctoral student include the following:[75]

- A sense of achievement during your candidature
- Increased motivation
- Feedback and critiques from peers, mentors, professors, and experts
- Benchmarking the quality of your work and joining the academic community in your discipline or areas of interest

  Long-term benefits include:

- Increasing future research opportunities
- Improving your competitiveness and eligibility for scholarships and fellowships
- Improving grant success
- Securing employment

**Recap** Research findings and scientific publications provide evidence that guides practice and contributes to efforts for improving patient care. The Academy of Nutrition and Dietetics has established groups and provides valuable resources to help students and professionals become more active in research. Becoming involved in research early in your career path will help you define your areas of interest and establish potential research collaborators.

## ▶ Chapter Summary

Research is the pursuit of knowledge with the hope that it will contribute to the betterment of society. Research findings and scientific publications provide evidence that guides practice and contributes to efforts for improving patient care and public-health outcomes. Nutrition research plays a central role in the health initiatives for creating guidelines and recommendations for meeting nutrient needs to promote health and well-being. The main purposes of research are to build knowledge and confirm previous scientific findings. Understanding different study approaches is essential when conducting a research project. Getting involved in interdisciplinary research teams creates collaboration among scholars and peers from other fields of science. Reading, understanding, interpreting, and appraising scientific research is an essential skill for healthcare professionals and nutrition practitioners.

## CASE STUDY

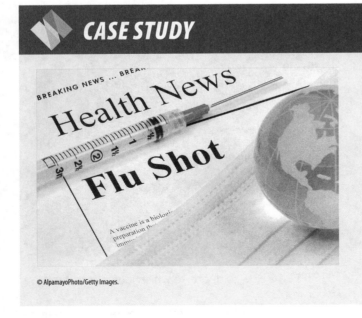

© AlpamayoPhoto/Getty Images.

### Social Aspects of the Responsible Conduct of Research

*Part I*

You are completing a post-doctoral fellowship and working under a well-known researcher. The investigation is studying potential risk factors for dementia. You are in charge of developing a report on the possible relationship between the flu vaccine and the development of dementia.

While revising the manuscript you realize that the information summarized on the data tables does not match the basic data gathered from the medical charts you have reviewed. The time elapsed since the last exposure to the flu vaccine and the date of initial dementia diagnosis for a few subjects is shorter than what your records state. A shorter period of time suggests a stronger association between the flu vaccine and dementia than would be noted otherwise.

You decide to meet with your research partner and principal investigator (PI) to discuss this issue. They explain that some statistical changes were made so they could "smooth" the data. Furthermore, they emphasize that the methods applied are standard and completely valid. They dismiss you and recommend not to be concerned about these data inconsistencies anymore.

**Questions:**
1. What are your responsibilities as first author?
   a. Should you investigate and question these data inconsistencies further?
   b. If so, what process would you follow?
2. Are there potential risks to you as a research fellow?
3. Should you be concerned that the data was purposely altered to produce more interesting findings?

**Part II**

Eventually, the study is published in a reputable scientific journal. A group of dementia research experts instantly disprove the study findings and conclusions. They proceed to request access to the raw data. This leads to the initiation of a formal National Institute of Health (NIH) misconduct investigation. The final report states that there is enough evidence that data was falsified and the paper must be withdrawn. Although the scientific community discredited the findings, the media had already interpreted the findings and spread the message that an increase in dementia in older adults is linked to receiving the flu vaccine. This impacted the general public and resulted in a decrease in flu vaccine compliance across all age groups.

**Questions:**
1. How does the media communicate scientific findings differently from what is published through scientific literature?
2. Are the authors of the study accountable for the future public dissemination of messages based on the original studies and journal publications?

Data from: Harvard Health Publications/ Harvard University; National Institutes of Health Office of Intramural Research
Research Cases for Use by the NIH Community https://oir.nih.gov/sourcebook/ethical-conduct/responsible-conduct-research-training/annual-review-ethics-case-studies/research-cases-use-nih-community#theme17 Date accessed 8.6.17.

# Learning Portfolio

## Key Terms

Advocacy research
Alternate hypothesis
Applied research
Basic research
Belmont Report of 1979
Beneficence
Bias
Carryover effects
Case-control studies
Cohort studies
Complete counterbalancing
Conflict of interest
Control condition
Controls
Counterbalancing
Crossover design
Cross-sectional studies
Cultural competence
Declaration of Helsinki of 1964
Dependent variable

Descriptive study
Double-blind study
Evidence-based nutrition practice
Exempt research
Experiment
Experimental research design
Factorial design
Factors
Familiarization
Greater than minimal risk
Health disparity
Health literacy
Hypothesis
Independent variable
Informed consent
Institutional review board (IRB)
Justice
Latin square
Literature review
Meta-analysis

Minimal-risk research
Multilevel randomized design
National Commission for the Protection of Human Subjects of Biomedical and Behavioral Research
National Institutes of Health Revitalization Act of 1993
National Research Act of 1974
Null hypothesis
Nuremberg Code
Nutrition Care Process (NCP)
Observational studies
Placebo

Placebo effect
Prospective study
Qualitative research
Quantitative research
Randomized assignment
Relative risk (RR)
Research
Research question
Respect for persons
Translational science
Vulnerable population

## Study Questions

1. Which of the following was a major violation to ethics committed by investigators conducting the Tuskegee study?
   a. Subjects did not receive economic compensation for their time and participation in the study.
   b. Participants were never given proper treatment for their disease.
   c. The study was done with vulnerable subjects.
   d. Education about syphilis was not provided before subjects were enrolled in the study.

2. Which of the following is true of the Nuremberg Code?
   a. It includes three ethical principles: respect for persons, beneficence, and justice.
   b. It was developed by the World Medical Association.
   c. It includes informed-consent procedures.
   d. None of the above.

3. Which of the following is not a requirement of informed consent?
   a. Information
   b. Compensation
   c. Comprehension
   d. Voluntariness

4. Which of the following is true of an institutional review board (IRB)?
   a. Oversees the ethical and safety aspect of the research study.
   b. Must review and approve the study protocol.
   c. Must be composed of faculty members and experts.
   d. Is appointed by the federal government.

5. Which of the following is considered the main secondary interest that could lead to a conflict of interest?
   a. Professional growth
   b. Financial gain
   c. Publication
   d. Gifts from a sponsor

6. In conjunction with following conflict-of-interest guidelines, the researcher must:
   a. openly declare research sponsorship.
   b. use a peer-review system.
   c. pay required fees to professional organizations.
   d. a and b.

7. Regarding bias in clinical research, which of the following is an example of bias in the pretrial stage?
   a. Selection bias
   b. Interviewer bias
   c. Confounding bias
   d. Performance bias

8. The National Institutes of Health Revitalization Act of 1993:
   a. established guidelines for inclusion of older adults in clinical research.
   b. established guidelines for inclusion of women and minorities in clinical research.
   c. established guidelines for inclusion of participants without health insurance in clinical research.
   d. established guidelines for inclusion of men and minorities in clinical research.

9. Which of the following is a major recruitment challenge in clinical research?
   a. Demographic changes
   b. High health literacy
   c. Language barrier
   d. Low health literacy

10. What is a health disparity?
    a. A health outcome difficult to understand in different populations
    b. A health outcome seen to a greater or lesser extent between different populations
    c. A health outcome seen to a greater extent between different populations
    d. A health outcome seen to a lesser extent between different populations

11. Which type of research is used to inform public policy, contribute to applied behavioral analysis, and support operational decision making?
    a. Nutrition research
    b. Applied research
    c. Basic research
    d. Translational research

12. Why is randomized assignment so important in an experimental design?
    a. Random assignment is a requirement for research funding.
    b. Random assignment increases control of the study.
    c. Random assignment limits bias.
    d. Random assignment makes the process of evaluation of results easier.

13. The *placebo effect* refers to:
    a. a sugar pill or cellulose pill given to a subject.
    b. simulation of an experimental drug.
    c. therapeutic procedure that has no physiological effect.
    d. a way of describing everything that surrounds the placebo treatment.

14. The "gold standard" in intervention-based research is a:
    a. double-blind study.
    b. crossover design study.
    c. descriptive study.
    d. translational study.

15. Which type of research is referred to as "bench to bedside"?
    a. Qualitative research
    b. Quantitative research
    c. Clinical research
    d. Translational research

16. True or false? The main responsibility of the Academy of Nutrition and Dietetics' Council on Research is to coordinate the academy's research efforts.
    a. True
    b. False

17. Which of the following provides food and nutrition professionals with a summary of the best available research on different nutrition topics?
    a. DPBRN
    b. Council on Research
    c. Eat Right Foundation
    d. Evidence Analysis Library

18. Which of the following factors must be considered when deciding to which journal to submit your work?
    a. Quality of the journal
    b. Page and word limit
    c. Impact factor
    d. a and c

19. How can presenting a poster or abstract improve a research project?
    a. It helps the authors identify strengths and weaknesses of their own project.
    b. It helps the authors network with other experts in the field.
    c. It helps the authors identify more funding opportunities to expand the project.
    d. It helps the authors secure scholarship opportunities.

20. A research hypothesis:
    a. is a prediction statement about what the investigators expect to happen during the study.
    b. the final take-away message from a research study.
    c. should be written as the last line of the study introduction.
    d. is required to be present in the study abstract when publishing in a scientific journal.
    e. is the question investigators are trying to answer while conducting their research study.

21. A research hypothesis should be which of the following?
    a. Measurable
    b. Specific about the population being studied
    c. Specific about the time frame when the study will take place
    d. Clear about the study variables and the control group
    e. All of the above

22. Performing a literature review:
    a. means searching the Internet on the topic.
    b. provides a basis for what is already known on the topic of interest.
    c. should be completed after the study is conducted but before the journal article is written for publication.
    d. is not necessary if funding for the research has already been secured.

23. Guidelines for writing a literature review includes all of the following except:
    a. starting with a clear introduction explaining how the review is organized and the purpose of the proposed research.
    b. an acknowledgement and respectful consideration of results and opinions that do not agree with the current thesis.

c.  intermittent references with direct quotes to present the ideas of others.

d.  a strong topic sentence that clearly states the main idea of each paragraph and transitional words and phrases to connect ideas between sentences and paragraphs.

24.  Critically evaluating scientific evidence means:

a.  criticizing and finding fault in each research article.

b.  conducting a systematic process to identify the strengths and limitations of a research article.

c.  summarizing your opinion of the research article.

d.  hosting an organized meeting or journal club meeting to discuss the article and its relevance to other published journal articles on the topic.

25.  Which study design is useful in establishing baseline data about prevalence of a disease or food intake, establishing associations among variables, and providing insight into areas of future research?

a.  Survey research

b.  Case study design

c.  Randomized controlled trials

d.  Intervention trials

26.  A limitation of cross-sectional study design is that:

a.  it cannot measure the prevalence of disease or exposure.

b.  it is not useful for identifying associations.

c.  it does not allow examination of a sequence of events.

d.  it is an expensive study design.

27.  When the study participants are observed and data are assessed over a long period of time, the study is considered:

a.  a repeated-measures cross-sectional design.

b.  a long-term intervention trial.

c.  a clinical trial.

d.  a longitudinal study.

28.  A cohort study design is:

a.  retrospective or prospective.

b.  quick and inexpensive to conduct.

c.  good for rare diseases.

d.  hard to assess in terms of its disease time frame or an outcome of interest.

29.  When an investigator is looking for an exposure to a known outcome, which study design should be used?

a.  Randomized trial

b.  Cross-sectional

c.  Survey

d.  Case control

e.  Descriptive

30.  The evidence analysis process for reviewing scientific research includes which one of the following steps?

a.  Looking up an evidence analysis question for a wide area of practice.

b.  Interviewing others who have conducted research in this area of practice.

c.  Critically appraising each article and evaluating it based on appropriateness of study design and the quality of how the study was conducted.

d.  Copying the summaries from each article into a checklist table to compare the key findings.

31.  Informational health literacy:

a.  enables providers to translate information about risk factors, diseases, and nutritional treatments to effectively communicate with patients, clients, and consumers.

b.  does not require healthcare practitioners to understand research methodology.

c.  involves understanding studies with complex statistical techniques that only a trained statistician can interpret.

d.  necessitates determining areas for future investigation that are novel and fundable to drive the profession of nutrition to the next level.

## Discussion Questions

1.  Mention and discuss examples of conflicts of interest that may arise within the dietetics field.

2.  Review the AND's code of ethics. What principles apply to RDNs who work for or with the food industry?

3.  Mention and discuss examples of conflicts of interest that may arise within the dietetics field.

4.  When would it be necessary or appropriate to conduct research with these populations? Think about examples in which nutrition and public-health research and interventions are needed.

5.  Consider the issue of living organ donors.

a.  Does a healthy donor have the right to consent to a potentially life-threatening procedure to benefit another person?

b.  Are the perceived psychological benefits of saving another person's life or improving his or her quality of life acceptable?

c.  How could you manage peer pressure or coercion from friends and family members?

## Activities

1. Select food- and nutrition-related scientific publications from each type of descriptive study. Identify which type of study it is and the advantages and limitations of each type.
2. Identify at least three possible sources of funding to support a thesis or dissertation research project. Explain to the rest of the class why the application or proposal should receive funding.
3. Discuss examples of additional safeguards needed when enrolling vulnerable populations.

## Online Resources

CDC Growth Charts. http://www.cdc.gov/growth-charts/who_charts.htm

Video: "10 Highly Unethical Medical Experiments." This video presents a series of 10 research studies around the world that followed unethical practices that were capable of harming human subjects. https://www.youtube.com/watch?v=ccB7rPnqzIE

National Institutes of Health: Research Ethics Timeline (1932–Present). This website presents a timeline involving the key events that affected research ethics starting in 1932 and up to 2016. https://www.niehs.nih.gov/research/resources/bioethics/timeline/

Declaration of Helsinki. This World Medical Association website includes a link to download the new version of the Helsinki Declaration published on the website of the *Journal of American Medical Association.* https://www.wma.net/what-we-do/medical-ethics/declaration-of-helsinki/

Dietitians' Food Industry Relationships: What Is Ethical and What Is Not? http://www.todaysdietitian.com/newarchives/031115p44.shtml

Academy of Nutrition and Dietetics Evidence Analysis Library. Nutrition Care Process introduction and tutorial. https://www.andeal.org/ncp

National Center for Advancing Translational Sciences at the National Institutes of Health. Inside the NCATS Laboratories. https://www.youtube.com/watch?v=FOp-lX3NY6E&feature=youtu.be

Cochrane. Cochrane is a global network of researchers who work to provide quality information to help those involved in health care make informed decisions: www.cochrane.org

PRISMA. The PRISMA group is an international group of researchers and clinicians who created a checklist of what should in included in a systematic review: http://www.prisma-statement.org/Default.aspx

Harvard Catalyst: Understanding the Spectrum of Translational Research. https://www.youtube.com/watch?v=rAblbUmyQgk

AND Foundation: Grants. http://eatrightfoundation.org/scholarships-funding/#Grants

American Society for Nutrition Funding Opportunities. https://nutrition.org/about-asn/awards/

Centers for Disease Control and Prevention: Grants. https://www.cdc.gov/grants/

USDA-NIFA: Grants. https://nifa.usda.gov/grants

## References

1. Monsen ER, Van Horn L, eds. *Research Successful Approaches.* 3rd ed. Chicago, IL: American Dietetics Association; 2008.
2. Forister JG, Blessing JD. *Introduction to Research and Medical Literature for Health Professionals.* 4th ed. Burlington, MA: Jones and Bartlett Learning; 2016.
3. Boushey C, Harris J, Bruemmer B, Archer SL, Van Horn L. Publishing nutrition research: A review of the study design, statistical analyses, and other key elements of manuscript preparation, Part 1. *J Am Diet Assoc.* 2006; 106(1):89–96.
4. Drummond KE, Murphy-Ryes A. *Nutrition Research Concepts and Applications.* Burlington, MA: Jones and Bartlett Learning; 2018.
5. Ware M., Mabe M. The STM Report. An overview of scientific and scholarly journal publishing. 4th ed. The Netherlands: International Association of Scientific, Technical and Medical Publishers Prins Willem Alexanderhof; 2015. http://www.stmassoc.org/2015_02_20_STM_Report_2015.pdf. Accessed July 5, 2017.
6. Dan Corlan A. Medline trend: Automated yearly statistics of PubMed results for any query, 2004. http://dan.corlan.net/medline-trend.html. Accessed July 5, 2017. http://dan.corlan.net/medline-trend.html.
7. Young JM, Solomon MJ. How to critically appraise an article. *Natl Clin Pract Gastroenterol Hepatol.* 2009; 6(2)89–91.
8. Cochrane. www.cochrane.org 7/21/17.
9. PRISMA. http://www.prisma-statement.org/Default.aspx. Accessed July 21, 2017.
10. Centers for Disease Control and Prevention. The Tuskegee Timeline. https://www.cdc.gov/tuskegee/timeline.htm. Accessed April 7, 2017.
11. Goldby S, Krugman S, Pappworth MH, Edsall G. The Willowbrook letters: Criticisms and defense. *Lancet*; 1971.
12. Fried AL, American Psychological Association. Chapter 3: Ethics in Psychological Research: Guidelines and Regulations by *APA Handbook of Research Methods in Psychology.* 2012; 55–73.

13. Holocaust Encyclopedia. Nazi Medical Experiments. https://www.ushmm.org/wlc/en/article.php?ModuleId=10005168. Accessed September 22, 2016.

14. *Trials of War Criminals before the Nuremberg Military Tribunals under Control Council Law.* Washington, DC: US Government Printing Office; 1949; 2(10);181–182.

15. WMA Declaration of Helsinki—Ethical principles for medical research involving human subjects. http://www.wma.net/en/30publications/10policies/b3/. Accessed September 22, 2016.

16. Presidential Commission for the Study of Bioethical Issues. History of Bioethics Commissions. https://bioethicsarchive.georgetown.edu/pcsbi/history.html. Accessed September 22, 2016.

17. US Department of Health and Human Services Office for Human Research Protections. *The Belmont Report.* https://www.hhs.gov/ohrp/regulations-and-policy/belmont-report/index.html.

18. Appelbaum PS, Grisso T. The MacArthur Treatment Competence Study: I. mental illness and competence to consent to treatment. *Law Hum Behav.* 1995; 19(2):105–126.

19. US Food and Drug Administration. Regulatory Information. http://www.fda.gov/RegulatoryInformation/Guidances/ucm126420.htm#IRBOrg. Accessed September 22, 2016.

20. Stone J. Conducting clinical research. A practice guide for physicians, nurses, study coordinators, and investigators. In: *Regulatory Issues.* 2nd ed. 2010; 123–124.

21. Office of the Institutional Review Board UT Health Science Center San Antonio. Glossary of Human Research Terms. http://research.uthscsa.edu/irb/glossary/IRB_glossary.PHP.

22. Office of the Institutional Review Board UT Health Science Center San Antonio. New Research Forms. http://research.uthscsa.edu/irb/forms_NewResearch.shtml.

23. Coughlin SS, Soskolne CL, Goodman KW. Case analysis and moral reasoning. In: *Case Studies in Public Health Ethics.* Washington, DC: American Public Health Association; 1997:1–18.

24. Institute of Medicine (US) Committee on Conflict of Interest in Medical Research, Education, and Practice. In: Lo B, Field MJ, eds. Washington, DC: National Academies Press; 2009.

25. Committee on Conflict of Interest in Medical Research, Education, and Practice. *Conflict of Interest in Medical Research, Education, and Practice.* Washington, DC: National Academies Press. https://www.ncbi.nlm.nih.gov/books/NBK22942/pdf/Bookshelf_NBK22942.pdf. Accessed October 5, 2016.

26. Federation of American Societies for Experimental Biology Conflict of Interest. Toolkit. http://faseb.org/coi/Tools/Societies.aspx. Accessed October 15, 2016.

27. Rowe S, Alexander N, Clydesdale FM, et al. Funding food science and nutrition research: Financial conflicts and scientific integrity. *Am J Clin Nutr.* 2009;89(5):1285–1291.

28. *Mosby's Pocket Dictionary of Medicine, Nursing & Health Professions.* 8th ed. St. Louis, MO: Elsevier; 2016.

29. IRB Guidebook at Chapter VI, the HHS Office for Human Research Protections. https://archive.hhs.gov/ohrp/irb/irb_chapter6.htm.

30. Health Literacy Interventions and Outcomes: An Updated Systematic Review. Available at http://www.ahrq.gov/downloads/pub/evidence/pdf/literacy/literacyup.pdf. Accessed December 28, 2016.

31. NIH Policy and Guidelines on the Inclusion of Women and Minorities as Subjects in Clinical Research—Amended, October 2001. https://grants.nih.gov/grants/funding/women_min/guidelines_amended_10_2001.htm. Accessed December 20, 2016.

32. US Department of Health and Human Services. 2000. *Healthy People 2010.* Washington, DC: US Government Printing Office. Originally developed for Ratzan SC, Parker RM. 2000. Introduction. In: Selden CR, Zorn M, Ratzan SC, Parker RM, eds. *National Library of Medicine Current Bibliographies in Medicine: Health Literacy.* NLM Pub. No. CBM 2000–1. Bethesda, MD: National Institutes of Health.

33. National Academies Press. Health Literacy: A Prescription to End Confusion http://www.nationalacademies.org/hmd/Reports/2004/Health-Literacy-A-Prescription-to-End-Confusion.aspx. April 8, 2004.

34. Newman SD, Andrews JO, Magwood GS, Jenkins C, Cox MJ, Williamson DC. Community advisory boards in community-based participatory research: A synthesis of best processes. *Prev Chronic Dis.* 2011; 8(3):A70. http://www.cdc.gov/pcd/issues/2011/may/10_0045.htm. Accessed October 1, 2016.

35. Office of Disease Prevention and Health Promotion. Determinants of Health. https://www.healthypeople.gov/2020/about/foundation-health-measures/Determinants-of-Health. Accessed October 16, 2017.

36. DePoy E, Gitlin L. Research as an important way of knowing. In: DePoy E, Gitlin L. eds. *Introduction to Research: Understanding and Applying Multiple Strategies.* 5th ed. St. Louis, MO: Elsevier; 2016:2–13.

37. Gaber J. Salkind NJ, ed. *Applied Research in Encyclopedia of Research Design.* Newbury Park, CA: Sage Publications; 2012.

38. Academy of Nutrition and Dietetics (AND). Research Philosophy and Structure: Making the Case for Research. http://www.eatrightpro.org/resources/research/philosophy-and-structure/making-the-case-for-research. Accessed March 5, 2017.

39. US Department of Health and Human Services. Office of Research Integrity. Module 2: Research Design. http://ori.hhs.gov/content/module-2-research-design#experimental-studies. Accessed November 13, 2016.

40. Grand Canyon University Center of Innovation in Research and Teaching. Quantitative Approaches Model. https://cirt.gcu.edu/research/developmentresources/research_ready/quantresearch/approaches. Accessed December 21, 2016.

41. Babbie ER. *The Practice of Social Research.* 12th ed. Belmont, CA: Wadsworth Cengage; 2010.

42. Food and Agriculture Organization. Quantitative and Qualitative approaches to Dietary Assessment. http://www.fao.org/docrep/008/y5825e/y5825e07.htm. Accessed December 20, 2016.

43. The Nurse's Health Study 3. http://www.nhs3.org/. Accessed July 21, 2017.

44. Interagency Board for Nutrition Monitoring and Related Research. Bialostosky K. ed. *Nutrition Monitoring in the United States: The Directory of Federal and State Nutrition Monitoring and Related Research Activities.* Hyattsville, MD: National Center for Health Statistics; 2000. https://www.cdc.gov/nchs/data/misc/direc-99.pdf. Accessed July 21, 2017.

45. Centers for Disease Control and Prevention. National Center for Health Statistics. National Health and Nutrition

Examination Survey. https://www.cdc.gov/nchs/nhanes/index.htm. Accessed July 6, 2017.

46. Brummer B, Harris J, Gleason P, et al. Publishing nutrition research: A a review of epidemiologic methods. *J Am Diet Assoc*. 2009; 109:1728–1737.

47. Thiese MS. Observational and interventional study design types: An overview. *Biochemia Medica*. 2014; 24(2):199–210. http://dx.doi.org/10.11613/BM.2014.022.

48. The Academy of Nutrition and Dietetics. About EAL; 2015. www.ANDEAL.org/study-designs. Accessed July 21, 2017.

49. The Academy of Nutrition and Dietetics. Evidence Analysis Library. Evidence Analysis Manual: Steps in the Academy Evidence Analysis Process; 2016; April. The manual is available in PDF format from the methodology section of the EAL (www.andeal.org).

50. Handu D, Moloney L, Wolfram T, Zigler P, Acosta A, Steiber A. Methodology for conducting systematic reviews for the Evidence Analysis Library *J Acad Nutr Dietet*. 2016. http://dx.doi.org/10.1016/j.jand.2015.11.008. Accessed July 11, 2017.

51. The Academy of Nutrition and Dietetics. Nutrition Care Process. Accessed July 11, 2017. https://ncpt.webauthor.com/nutrition-care-process.

52. The Academy of Nutrition and Dietetics. ADNHII http://www.eatrightpro.org/resources/practice/nutrition-care-process/andhii. Accessed July 12, 2017.

53. US Department of Health and Human Services Office of Research Integrity. https://ori.hhs.gov/content/module-2-research-design.

54. Cooper H, Camic PM, Long DL, Panter AT, Rindskopf D, Sher KJ. eds. Research designs: quantitative, qualitative, neuropsychological, and biological. In: *APA Handbook of Research Methods in Psychology*. Washington, DC: 2012; 2:469–488.

55. National Center for Complementary and Integrative Health. What is a placebo? 2015; December 10. https://nccih.nih.gov/health/placebo. Accessed December 20, 2016.

56. Mosby's Medical Dictionary. Double-blind study. http://medical-dictionary.thefreedictionary.com/double-blind+study. Accessed November 6, 2016.

57. Research Methods II. Chapter 9. Analysis of intervention studies III factorial designs. *Oxford Journals*. http://www.oxfordjournals.org/our_journals/tropej/online/ma_chap9.pdf. Accessed December 11, 2016.

58. National Institute of Health. Cross-over design. https://clinicaltrials.gov/ct2/about-studies/glossary#C. Accessed January 2, 2017.

59. Wellek S, Blettner M. On the proper use of the crossover design in clinical trials: Part 18 of a series on evaluation of scientific publications. *Deutsches Ärzteblatt Int*. 2012; 109(15):276–281.

60. Mitchell ML, Jolley JM. Matched pairs, within-subjects, and mixed designs. In: *Research Design Explained*. 8th ed. Belmont, CA: Cengage Learning; 2012: 541.

61. Cozby P, Bates S. Experimental design. In: *Methods in Behavioral Research*. 12th ed. New York, NY: McGraw-Hill; 2012;161–177.

62. McArdle JJ, Woodcock JR. Expanding test–rest designs to include developmental time-lag components. *Psychol Meth*. 1997; 2:403–435.

63. National Center for Advancing Translational Sciences. Translational science spectrum. https://ncats.nih.gov/translation/spectrum. Accessed January 2, 2017.

64. Boushey CJ, Harris J, Bruemmer B, Archer SL. Publishing nutrition research: A review of sampling, sample size, statistical analysis, and other key elements of manuscript preparation, part 2. *J Am Diet Assoc*. 2008; 108:679–688.

65. Pelletier DL, Porter CM, Aarons GA, Wuehler SE, Neufeld LM. Expanding the frontiers of population nutrition research: New questions, new methods and new approaches. *Adv Nutr*. 2013; 4:92–114.

66. Bartkowski JP, Deem CS, Ellison CG. Publishing in academic journal strategic advice for doctoral students and academic mentors. *Am Soc*. 2015; 46:99–115.

67. Academy of Nutrition and Dietetics. Council on Research. https://www.eatrightpro.org/resource/leadership/volunteering/committees-and-task-forces/council-on-research. Accessed January 30, 2017.

68. AND. Structure for research activities at the Academy. http://www.eatrightpro.org/resources/research/philosophy-and-structure/structure-for-research-activities-at-the-academy. Accessed January 29, 2017.

69. Conducting Research to Influence Policy. Community Tool Box. Chapter 31. Section 10. http://ctb.ku.edu/en/table-of-contents/advocacy/advocacy-research/influence-policy/main.

70. The Academy of Nutrition and Dietetics. Applied practice. http://www.eatrightpro.org/resources/research/applied-practice. Accessed January 30, 2017.

71. The Academy of Nutrition and Dietetics. Evidence Analysis Library. Orientation tutorial. https://www.andeal.org/tutorials date. Accessed August 6, 2017.

72. The Academy of Nutrition and Dietetics. Evidence Analysis Library. https://www.andeal.org/. Accessed January 30, 2017.

73. The Academy of Nutrition and Dietetics. Dietetics practice based research network. http://www.eatrightpro.org/resources/research/evidence-based-resources/dpbrn. Accessed January 30, 2017.

74. The Academy of Nutrition and Dietetics Foundation. Research. http://eatrightfoundation.org/why-it-matters/research/. Accessed September 22, 2017.

75. Pickering C., Griffith University. Why publish papers during your PhD? https://www.youtube.com/watch?v=EvT71knryYc&t=14s.

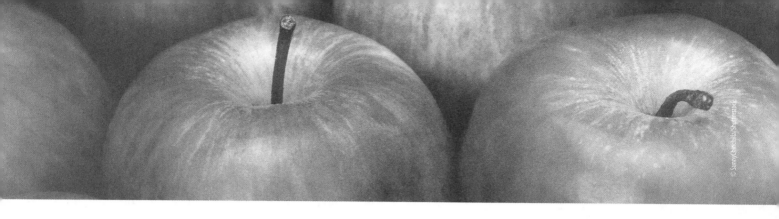

# CHAPTER 3

# Standards for Desirable Nutrient Intake

**Jessica Pearl**, MS, RD, CSSD, CSCS, CLT, CDN, FAND

## CHAPTER OUTLINE

- Introduction
- Historical Perspective for Dietary Standards and Recommendations
- Dietary Reference Intake (DRI)
- Tolerable Upper Intake Level (UL)

- Energy Requirements
- Macronutrient Recommendations
- Nutrient Density and Nutritional Rating
- Diet Quality Indicators

- *Dietary Guidelines for Americans 2015*
- Food Labeling and Nutrition
- Food Guides (MyPlate Food Exchange)
- Chapter Summary

## LEARNING OBJECTIVES

After reading this chapter, the learner will be able to:

1. Describe the process that led to the formation of the *Dietary Guidelines* and the Dietary Reference Intakes (DRIs).
2. Identify the main USDA food guides.
3. Explain why the DRIs were developed and what purpose each value is intended to serve.
4. Identify the components of total energy expenditure and the methods used to measure energy expenditure.
5. Summarize the intake recommendations for protein, fat, and carbohydrates as established by the Recommended Dietary Allowance (RDA), Estimated Average Requirement (EAR), tolerable upper intake level (UL), and Acceptable Macronutrient Distribution Range (AMDR).
6. Explain the profiling tools most commonly used to guide consumer food choices.
7. Summarize the purpose of the Healthy Eating Index and food pattern modeling analysis.
8. Summarize the process for developing the *Dietary Guidelines for Americans* and MyPlate, including the key recommendations of the *Dietary Guidelines for Americans 2015*.
9. Explain the reasoning for the major changes to the Nutrition Facts Label.

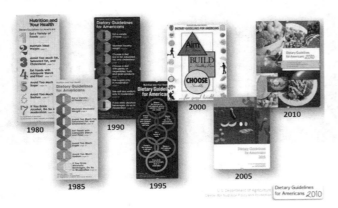

Reproduced from Academy of Nutrition and Dietetics (2015). Updating the *Dietary Guidelines for Americans*: Status and Looking Ahead, Figure 1 *Dietary Guidelines for Americans*, 1980-2010. *Journal of the Academy of Nutrition and Dietetics.* Rahavi, E., Stoody, E. E., Rihane, C., Casavale, K. O., Olson, R. 115/2/181. http://www.andjrnl.org/article/S2212-2672(14)01770-5/pdf.

## ▶ Introduction

Throughout the past century, as our understanding of the relationship between food intake and health evolved, so did the eating habits of individuals. As a result, the standards of desirable nutrient intake and eating patterns also transitioned. These standards, established by government agencies including the United States Department of Agriculture (USDA) and the Department of Health and Human Services (HHS), are meant to encourage optimal eating behaviors throughout the population. The first USDA food guide was developed in 1916 with "Food for Young Children" and "How to Select Food" using food groups and household measures to encourage proper intake. Today the food guide has taken the form of MyPlate, a graphic image created to support conformance to the *Dietary Guidelines for Americans* (*Dietary Guidelines*). Since it was first issued in 1980, the *Dietary Guidelines* has served as the basis for the USDA food guides. The guidelines are updated every five years to reflect current scientific data, and food guides are revised as necessary to best reflect the message of the *Dietary Guidelines* and most effectively resonate with the public.

## ▶ Historical Perspective for Dietary Standards and Recommendations

**Preview**   The *Dietary Guidelines for Americans*, Dietary Reference Intakes, and USDA food guides have collectively evolved over the past century to guide the intake of the American population.

## History of the *Dietary Guidelines*

In 1977, the US Senate Select Committee on Nutrition and Human Needs recommended that dietary goals be established for the American people. The goals consisted of complementary nutrient based and food-based recommendations. Since 1980, the *Dietary Guidelines for Americans* has been the authoritative source of nutrition advice for people 2 years of age and older and serve as the basis for federal food and nutrition education programs.[1] The *Dietary Guidelines* are revised and published every five years by the HHS Office of Disease Prevention and Health Promotion and the USDA's Center for Nutrition Science and Policy, along with the Agriculture Research Service (**TABLE 3.1**). Since the first dietary goals were established, the *Dietary Guidelines* has changed in important ways to reflect available scientific evidence, but the guidelines have also been consistent in their recommendations of the components needed to follow a healthy diet (**TABLE 3.2**).

## Development of the *Dietary Guidelines*

Table 3.2 summarizes the key recommendations of the *Dietary Guidelines* for each year they have been issued.

Many landmark changes have been added to each edition of the *Dietary Guidelines*[1]:

- First edition (1980): *Dietary Guidelines* recommendations are developed and released by the federal government.
- Second edition (1985): For the first time, the *Dietary Guidelines* advisory committee presented a report of recommendations to the federal government based on nutrition science evidence. This report was then used to inform the *Dietary Guidelines 1985*.
- Third edition (1990): The definition of "healthy" weight considers body mass index, waist-to-hip ratio, and weight-related health problems. Numerical goals are suggested for total fat and saturated fat in the diets of adults.
- Fourth edition (1995): Estimated Average Requirement (EAR), Recommended Dietary Allowance (RDA), and Estimated Energy Requirement (EER) are defined by specific criteria of nutrient adequacy. Tolerable upper intake level (UL) is set according to a specific endpoint.
- Fifth edition (2000): Ten key messages are established and split into three groups instead of seven key messages. The emphasis of this issue was "nutrition and your health."
- Sixth edition (2005): This was the first time a policy document intended primarily for policy

**TABLE 3.1** Historical Timeline: *The Dietary Guidelines for Americans*

| | |
|---|---|
| **1977** | *Dietary Goals for the United States* is issued.<br>Shift in focus from ensuring adequate nutrient intake to avoiding excessive intake of nutrients potentially linked to chronic disease.<br>Goals were met with controversy from nutrition professionals and others who had concerns. |
| **1979** | *Healthy People: The Surgeon General's Report on Health Promotion and Disease Prevention* is released.<br>Reports findings from a panel assembled by the American Society for Clinical Nutrition to study the relationship between dietary practice and health outcomes. |
| **1980** | *Nutrition and Your Health: Dietary Guidelines for Americans* released by the USDA and HHS. Contained seven principles for a healthy diet.<br>US Senate Committee on Appropriations report calls for establishment of a committee to review scientific evidence and recommend revisions to the 1980 nutrition guidelines. |
| **1983** | *The Dietary Guidelines* reviewed by federal advisory committee.<br>A federal advisory committee composed of nine nutrition scientists is formed to review the guidelines and report recommendations to the HHS and USDA. |
| **1985** | *The Dietary Guidelines for Americans* (2nd ed.) released by the HHS and USDA.<br>Main amendments made were for clarification and modification of scientific knowledge to reflect new findings of relationship between diet and chronic disease. |
| **1987** | *Conference Report of the House Committee on Appropriations* specifies that the *Dietary Guidelines* are to be reviewed periodically. |
| **1989** | Federal advisory group reviews *1985 Dietary Guidelines* to assess need for modifications or updates. |
| **1990** | *The Dietary Guidelines for Americans* (3rd ed.) released by the HHS and the USDA.<br>Focus on total diet and specifics on food selection. First edition containing numerical recommendations for dietary fat and saturated fat intake.<br>National Nutrition Monitoring and Related Research Act requires that the *Dietary Guidelines for Americans* be published every five years. |
| **1993** | The 1995 *Dietary Guidelines* committee is established by the HHS and the USDA. |
| **1994** | The secretaries of the HHS and USDA appoint an 11-member *Dietary Guidelines* advisory committee to review the third edition of the *Dietary Guidelines for Americans* and assess the need for changes and make recommendations as necessary. |
| **1995** | The report of the *Dietary Guidelines* advisory committee was published, serving as the basis for the fourth edition of *Nutrition and Your Health: Dietary Guidelines for Americans*.<br>The *Dietary Guidelines for Americans* (4th ed.) released by the HHS and the USDA.<br>Changes to this edition were inclusion of the Food Guide Pyramid, Nutrition Facts Label boxes highlighting good food sources of key nutrients, and a chart representing three weight ranges in relation to height. |
| **1997** | The 2000 *Dietary Guidelines* advisory committee is established by the USDA charter. |
| **1998** | The secretaries of the HHS and the USDA appoint an 11-member *Dietary Guidelines* advisory committee to again review the latest edition of the *Dietary Guidelines for Americans* and recommend any needed changes. |
| **2000** | The *Dietary Guidelines for Americans* (5th ed.) is issued by the president, the HHS, and the USDA.<br>Changes to this document include 10 statements instead of seven; this was accomplished by separating physical activity from weight guidelines, separating grains from fruits and vegetables, and adding a new guideline on safe food handling. |

*(continues)*

**TABLE 3.1** *(continued)*

| | |
|---|---|
| **2003** | The 2005 *Dietary Guidelines* advisory committee is established by the HHS charter.<br>The secretaries of the HHS and the USDA appoint a 13-member *Dietary Guidelines* advisory committee to once again review the latest edition of the *Dietary Guidelines for Americans* and make recommendations for revisions. |
| **2003–2004** | Committee members systematically reviewed the scientific literature to address issues include the relationship between diet and physical activity and health promotion and chronic disease prevention.<br>Resources consulted include reports from the Institute of Medicine (Dietary Reference Intake), the Agency for Healthcare Research and Quality, and the World Health Organization.<br>The USDA completed food intake pattern modeling analyses and the Committee analyzed national data sets as well as the input of experts. |
| **2004** | The committee submits its report to the secretaries of the HHS and the USDA; the report serves as the basis for the *Nutrition and Your Health: Dietary Guidelines for Americans* (6th ed.). |
| **2005** | The *Dietary Guidelines for Americans* (6th ed.) released by the HHS and the USDA.<br>Intended for use primarily by policy makers, healthcare providers, nutritionists, and nutrition educators.<br>Composed of nine main messages that specified 41 key recommendations; 23 for the general public and 18 for special populations. Examples of eating patterns used to exemplify the *Dietary Guidelines* include the USDA food guide and DASH eating plan.<br>A supplementary brochure, *Finding Your Way to a Healthier You*, was provided to advise consumers in their food choices. The USDA released the MyPyramid food-guidance system, an update of the Food Guide Pyramid containing additional advice for consumers. |
| **2008** | The 2010 Dietary Guidelines advisory committee is established by the USDA charter.<br>The secretaries of HHS and USDA appoint a 13-member *Dietary Guidelines* advisory committee to review the sixth edition of the *Dietary Guidelines for Americans* and make recommendations for revisions. |
| **2009** | The Nutrition Evidence Library is established by the USDA to review scientific literature. |
| **2010** | The committee submits its report to the secretaries of the HHS and the USDA, and it serves as the basis for the seventh edition of the *Dietary Guidelines for Americans*. |

Data from Dietary Guidelines Advisory Committee. (2010). Report of the Dietary Guidelines Advisory Committee on the *Dietary Guidelines for Americans*, 2010, to the Secretary of Agriculture and the Secretary of Health and Human Services. Appendix E-4: History of the Dietary Guidelines for Americans. Pages 434-437. https://www.cnpp.usda.gov/sites/default/files/dietary_guidelines_for _americans/2010DGACReport-camera-ready-Jan11-11.pdf.

makers, healthcare professionals, nutritionists, and nutrition educators was prepared. The *Dietary Guidelines* included 41 key recommendations, 23 of which were for the general population and 18 for specific populations. The USDA food guide and the Dietary Approaches to Stop Hypertension (DASH) were used as examples of eating patterns consistent with the *Dietary Guidelines*. The USDA MyPyramid Food Guidance System replaced the Food Guide Pyramid.

■ Seventh edition (2011): This version encompassed the overarching concepts of consuming nutrient-dense foods and beverages and maintaining calorie balance to achieve and sustain a healthy weight. For this edition, the eating patterns were updated to assist individuals in building healthful diets based on the *Dietary Guidelines*. MyPlate was released to serve as a visual icon to help consumers follow the *Dietary Guidelines*.

■ Eighth edition (2015): The most recent version of the guidelines is designed to help Americans eat a healthier diet. This issue of the *Dietary Guidelines* emphasizes the importance of following an overall healthy eating pattern to reduce the risk of diseases and maintain health by making favorable shifts in food choices.

**TABLE 3.2** Evolution of the *Dietary Guidelines for Americans*

| | 1980 | 1985 | 1990 | 1995 | 2000 | |
|---|---|---|---|---|---|---|
| 1 | Eat a variety of foods. | Eat a variety of foods. | Eat a variety of foods. | Eat a variety of foods. | Aim for a healthy weight. | Aim for fitness. |
| 2 | Maintain ideal weight. | Maintain desirable weight. | Maintain healthy weight. | Balance the food you eat with physical activity. | Be physical active every day. | |
| 3 | Avoid fat, saturated fat, and cholesterol. | Avoid fat, saturated fat, and cholesterol. | Choose a diet low in fat, saturated fat, and cholesterol. | Choose a diet with plenty of grain products, vegetables, and fruits. | Let the Food Pyramid guide your food choices. | Build a healthy base. |
| 4 | Eat foods with adequate starch and fiber. | Eat foods with adequate starch and fiber. | Choose a diet with plenty of vegetables, fruits, and grain products. | Choose a diet low in fat, saturated fat, and cholesterol. | Choose a variety of grains daily, especially whole grains. | |
| 5 | Avoid sugar. | Avoid sugar. | Use sugars only in moderation. | Choose a diet moderate in sugars. | Choose a variety of fruits and vegetables daily. | |
| 6 | Avoid sodium. | Avoid sodium. | Use salt and sodium only in moderation. | Choose a diet moderate in salt and sodium. | Keep food safe to eat. | |
| 7 | If you drink alcohol, do so in moderation. | If you drink alcoholic beverages, do so in moderation. | If you drink alcoholic beverages, do so in moderation. | If you drink alcoholic beverages, do so in moderation. | Choose a diet low in saturated fat and cholesterol and moderate in total fat. | |
| 8 | | | | | Choose beverages and foods to moderate your intake of sugars. | Choose sensibly. |
| 9 | | | | | Choose and prepare foods with less salt. | |
| 10 | | | | | If you drink alcoholic beverages, do so in moderation. | |

*(continues)*

**TABLE 3.2**  (continued)

| | 2005 | 2010 | 2015 |
|---|---|---|---|
| 1 | Consume a variety of foods within and among the basic food groups while staying within energy needs | Maintain calorie balance over time to achieve and sustain a healthy weight | Follow a healthy eating pattern across the life span |
| 2 | Control calorie intake to manage body weight | Focus on consuming nutrient-dense foods and beverages | Focus on variety, nutrient density, and amount |
| 3 | Be physically active every day | | Limit calories from added sugars and saturated fat and reduce sodium intake |
| 4 | Increase daily intake of fruits and vegetables, whole grains, and nonfat or low-fat milk and milk products | | Shift to healthier food and beverage choices |
| 5 | Choose fats wisely for good health | | Support healthy eating patterns for all |
| 6 | Choose carbohydrates wisely for good health | | |
| 7 | Choose and prepare foods with little salt | | |
| 8 | If you drink alcohol, do so in moderation | | |
| 9 | Keep food safe to eat | | |

Data from US Department of Agriculture (USDA), US Department of Health and Human Services (HHS), Dietary Guidelines for Americans (HHS), Dietary Guidelines for Americans 1980–2015. Retrieved from: https://health.gov/dietaryguidelines.
USDA, HHS. *Nutrition and Your Health: Dietary Guidelines for Americans.* Washington, DC: US Government Printing Office; 1980.
USDA, HHS. *Nutrition and Your Health: Dietary Guidelines for Americans 2nd ed.* Washington, DC: U. S. Government Printing Office, 1985.
USDA, HHS. *Dietary Guidelines for Americans 3rd ed.* Washington, DC: US Government Printing Office; 1990.
USDA, HHS. *Dietary Guidelines for Americans 4th ed.* Washington, DC: US Government Printing Office; 1995.
USDA, HHS. *Dietary Guidelines for Americans 5th ed.* Washington, DC: US Government Printing Office; 2000.
USDA, HHS. *Dietary Guidelines for Americans 6th ed.* Washington, DC: US Government Printing Office; 2005.
USDA, HHS. *Dietary Guidelines for Americans, 2010* 7th ed. Washington, DC: US Government Printing Office; 2010.
USDA, HHS. *2015–2020 Dietary Guidelines For Americans 8th ed.* Washington, DC: US Government Printing Office; 2015.

## History of the Dietary Reference Intakes

The **Dietary Reference Intakes (DRIs)** are the reference values used to guide nutrient assessment and planning in the United States and Canada. The DRIs replace the Recommended Dietary Allowances that were issued periodically from 1941 to 1989 by the National Academy of Sciences and the Recommended Nutrient Intakes (RNIs) published by the Canadian government. The Dietary Reference Intakes are a set of reference values for specific nutrients established in 1994; each DRI category has a special use. Since the RDAs were originally established, there has been significant growth in the research basis relevant to the defining and understanding of nutrient requirements and food constituents and the relationship to various aspects of health. There was a need for developing DRIs for diet planning, nutrition assessment, food labeling, and nutrition policy development.[2] The historical timeline of the establishment of DRIs is shown in TABLE 3.3. From 1997 to 2004, the first DRI reports were based on the work of nutrient expert committees to define and set the DRI values, set chronic disease endpoints, review available data on requirements for children, and assess the health benefits of nonessential substances in foods.[3] Many applications such as the *Dietary Guidelines for Americans* and other food-guidance programs are based on the DRI nutrient values necessitating current and accurate evidence for their ongoing utility and application.

## Historical Timeline of USDA Food Guides

As early as 1916 and into the 1930s, *Food for Young Children* and *How to Select Food* established guidance for Americans based on food groups and household measures and focused on "protective foods."

In the 1940s, *A Guide to Good Eating (Basic Seven)* highlighted the foundation diet for nutrient adequacy. It included the daily number of servings

| **TABLE 3.3** Historical timeline: Dietary reference intakes | |
| --- | --- |
| **1941** | Recommended Dietary Allowances (RDAs) are published by the National Academy of Medicine. They serve as the primary components for nutrition policy in the United States, with the Dietary Standards/Recommended Nutrient Intakes (RNIs) serving that role in Canada. <br> As nutrition science continues to advance in the coming years, the RDIs and RDAs continually change to reflect the progressive increase in knowledge and transition in consumer eating behaviors. |
| **1990s** | Scientific knowledge of the link between diet, health, and chronic disease increases. Additional advancements made in technology allow for measurement of small changes in individual adaptations to several nutrients. <br> Eating behaviors shift to include increased consumption of nutrients in their pure form as well as fortified and enriched products. The risk for excess nutrient intake warrants investigation of possible effects. |
| **1994** | The Food and Nutrition Board of the National Academies' Institute of Medicine is supported by the American and Canadian governments in their quest to develop a new, broader set of dietary reference values. This become the Dietary Reference Intakes (DRIs). |
| **1997–2005** | The *Dietary Reference Intakes* report is published. <br> RDAs and RNIs have been replaced with four values of categories aimed at helping individuals optimize health, prevent disease, and avoid overconsumption of any nutrients. |
| **2005–Present** | The Food and Nutrition Board and Health Canada jointly release *Dietary Reference Intakes: The Essential Guide to Nutrient Requirements*. <br> Rooted in the key concepts and primary recommendations introduced by the DRI series, this resource provides a practical, hands-on reference to facilitate in the education of individuals, groups, and students by health care professionals. |

Data from Institute of Medicine of the National Academies (2006). *Dietary Reference Intakes: The Essential Guide to Nutrient Requirements*. Otten, J. J., Hellwig, J. P., Meyers, L. D. Pages 1, 5. https://www.nap.edu/catalog/11537/dietary-reference-intakes-the-essential-guide-to-nutrient-requirements. Accessed July 27, 2016.

needed from each of seven food groups, but it lacked serving sizes and was considered too complex. *Food for Fitness, A Daily Food Guide (Basic Four)* from 1956 to the 1970s continued with the foundation diet approach and gave goals for nutrient adequacy, with specified amounts from four food groups. It did not provide guidance on appropriate amounts of fat, sugar, and calories. The *Hassle-Free Daily Food Guide* was developed in 1979 after the 1977 dietary goals for the United States were released. They were again based on the basic four but included an additional fifth group to impress the need for Americans to moderate their intake of fat, sweets, and alcohol. In 1984, the *Food Wheel: A Pattern for Daily Food Choices* was created to give a total diet approach, including goals for both nutrient adequacy and moderation. Five food groups formed the basis for

the Food Guide Pyramid, with daily amounts of food specified at three calorie levels. It was originally illustrated as a food wheel for an American Red Cross nutrition course. The Food Guide Pyramid, which was developed in 1992, again provided a graphic illustration of the total diet approach, with goals for both nutrient adequacy and moderation. It was developed using consumer research for the purpose of bringing awareness about the new food patterns. The visual focused on variety, moderation, and proportion by depicting images of added fats and sugars and a range for daily amounts of food for three calorie levels. The Food Guide Pyramid is shown in **FIGURE 3.1**.

In 2005, the MyPyramid food guidance system was introduced again with an update to the Food Guide Pyramid food patterns for the *2005*

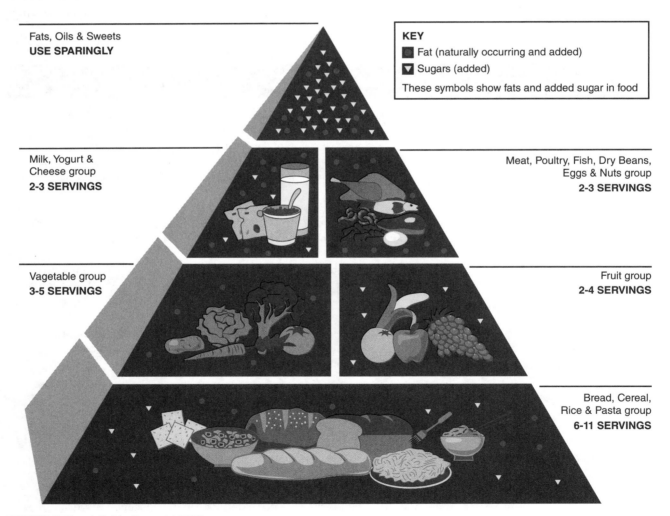

**FIGURE 3.1** Food Guide Pyramid 1992

*Dietary Guidelines for Americans,* and included daily amounts of food at 12 calorie levels. The information remained in a pyramid shape but with simplified illustrations and a band added for oils and physical activity. Further details are made available on MyPyramid.gov. Concepts represented include variety, moderation, and proportion. The MyPyramid visual is represented in **FIGURE 3.2**.

MyPlate was introduced in 2011 along with an update of the USDA food patterns for the *2010 Dietary Guidelines.* The shape was changed, with icons serving as reminders for healthy eating but without any specific messages provided. The plate visual is meant to be a familiar mealtime symbol for consumers and links

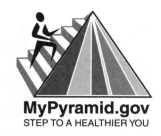

**FIGURE 3.2** MyPyramid food-guidance system

Reproduced from U.S. Department of Agriculture, U.S. Department of Health and Human Services (1995). MyPyramid. https://www.cnpp.usda.gov/sites/default/files/archived_projects/MyPyramid.psd.

to food.[4] A historical review of USDA food guides is summarized in **TABLE 3.4**. The MyPlate graphic can be seen in **FIGURE 3.3**.

| **TABLE 3.4** Historical timeline: Summary of USDA food guides | |
|---|---|
| **1916–1930s** | *Food for Young Children* and *How to Select Food* establish guidance based on food groups and household measures. They are focused on "protective foods." |
| **1940s** | *A Guide to Good Eating (Basic Seven)* highlights the foundation diet for nutrient adequacy. It included the daily number of servings needed from each of seven food groups, but it lacked serving sizes and was considered too complex. |
| **1956–1970s** | *Food for Fitness, A Daily Food Guide (Basic Four)* continues with the foundation diet approach and gives goals for nutrient adequacy with specified amounts from four food groups. It did not provide guidance on appropriate amounts of fat, sugar, and calories. |
| **1979** | *Hassle-Free Daily Food Guide* was developed after the 1977 Dietary Goals for the United States were released. They were again based on the basic four but included an additional fifth group to impress the need to moderate intake of fats, sweets, and alcohol. |
| **1984** | *Food Wheel: A Pattern for Daily Food Choices* gives a total diet approach, including goals for both nutrient adequacy and moderation. Five food groups and amounts formed the basis for the Food Guide Pyramid, with daily amounts of food specified at three calorie levels. It was originally illustrated as a food wheel for an American Red Cross nutrition course. |
| **1992** | Food Guide Pyramid again gives a total diet approach with goals included for both nutrient adequacy and moderation. It was developed using consumer research for the purpose of bringing awareness to the new USDA Food Patterns. The visual focused on variety, moderation, and proportion, depicting images of added fats and sugars and a range for daily amounts of food for three calorie levels. |
| **2005** | MyPyramid food-guidance system is introduced again with an update of the Food Guide Pyramid Food Patterns for the *2005 Dietary Guidelines for Americans,* which includes daily amounts of food at 12 calorie levels. Information is again presented in a "pyramid" shape but with simplified illustration and a band added for oils and physical activity. Further details are made available on MyPyramid.gov. Concepts represented include variety, moderation, and proportion. |
| **2011** | MyPlate is introduced along with an update of the USDA Food Patterns for the *2010 Dietary Guidelines for Americans.* The shape is changed, with icons serving as reminders for healthy eating, not providing specific messages. The plate visual is meant to be a familiar mealtime symbol for consumers and links to food. |

Modified from U.S. Department of Agriculture. A Brief History of USDA Food Guides. USDA Choose MyPlate. https://www.choosemyplate.gov/content/brief-history-usda-food-guides. Updated January 25, 2017. Accessed September 28, 2016.

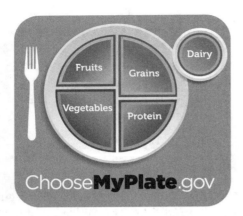

**FIGURE 3.3**  Choose MyPlate

Reproduced from United States Department of Agriculture. Choose MyPlate. choosemyplate.gov. https://choosemyplate-prod
.azureedge.net/sites/default/files/printablematerials/myplate_green.jpg

> **Recap**    The progression of dietary standards since the first food guides were established in 1916 have led to a current nutritional guidance landscape consisting of *Dietary Guidelines* that are updated and issued every five years. Current nutrient guidance includes four nutrient standard values known as the Dietary Reference Intakes and the MyPlate food guide, which was established to show healthy eating choices.

## ▶ Dietary Reference Intake

> **Preview**    The Dietary Reference Intakes are a widely applicable and complete set of nutrient intake standards that have been set to guide the population's intake according to the most accurate scientific information available.

The DRIs are a nutrient-based reference values that have replaced the former Recommended Dietary Allowances in the United States and the RNIs in Canada. The DRIs encompass a more complete set of values that were developed in response to the increasingly widespread use of quantitative reference values as well as the development of more advanced approaches to dietary planning and assessment. Four nutrient-based values are included in the DRI: (1) the Estimated Average Requirement, the Recommended Dietary Allowance, Adequate Intake, and Tolerable Upper Intake Level (UL).

The DRIs represented a shift from the focus of the RDAs and RNIs to reduce the incidence of diseases of deficiency to help people optimize their health and prevent disease as well as avoid overconsuming any nutrient. There are other key ways in which the DRIs differ from the previous intake standards. Data on a nutrient's safety and role in health are considered in the formulation of a recommendation—specifically, the potential reduction in risk of chronic disease. Probability and risk are assessed in the process of determining the DRIs. Emphasis is on the distribution of nutrient requirements within a population rather than on just a single value. ULs of nutrient intake are established to addresses the risk of adverse effects. And components of food that are not natural but may introduce health risks or benefits are reviewed, and standards are established for those with available data.

The primary purposes served by these standards are to assess the intakes of individuals and population groups, as well as plan diets for individuals and groups. In addition, the DRIs are used in dietary-planning activities such as dietary guidance, institutional food planning, military food and nutrition planning, planning for food assistance programs, food labeling, food fortification, developing new or modified food products, and food safety assurance.[5]

## DRI Review and Update Process

The American and Canadian governments have both established federal DRI committees that collaborate to identify DRI needs and procure government sponsorship of DRI reviews and related activities. The DRIs have been developed under the sponsorship of the Institute of Medicine with financial support from the American and Canadian governments. The DRIs represent nutrient reference values that are fundamental to national nutrition policies and important to professionals working in nutrition and health.

Nutrients nominated for review must be submitted with a cover letter and literature search. The cover letter contains the rationale and description of why a review is warranted as well as how it would address a current public health concern. The literature search gives a description of the search strategy and lists new, relevant literature published since the last DRI review. The two government DRI committees prioritize nutrients for government-funded reviews and commission expert reviews to establish reference values. New reviews are established based on current public health concerns along with significant, new, and relevant data since the previous DRI review. The DRI committees also determine whether any methodological issues identified as possible impedances to a new review have been resolved. Procuring funds also plays a factor in the initiation of new reviews.

Significant, new, and relevant data are defined by the following criteria:

- *Significant*: The overall scientific quality of the evidence, the number of new studies, the consistency of the results, and whether the new study results expand the DRI-related information available to the original DRI expert panel. Randomized controlled trials of high scientific quality are of particular interest.

- *New*: Research that was unlikely to have been available to the previous DRI expert panel.
- *Relevant*: Study results are generalizable to the North American population and to DRI development.

The DRI committees consider input from both individuals and organizations within and outside the government when making future prioritization decisions. The committees established a nomination process to assist in planning for new DRI reviews of nutrition and related substances to be renewed from previous DRI reports. Nominations have been made for various nutrients including: arachidonic acid, choline, chromium, docosahexaenoic acid (DHA), eicosapentaenoic acid (EPA), fiber, magnesium, niacin, potassium, protein, saturated fat, sodium, stearic acid, vitamin $B_6$, vitamin E, and zinc. The DRI committee for each country is prompted to select its top three priority nutrients based on public health or public policy. Omega-3 fatty acids, sodium, magnesium, and vitamin E were selected for further consideration based on these submissions. Nutrient-assessment working groups were established with staff from the United States and Canada. Each group was to determine if any new science had been published since the last DRI review. Government agencies jointly prioritized the nutrients and came to the conclusion that a workshop on the potential use of chronic disease endpoints in setting DRI values was necessary before a proper nutrient DRI review would be conducted. A workshop commissioned by the federal government took place in March 2015 to address if and how chronic disease outcomes can be incorporated into setting DRI values. This is expected to be the foundation for an expert report on this facet of public health.[5]

The Panel on Micronutrients, Panel on the Definition of Dietary Fiber, Subcommittee on Upper Reference Levels of Nutrients (UL Subcommittee), Subcommittee on Interpretation and Uses of Dietary Reference Intakes (Uses Subcommittee), and the Standing Committee on the Scientific Evaluation of Dietary Reference Intakes (DRI committee) analyzed evidence on the risks and benefits of nutrients and other components to determine the appropriate reference levels. DRI values were determined primarily from scientific data from observational and experimental studies in peer-reviewed journals.[6]

## Estimated Average Requirement

The **Estimated Average Requirement (EAR)** is the average daily nutrient-intake level estimated to meet the requirements of half of the healthy individuals in a particular life stage or gender group. It represents an estimated median requirement. This means the EAR exceeds the needs of half of the group and is unable to meet the needs of the other half.[5] The main purposes of the EAR are to assess the adequacy of population intakes and to be used as the basis for calculating Recommended Dietary Allowances. It was not itself designed to be used as a goal for daily intake by individuals.[6] **TABLE 3.5** shows the EAR for all nutrients. EARs have not been established for vitamin D, vitamin K, pantothenic acid, biotin, choline, calcium, chromium, fluoride, manganese, and other nutrients not yet evaluated by the DRI committee.[5] For further detail on the EAR for macronutrients, see the section titled "Macronutrient Recommendations."

## Recommended Dietary Allowance and Adequate Intake

The **Recommended Dietary Allowance (RDA)** is the average daily dietary nutrient-intake level sufficient to meet the nutrient requirements of nearly all (approximately 98%) of healthy individuals in a particular life stage and gender group. The RDA therefore exceeds the requirements of almost all members of the group. The RDA serves as a guide for daily intake by individuals and it is not intended to be used to assess the intake of groups. Because it exceeds the requirements for almost all individuals, intake at RDA levels is unlikely to be inadequate.[5]

If an EAR cannot be set because of data limitations, no RDA will be established. For those nutrients with a statistically normal requirement distribution, the RDA is set by adding two standard deviations (SDs) to the EAR:

$$RDA = EAR + 2 \times SD$$

In the event an RDA cannot be determined, the **adequate intake (AI)** value is used to set the reference level. AI is a recommended average daily intake level based on observed or experimentally determined approximations or estimates of nutrient intake by a group of individuals who appear to be healthy and are assumed to be in adequate nutritional state. It is expected to at least meet the needs of most individuals in a specific life stage and gender group. For healthy breastfed infants, the AI is the mean intake. As for other life stages and gender groups, although AIs are assumed to cover the needs of all healthy individuals, the limited data available prevent definitive determination of what percentage it actually covers. The AI is ultimately not particularly useful in assessments.[5]

The RDAs for macronutrients can be found in **TABLE 3.6**; see "Macronutrient Recommendations" for more information on these RDAs. RDAs for micronutrients are presented in **TABLE 3.7**.

**TABLE 3.5** Estimated average requirement

| | Infants (Months) | Children (Years) | | | Males (Years) | | | | | Females (Years) | | | | | | Pregnancy (Years) | | | Lactation (Years) | | |
|---|---|---|---|---|---|---|---|---|---|---|---|---|---|---|---|---|---|---|---|---|---|
| | 7–12 | 1–3 | 4–8 | 9–13 | 14–18 | 19–30 | 31–50 | 50–70 | >70 | 9–13 | 14–18 | 19–30 | 31–50 | 50–70 | >70 | 14–18 | 19–30 | 31–50 | 14–18 | 19–30 | 31–50 |
| **Carbohydrate (g/d)** | | 100 | 100 | 100 | 100 | 100 | 100 | 100 | 100 | 100 | 100 | 100 | 100 | 100 | 100 | 135 | 135 | 135 | 160 | 160 | 160 |
| **Protein (g/kg/d)** | 1.0 | 0.87 | 0.76 | 0.76 | 0.73 | 0.66 | 0.66 | 0.66 | 0.66 | 0.76 | 0.71 | 0.66 | 0.66 | 0.66 | 0.66 | 0.88 | 0.88 | 0.88 | 1.05 | 1.05 | 1.05 |
| **Vitamin A (µg/d)** | | 210 | 275 | 445 | 630 | 625 | 625 | 625 | 625 | 420 | 485 | 500 | 500 | 500 | 500 | 530 | 550 | 550 | 885 | 900 | 900 |
| **Vitamin C (mg/d)** | | 13 | 22 | 39 | 63 | 75 | 75 | 75 | 75 | 39 | 56 | 60 | 60 | 60 | 60 | 66 | 70 | 70 | 96 | 100 | 100 |
| **Vitamin E (mg/d)** | | 5 | 6 | 9 | 12 | 12 | 12 | 12 | 12 | 9 | 12 | 12 | 12 | 12 | 12 | 12 | 12 | 12 | 16 | 16 | 16 |
| **Thiamin (mg/d)** | | 0.4 | 0.5 | 0.7 | 1.0 | 1.0 | 1.0 | 1.0 | 1.0 | 0.7 | 0.9 | 0.9 | 0.9 | 0.9 | 0.9 | 1.2 | 1.2 | 1.2 | 1.2 | 1.2 | 1.2 |
| **Riboflavin (mg/d)** | | 0.4 | 0.5 | 0.8 | 1.1 | 1.1 | 1.1 | 1.1 | 1.1 | 0.8 | 0.9 | 0.9 | 0.9 | 0.9 | 0.9 | 1.2 | 1.2 | 1.2 | 1.3 | 1.3 | 1.3 |
| **Niacin (mg/d)** | | 5 | 6 | 9 | 12 | 12 | 12 | 12 | 12 | 9 | 11 | 11 | 11 | 11 | 11 | 14 | 14 | 14 | 13 | 13 | 13 |
| **Vitamin B$_6$ (mg/d)** | | 0.4 | 0.5 | 0.8 | 1.1 | 1.1 | 1.1 | 1.4 | 1.4 | 0.8 | 1.0 | 1.1 | 1.1 | 1.3 | 1.3 | 1.6 | 1.6 | 1.6 | 1.7 | 1.7 | 1.7 |
| **Folate (µg/d)** | | 120 | 160 | 250 | 330 | 320 | 320 | 320 | 320 | 250 | 330 | 320 | 320 | 320 | 320 | 520 | 520 | 520 | 450 | 450 | 450 |
| **Vitamin B$_{12}$ (µg/d)** | | 0.7 | 1.0 | 1.5 | 2.0 | 2.0 | 2.0 | 2.0 | 2.0 | 1.5 | 2.0 | 2.0 | 2.0 | 2.0 | 2.0 | 2.2 | 2.2 | 2.2 | 2.4 | 2.4 | 2.4 |
| **Copper (µg/d)** | | 260 | 340 | 540 | 685 | 700 | 700 | 700 | 700 | 540 | 685 | 700 | 700 | 700 | 700 | 785 | 800 | 800 | 985 | 1000 | 1000 |
| **Iodine (µg/d)** | | 65 | 65 | 73 | 95 | 95 | 95 | 95 | 95 | 73 | 95 | 95 | 95 | 95 | 95 | 160 | 160 | 160 | 209 | 209 | 209 |
| **Iron (mg/d)** | 6.9 | 3.0 | 4.1 | 5.9 | 7.7 | 6 | 6 | 6 | 6 | 5.7 | 7.9 | 8.1 | 8.1 | 5 | 5 | 23 | 22 | 22 | 7 | 6.5 | 6.5 |
| **Magnesium (mg/d)** | | 65 | 110 | 200 | 340 | 330 | 350 | 350 | 350 | 200 | 300 | 255 | 265 | 265 | 265 | 335 | 290 | 300 | 300 | 255 | 265 |
| **Molybdenum (µg/d)** | | 13 | 17 | 26 | 33 | 34 | 34 | 34 | 34 | 26 | 33 | 34 | 34 | 34 | 34 | 40 | 40 | 40 | 35 | 36 | 36 |
| **Phosphorus (mg/d)** | | 380 | 405 | 1055 | 1055 | 580 | 580 | 580 | 580 | 1055 | 1055 | 580 | 580 | 580 | 580 | 1055 | 580 | 580 | 1055 | 580 | 580 |
| **Selenium (µg/d)** | | 17 | 23 | 35 | 45 | 45 | 45 | 45 | 45 | 35 | 45 | 45 | 45 | 45 | 45 | 49 | 49 | 49 | 59 | 59 | 59 |
| **Zinc (mg/d)** | 2.5 | 2.5 | 4.0 | 7.0 | 8.5 | 9.4 | 9.4 | 9.4 | 9.4 | 7.0 | 7.3 | 6.8 | 6.8 | 6.8 | 6.8 | 10.5 | 9.5 | 9.5 | 10.9 | 10.4 | 10.4 |

Adapted from Institute of Medicine of the National Academies (2006). *Dietary Reference Intakes: The Essential Guide to Nutrient Requirements.* Otten, J. J., Hellwig, J. P., Meyers, L. D. Pages 530–531. https://www.nap.edu/catalog/11537/dietary-reference-intakes-the-essential-guide-to-nutrient-requirements. Accessed July 27, 2016.

**TABLE 3.6** Recommended Dietary Allowances (RDAs) for macronutrients

| | Infant (Months) | | Children (Years) | | Males (Years) | | | | | | Females (Years) | | | | | |
|---|---|---|---|---|---|---|---|---|---|---|---|---|---|---|---|---|
| | 0–6 | 7–12 | 1–3 | 4–8 | 9–13 | 14–18 | 19–30 | 31–50 | 50–70 | >70 | 9–13 | 14–18 | 19–30 | 31–50 | 50–70 | >70 |
| Carbohydrate (g/d) | 60 | 95 | 130 | 130 | 130 | 130 | 130 | 130 | 130 | 130 | 130 | 130 | 130 | 130 | 130 | 130 |
| Fiber (g/d) | ND | ND | 19 | 25 | 31 | 38 | 38 | 38 | 30 | 30 | 26 | 26 | 25 | 25 | 21 | 21 |
| Fat (g/d) | 31 | 30 | ND | ND | ND | ND | ND | ND | ND | ND | ND | ND | ND | ND | ND | ND |
| Linoleic Acid (g/d) | 4.4 | 4.6 | 7 | 10 | 12 | 16 | 17 | 17 | 14 | 14 | 10 | 11 | 12 | 12 | 11 | 11 |
| α-Linoleic Acid (g/d) | 0.5 | 0.5 | 0.7 | 0.9 | 1.2 | 1.6 | 1.6 | 1.6 | 1.6 | 1.6 | 1/0 | 1.1 | 1.1 | 1.1 | 1.1 | 1.1 |
| Protein | 9.1 | 11.0 | 13 | 19 | 34 | 52 | 56 | 56 | 56 | 56 | 34 | 46 | 46 | 46 | 46 | 46 |

| | Pregnancy (Years) | | | Lactation (Years) | | |
|---|---|---|---|---|---|---|
| | ≤18 | 19–30 | 31–50 | ≤18 | 19–30 | 31–50 |
| Carbohydrate (g/d) | 175 | 175 | 175 | 210 | 210 | 210 |
| Fiber (g/d) | 28 | 28 | 28 | 29 | 29 | 29 |
| Fat (g/d) | ND | ND | ND | ND | ND | ND |
| Linoleic Acid (g/d) | 13 | 13 | 13 | 13 | 13 | 13 |
| α-Linoleic Acid (g/d) | 1.4 | 1.4 | 1.4 | 1.3 | 1.3 | 1.3 |
| Protein (g/d) | 71 | 71 | 71 | 71 | 71 | 71 |

AI
RDA

Adapted from Institute of Medicine of the National Academies (2002/2005). Dietary Reference Intakes for Energy, Carbohydrate, Fiber, Fat, Fatty Acids, Cholesterol, Protein, and Amino Acids (Macronutrients). Panel on Macronutrients, Panel on the Definition of Dietary Fiber, Subcommittee on Upper Reference Levels of Nutrients, Subcommittee on Interpretation and Uses of Dietary Reference Intakes, and the Standing Committee on the Scientific Evaluation of Dietary Reference Intakes. Page 1324. https://www.nap.edu/catalog/10490/dietary-reference-intakes-for-energy-carbohydrate-fiber-fat-fatty-acids-cholesterol-protein-and-amino-acids-macronutrients. Accessed July 27, 2016.

**TABLE 3.7** Recommended Dietary Allowances (RDAs) for micronutrients

| | Infant (Months) | | Children (Years) | | Males (Years) | | | | | | Females (Years) | | | | | | Pregnancy (Years) | | | Lactation (Years) | | |
|---|---|---|---|---|---|---|---|---|---|---|---|---|---|---|---|---|---|---|---|---|---|---|
| | 0–6 | 7–12 | 1–3 | 4–8 | 9–13 | 14–18 | 19–30 | 31–50 | 50–70 | >70 | 9–13 | 14–18 | 19–30 | 31–50 | 50–70 | >70 | ≤18 | 19–30 | 31–50 | ≤18 | 19–30 | 31–50 |
| Vitamin A (µg/d) | 400 | 500 | 300 | 400 | 600 | 900 | 900 | 900 | 900 | 900 | 600 | 700 | 700 | 700 | 700 | 700 | 750 | 770 | 770 | 1200 | 1300 | 1300 |
| Vitamin C (mg/d) | 40 | 50 | 15 | 25 | 45 | 75 | 90 | 90 | 90 | 90 | 45 | 65 | 75 | 75 | 75 | 75 | 80 | 85 | 85 | 115 | 120 | 120 |
| Vitamin D (µg/d) | 5 | 5 | 5 | 5 | 5 | 5 | 5 | 5 | 10 | 15 | 5 | 5 | 5 | 5 | 10 | 15 | 5 | 5 | 5 | 5 | 5 | 5 |
| Vitamin E (mg/d) | 4 | 5 | 6 | 7 | 11 | 15 | 15 | 15 | 15 | 15 | 11 | 15 | 15 | 15 | 15 | 15 | 15 | 15 | 15 | 19 | 19 | 19 |
| Vitamin K (µg/d) | 2.0 | 2.5 | 30 | 55 | 60 | 75 | 120 | 120 | 120 | 120 | 60 | 75 | 90 | 90 | 90 | 90 | 75 | 90 | 90 | 75 | 90 | 90 |
| Thiamin (mg/d) | 0.2 | 0.3 | 0.5 | 0.6 | 0.9 | 1.2 | 1.2 | 1.2 | 1.2 | 1.2 | 0.9 | 1.0 | 1.1 | 1.1 | 1.1 | 1.1 | 1.4 | 1.4 | 1.4 | 1.4 | 1.4 | 1.4 |
| Riboflavin (mg/d) | 0.3 | 0.4 | 0.5 | 0.6 | 0.9 | 1.3 | 1.3 | 1.3 | 1.3 | 1.3 | 0.9 | 1.0 | 1.1 | 1.1 | 1.1 | 1.1 | 1.4 | 1.4 | 1.4 | 1.6 | 1.6 | 1.6 |
| Niacin (mg/d) | 2 | 4 | 6 | 8 | 12 | 16 | 16 | 16 | 16 | 16 | 12 | 14 | 14 | 14 | 14 | 14 | 18 | 18 | 18 | 17 | 17 | 17 |
| Vitamin $B_6$ (mg/d) | 0.1 | 0.3 | 0.5 | 0.6 | 1.0 | 1.3 | 1.3 | 1.3 | 1.7 | 1.7 | 1.0 | 1.2 | 1.3 | 1.3 | 1.5 | 1.5 | 1.9 | 1.9 | 1.9 | 2.0 | 2.0 | 2.0 |
| Folate (µg/d) | 65 | 80 | 150 | 200 | 300 | 400 | 400 | 400 | 400 | 400 | 300 | 400 | 400 | 400 | 400 | 400 | 600 | 600 | 600 | 500 | 500 | 500 |
| Vitamin $B_{12}$ (µg/d) | 0.4 | 0.5 | 0.9 | 1.2 | 1.8 | 2.4 | 2.4 | 2.4 | 2.4 | 2.4 | 1.8 | 2.4 | 2.4 | 2.4 | 2.4 | 2.4 | 2.6 | 2.6 | 2.6 | 2.8 | 2.8 | 2.8 |
| Pantothenic Acid (mg/d) | 1.7 | 1.8 | 2 | 3 | 4 | 5 | 5 | 5 | 5 | 5 | 4 | 5 | 5 | 5 | 5 | 5 | 6 | 6 | 6 | 7 | 7 | 7 |
| Biotin (µg/d) | 5 | 6 | 8 | 12 | 20 | 25 | 30 | 30 | 30 | 30 | 20 | 25 | 30 | 30 | 30 | 30 | 30 | 30 | 30 | 35 | 35 | 35 |
| Choline (mg/d) | 125 | 150 | 200 | 250 | 375 | 550 | 550 | 550 | 550 | 550 | 375 | 400 | 425 | 425 | 425 | 425 | 450 | 450 | 450 | 550 | 550 | 550 |
| Calcium (mg/d) | 210 | 270 | 500 | 800 | 1300 | 1300 | 1000 | 1000 | 1200 | 1200 | 1300 | 1300 | 1000 | 1000 | 1200 | 1200 | 1300 | 1000 | 1000 | 1300 | 1000 | 1000 |
| Chromium (µg/d) | 0.2 | 5.5 | 11 | 15 | 25 | 35 | 35 | 35 | 30 | 30 | 21 | 24 | 25 | 25 | 20 | 20 | 29 | 30 | 30 | 44 | 45 | 45 |
| Copper (µg/d) | 200 | 220 | 340 | 440 | 700 | 890 | 900 | 900 | 900 | 900 | 700 | 890 | 900 | 900 | 900 | 900 | 1000 | 1000 | 1000 | 1300 | 1300 | 1300 |
| Fluoride (mg/d) | 0.01 | 0.5 | 0.7 | 1 | 2 | 3 | 4 | 4 | 4 | 4 | 2 | 3 | 3 | 3 | 3 | 3 | 3 | 3 | 3 | 3 | 3 | 3 |
| Iodine (µg/d) | 110 | 130 | 90 | 90 | 120 | 150 | 150 | 150 | 150 | 150 | 120 | 150 | 150 | 150 | 150 | 150 | 220 | 220 | 220 | 290 | 290 | 290 |
| Iron (mg/d) | 0.27 | 11 | 7 | 10 | 8 | 11 | 8 | 8 | 8 | 8 | 8 | 15 | 18 | 18 | 8 | 8 | 27 | 27 | 27 | 10 | 9 | 9 |
| Magnesium (mg/d) | 30 | 75 | 80 | 130 | 240 | 410 | 400 | 420 | 420 | 420 | 240 | 360 | 310 | 320 | 320 | 320 | 400 | 350 | 360 | 360 | 310 | 320 |
| Manganese (mg/d) | 0.0003 | 0.6 | 1.2 | 1.5 | 1.9 | 2.2 | 2.3 | 2.3 | 2.3 | 2.3 | 1.6 | 1.6 | 1.8 | 1.8 | 1.8 | 1.8 | 2.0 | 2.0 | 2.0 | 2.6 | 2.6 | 2.6 |
| Molybdenum (µg/d) | 2 | 3 | 17 | 22 | 34 | 43 | 45 | 45 | 45 | 45 | 34 | 43 | 45 | 45 | 45 | 45 | 50 | 50 | 50 | 50 | 50 | 50 |
| Phosphorus (mg/d) | 100 | 275 | 460 | 500 | 1250 | 1250 | 700 | 700 | 700 | 700 | 1250 | 1250 | 700 | 700 | 700 | 700 | 1250 | 700 | 700 | 1250 | 700 | 700 |
| Selenium (µg/d) | 12 | 20 | 20 | 30 | 40 | 55 | 55 | 55 | 55 | 55 | 40 | 55 | 55 | 55 | 55 | 55 | 60 | 60 | 60 | 70 | 70 | 70 |
| Zinc (mg/d) | 2 | 3 | 3 | 5 | 8 | 11 | 11 | 11 | 11 | 11 | 8 | 9 | 8 | 8 | 8 | 8 | 12 | 11 | 11 | 13 | 12 | 12 |
| Potassium (g/d) | 0.4 | 0.7 | 3.0 | 3.8 | 4.5 | 4.7 | 4.7 | 4.7 | 4.7 | 4.7 | 4.5 | 4.7 | 4.7 | 4.7 | 4.7 | 4.7 | 4.7 | 4.7 | 4.7 | 5.1 | 5.1 | 5.1 |
| Sodium (g/d) | 0.12 | 0.37 | 1.0 | 1.2 | 1.5 | 1.5 | 1.5 | 1.5 | 1.3 | 1.2 | 1.5 | 1.5 | 1.5 | 1.5 | 1.3 | 1.2 | 1.5 | 1.5 | 1.5 | 1.5 | 1.5 | 1.5 |
| Chloride (g/d) | 0.18 | 0.57 | 1.5 | 1.9 | 2.3 | 2.3 | 2.3 | 2.3 | 2.0 | 1.8 | 2.3 | 2.3 | 2.3 | 2.3 | 2.0 | 1.8 | 2.3 | 2.3 | 2.3 | 2.3 | 2.3 | 2.3 |

AI ▢    RDA ▢

Adapted from Institute of Medicine of the National Academies (2002/2005). Dietary Reference Intakes for Energy, Carbohydrate, Fiber, Fat, Fatty Acids, Cholesterol, Protein, and Amino Acids (Macronutrients). Panel on Micronutrients, Panel on the Definition of Dietary Fiber, Subcommittee on Upper Reference Levels of Nutrients, Subcommittee on Interpretation and Uses of Dietary Reference Intakes, and the Standing Committee on the Scientific Evaluation of Dietary Reference Intakes. Page 1320-1323. https://www.nap.edu/catalog/10490/dietary-reference-intakes-for-energy-carbohydrate-fiber-fat-fatty-acids-cholesterol-protein-and-amino-acids-macronutrients. Accessed July 27, 2016.

# Tolerable Upper Intake Level

The **tolerable upper intake level (UL)** is the highest average daily nutrient-intake level likely to pose no risk of adverse health effects for almost all individuals in a particular group. It represents the highest intake level that can be tolerated without the possibility of undesirable health effects and was established in response to the growing number of foods with nutrient fortification and increased amount of dietary supplementation usage. In groups, it is used to estimate the percentage of the population at risk for adverse effects from excessive nutrient intake. As intake increases above the UL, the risk increases for potential adverse events.

The tolerable upper level is derived using a risk-assessment model consisting of a systematic series of scientific considerations and judgments. The UL value represents the total daily intake of a nutrient from all available sources (food, water, supplements) if potential harmful effects have been identified.[5] **TABLE 3.8** shows the UL for micronutrients. Macronutrient standards were unable to be established because of insufficient data.

# Energy Requirements

The **Estimated Energy Requirement (EER)** is the average dietary energy intake predicted to maintain energy balance in a healthy adult of a defined age, gender, weight, height, and level of physical activity consistent with good health. For children and pregnant or lactating women, the EER includes energy needs required for the deposition of tissue or secretion of milk at rates consistent with good health.[5] Because the variability of measured energy intake between individuals is greater than that of energy expenditure, there is an impedance to measuring energy intake without accounting for intake behaviors. Therefore, energy requirement is more precisely estimated from energy expenditure than from energy intake.

## Components of Total Energy Expenditure

Energy is expended in the body in the form of Basal Energy Expenditure (Resting Energy Expenditure), Thermic Effect of Food, and Activity Thermogenesis (physical activity and activities of daily living). These three factors make up an individual's total daily energy expenditure. The percent contribution of each to total energy expenditure is depicted in **FIGURE 3.4**.

**Basal Energy Expenditure (BEE)** is the minimum amount of energy expended that is compatible with life. It typically represents 60% to 70% total energy

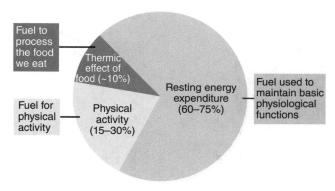

**FIGURE 3.4** Components of total energy expenditure

**TABLE 3.8** The UL for certain micronutrients

| | Infant (Months) | | Children (Years) | | | Males/Females (Years) | | | Pregnancy (Years) | | Lactation (Years) | |
|---|---|---|---|---|---|---|---|---|---|---|---|---|
| | 0–6 | 7–12 | 1–3 | 4–8 | 9–13 | 14–18 | 19–70 | >70 | 14–18 | 19–50 | 14–18 | 19–50 |
| **Vitamin A (µg/d)** | 600 | 600 | 600 | 900 | 1700 | 2800 | 3000 | 3000 | 2800 | 3000 | 2800 | 3000 |
| **Vitamin C (mg/d)** | ND | ND | 400 | 650 | 1200 | 1800 | 2000 | 2000 | 1800 | 2000 | 1800 | 2000 |
| **Vitamin D (µg/d)** | 25 | 25 | 50 | 50 | 50 | 50 | 50 | 50 | 50 | 50 | 50 | 50 |
| **Vitamin E (mg/d)** | ND | ND | 200 | 300 | 600 | 800 | 1000 | 1000 | 800 | 1000 | 800 | 1000 |
| **Vitamin K** | ND | ND | ND | ND | ND | ND | ND | ND | ND | ND | ND | ND |
| **Thiamin** | ND | ND | ND | ND | ND | ND | ND | ND | ND | ND | ND | ND |
| **Riboflavin** | ND | ND | ND | ND | ND | ND | ND | ND | ND | ND | ND | ND |
| **Niacin (mg/d)** | ND | ND | 10 | 15 | 20 | 30 | 35 | 35 | 30 | 35 | 30 | 35 |
| **Vitamin B$_6$ (mg/d)** | ND | ND | 30 | 40 | 60 | 80 | 100 | 100 | 80 | 100 | 80 | 100 |
| **Folate (µg/d)** | ND | ND | 300 | 400 | 600 | 800 | 1000 | 1000 | 800 | 1000 | 800 | 1000 |
| **Vitamin B$_{12}$** | ND | ND | ND | ND | ND | ND | ND | ND | ND | ND | ND | ND |
| **Pantothenic Acid** | ND | ND | ND | ND | ND | ND | ND | ND | ND | ND | ND | ND |
| **Biotin** | ND | ND | ND | ND | ND | ND | ND | ND | ND | ND | ND | ND |
| **Choline (g/d)** | ND | ND | 1.0 | 1.0 | 2.0 | 3.0 | 3.5 | 3.5 | 3.0 | 3.5 | 3.0 | 3.5 |
| **Carotenoids** | ND | ND | ND | ND | ND | ND | ND | ND | ND | ND | ND | ND |
| **Arsenic** | ND | ND | ND | ND | ND | ND | ND | ND | ND | ND | ND | ND |
| **Boron (mg/d)** | ND | ND | 3 | 6 | 11 | 17 | 20 | 20 | 17 | 20 | 17 | 20 |
| **Calcium (g/d)** | ND | ND | 2.5 | 2.5 | 2.5 | 2.5 | 2.5 | 2.5 | 2.5 | 2.5 | 2.5 | 2.5 |
| **Chromium** | ND | ND | ND | ND | ND | ND | ND | ND | ND | ND | ND | ND |

**TABLE 3.8** *(continued)*

| | Infant (Months) | | Children (Years) | | | Males/Females (Years) | | | Pregnancy (Years) | | Lactation (Years) | |
|---|---|---|---|---|---|---|---|---|---|---|---|---|
| | 0–6 | 7–12 | 1–3 | 4–8 | 9–13 | 14–18 | 19–70 | >70 | 14–18 | 19–50 | 14–18 | 19–50 |
| **Copper (µg/d)** | ND | ND | 1000 | 3000 | 5000 | 8000 | 10,000 | 10,000 | 8000 | 10,000 | 8000 | 10,000 |
| **Fluoride (mg/d)** | 0.7 | 0.9 | 1.3 | 2.2 | 10 | 10 | 10 | 10 | 10 | 10 | 10 | 10 |
| **Iodine (µg/d)** | ND | ND | 200 | 300 | 600 | 900 | 1100 | 1100 | 900 | 1100 | 900 | 1100 |
| **Iron (mg/d)** | 40 | 40 | 40 | 40 | 40 | 45 | 45 | 45 | 45 | 45 | 45 | 45 |
| **Magnesium (mg/d)** | ND | ND | 65 | 110 | 350 | 350 | 350 | 350 | 350 | 350 | 350 | 350 |
| **Manganese (mg/d)** | ND | ND | 2 | 3 | 6 | 9 | 11 | 11 | 9 | 11 | 9 | 11 |
| **Molybdenum (µg/d)** | ND | ND | 300 | 600 | 1100 | 1700 | 2000 | 2000 | 1700 | 2000 | 1700 | 2000 |
| **Nickel (mg/d)** | ND | ND | 0.2 | 0.3 | 0.6 | 1.0 | 1.0 | 1.0 | 1.0 | 1.0 | 1.0 | 1.0 |
| **Phosphorus (g/d)** | ND | ND | 3.0 | 3.0 | 4.0 | 4.0 | 4.0 | 3.0 | 3.5 | 3.5 | 4.0 | 4.0 |
| **Potassium** | ND | ND | ND | ND | ND | ND | ND | ND | ND | ND | ND | ND |
| **Selenium (µg/d)** | 45 | 60 | 90 | 150 | 280 | 400 | 400 | 400 | 400 | 400 | 400 | 400 |
| **Silicon** | ND | ND | ND | ND | ND | ND | ND | ND | ND | ND | ND | ND |
| **Sulfate** | ND | ND | ND | ND | ND | ND | ND | ND | ND | ND | ND | ND |
| **Vanadium (mg/d)** | ND | ND | ND | ND | ND | ND | 1.8 | 1.8 | ND | ND | ND | ND |
| **Zinc (mg/d)** | 4 | 5 | 7 | 12 | 23 | 34 | 40 | 40 | 34 | 40 | 34 | 40 |
| **Sodium (g/d)** | ND | ND | 1.5 | 1.9 | 2.2 | 2.3 | 2.3 | 2.3 | 2.3 | 2.3 | 2.3 | 2.3 |
| **Chloride (g/d)** | ND | ND | 2.3 | 2.9 | 3.4 | 3.6 | 3.6 | 3.6 | 3.6 | 3.6 | 3.6 | 3.6 |

ND: Not determinable as limited data exists on adverse effects in regards to inability to handle excess amounts for this age group

Adapted from Institute of Medicine of the National Academies (2002/2005), Dietary Reference Intakes for Energy, Carbohydrate, Fiber, Fat, Fatty Acids, Cholesterol, Protein, and Amino Acids (Macronutrients), Panel on Micronutrients, Panel on the Definition of Dietary Fiber, Subcommittee on Upper Reference Levels of Nutrients, Subcommittee on Interpretation and Uses of Dietary Reference Intakes, and the Standing Committee on the Scientific Evaluation of Dietary Reference Intakes. Page 1320–1323. https://www.nap.edu/catalog/10490/dietary-reference-intakes-for-energy-carbohydrate-fiber-fat-fatty-acids-cholesterol-protein-and-amino-acids-macronutrients. Accessed July 27, 2016.

expenditure. **Resting Energy Expenditure (REE)** is the amount of energy expended by a resting individual in a thermoneutral environment without the effects of meal consumption, physical activity, or other physiological or mental stress. The value can be as much as 10% to 20% higher than the true basal metabolic rate, which is measured in the morning after 12–18 hours of rest. Interindividual variations exist between individuals with regard to REE, depending on age, gender, height, and weight within the range of 7.5% to 17.9%. Energy expended at rest is generated from many sources including maintaining the biochemical and structural integrity of the body and the cost of cellular work, ion pumps, synthesis and degradation of cell constituents, and biochemical cycles.

To measure energy adequately, several conditions must be met. Subjects should be awake but at rest, lying in a supine position in a physically comfortable test site (thermoneutral) that is quiet and not brightly lit. The subjects should be fasting and not consume food, energy-containing beverages, or drugs that artificially increase energy expenditure (such as ethanol or nicotine) for at least four hours before the energy assessment. The assessment should be performed at least two hours after meal consumption, with the exemption of those patients who are receiving continuous nutritional support. Subjects should be given adequate time to recover from activities of daily living such as getting dressed and traveling to the testing location; at least 20 minutes is recommended. Individuals should not engage in physical activity in the previous four to six hours before testing. Medically strenuous activities such as a wound dressing change, chest physiotherapy, or physical therapy should be avoided for 60 minutes prior to measuring energy expenditure. The procedure should not be performed within 24 hours of a hemodialysis session. During the test, subjects should lay motionless and refrain from talking or engaging in any other stimulating distractions. The measurement period should last until a steady state is achieved—which is characterized by five consecutive minute measurements of $VO_2$ within 10% of each other and corresponding respiratory quotients within 5% of each other). The measurement period should be no longer than 20 to 30 minutes.

The **thermic effect of food (TEF)** is the increase in energy expenditure immediately following meal digestion. It is also referred to as *diet-induced thermogenesis* and *specific dynamic action*. The primary determinants of TEF are the nutrient composition and energy content of the food consumed. Protein has been found to elicit the greatest increase in metabolic rate, followed by a mixed-nutrient meal, glucose, and then fat. The magnitude of the TEF is found to closely reflect the energy load contained in the test meal. The components of TEF include obligatory and facultative thermogenesis. Obligatory thermogenesis is the energy expended absorbing, processing, and storing nutrients. Facultative thermogenesis involves sympathetic nervous system activation and is otherwise not as well understood.

The **thermic effect of activity (TEA)** is the energy expended above the resting level both during and after physical activity. Activity thermogenesis is divided into exercise and nonexercise activity thermogenesis. Exercise activity thermogenesis contributes approximately 15% to 30% of total daily energy expenditure for those who exercise regularly. The intensity and duration of activity determine the contribution of exercise to total energy expenditure. The rate of energy expenditure for the duration of activity may be from 1.5 × resting metabolic rate (RMR) (such as with clerical work) to 15 × RMR (such as with running). Research has found that exercise has no effect on RMR unless it is prolonged or severe. The contribution of exercise to energy balance is demonstrated in several ways. First, thermogenesis is retained by maintaining fat-free mass. Second, energy expenditure is increased by exercise. Finally, excess postexercise oxygen consumption may increase energy expenditure in relation to the duration and intensity of activity.

Nonexercise activity thermogenesis (NEAT) is the energy expenditure of spontaneous physical activity, including the combined energy costs of the physical activities of daily living, fidgeting, spontaneous muscle contraction, and maintaining posture when not recumbent. NEAT accounts for the remainder of the total daily energy expenditure and explains the variation in activity thermogenesis in adults of similar size. Its major determinants include occupation and leisure time, which varies from 15% to more than 50% of total daily energy expenditures. Occupational NEAT can vary from 700 to 2,300 kcal/day, depending on strenuous level of work activities. Variation in leisure activities may reach 1,000 kcal/day. Altering energy balance in individuals is possible by changing the factor of NEAT to become more active. NEAT may also be influenced by biological, genetic, and environmental changes attributed to the human population over the last century and a half, primarily as a decrease.[7]

## Methods of Measuring Energy Expenditure

The methods of measuring energy expenditure are summarized in **FIGURE 3.5** and include calorimetric and noncalorimetric techniques. Calorimetric techniques include direct and indirect calorimetry.

| Approach and type of calorimeter | Indirect calorimeter | | | | | Direct calorimeter | Non-calorimetric methods |
|---|---|---|---|---|---|---|---|
| | Room open-air circuit | Hood/canopy open-circuit | Open-circuit expiratory collection | Doubly labelled water | Total collection Douglas bag | | |
| Basal metabolic rate and resting metabolic rate | Y | Y | Y* | N | Y | Y | N |
| Thermic effect of food | Y | Y | Y* | N | Y* | Y | N |
| Activity related energy expenditure | Y | Y | Y | N | Y | Y | N |
| Total daily energy expenditure | Y# | N | Y* | Y | N | Y# | E |

Y= "yes" a technique can be used to perform the measurement
N= 'No' it cannot be used to perform the measurement
E= estimated
* indicates that precision maybe unreliable
# indicates a confined subject

**FIGURE 3.5** Techniques used to measure energy expenditure in humans

Data from Academy of Nutrition and Dietetics. Measurement of Energy Expenditure. Nutrition Care Manual. https://www.nutritioncaremanual.org/topic.cfm?ncm_category_id=11&lv1=144882&lv2=144900&ncm_toc_id=144900&ncm_heading=&. Accessed July 27, 2016.

Noncalorimetric techniques include the isotope-dilution method (doubly labeled water) DLW, kinematics recordings (mechanical activity meters), human observations and records (time and motion studies), and physiologic measurements (heart rate, energy intake, and electromyography).[8]

## Direct Calorimetry

Direct measurement of metabolic rate is performed by assessing heat loss. The sum of convective, conductive, and evaporative heat transfer and radiant heat exchange are measured, with the total heat loss equaling the rate of energy use when body temperature is constant. This method is based purely on conservation of energy and does not involve any assumptions made about the physiology of energy metabolism. The subject is placed in a thermically isolated chamber, and the heat dissipated by the individual is collected and measured.

Several limitations exist that prevent direct calorimetry from being widely used. These include the confining nature of the testing environment, the inability to use calorimetry in measuring short-term effects of thermogenic stimuli (i.e., food) on heat exchange because of the body's large heat-storage capacity, and the costly nature of the instruments required.[9]

## Indirect Calorimetry

Indirect calorimetry involves estimating the metabolic rate from measurements of oxygen consumption and carbon dioxide production using a set of assumptions and equations. It is assumed that all oxygen consumed ($VO_2$) is used to oxidize degradable fuels and that all carbon dioxide expended ($VCO_2$) is recovered. Eventually, all energy is converted into heat, so direct and indirect calorimetry provide identical rates of energy expenditure within steady-state conditions. The percentage of error for indirect calorimetry (respiratory gas exchange) is 2% compared to direct calorimetry.[9]

Energy expenditure from $VO_2$ and $VCO_2$ is calculated using the Weir equation:

$$\text{Energy expenditure} = (3.94 \times VO_2) + (1.11 \times VCO_2)$$

Use of indirect calorimetry is indicated under the following conditions:

- Clinical disorders that significantly alter REE
- Failure of an individual to respond to adequate nutrition support
- Individualizing nutrition support in an intensive care unit
- Individualizing nutrition program for healthy or ambulatory individuals receiving nutrition therapy for a disease such as diabetes

Estimating an individual's energy needs involves three steps. First, determine whether REE should be estimated or measured. Second, use critical thinking skills to evaluate REE. Third, determine when REE should be reevaluated.

## Doubly Labeled Water

The DLW method of measuring energy expenditure assumes that the oxygen in respiratory $CO_2$ is in isotopic-exchange equilibrium with the oxygen contained in body water. Two isotopes of water are given, and their disappearance rates from the body (through urine and other bodily fluids) are monitored for one to three half-lives for isotope disappearance.[9]

## Estimating Calorie Needs

The total number of calories a person needs daily varies by age, gender, weight, and level of physical activity. A need or desire to lose, maintain, or gain weight, among other factors, affects the total number of calories that should be consumed.[10,11] The estimated amounts of calories needed to maintain caloric balances for different age and gender groups across three levels of physical activity are provided in **TABLE 3.9**.

The estimates in Table 3.9 are based on the EER equations, using reference average heights and healthy weights for the different age and gender groups. Reference height and weight vary for children and adolescents. The adult reference height and weights are 5′10″ and 154 pounds for men and 5′4″ and 126 pounds for women. Estimates range from 1,600–2,400 calories per day for adult women and 2,000–3,000 calories per day for adult men. The lower end is of each range is designated for those individuals who are more sedentary, and the higher end is for those who are more active. Calorie needs decrease for adults with age, as basal metabolic rate steadily declines, therefore necessitating a lower energy intake.

Estimates range from 1,000–2,000 calories per day for young children and 1,400–3,200 calories per day for older children and adolescents. In general, boys have higher calorie needs than girls. Approximations of calorie needs can be determined on a more individual basis at www.supertracker.usda.gov.[10,11]

## Predictive Equations

Energy requirements are traditionally estimated based on multiples of REE, which are known as *physical activity levels* (PALs). More recently, the regression approach, which is based on data of total energy expenditure from DLW studies, has formed the basis for the Dietary Reference Intakes for energy.[5,12] The Dietary Reference Intake EERs can be found in **Table 3.10**. Several predictive equations have been developed for estimating resting energy expenditure with applications for multiple settings. RDNs working with the healthcare team complete a full nutrition assessment that includes an estimate of energy expenditure using the appropriate predictive formula based on clinical and individual considerations. The equation most commonly used in the clinical setting is Mifflin St.-Jeor because it is the most accurate.

**Recap** Energy requirements vary based on age, gender, and level of physical activity, among other factors. Individual requirements are typically calculated using energy expenditure based on a series of estimates and reference equations.

# ▶ Macronutrient Recommendations

**Preview** The recommendations for carbohydrate, protein, and fat are each determined by different means and are dependent on availability and their metabolic functions within the body.

## Estimated Average Requirement for Macronutrients

The EAR for carbohydrates is established based on the average amount of glucose used by the brain. No EAR is set for fat because the percent of energy derived from fat varies, yet it still can meet daily energy needs. Furthermore, no EAR exists for saturated fatty acids, monounsaturated fatty acids, or cholesterol because they are produced by the body and pose no benefit in the prevention of chronic disease.[13] For energy, an EER is provided.[5] (See the previous section titled "Energy Requirements.") The EAR and other DRIs for macronutrients are summarized in **TABLE 3.11**.

## Recommended Dietary Allowance (RDA) for Macronutrients

The RDA for carbohydrates is 130 grams per day for adults and children. No RDA exists for fats, including saturated fatty acids, monounsaturated fatty acids, or cholesterol, because they are produced by the body and pose no benefit in preventing chronic disease. The RDA for protein is 0.8 grams per kilogram body weight per day for both men and women. It is established based on meta-analysis of nitrogen balance studies.[6] The RDAs for macronutrients can be found in Table 3.6.

Research has shown that consuming an imbalance of macronutrients may increase the risk of chronic disease. In response to this, the **acceptable macronutrient distribution range (AMDR)** for

| TABLE 3.9 Estimated calorie needs per day by age, sex, and physical activity level | | | | | | |
|---|---|---|---|---|---|---|
| | **Males** | | | **Females** | | |
| **Age** | **Sedentary** | **Moderately Active** | **Active** | **Sedentary** | **Moderately Active** | **Active** |
| 2 | 1000 | 1000 | 1000 | 1000 | 1000 | 1000 |
| 3 | 1000 | 1400 | 1400 | 1000 | 1200 | 1400 |
| 4 | 1200 | 1400 | 1600 | 1200 | 1400 | 1400 |
| 5 | 1200 | 1400 | 1600 | 1200 | 1400 | 1600 |
| 6 | 1400 | 1600 | 1800 | 1200 | 1400 | 1600 |
| 7 | 1400 | 1600 | 1800 | 1200 | 1600 | 1800 |
| 8 | 1400 | 1600 | 2000 | 1400 | 1600 | 1800 |
| 9 | 1600 | 1800 | 2000 | 1400 | 1600 | 1800 |
| 10 | 1600 | 1800 | 2200 | 1400 | 1800 | 2000 |
| 11 | 1800 | 2000 | 2200 | 1600 | 1800 | 2000 |
| 12 | 1800 | 2200 | 2400 | 1600 | 2000 | 2200 |
| 13 | 2000 | 2200 | 2600 | 1600 | 2000 | 2200 |
| 14 | 2000 | 2400 | 2800 | 1800 | 2000 | 2400 |
| 15 | 2200 | 2600 | 3000 | 1800 | 2000 | 2400 |
| 16–18 | 2400 | 2800 | 3200 | 1800 | 2000 | 2400 |
| 19–20 | 2600 | 2800 | 3000 | 2000 | 2200 | 2400 |
| 21–25 | 2400 | 2800 | 3000 | 2000 | 2200 | 2400 |
| 26–30 | 2400 | 2600 | 3000 | 1800 | 2000 | 2400 |
| 31–35 | 2400 | 2600 | 3000 | 1800 | 2000 | 2200 |
| 36–40 | 2400 | 2600 | 2800 | 1800 | 2000 | 2200 |
| 41–45 | 2200 | 2600 | 2800 | 1800 | 2000 | 2200 |
| 46–50 | 2200 | 2400 | 2800 | 1800 | 2000 | 2200 |
| 51–55 | 2200 | 2400 | 2800 | 1600 | 1800 | 2200 |
| 56–60 | 2200 | 2400 | 2600 | 1600 | 1800 | 2200 |
| 61–65 | 2000 | 2400 | 2600 | 1600 | 1800 | 2000 |
| 66–70 | 2000 | 2200 | 2600 | 1600 | 1800 | 2000 |
| 71–75 | 2000 | 2200 | 2600 | 1600 | 1800 | 2000 |
| 76+ | 2000 | 2200 | 2400 | 1600 | 1800 | 2000 |

*Sedentary*: a lifestyle that includes only the physical activity of independent living.

*Moderately active*: a lifestyle that includes physical activity equivalent to walking 1.5–3 miles per day at 3–4 miles per hour in addition to activities of independent living.

*Active*: a lifestyle that includes physical activity equivalent to walking more than 3 miles per day at 3–4 miles per hour in addition to the activities of independent living.

Estimates for females do not include women who are pregnant or breastfeeding.

Reproduced from U.S. Department of Health and Human Services and U.S. Department of Agriculture (2015). 2015-2020 *Dietary Guidelines For Americans* 8th Edition. Appendix 2. Estimated Calorie Needs per Day, by Age, Sex and Physical Activity Level. Pages 77-78/ https://health.gov/dietaryguidelines/2015/guidelines/appendix-2/. Accessed July 27, 2016.

**TABLE 3.10A** Equations used to predict EER: Dietary Reference Intake Estimated Energy Requirements

| Infants and Children | **Months** | EER = Total Energy Expenditure + Energy Deposition |
|---|---|---|
| | 0–3 | EER = (89 x weight – 100) + 175 |
| | 4–6 | EER = (89 x weight – 100) + 56 |
| | 7–12 | EER = (89 x weight – 100) + 22 |
| | 13–35 | EER = (89 x weight – 100) + 20 |
| Children and Adolescents | **Years** | EER = Total Energy Expenditure + Energy Deposition |
| | Boys 3–8 | EER = 88.5 – (61.9 x age) + PA x [(26.7 x weight) + (903 x height)] + 20 |
| | Boys 9–18 | EER = 88.5 – (61.9 x age) + PA x [(26.7 x weight) + (903 x height)] + 25 |
| | Girls 3–8 | EER = 135.3 – (30.8 x age) + PA x [(10.0 x weight) + (934 x height)] + 20 |
| | Girls 9–18 | EER = 135.3 – (30.8 x age) + PA x [(10.0 x weight) + (934 x height)] + 25 |
| Adults 19+ | **Gender** | EER = Total Energy Expenditure |
| | Men | EER = 662 – (9.53 x age) + PA x [(15.91 x weight) + (539.6 x height)] |
| | Women | EER = 354 – (6.91 x age) + PA x [(9.36 x weight) + (726 x height)] |
| Pregnancy | **Trimester** | EER = Nonpregnant EER + Pregnancy Energy Deposition |
| | First | EER = Nonpregnant EER + 0 |
| | Second | EER = Nonpregnant EER + 340 |
| | Third | EER = Nonpregnant EER + 452 |
| Lactation | **Months Postpartum** | EER = Nonpregnant EER + Milk Energy Output – Weight Loss |
| | 0–6 | EER = Nonpregnant EER + 500 – 170 |
| | 7–12 | EER = Nonpregnant EER + 400 – 0 |

**TABLE 3.10B** Equations used to predict EER: Physical Activity Coefficients for EER Equations

| | **Males (Years)** | | **Females (Years)** | | |
|---|---|---|---|---|---|
| | **3–18** | **19+** | **3–18** | **19+** | |
| Sedentary (PAL 1.0–1.39) | 1.00 | 1.00 | 1.00 | 1.00 | Typical ADL (activities of daily living) |
| Low Active (PAL 1.4–1.59) | 1.13 | 1.11 | 1.16 | 1.12 | Typical ADL + 30–60 minutes daily moderate activity (e.g., walking at 5–7 km/h) |
| Active (PAL 1.6–1.89) | 1.26 | 1.25 | 1.31 | 1.27 | Typical ADL + ≥ 60 minutes daily moderate activity |
| Very Active (PAL 1.9–2.5) | 1.42 | 1.48 | 1.56 | 1.45 | Typical ADL + ≥ 60 minutes daily moderate activity + 60 minutes vigorous activity or 120 minutes moderate activity |

**TABLE 3.10C** Equations used to predict EER: Predictive Equations for Estimating REE

| | | |
|---|---|---|
| Harris-Benedict | Men | RMR = 66.47 + (13.75 × weight) + (5 × height) − (6.76 × age) |
| | Women | RMR = 655.1 + (9.56 × weight) + (1.7 × height) − (4.7 × age) |
| Mifflin-St Jeor | Men | RMR = (9.99 × weight ) + (6.25 × height) − (4.92 × age) + 5 |
| | Women | RMR = (9.99 × weight) + (6.25 × height) − (4.92 × age) − 161 |
| Owen | Men | RMR = 879 + (10.2 × weight) |
| | Women | RMR = 795 + (7.18 × weight) |
| Ireton-Jones Energy Equation | Breathing | (s) = 629 − (11 × age) + (25 × weight) − (609 × O) |
| | Ventilator | (v) = 1925 − 10(A) + 5(W) + 281(S) + 292(T) + 851(B) |
| World Health Organization | Age: 18–30 years old | |
| | Men | RMR = 15.3 × weight + 679 |
| | | RMR = 15.4 × weight − 27 × height + 717 |
| | Women | RMR = 14.7 × weight + 496 |
| | | RMR = 13.3 × weight + 334 × height + 35 |
| | Age: 31–60 years old | |
| | Men | RMR = 11.6 × weight + 879 |
| | | RMR = 11.3 × weight + 16 × height + 901 |
| | Women | RMR = 8.7 × weight + 829 |
| | | RMR = 8.7 × weight − 25 × height + 865 |
| | Age: 60+ years old | |
| | Men | RMR = 13.5 × weight + 487 |
| | | RMR = 8.8 × weight + 1128 × height + 1071 |
| | Women | RMR = 10.5 × weight + 596 |
| | | RMR = 9.2 × weight + 637 × height − 302 |

Adapted from Institute of Medicine of the National Academies (2006). *Dietary Reference Intakes: The Essential Guide to Nutrient Requirements*. Otten, J. J., Hellwig, J. P., Meyers, L. D. Page 82. https://www.nap.edu/catalog/11537/dietary-reference-intakes-the-essential-guide-to-nutrient-requirements. Accessed July 27, 2016.

Note: Weight in kilograms, height in centimeters, age in years for equations below unless otherwise indicated.
Adapted from Institute of Medicine of the National Academies (2006). *Dietary Reference Intakes: The Essential Guide to Nutrient Requirements*. Otten, J. J., Hellwig, J. P., Meyers, L. D. Page 84. https://www.nap.edu/catalog/11537/dietary-reference-intakes-the-essential-guide-to-nutrient-requirements. Accessed July 27, 2016.

Adapted from Academy of Nutrition and Dietetics. Equations. Nutrition Care Manual. https://www.nutritioncaremanual.org/topic.cfm?ncm_category_id=11&lv1=255519&ncm_toc_id=255519&ncm_heading=&. Accessed July 27, 2016.

**TABLE 3.11** Standards of nutrient intake for macronutrients

| | Recommended Dietary Allowance (RDA) | Estimated Average Requirement (EAR) | Upper Tolerable Intake Level (UL) |
|---|---|---|---|
| Carbohydrate | 130 g per day for adults | Established based on average amount of glucose used by the brain | Insufficient data to set for added sugars Recommended maximum level ≤25% total energy |
| Fat | No RDA for saturated, monounsaturated fatty acids, or cholesterol; these nutrients are produced by the body and do not play any role in the prevention of chronic disease | Not set; % energy derived from fat varies yet can still meet daily energy needs | Insufficient data for fat, monounsaturated fatty acids, n-6 and n-3 polyunsaturated fatty acids |
| Protein | 0.8 g/kg body weight for men and women | | Insufficient data for protein and amino acids |

Data from Dietary Reference Intakes for Energy, Carbohydrate, Fiber, Fat, Fatty Acids, Cholesterol, Protein, and Amino Acids (Macronutrients), www.nap.edu.

macronutrients has been established (**TABLE 3.12**). AMDR is the range of intake of an energy source that correlates to a reduced risk of chronic disease and is able to provide adequate amounts of essential nutrients. It is presented as a percentage of total energy intake, giving a range; numbers below or above that percentage represent an elevated risk of chronic disease.[5]

**TABLE 3.13** lists additional macronutrient recommendations.

**TABLE 3.12** Acceptable macronutrient distribution ranges

| | Children, 1–3 yo (%) | Children, 4–18 yo (%) | Adults (%) |
|---|---|---|---|
| Fat | 30–40 | 25–35 | 20–35 |
| n-6 polyunsaturated fatty acids* (linoleic acid) | 5–10 | 5–10 | 5–10 |
| n-3 polyunsaturated fatty acids* (α-linoleic acid) | 0.6–1.2 | 0.6–1.2 | 0.6–1.2 |
| Carbohydrate | 45–65 | 45–65 | 45–65 |
| Protein | 5–20 | 10–30 | 10–35 |

*Approximately 10% of the total can come from longer-chain n-3 or n-6 fatty acids.
Adapted from Institute of Medicine of the National Academies (2002/2005). Dietary Reference Intakes for Energy, Carbohydrate, Fiber, Fat, Fatty Acids, Cholesterol, Protein, and Amino Acids (Macronutrients). Panel on Micronutrients, Panel on the Definition of Dietary Fiber, Subcommittee on Upper Reference Levels of Nutrients, Subcommittee on Interpretation and Uses of Dietary Reference Intakes, and the Standing Committee on the Scientific Evaluation of Dietary Reference Intakes. Page 1325. https://www.nap.edu/catalog/10490/dietary-reference-intakes-for-energy-carbohydrate-fiber-fat-fatty-acids-cholesterol-protein-and-amino-acids-macronutrients. Accessed July 27, 2016.

| TABLE 3.13 Additional macronutrient recommendations | |
|---|---|
| **Macronutrient** | **Recommendation** |
| Dietary cholesterol | As low as possible while consuming a nutritionally adequate diet |
| Trans fatty acids | As low as possible while consuming a nutritionally adequate diet |
| Saturated fatty acids | As low as possible while consuming a nutritionally adequate diet |
| Added sugars* | Limit to no more than 25% of total energy |

*Not a recommended intake. A daily intake of added sugars that individuals should aim for to achieve a healthful diet was not set.
Adapted from Institute of Medicine of the National Academies (2002/2005). Dietary Reference Intakes for Energy, Carbohydrate, Fiber, Fat, Fatty Acids, Cholesterol, Protein, and Amino Acids (Macronutrients). Panel on Micronutrients, Panel on the Definition of Dietary Fiber, Subcommittee on Upper Reference Levels of Nutrients, Subcommittee on Interpretation and Uses of Dietary Reference Intakes, and the Standing Committee on the Scientific Evaluation of Dietary Reference Intakes. Page 1325. https://www.nap.edu /catalog/10490/dietary-reference-intakes-for-energy-carbohydrate-fiber-fat-fatty-acids -cholesterol-protein-and-amino-acids-macronutrients. Accessed July 27, 2016.

## Tolerable Upper Intake Level for Macronutrients

The data for UL typically proves insufficient to set the levels for macronutrients. A maximal intake level of 25% or less of total calories from added sugars is suggested. This amount is deemed adequate to avoid displacement of foods that serve as major sources of essential micronutrients. As for fat, the data were not sufficient enough for total fat, monounsaturated fatty acids, and omega polyunsaturated fatty acids to use the model of risk assessment to set values for these nutrients. As for saturated fatty acids, trans fatty acids and cholesterol, the level at which risk increases is relatively low and unlikely to be achieved by usual diets that still have adequate intakes of other required nutrients. The consumption of these nutrients is recommended to be as low as possible when consuming a nutritionally adequate diet. Data was insufficient for protein to establish any UL.[6]

**Recap** The amount of dietary intake recommended per day for each macronutrient is primarily based on its chronic disease prevention qualities and the optimal level known to reduce risk.

## ▶ Nutrient Density and Nutritional Rating

**Preview** Nutrient-dense foods have a high nutrient value per amount of food, whereas energy-dense foods have a high calorie content per amount of food. An eating pattern that contains more nutrient-dense foods is more nutritious, promotes health, is better at reducing the risk of chronic degenerative conditions, and supports a healthy body weight.

**Nutrient density** is a characteristic of foods and beverages that provide vitamins, minerals, and other substances that contribute to adequate nutrient intake or otherwise have positive health effects. Nutrient-dense food items contain little or no solid fats, added sugars, refined starches, or sodium. They are ideally in forms that retain naturally occurring components such as dietary fiber.[10] The underlying concept of nutrient density is the concentration of nutrients per amount of food or caloric contribution of that food.[14] All vegetables, fruits, whole grains, seafood, eggs, beans and peas, unsalted nuts and seeds, fat-free and low-fat dairy products, and lean meats and poultry are nutrient dense—granted they are prepared with little or no added solid fats, sugars, refined starches, or sodium.[10]

Nutrient-dense items contribute to meeting food group recommendations within calorie and sodium limits. Nutrients and other beneficial substances in a nutrient-dense food have not been "diluted" by extra calories from added solid fats, sugars, or refined starches or by solid fats naturally present in the food. Foods in nutrient-dense forms contain essential vitamins and minerals as well as dietary fiber and other naturally occurring substances with positive health effects.[10] A diet consisting of nutrient-dense items includes whole grains, low-fat dairy products, fruits and vegetables. Regular intake of all these foods promotes the prevention of chronic disease.[14]

## Adopting Nutrient-Dense Eating Patterns

The *Dietary Guidelines* emphasize substituting less healthy options with nutrient-dense foods and beverages. To increase dietary intake of these foods, the *Dietary Guidelines* suggests shifting common food and beverage choices from those containing solid fats, added sugars, refined starches, or sodium to foods that are more nutrient dense.[10] **FIGURE 3.6** includes examples of nutrient-dense foods and beverages.

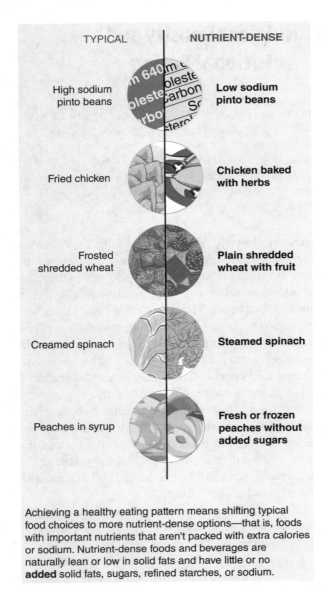

Achieving a healthy eating pattern means shifting typical food choices to more nutrient-dense options—that is, foods with important nutrients that aren't packed with extra calories or sodium. Nutrient-dense foods and beverages are naturally lean or low in solid fats and have little or no **added** solid fats, sugars, refined starches, or sodium.

**FIGURE 3.6** Typical versus nutrient-dense foods and beverages

Reproduced from U.S. Department of Health and Human Services and U.S. Department of Agriculture (2015). 2015-2020 *Dietary Guidelines For Americans* 8th Edition. Figure 2-8 Typical Versus Nutrient–Dense Foods & Beverages. Page 53. https://health.gov /dietaryguidelines/2015/guidelines. Accessed July 27, 2016.

## Rating Nutrient Density of Foods

Systematic ranking and classification structures have been developed to rate the nutrient density of food. Established algorithms are used to assign each food a score based on the presence or absence of specific nutrients, using specific criteria. The resulting score is converted into a practical tool for consumers to use in choosing foods with a balance of essential nutrients versus those foods considered less healthy and linked to poor health outcomes—for example, those containing added sugars, saturated fat, trans fat, and sodium. More than a dozen nutrient-density

rating tools have been developed for and tested with the public to help consumers differentiate between similar, less-healthful products and make smart, nutrient-dense choices.[14] The tools created in both the United States and internationally are summarized in **TABLES 3.14** and **3.15**.

Although the tools are useful they have limitations. Nutrient-density profiling tools tend to consider both beneficial nutrients as well as those identified as having negative effects on health when consumed in excessive amounts. Certain tools are more specific to essential nutrients. In addition, several nutrient-density ranking tools highlight nutrients based on their known influences on primary health outcomes. For instance, scores in the NuVal system reflect what is known about relationships between saturated fatty acids, *n*-3 fatty acids, and cardiovascular disease, and therefore, they promote *n*-3 fatty acids as beneficial for preventing cardiovascular disease. Each nutrition-profiling system uses different methods to present similarly directed information. The Guiding Stars program, for example, assigns foods one to three stars to denote how nutrient dense they are, whereas the NuVal scale ranges from 1 to 100.

Front-of-package (FOP) labeling presents a symbol or logo on food packaging to indicate the nutritional quality of the food and communicate any health claims. It restates facts already included on the Nutrition Facts Panel such as calories, nutrients, and their percentage Daily Value (DV) per serving. Foods are ranked as high or low in certain nutrients based on predetermined criteria, and this ranking is communicated to consumers through logos, symbols, or colors. This tool is effective because consumers have been shown to respond to visuals on packaging. The US Facts Up Front campaign is one example of FOP labeling. The Grocery Manufacturers Association and Food Marketing Institute joined together to direct consumers' attention to calories per serving; saturated fat, sodium, and sugar (which have specified limits); and fiber, potassium, calcium, iron, protein, vitamin C, vitamin A, and vitamin D (which people are encouraged to consume). The aforementioned nutrients would only appear on packaging when the product contained ≥10% of the daily value per serving. Facts Up Front packaging is not mandatory and carries a fee for manufacturers who choose to use this particular labeling. The Healthy Eating System is the most widely used FOP labeling tool and was found to resonate best with consumers. This nutrient-density profiling tool provides guidance to consumers on how frequently they should consume specific foods to meet dietary guidelines.

| Tool | Description | Characteristics |
|---|---|---|
| NuVal Nutrition Scoring System (previously Overall Nutritional Quality Index) | Helps consumers understand the nutrient density of the food they purchase. Generates a summative score based on presence of absence of > 30 nutrients. Uses Institute of Medicine Dietary Reference Index and Dietary Guidelines for Americans. Scores range from 1 to 100. | Scores correlate with health outcomes. Incorporates measures for quality of proteins, fats, and carbohydrates. Measures calories and *n*-3 fatty acid content and then distinguishes between nutrient consumption to be encouraged (vitamins, minerals) and nutrient consumption to be limited (added sugar, sodium, cholesterol). |
| Nutrient Rich Foods Index | Validated index is a sum of percent daily values for nine nutrients to encourage minus the sum of percent daily values for three nutrients to limit. All daily values calculated per serving size. | Distinguishes between nutrients to encourage and limit. Versatile across individual foods, total diet, and menus. Allows calculation of nutritional value of food per unit cost. |
| Affordable Nutrition Index | Scoring system based on Nutrient Rich Foods Index. Produces a nutritional value per dollar score to help consumers identify low-cost, nutritious foods. | Provides nutrition value per dollar tool to help clients of federal food-assistance programs distinguish between nutrients to encourage and limit. |

**TABLE 3.14** Nutrient-density profiling tools, United States

Reproduced from Academy of Nutrition and Dietetics (2016). Practice Paper of the Academy of Nutrition and Dietetics: Selecting Nutrient-Dense Foods for Good Health, Figure 1 Nutrient density profiling tools, United States. *Journal of the Academy of Nutrition and Dietetics*. Hingle, M. D., Kandiah, J., Maggi, A. 116/9/1474. http://www.andjrnl.org/article/S2212-2672(16)30784-5/pdf.

Research in the United States and Canada has found that more than 50% of consumers prefer government-regulated FOP labeling. It has been established as an effective way to help consumers select healthier foods. For food manufacturers to sell their products in the European Union, they must meet three criteria when it comes to FOP labeling: (1) it must help consumers meet dietary guidelines, (2) it must be used to guide or inform public policy, and (3) it must help prevent the development of chronic diseases for diverse populations throughout the life span. The nutrient-profile model has been proposed by the Pan American Health Organization to assess the nutrient density of foods and guide consumers to identify which products contain added sugars, sodium, total fat, saturated fat, and trans fat. The purpose is to promote less consumption of these undesirable nutrients and is geared toward promoting polices and regulations, including FOP labeling and nutrition guidelines, that will help the school food environment.

The underlying considerations of these nutrition tools is that they be grounded in science, be validated against objective measures of diet quality, and be able to effectively translate recommendations into actionable strategies. In short, they should be user-friendly and allow for easy identification of nutrient-dense foods. In terms of terminology, *nutrient rich* and *rich in nutrients* were found to resonate more with consumers than does *nutrient dense*.[14]

## Energy Density

**Energy density** is the amount of energy per weight of food or beverage. Foods low in energy density have

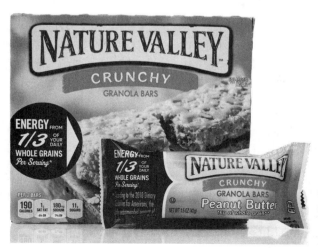

**TABLE 3.15** Nutrient-density profiling tools, international

| Tool | Description | Characteristics |
|---|---|---|
| Guiding Stars | Uses information from the Nutrition Facts Panel and ingredient list to rate nutritional quality.<br>Foods are rated on a scale of zero to three stars based on credits (those nutrients encouraged) and debits (those food components discouraged).<br>High nutrient density → more stars (1 = good, 2 = better, 3 = best). | First storewide nutrition-related guidance system developed by retail stores for foods and beverages.<br>Tiered star icon system distinguishes between nutritious and nonnutritious foods.<br>Each product must provide 5 kcal/serving or more to be rated.<br>Limitation: 100 kcal standard serving may result in over- or underestimation of nutrient density. |
| Healthy eating systems | FOP system derived from Traffic Light and Guideline Daily Amounts.<br>Jointly developed by Sanitarium Health & Wellbeing Company and Australia's Public Health Association. | Color coding based on recommendations from Food Standards of Australia New Zealand.<br>Provides guidance on how frequently to eat foods to meet dietary guidelines: often, occasionally, or sparingly. |
| International Choices Programme | Uses FOP labeling model that incorporates >20 countries' dietary guidance.<br>Focuses on basic and essential nutrients (vitamins, minerals, water) and those detrimental to health (added sugar, sodium, trans and saturated fat). | Publicly available data underline the algorithm.<br>Reassessment of the system is conducted every three years by a panel of international scientific committee members. |
| Nutrient Density Climate Index | Based on Nordic Nutrition Recommendations for 21 essential nutrients.<br>Uses greenhouse gas emissions presented in grams of $CO_2$ to assess whether nutrient density of beverages can change or offset emissions cost.<br>Beverages with highest emissions have highest Nutrient Density Climate Index score.<br>Nutrient density of beverages was calculated based on presence of proteins, carbohydrates, fats, and 18 vitamins and minerals. | Limitation: Does not consider bioavailability of foods or quality of carbohydrates, proteins, or fats. |
| Powerhouse Fruits and Vegetables | Used by the UN's Food and Agriculture Organization and the Institute of Medicine.<br>Related to consumption of "powerhouse" fruits and vegetables that provide an average of ≥ 10% daily value per 100 kcal of 17 nutrients. | Limitations: Excludes other food groups that could also be nutrient dense.<br>Phytochemicals not considered in calculation of nutrient density score. |

Reproduced from Academy of Nutrition and Dietetics (2016). Practice Paper of the Academy of Nutrition and Dietetics: Selecting Nutrient-Dense Foods for Good Health, Figure 2 International nutrient density profiling tools. *Journal of the Academy of Nutrition and Dietetics.* Hingle, M. D., Kandiah, J., Maggi, A. 116/9/1476-7. http://www.andjrnl.org/article/S2212-2672(16)30784-5/pdf

a high proportion of fiber and water, which contribute weight and volume without adding excess calories. These food items are often also low in saturated fat and added sugar, making them high in nutrient density. This supports the supposition that low energy-dense foods promote weight loss and weight maintenance in adults. The *Dietary Guidelines* advise staying within individual energy requirements and also suggest meeting nutrition needs from a selection of nutrient-dense foods to maintain caloric balance. Foods with added sugars, refined grains, and solid fats should be limited because of their high energy density and low nutrient density. One concern in recommending nutrient-dense foods is that some are also energy-dense foods—olive oil, avocado, nuts, and seeds, for example. Consumers are now being urged to make shifts within each food group to nutrient-dense choices and strike a balance of intake and calories.[14]

**Recap** The *Dietary Guidelines* aim to influence consumers to choose nutrient-dense items because they contain high quantities of nutrients per amount of calories. Nutrient-density profiling tools have been created to help the public identify optimal food options.

▶ # Diet Quality Indicators

**Preview** Measuring diet quality provides information about the nutritional adequacy of a population or a population group's dietary intake and identifies nutrients and groups to target for improvement.

## Healthy Eating Index

**The Healthy Eating Index (HEI)** is a measure of diet quality that assesses adherence to the *Dietary Guidelines for Americans*.[15] Its primary use is in monitoring the diet quality of the American population and low-income subpopulations using data, specifically 24-hour dietary recalls, from the National Health and Nutrition Examination Survey (NHANES). The tool is also used to assess relationships between diet and health-related outcomes as well as the quality of food-assistance packages, menus, and the food supply.[15] The key features of the HEI are outlined in **FIGURE 3.7**.

HEI standards are based on the USDA food patterns, which translate key recommendations from the *Dietary Guidelines* into specific food types and amounts people should be eating per calorie level.

| Feature | Rationale |
|---|---|
| Assesses diet quality with regard to recommendations of the Dietary Guidelines for Americans (DGA) | • The DGA are the nutrition policy of the US government and are evidence based |
| Assesses diet—foods and beverages and nutrients from them—and not supplement intake | • Is consistent with fundamental premise of DGA to meet nutrient needs primarily from foods and beverages |
| Captures balance among food groups, including foods to encourage and foods to reduce | • Reflects DGA<br>• Considers gaps between intakes and recommendations |
| Uncouples dietary quality from quantity, employing a density-based approach | • Indicates appropriate mix of, or balance among, food groups<br>• Overcomes limitations of diet and physical activity data, which do not adequately capture energy intake and expenditure, respectively<br>• Enables application to various levels, including groups of people, environments, food supply |
| Employs a least-restrictive approach to setting standards for maximum scores by using the recommendations that are easiest to achieve among those that vary by age and sex | • Results in highest possible scores<br>• Potential error is in the same direction for everyone; however, because very high scores for most components are rare among the US population, the score is optimized for sensitivity to improvement |
| Requires no single food or commodity to be indispensible to a perfect score | • Accommodates a variety of eating patterns, reflecting cultural, ethnic, traditional and personal preferences and tolerances and food costs and availability |
| **Guiding principles for the 2010 update to the HEI** | |
| **Principle** | **Rationale** |
| Focus on key recommendations of the DGA, making only changes to the index that have a strong rationale | • Stability of the HEI should reflect consistency of recommendations over time<br>• Unsubstantiated changes in the HEI may imply emergence of new evidence that does not exist |
| Limit the number of components | • Each component should assess a critical aspect of diet quality |
| Avoid an unduly complex algorithm | • The index should be transparent and straightforward to explain and apply |

**FIGURE 3.7** Key features of the Healthy Eating Index (HEI)

Reproduced from Guether, P. M., Casavale, K. O., Reedy, J., Kirkpatrick, S. I., Hiza, H. A. B., Kuczynski, K. J., Kahle, L. L., Krebs-Smith, S.M. (2013). Update of the Healthy Eating Index: HEI-2010. *Journal of the Academy of Nutrition and Dietetics*. 113/4/570.

The HEI helps nutrition practitioners understand and keep tabs on public eating habits and discern which areas need improvement. Diet quality is scored on a 100-point scale. A score of 100 indicates complete fulfillment of the *Dietary Guidelines* recommendations.[16] An HEI score of >80 suggests a good diet, a score of 51–80 implies the quality of diet needs improvement, and a score <51 indicates the diet is poor.

Data from NHANES (2009–2010) determined that the HEI score the of the American population was 57, thus putting the nation's overall diet into the "needs improvement" range. Although better than the previous score of 52 from 2001–2002, diet quality did not improve significantly in the interim years. The conclusion was that Americans are "eating too little fruits, too few vegetables, not enough whole grains and not enough low-fat dairy and fish and seafood." Also noted was an "overconsumption of empty calories . . . such as refined grains." Dietitians and other healthcare professionals are tasked with supporting a score close to 80 and to help reverse the trend of diet-related diseases. The 2009–2010 HEI total and component scores for 2010 are shown in **FIGURE 3.8**.

The HEI was established by the USDA's Center for Nutrition Policy and Promotion (CNPP) in 1995 and is continually updated as revisions are made to the *Dietary Guidelines*.[14] The HEI has several important uses in public health and nutrition policy. Examining relationships between diet and outcomes of public health concern, evaluating the food environment, and determining the relationship between diet cost and diet quality are primary uses of HEI data. HEI findings can be used to assessing the quality of food-assistance packages, menus, and the American food supply, and evaluating intervention trials, and assessing dietary patterns.[16] The USDA's consumer website contains interactive tools to help individuals use the *Dietary Guidelines* to improve the quality of their diets.[16]

## Food Pattern Modeling Analysis

The purpose of food pattern modeling analysis is to determine whether the USDA food patterns continue to meet nutritional goals for adequacy and moderation while staying within the established calorie targets. This type of analysis uses the food patterns presented in the 2010 *Dietary Guidelines*, with updated food group nutrient profiles based on the most recent food consumption and nutrient-composition data. As part of the assessment, all foods reported in the What We Eat in America/National Health and National Health and

| HEI-2010 Dietary Component (maximum score) | Children 2–17 years (n = 2,990) | Adults 18–64 years (n = 4,673) | Older Adults ≥ 65 years (n = 1,379) |
|---|---|---|---|
| | | Mean score (standard error) | |
| Total fruit (5) | 3.82 (0.19) | 2.93 (0.08) | 4.40 (0.13) |
| Whole fruit (5) | 4.77 (0.22) | 3.92 (0.12) | 5.00 (0.00) |
| Total vegetables (5) | 2.10 (0.05) | 3.49 (0.07) | 4.21 (0.11) |
| Greens and beans (5) | 0.56 (0.07) | 2.92 (0.12) | 3.37 (0.31) |
| Whole grains (10) | 2.22 (0.08) | 2.47 (0.13) | 3.52 (0.16) |
| Dairy (10) | 9.23 (0.19) | 6.23 (0.12) | 6.19 (0.20) |
| Total protein foods (5) | 4.59 (0.14) | 5.00 (0.00) | 5.00 (0.00) |
| Seafood and plant proteins (5) | 2.90 (0.23) | 4.03 (0.23) | 4.98 (0.06) |
| Fatty acids (10) | 3.08 (0.10) | 4.39 (0.14) | 4.69 (0.15) |
| Refined grains (10) | 4.54 (0.21) | 6.35 (0.16) | 7.29 (0.20) |
| Sodium (10) | 4.50 (0.17) | 3.57 (0.13) | 3.30 (0.26) |
| Empty calories (20) | 11.17 (0.23) | 12.04 (0.26) | 13.94 (0.33) |
| **Total HEI score (100)** | **53.47 (0.77)** | **57.34 (0.86)** | **65.90 (0.56)** |

[1]Calculated using the population ratio method.

**FIGURE 3.8** HEI-2010 total and component scores for children, adults, and older adults during 2009–2010

Reproduced from United States Department of Agriculture. Healthy Eating Index. USDA Center for Nutrition Policy and Promotion. https://www.cnpp.usda.gov/healthyeatingindex. Accessed September 28, 2016.

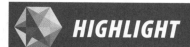

**HIGHLIGHT**

### Applications of the Healthy Eating Index (HEI)

The Healthy Eating Index has been used for more than simply assessing diet quality. Applications of the HEI in literature encompass epidemiology, population monitoring, nutrition intervention, the relationship between diet quality and biomarkers, and diet quality of a specific set of foods in the food environment.

#### Diet and Chronic Disease

The HEI is effective in assessing diet quality and health outcomes in populations with existing diagnoses: for example, diet quality and risk for cardiovascular disease deaths and diet quality among cancer survivors. The impact of dietary intervention is also assessed for diet quality and glycemic index improvement in individuals with type 2 diabetes.

#### Population Estimates of Diet Quality

In addition to monitoring the diet quality of the entire American population, the HEI is also effective for analyzing subgroups, including children and adolescents, older adults, and specific races and ethnicities.

The National Healthy and Nutrition Examination Survey (NHANES) incorporates a section titled "What We Eat," a data set useful for assessing diet quality in the American population. NHANES data are frequently referenced to provide insight about diet quality—specifically its association with health outcomes, health behaviors, and biomarkers of disease risk.

#### Children

Research studies incorporating the HEI assess the diet quality of children and adolescents in regard to its association with television viewing time, dental caries, and food away from home. The diet quality of children enrolled in federal nutrition programs is also explored.

#### Federal Nutrition Programs

The HEI serves as a measuring tool to ascertain the diet quality of the foods made available by federal nutrition programs (guided by the *Dietary Guidelines for Americans*) and the diet quality of the groups assisted by the program. The Supplemental Nutrition Assistance Program, the National School Lunch Program, and the Supplemental Nutrition Program for Women, Infants, and Children were investigated. These programs generally are targeted toward food-insecure and vulnerable population groups, providing valuable data regarding disparities in diet quality among income groups, education levels, and additional sociodemographic indicators.

#### Food Environment

The HEI scores of restaurant menus, grocery store flyers, and the entire American supply are compared against the *Dietary Guidelines for Americans* to determine how well the food supply aligns with the recommendations. The analysis is effective in identifying which aspects of food availability require improvement.

#### Global Applications

The HEI lends support to other countries because its framework serves as a model on which they can base their own diet quality indexes; adjustments are made for their own specific populations. This is possible because the 12 components of the HEI represent basic food groups that are culturally neutral.

Further information on the HEI is available on the websites of the Center for Nutrition Policy and Promotion (cnpp.usda.gov) and the National Cancer Institute (www.epi.grants.cancer.gov/hei/). The sites include updated scores for population levels, research tools, and fact sheets.

Modified from Healthy Eating Index – beyond the score. *J Acad Nutr Diet*. 2017; 117(4):519-521.

Nutrition Examination Survey (WWEIA NHANES) 2009–2010 were assigned to appropriate item clusters. Then the nutrient profiles were calculated for each food group or subgroup using the nutrient data for representative foods and the proportional consumption of each item cluster from the group composite. The existing recommended intake amounts for each food group and energy levels for the patterns were compared to the usual intake distributions. The calories and nutrients provided by each pattern were calculated from the nutrient profile and recommended intake amounts. Then nutrients in each pattern were compared with nutrient recommendations, and then nutritional goals that were or were not met for age and gender groups were identified at each calorie level.[17]

## Alternative Healthy Eating Index

The Alternative Healthy Eating Index (AHEI) incorporates some aspects of the original HEI as well as some components corresponding to the existing *Dietary Guidelines*. The AHEI's six components are (1) vegetables, (2) fruit, (3) nuts and soy, (4) cereal fiber, (5) polyunsaturated fatty acids and saturated fatty acids, and (6) white and red meat. Alcohol and trans fats are also assessed.[18] Other diet quality indicators that have been used include the Diet Quality Index, Programme National Nutrition Santé Guideline Score, DASH food group score, Mediterranean Diet Score, relative Med Diet Score, and Mediterranean-Style Pattern Score.

> **Recap** The Healthy Eating Index and other indicators of diet quality serve to inform policy makers of the healthfulness of our population's diet and identify which aspects need improvement.

# ▶ *Dietary Guidelines for Americans 2015*

> **Preview** The *Dietary Guidelines for Americans* are reissued by the HHS and USDA every five years to reflect the most current nutrition science research and update the recommendations established to guide the population toward optimal health.

## Purpose

The *Dietary Guidelines* are the evidence-based foundation for nutrition guidance created for the public by the federal government. The purpose is to direct professionals in their work with all individuals age 2 years and older and their families to support the consumption of healthy, nutritionally adequate diets. The *Dietary Guidelines* are published every five years as mandated by the National Nutrition Monitoring and Related Research Act (1990). Under the legislature, the Department of Health and Human Services and the Department of Agriculture must jointly publish a report consisting of nutrition and dietary guidelines and information for the general public. They strive to make recommendations regarding components of a healthy and nutritionally adequate diet that will both promote health and prevent chronic disease for current and future generations.[10]

The recommendations provided in the *Dietary Guidelines* aim to promote health, prevent chronic disease, and help people reach and maintain a healthy body weight. The *Dietary Guidelines* significantly affect nutrition in the United States because they form the basis of federal nutrition and policy programs; help local, state, and national health promotion and disease prevention initiatives; and inform numerous organizations and industries (i.e., products developed and marketed by the food and beverage industry). Public health agencies, healthcare providers, and educational institutions all base their fundamentals on the strategies, recommendations, and messages dictated in the *Dietary Guidelines*.[19]

## Process

The main objective of the *Dietary Guidelines* is to help individuals maintain their overall health and reduce the prevalence of disease. The process for developing the *Dietary Guidelines* is summarized in **FIGURE 3.9** and includes a review of the science, development and implementation of the *Dietary Guidelines*.[20] The HHS and USDA assemble a *Dietary Guidelines* advisory

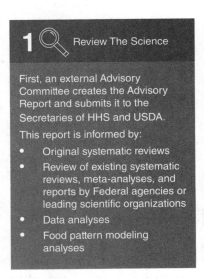
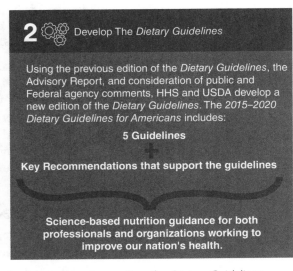
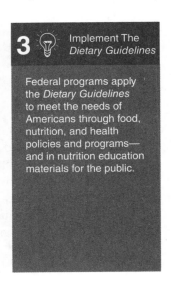

**1** Review The Science

First, an external Advisory Committee creates the Advisory Report and submits it to the Secretaries of HHS and USDA.

This report is informed by:
- Original systematic reviews
- Review of existing systematic reviews, meta-analyses, and reports by Federal agencies or leading scientific organizations
- Data analyses
- Food pattern modeling analyses

**2** Develop The *Dietary Guidelines*

Using the previous edition of the *Dietary Guidelines*, the Advisory Report, and consideration of public and Federal agency comments, HHS and USDA develop a new edition of the *Dietary Guidelines*. The *2015–2020 Dietary Guidelines for Americans* includes:

**5 Guidelines**

**+**

**Key Recommendations that support the guidelines**

**Science-based nutrition guidance for both professionals and organizations working to improve our nation's health.**

**3** Implement The *Dietary Guidelines*

Federal programs apply the *Dietary Guidelines* to meet the needs of Americans through food, nutrition, and health policies and programs— and in nutrition education materials for the public.

**FIGURE 3.9** Process for reviewing, developing, and implementing the *Dietary Guidelines*

# VIEWPOINT

## Product Development Process

*Lauren Grosskopf, MS*

Ever wondered how much work goes into putting a new food product on the grocery shelf? To give you an overview, let's discuss the four-step process of product development used by a major food manufacturer.

1. Come up with an *idea* for a product.
   - During this phase, a few characteristics will be identified and defined: What is the product? What does the product look like? Does another manufacturer currently produce something like it? This is the blue-sky phase when the product has no limits.

2. Next comes *scoping*, which is background investigation.
   - After the idea is defined, it is time to shop grocery stores, natural food stores, convenience stores, and so on. Exploring a variety of stores allows developers to understand the competitive landscape. Using information from competitors will also allow developers to get an idea of the flavors, textures, and other thought starters to help execute the idea. Team tastings are typically used during this phase to get feedback from cross-functional teams and understand general preferences. Many questions will be asked during this phase to gain the appropriate knowledge to move the idea forward. At the end of this phase, a gold standard should be identified— the ideal product , flavor, or texture that the developer should be targeting.

3. The most involved part of the process is the product *development*.
   - This part of the process typically starts with benchtop development and then moves to small-scale development in a pilot plant setting before final large-scale development in a full plant trial. All raw materials, packaging, and manufacturing plants must be quality audited and approved. In between each phase of a trial, different levels of consumer research may be completed, ranging from concept testing to heat maps, central location tests, in-home use testing, and so on. Each phase gets the developer closer to the ideal product by learning more about what aspects of the product or packaging pleases consumers. After the product, package, and process have been finalized, several pieces need to fall in place. A shelf-life study should be implemented to understand the expected life span of the product under actual product storage conditions. In addition, regulatory, microbiological, quality, and legal groups will review the product as a whole. They will ensure that the product meets all quality and food safety standards and that Nutrition Fact Panels, ingredient line statements, and claims are all appropriately generated and substantiated with credible documentation.

4. Now it's time to get the product into the hands of consumers. This stage is called *execution*.
   - The product-development process is different for everyone. It can take anywhere from six months to several years to get a product on the shelf. Product approval requires alignment from many different business team partners, including research and development, marketing, operations, sales, and quality control. Once the business team is aligned with the product, then the team can move forward with first production. In this final step, products are manufactured to defined manufacturing and packaging specifications and established quality standards. The finished product is then shipped to distribution centers, where customers can begin to place orders to stock their store shelves. Ongoing quality reviews, confirmatory shelf-life studies, and consumer comment trackers are established and monitored for an extended period of time after initial production to ensure that the product continues to meet consumer expectations.

© TaLaNoVa/Shutterstock.

committee of nationally recognized nutrition and medical researchers, academics, and practitioners to review the current nutrition science. The committee holds a series of public meetings, one of them with the purpose of receiving oral comments from the public. Members of the public are also permitted to submit written comments to the advisory committee during the review process. The committee generates an advisory report comprising current scientific and medical evidence in nutrition. Within the report, science-based recommendations to the federal government are outlined for development of the new edition of the *Dietary Guidelines*.

First, an external advisory committee creates an advisory report that is submitted to the secretaries of the HHS and the USDA. Data and food pattern modeling are analyzed. The new edition is created by the HHS and the USDA with consideration of the previous *Dietary Guidelines* edition as well as input from the public and federal agencies. The guidelines are implemented by federal programs to meet the needs of Americans through food, health policies and programs, and nutrition education materials. A peer-review process is also completed, with nonfederal experts conducting a confidential review of the draft policy document. After the advisory report is completed, the public is again given the opportunity to respond orally or with written comments via the website. The information from the advisory report along with comments from the public and federal agents are used by the HHS and the USDA for the formation of the new edition of the *Dietary Guidelines*.[20]

## Evolution

The *Dietary Guidelines* was first released in 1980. In 1990, Congress passed the National Nutrition Monitoring and Related Research Act, which required that the HHS and the USDA review, update, and jointly publish the *Dietary Guidelines* every five years. The guidelines have evolved to address shifting public health concerns and nutritional needs of specific populations. This is demonstrated in the fact that the *Dietary Guidelines* have typically focused on Americans ages 2 years and older, although newer science shows that dietary intake from birth—and even the mother's diet during gestation—may have lasting effects on a child's health and, therefore, should be included in the recommendations. In response, the federal government has pioneered a project to begin evaluating the scientific evidence available, with the potential to support dietary guidance in the future for infants and toddlers, from birth to 24 months of age, as well as women who are pregnant. The *Dietary Guidelines* are projected to include these special populations by 2020. Information on the Pregnancy and Birth to 24 Months Project is available at www.cnpp.usda.gov/birthto24months.[21]

## The *Dietary Guidelines* for Americans 2015

In contrast to previous editions, which centered around individual dietary components including food groups and nutrients, the *Dietary Guidelines 2015* focuses on eating patterns and their food and nutrient characteristics. The DAG encourage a shift in eating behavior to

**The Guidelines**

1. **Follow a healthy eating pattern across the lifespan.** All food and beverage choices matter. Choose a healthy eating pattern at an appropriate calorie level to help achieve and maintain a healthy body weight, support nutrient adequacy, and reduce the risk of chronic disease.

2. **Focus on variety, nutrient density, and amount.** To meet nutrient needs within calorie limits, choose a variety of nutrient-dense foods across and within all food groups in recommended amounts.

3. **Limit calories from added sugars and saturated fats and reduce sodium intake.** Consume an eating pattern low in added sugars, saturated fats, and sodium. Cut back on foods and beverages higher in these components to amounts that fit within healthy eating patterns.

4. **Shift to healthier food and beverage choices.** Choose nutrient-dense foods and beverages across and within all food groups in place of less healthy choices. Consider cultural and personal preferences to make these shifts easier to accomplish and maintain.

5. **Support healthy eating patterns for all.** Everyone has a role in helping to create and support healthy eating patterns in multiple settings nationwide, from home to school to work to communities.

**FIGURE 3.10** The five guidelines of the 2015–2020 *Dietary Guidelines for Americans*

patterns that promote the intake of foods that provide adequate nutrients to meet requirements and promote improved health overall. In summary, the key recommendations are to "consume a healthy eating pattern that accounts for all foods and beverages within the appropriate calorie level."[13] *The Dietary Guidelines for Americans 2015–2020* are summarized in **FIGURE 3.10**.

The *Dietary Guidelines 2015* emphasizes choosing nutrient-dense foods and beverages in favor of less healthy options. The main objective of the *Dietary Guidelines* is to help individuals maintain overall health and reduce the prevalence of disease. Described in the *Dietary Guidelines* are the healthy eating patterns that have been found to support overall health (including body weight and chronic disease risk) throughout the life span, in accordance with Key Recommendations, including:

- An eating pattern that represents the totality of all foods and beverages consumed
- Meeting nutritional needs primarily from foods
- Having adaptable healthy eating patterns

The healthy eating patterns are the result of a combination of three evaluative measures: systematic reviews

**Consume a healthy eating pattern that accounts for all foods and beverages within an appropriate calorie level.**

**A healthy eating pattern includes:**[1]

- A variety of vegetables from all of the subgroups—dark green, red and orange, legumes (beans and peas), starchy, and other
- Fruits, especially whole fruits
- Grains, at least half of which are whole grains
- Fat-free or low-fat dairy, including milk, yogurt, cheese, and/or fortified soy beverages
- A variety of protein foods, including seafood, lean meats and poultry, eggs, legumes (beans and peas), and nuts, seeds, and soy products
- Oils

**A healthy eating pattern limits:**

- Saturated fats and *trans* fats, added sugars, and sodium

Key Recommendations that are quantitative are provided for several components of the diet that should be limited. These components are of particular public health concern in the United States, and the specified limits can help individuals achieve healthy eating patterns within calorie limits:

- Consume less than 10 percent of calories per day from added sugars[2]
- Consume less than 10 percent of calories per day from saturated fats[3]
- Consume less than 2,300 milligrams (mg) per day of sodium[4]
- If alcohol is consumed, it should be consumed in moderation—up to one drink per day for women and up to two drinks per day for men—and only by adults of legal drinking age.[5]

In tandem with the recommendations above, Americans of all ages—children, adolescents, adults, and older adults—should meet the Physical Activity Guidelines for Americans to help promote health and reduce the risk of chronic disease. Americans should aim to achieve and maintain a healthy body weight. The relationship between diet and physical activity contributes to calorie balance and managing body weight. As such, the Dietary Guidelines includes a Key Recommendation to:

- Meet the *Physical Activity Guidelines for Americans*.[6]

[1] Definitions for each food group and subgroup are provided throughout the chapter and are compiled in Appendix 3. USDA Food Patterns: Healthy U.S.-Style Eating Pattern.

[2] The recommendation to limit intake of calories from added sugars to less than 10 percent per day is a target based on food pattern modeling and national data on intakes of calories from added sugars that demonstrate the public health need to limit calories from added sugars to meet food group and nutrient needs within calorie limits. The limit on calories from added sugars is not a Tolerable Upper Intake Level (UL) set by the Institute of Medicine (IOM). For most calorie levels, there are not enough calories available after meeting food group needs to consume 10 percent of calories from added sugars and 10 percent of calories from saturated fats and still stay within calorie limits.

[3] The recommendation to limit intake of calories from saturated fats to less than 10 percent per day is a target based on evidence that replacing saturated fats with unsaturated fats is associated with reduced risk of cardiovascular disease. The limit on calories from saturated fats is not a UL set by the IOM. For most calorie levels, there are not enough calories available after meeting food group needs to consume 10 percent of calories from added sugars and 10 percent of calories from saturated fats and still stay within calorie limits.

[4] The recommendation to limit intake of sodium to less than 2,300 mg per day is the UL for individuals ages 14 years and older set by the IOM. The recommendations for children younger than 14 years of age are the IOM age- and sex-appropriate ULs (see Appendix 7. Nutritional Goals for Age-Sex Groups Based on Dietary Reference Intakes and Dietary Guidelines Recommendations).

[5] It is not recommended that individuals begin drinking or drink more for any reason. The amount of alcohol and calories in beverages varies and should be accounted for within the limits of healthy eating patterns. Alcohol should be consumed only by adults of legal drinking age. There are many circumstances in which individuals should not drink, such as during pregnancy. See Appendix 9. Alcohol for additional information.

[6] U.S. Department of Health and Human Services. 2008 Physical Activity Guidelines for Americans. Washington (DC): U.S. Department of Health and Human Services; 2008. ODPHP Publication No. U0036. Available at: http://www.health.gov/paguidelines. Accessed August 6, 2015.

**FIGURE 3.11** Key Recommendations provide further guidance on how individuals can follow the five Guidelines. The Dietary Guidelines' Key Recommendations for healthy eating patterns should be applied in their entirety, given the interconnected relationship that each dietary component can have with others.

# VIEWPOINT

## Food Service Perspectives

*Linda S. Eck Mills, MBA, RDN, LDN, FADA*

At the center of the seal for the Academy of Nutrition and Dietetics are three symbols that represent the profession's principal characteristics: a balance scale to represent science as the foundation and equality, a caduceus to represent the close relationship between dietetics and medicine, and a cooking vessel to represent cookery and food preparation.[1]

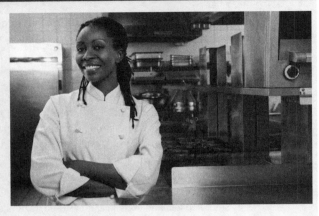

© sirtravelalot/Shutterstock.

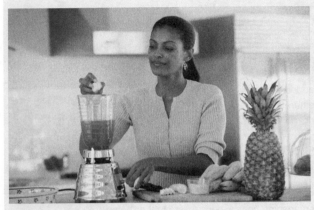

© Ariel Skelley/Getty Images.

During my career as a registered dietitian nutritionist, I have seen firsthand many changes to the "cooking vessel" and those who work in the food-service portion of the healthcare profession. My top-five list of changes in healthcare food service are the following:

1. *Dress of Dietitians.* We have gone from wearing white uniforms, white shoes, beige stockings, and a white nurses'-style cap in 1932 to wearing profession business attire and even position-appropriate clothing if working as a certified personal trainer. In 1932, dietitians wore dresses. Today, many dietitians wear pants.

2. *Tube Feedings.* In 1975, the *Simplified Diet Manual with Meal Patterns*, 4th ed., by the Nutrition Section of the Iowa State Department of Health in cooperation with the Iowa Dietetic Association, provided a nutritionally adequate formula for tube feeding.[2] Today, commercial products are able to meet the needs of a variety of medical complications requiring oral or tube feeding.

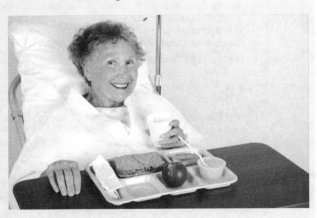

© Lisa F. Young/Shutterstock.

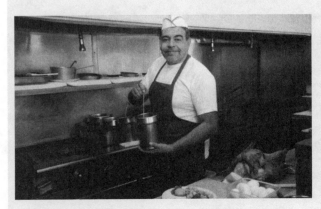

© Hill Street Studios/Blend Images/Thinkstock/Getty Images.

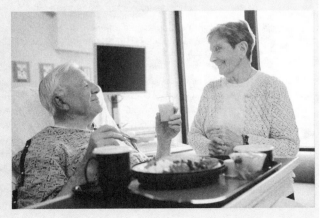

© Monkey Business Images/Shutterstock.

3. *Methods of Cooking and Production Equipment.* Naturally, cooking methods have changed over time. Cook-chill systems have been used in large facilities where foods are prepared as many as five days in advance and then rapidly chilled and held in refrigeration until they can be plated and rethermalized before serving.[3,4,5] Some facilities are now using short-order cooking with their room-service systems.

   For decades, the standard kitchen equipment was a stove top, an oven, and a steamer. Now when you walk into a kitchen, you might see convection and conduction ovens and multifunction pieces of equipment. The trade show of the North American Food Equipment Manufacturers (NAFEM) show held in odd-numbered years is one of the best places to see the latest in food-service equipment.[6,7]

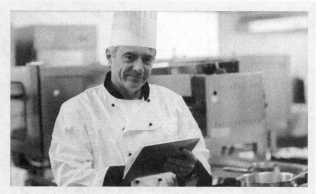
© ESB Professional/Shutterstock.

5. *Food-Service Management and Budgets.* Today's food-service management is increasingly being done by certified dietary managers instead of dietitians as we give up yet another piece of our scope of practice.[10]

   Change is inevitable in all aspects of our professional lives, and healthcare food service is no exception. Consumer demands and trends in this industry will continue to evolve, and as food and nutrition professionals we will need to keep up with these changes.[11]

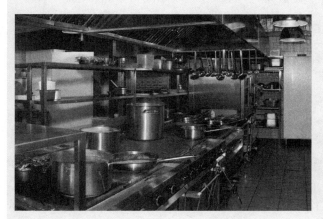
© Kondor83/Shutterstock.

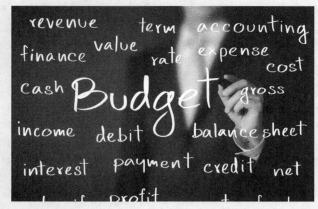
© Dusit/Shutterstock.

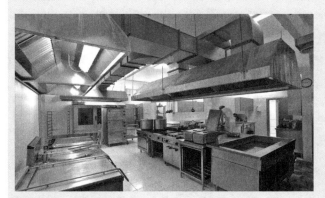
© Dalibor Sevaljevic/Shutterstock.

4. *Menus and Types of Meal Service.* As the length of stay and customer demands have changed over the years, menus have evolved from the nonselective menu, to a main meal with an alternate entrée, to restaurant-style items ordered from a menu.[8] Cultural change has transformed the institutional model for patient care in many ways, including meal service.[9] Restaurant-style menus are now common in health care.

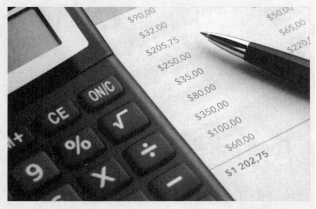
© Peter Kotoff/Shutterstock.

### References

1. Academy of Nutrition and Dietetics. http://www.eatrightpro.org/. Accessed March 13, 2017.
2. Nutrition Section of the Iowa State Department of Health in cooperation with the Iowa Dietetic Association. *Simplified Diet Manual with Meal Patterns*. 4th ed. Ames, IA: Iowa State University Press; 1975.
3. Williams Refrigeration. Guide to Cook Chill. http://www.williams-refrigeration.com.hk/guides/the-cook-chill-process-explained. Accessed March 13, 2017.
4. Williams Refrigeration. Guide to Cook Chill. https://www.chefservicesgroup.com/services/cook-chill.html. Accessed March 13, 2017.
5. Nummer B. Cook-chill reduced-oxygen packaging in retail and foodservice operations. http://www.foodsafetymagazine.com/magazine-archive1/junejuly-2010/cook-chill-reduced-oxygen-packaging-in-retail-and-foodservice-operations/. Accessed March 13, 2017.
6. North American Food Equipment Manufacturers (NAFEM). https://www.nafem.org/. Accessed March 13, 2017.
7. NAFEM Show. https://www.thenafemshow.org/. Accessed March 13, 2017.
8. Hospitality School. Types of menus. http://www.hospitality-school.com/types-menus-restaurant. Accessed March 13, 2017.
9. Pioneer Network. Changing the culture of aging in the 21st century. https://www.pioneernetwork.net/. Accessed March 13, 2017.
10. Association of Nutrition and Foodservice Professionals. http://www.anfponline.org/
11. Keller M. That's progress—Advancements in hospital foodservice. *Today's Diet*. 2009; 11:28. http://www.todaysdietitian.com/newarchives/072709p28.shtm. Accessed March 13, 2017.

### Publications

FoodService Director. http://www.foodservicedirector.com/.

Food-Service Equipment and Supplies. http://www.fesmag.com/.

Food Management. http://www.food-management.com/news-trends/business-industry.

of scientific research, food pattern modeling, and analysis of the food intake of the current American population. The integration of these three factors provides the evidence-based foundation for regulations to reduce the risk of diet-associated chronic disease and support nutrient adequacy.[10]

The *Dietary Guidelines* recommended food guides provide further information regarding healthy eating pattern as well as other tools to help the population meet its nutritional requirements through proper food choices.

**Recap** The *Dietary Guidelines* serve as a road map to help Americans reach their optimal health status and avoid common diseases and conditions associated with an unhealthy lifestyle. The development process is designed to ensure the information is current and relevant and the goals realistic and achievable.

## ▶ Food Labeling and Nutrition

**Preview** The Nutrition Facts Label has been revised to more appropriately reflect consumer preferences as well as current nutrition sciences in relation to fats, sugar, fiber, and certain vitamins and minerals.

## The New Food Label

The US Food and Drug Administration released the new Nutrition Facts Label in 2016, making it easier for consumers to make informed food choices. The changes were made to represent the most current scientific data, specifically the links between diet and chronic diseases such as obesity and heart disease. Manufacturers will need to use the new food label by July 26, 2018; small businesses will have an additional year to comply.

The new food label has a refreshed design (**FIGURE 3.12**).[22] The size of print showing calories, servings per container, and serving size has been increased. Bold type is used for calories and serving sizes. Manufacturers must provide the actual amounts and percentage daily values of vitamin D, calcium, iron, and potassium. They are given the option to declare the gram amount of other vitamins and minerals on a voluntary basis, and the footnote has been changed to clarify what percent daily value means. A footnote now states: "The % daily value tells you how much a nutrient in a serving of food contributes to a daily diet. 2,000 calories a day is used for general nutrition advice."[23] The changes to the Nutrition Facts Label are highlighted in **FIGURE 3.13**.

In addition, the new food label reflects updated information about nutrition science. Added sugars are included on the label in grams and percent daily

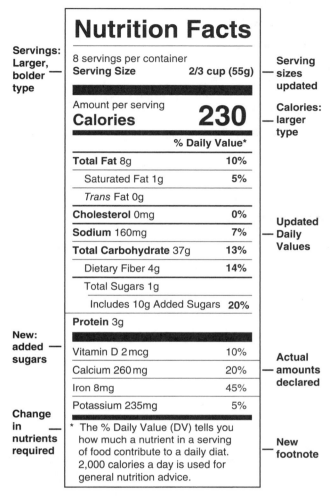

**NEW LABEL: WHAT'S DIFFERENT**

**Servings: Larger, bolder type** —

**Nutrition Facts**

8 servings per container

**Serving Size** 2/3 cup (55g)

— **Serving sizes updated**

Amount per serving

**Calories** **230**

— **Calories: larger type**

% Daily Value*

| | |
|---|---|
| **Total Fat** 8g | **10%** |
| Saturated Fat 1g | **5%** |
| *Trans* Fat 0g | |
| **Cholesterol** 0mg | **0%** |
| **Sodium** 160mg | **7%** |
| **Total Carbohydrate** 37g | **13%** |
| Dietary Fiber 4g | **14%** |
| Total Sugars 1g | |
| Includes 10g Added Sugars | **20%** |
| **Protein** 3g | |

**New: added sugars** —

| | |
|---|---|
| Vitamin D 2mcg | 10% |
| Calcium 260mg | 20% |
| Iron 8mg | 45% |
| Potassium 235mg | 5% |

**Change in nutrients required** —

**Updated Daily Values** —

**Actual amounts declared** —

\* The % Daily Value (DV) tells you how much a nutrient in a serving of food contribute to a daily diat. 2,000 calories a day is used for general nutrition advice.

— **New footnote**

**FIGURE 3.12** Changes to the Nutrition Facts Label

Reproduced from U. S. Food & Drug Administration. Changes to the Nutrition Facts Label. fda.gov. https://www.fda.gov/Food /GuidanceRegulation/GuidanceDocumentsRegulatoryInformation/LabelingNutrition/ucm385663.htm. Last updated 2/10/2017. Accessed September 6, 2016.

value. It is in accordance with the *Dietary Guidelines for Americans 2015–2020*, which notes the difficulty of meeting nutrient needs and staying within calorie limits if >10% of total daily calories are from added sugar. Additionally, the list of nutrients required to appear on the label has changed. Calcium and iron remain required, and vitamin D and potassium now mandated as well. Vitamins A and C are longer be required, and are now optional. Calories from fat will be removed because research has shown that the type of fat is more important than the amount. Therefore, total fat, saturated fat, and trans fat will remain on the label. Daily values for sodium, dietary fiber, and vitamin D are being updated based on newer scientific evidence from the National Academy of Medicine, the *Dietary*

*Guidelines* advisory committee report, and other sources. Daily values are reference amounts of nutrients to consume or avoid overconsuming and are used to calculate the percent daily value—listed as "%DV"— that manufacturers put on labels. This reference value aids in consumer understanding of the nutrition information provided in the context of total daily diet.

Updated serving sizes and labeling requirements for certain package sizes are also required on the new label. Serving sizes are specified by law to be based on amounts of foods and beverages that people actually eat, not what they are recommended to be eating. The amounts people consume has changed, with a marked increase, since the previous serving size standards were established in 1993. Serving size references have changed from ½ cup to 1 cup of ice cream and 8 ounces to 12 ounces of soda, for example. For packages between one and two servings (e.g., a 20-ounce can of soda, a 15-ounce can of soup), the calories and other nutrients on the label will be indicated as one serving, because people typically consume the entire item in one sitting. It has been noted that package size affects how much people eat. Products that are more than one serving but could be consumed in one or multiple sittings will have a dual column label to address the amount of calories and nutrients per serving and per package or unit.

## Compliance and Dates

As previously noted, manufacturers are required to transition to the new label by July 26, 2018. Those companies with less than $10 million in annual food sales are given an additional year to comply. Manufacturers also must ensure that by June 18, 2018, their products will contain no partially hydrogenated oils for uses other than those authorized by the Food and Drug Administration (FDA). Vending machine operators with glass-front vending machines must comply with all requirements of the vending machine labeling rule by July 26, 2018. The calorie declaration requirement has been delayed for certain food products sold in glass-front vending machines partly to maintain consistency with the compliance date for the new Nutrition Facts Label requirements. This allows manufacturers to make changes to FOP labeling for products they supply to vending operators at the same time they make changes to the Nutrition Facts Label. Food establishments covered by the menu-labeling rule must comply with menu labeling requirements by May 7, 2018. Targets for sodium reduction being developed by the FDA are voluntary and therefore do not have a compliance date. However, companies

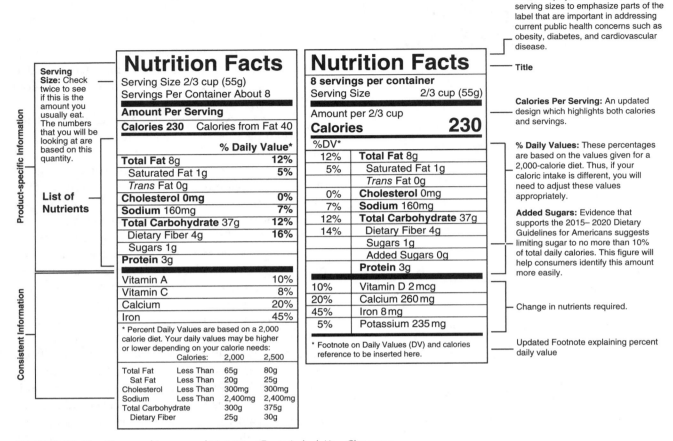

**FIGURE 3.13** The New and Improved Nutrition Facts Label: Key Changes

Reproduced from U.S. Food and Drug Administration. The New and Improved Nutrition Facts Label- Key Changes https://www.fda.gov/downloads/food/ingredientspackaginglabeling/labelingnutrition/ucm511646.pdf

that choose to implement the targets do have recommended time frames by which to implement them. The FDA has published voluntary targets for reducing sodium in commercially produced and prepared foods for both the short and long terms (2 years and 10 years, respectively).[23]

> **Recap** The updated Nutrition Facts Label is designed to highlight the key nutrition information consumers should pay attention to when considering food choices. With larger font, bold type, and revised requirements, the focus shifts to those parameters that have the largest effects on health.

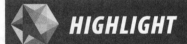

## Best if Used By...

In addition to targeting the Nutrition Facts Label, the USDA, along with the Food Safety and Inspection Service (FSIS), have issued updated guidance regarding date labeling.

The Nutrition Facts Label is not the only packaging component to undergo review. The USDA and the FSIS have issued new guidance aimed at reducing food waste. As the new Nutrition Facts Label is designed to best resonate with the consumer, so too is the revised product dating. Product dating is not a federal requirement on any item other than infant formula. It turns out that the "Sell By" and "Use By" dates are confusing to consumers and result in perfectly usable and safe food products being thrown out. The USDA and FSIS thus recommend that manufacturers use "Best If Used By" to communicate quality to consumers. Adoption of this practice may help the USDA and EPA meet their 2015 goal of reducing national food waste 50% by 2030. The agencies have also taken steps to facilitate the donation of food, bringing about the allocation of 2.6 million pounds of products to establishments such as food banks in 2016.

Modified from USDA Food Safety and Inspection Service. USDA Revises Guidance on Date Labeling to Reduce Food Waste. fsis.usda.gov. https://www.fsis.usda.gov/wps/portal/fsis/newsroom/news-releases-statements-and-transcripts/news-release-archives-by-year/archive/2016/nr-121416-01. Accessed December 24, 2016.

## HIGHLIGHT

### Gluten-Free and Food Allergy Labeling

With continued updates in food-labeling requirements comes revised legislation regarding gluten-free claims. As of September 4, 2013, foods labeled as *gluten free*—including the variations *no gluten, free of gluten*, and *without gluten*—must either inherently not contain gluten or comply with all of the following requirements:

- They cannot contain any gluten-containing grain in any product ingredient.
- They cannot contain an ingredient derived from a gluten-containing grain that has not been processed to remove gluten.
- They cannot contain an ingredient that is derived from a gluten-containing grain that has been processed to remove gluten if that ingredient causes

the final food product to contain 20 parts per million or more of gluten.

#### *"May Contain" Statements*

"May Contain" statements, referred to as allergy advisory statements, differ from "contains" statements. Of primary distinction is that "contains" statements are regulated under the Food Allergen Labeling and Consumer Protection Act, and "may contain" statements do not fall under any federal regulations.

"Manufactured in a facility that also contains wheat," another allergy advisory statement, provides information for consumers regarding food-processing procedures. However, these regulations are neither regulated nor mandatory, so they are not used by all manufacturers. Products were required to be in compliance with the gluten-free label ruling by August 5, 2014.

Modified from the gluten-free labeling rule: What registered dietitian nutritionists need to know to help clients with gluten-related disorders. *J Acad Nutr Diet*. 2015; 115(1):13-16.

## ▶ Food Guides (MyPlate Food Exchange)

**Preview**  In conjunction with the *Dietary Guidelines*, food guides serve as a tool to help Americans decide what types and amounts of foods to consume. The USDA has developed several food guides throughout the years to identify which patterns of eating would meet known nutrient needs at the time, as well as balance intake from various food groups. A timeline of these food guides was discussed previously in this chapter. Two of the contemporary remaining guides are MyPlate and the USDA Food Patterns.

## MyPlate

MyPlate serves as a vehicle that reminds the public to create healthy eating patterns by making healthy choices in line with the *Dietary Guidelines*. MyPlate is used by federal and nonfederal programs to encourage Americans to make shifts in their daily food and beverage choices as dictated by the *Dietary Guidelines*.[10] MyPlate focuses on building the right mix of food to promote optimal health for the present and future.

Specifically, the main ideas focus on variety, amount, and nutrition. Individuals are encouraged to consume food from all five food groups—fruits, vegetables,

grains, proteins, and dairy products—to receive adequate nutrients to meet their needs. Calories should be adequate based on their age, gender, height, weight, and level of physical activity. Adopting this healthy eating pattern should promote health, specifically with reduced risk of causing or exacerbating conditions such as heart disease, diabetes, cancer and obesity.

Americans are encouraged to choose foods and beverages with less saturated fat, sodium, and added sugars. Eating fewer calories from foods high in saturated fat and added sugars helps manage overall calorie intake and prevent overweight and obesity. Eating foods with less sodium reduces the risk of hypertension. To put these recommendations into practice, the guidelines emphasize starting with small changes to build healthier eating styles. These include covering half the plate with fruits and vegetables and half with whole grains and choosing fat-free dairy products in favor of low-fat, a variety of protein sources, and eating and drinking the appropriate amount per individual. Supporting healthy eating for everyone entails creating settings in which healthy choices are available and affordable for the community.[24]

## Food Groups

Fruit for consumption is defined as fresh, canned, frozen, dried, whole, cut up, puréed, or 100% fruit juice. The specific amount needed per individual depends on age, gender, and level of physical activity. For recommended daily amounts of fruit as well as from other food groups, see **TABLE 3.16**. At least half the recommended amount of fruit should come from whole fruit because juice is lower in fiber and may contribute excess calories. If consumed, juices should be 100% whole juice. Canned fruit should contain no added sugars.[25]

Any vegetable—raw, cooked, fresh, frozen, canned, dried, whole, cut up, mashed, or as 100% vegetable juice—counts as a vegetable source. Vegetables are organized into five subgroups—dark green, starchy, red and orange, beans and peas, and other vegetables—based on nutrient content. As with fruit, the amount needed per individual depends on age, gender, and level of physical activity.[26] See Table 3.16 for recommended daily amounts of vegetables and the five other food groups. Recommended weekly amounts from each vegetable subgroup are found in **TABLE 3.17**.

The category of grains is characterized as food made from wheat, rice, oats, cornmeal, barley, or other cereal grains. The amount of grains needed depends on age, gender, and physical activity level. See Table 3.16 for specific recommendations per age group.[27] In addition to the daily recommendation, daily minimum amounts have also been established for whole grains.

Grains are divided into two subgroups: whole and refined. Whole grains contain the entire grain kernel—bran, germ, and endosperm. Examples include whole-wheat flour, bulgur, oatmeal, whole cornmeal, and brown rice. In contrast, refined grains have been milled, a process that removes the bran and germ and gives the resulting products finer texture and extended shelf life. Refining grains, however, removes dietary fiber, iron, and the B vitamins. Most refined grains are therefore enriched with some of the B vitamins (thiamin, riboflavin, niacin, folic acid) as well as iron, which is added after processing. Examples of refined grains include white flour, degermed cornmeal, white bread, and white rice. See **TABLE 3.18**.

The protein group constitutes foods made from meat, poultry, seafood, legumes, eggs, processed soy products, nuts, and seeds. Note that legumes, for example beans and peas, are classified in the vegetable group as well. A variety of protein foods intake is recommended for improved nutrient intake and overall health, including at least 8 ounces of cooked seafood per week. Young children need less, depending on age and calorie needs.[28] See Table 3.16 for protein recommendations based on age. With similar nutrient profiles to both proteins and vegetables, legumes can be counted toward the intake of either the protein or vegetable group.[10]

All fluid milk products and several foods made from milk are part of the dairy group. It is recommended that the majority of choices from the dairy group be fat-free or low-fat. Foods made from milk that retain their calcium are considered part of this group; foods made from milk that contains little to no calcium—cream cheese, cream, and butter—are not. Calcium-fortified soymilk and nut-milks are included in the dairy group. The amount of dairy needed depends on age.[29] See Table 3.16.

Fats that are liquid at room temperature count as oils. For example, vegetable oils used in cooking such as canola, olive, safflower, sunflower, and corn are considered oils. Although not considered a food group, oils provide essential nutrients and therefore are an integral part of the USDA Food Patterns. Nuts, olives, avocado, and certain fish are examples of foods naturally high in oils.[30]

## USDA Food Patterns

The USDA Food Patterns are designed to meet food group and nutrient recommendations while remaining within calorie needs. Patterns are based on consuming foods in nutrient-dense forms. The Healthy US-Style Eating Pattern, the basis for the USDA Food Pattern, was created around the types and proportions of foods typically consumed by Americans, although in nutrient-dense forms and in appropriate amounts. The design focuses on consumers achieving nutrient needs without exceeding calorie requirements and staying within the limits for excessively consumed dietary components.

The Healthy US-Style Eating Pattern demonstrates the specific amounts and limits for food groups and other dietary components that form healthy eating patterns. It was formulated to comply with the RDA, AI, and AMDR established by the Food and Nutrition Board of the National Academy of Medicine. The guidance for healthy eating provided by the tool ensures success in meeting nutritional goals for almost all nutrients. Cup and ounce equivalents for foods with similar nutritional content are provided for each of the five food groups and allows consumers to easily identify which amount of food will be adequate to meet their goals. Amounts of each food group and subgroup are modified as needed to ensure they meet recommendations for nutrient intake and the *Dietary Guidelines* while staying within both the typical consumption range and the limits for calories and over-consumed dietary components. See **TABLE 3.19** for cup and ounce equivalents.

The standards for nutrient adequacy are set to reach the RDA, which is able to account for the needs

**TABLE 3.16** MyPlate intake recommendations

| Food Group | Children (Years) | | Girls (Years) | | Boys (Years) | | Women (Years) | | | Men (Years) | | |
|---|---|---|---|---|---|---|---|---|---|---|---|---|
| | 2–3 | 4–8 | 9–13 | 14–18 | 9–13 | 14–18 | 19–30 | 31–50 | 51+ | 19–30 | 31–50 | 51 |
| Fruit (cups) | 1 | 1–1.5 | 1.5 | 1.5 | 1.5 | 2 | 2 | 1.5 | 1.5 | 2 | 2 | 2 |
| Vegetables (cups) | 1 | 0.5 | 2 | 2.5 | 2.5 | 3 | 2.5 | 2.5 | 2 | 3 | 3 | 2.5 |
| Grains (oz. equiv) | 3 | 5 | 5 | 6 | 6 | 8 | 6 | 6 | 5 | 8 | 7 | 6 |
| Protein (oz. equiv) | 2 | 4 | 5 | 5 | 5 | 6.5 | 5.5 | 5 | 5 | 6.5 | 6 | 5.5 |
| Dairy (cups) | 2 | 2.5 | 3 | 3 | 3 | 3 | 3 | 3 | 3 | 3 | 3 | 3 |
| Oils (tsp) | 3 | 4 | 5 | 5 | 5 | 6 | 6 | 5 | 5 | 7 | 6 | 6 |

Note: The amounts provided are specific to individuals with a physical activity level of <30 minutes per day of moderate activity, above activities of daily living (ADL). Those with increased activity may consume greater amounts, while staying within their estimated calorie needs.
Adapted from USDA Choose MyPlate. choosemyplate.gov. https://www.choosemyplate.gov. Accessed September 28, 2016.

**TABLE 3.17** Weekly vegetable subgroup recommendations

| Vegetable | Children (Years) | | Girls (Years) | | Boys (Years) | | Women (Years) | | | Men (Years) | | |
|---|---|---|---|---|---|---|---|---|---|---|---|---|
| | 2–3 | 4–8 | 9–13 | 14–18 | 9–13 | 14–18 | 19–30 | 31–50 | 51+ | 19–30 | 31–50 | 51+ |
| Dark green (cups) | 0.5 | 1 | 1.5 | 1.5 | 1.5 | 2 | 1.5 | 1.5 | 1.5 | 2 | 2 | 1.5 |
| Red, orange (cups) | 2.5 | 3 | 4 | 5.5 | 5.5 | 6 | 5.5 | 5.5 | 4 | 6 | 6 | 5.5 |
| Beans, peas (cups) | 0.5 | 0.5 | 1 | 1.5 | 1.5 | 2 | 1.5 | 1.5 | 1 | 2 | 2 | 1.5 |
| Starchy (cups) | 2 | 3.5 | 4 | 5 | 5 | 6 | 5 | 5 | 4 | 6 | 6 | 5 |
| Other (cups) | 1.5 | 2.5 | 3.5 | 4 | 4 | 5 | 4 | 4 | 3.5 | 5 | 5 | 4 |

Adapted from USDA Choose MyPlate. Vegetables. ChooseMyPlate.gov. https://www.choosemyplate.gov/vegetables. Last updated July 26, 2016. Accessed September 28, 2016.

**TABLE 3.18** Daily minimum amount of whole grains (in oz. equivalents)

| Children (Years) | | Girls (Years) | | Boys (Years) | | Women (Years) | | | Men (Years) | | |
|---|---|---|---|---|---|---|---|---|---|---|---|
| 2–3 | 4–8 | 9–13 | 14–18 | 9–13 | 14–18 | 19–30 | 31–50 | 51+ | 19–30 | 31–50 | 51+ |
| 1.5 | 2.5 | 3 | 3 | 3 | 4 | 3 | 3 | 3 | 4 | 3.5 | 3 |

Modified from USDA Choose MyPlate. Grains. ChooseMyPlate.gov. https://www.choosemyplate.gov/grains. Last updated October 18, 2016. Accessed September 28, 2016.

of the majority of the population (approximately 98%), and adequate intake, the level used in the event average nutrient requirement is unable to be determined. Although the pattern does successfully cover the requirements for most nutrients, a few—vitamin D, vitamin E, potassium, and choline—have fallen marginally below the RDA or AI recommendations. However, inadequate intake for these nutrients has not been determined to be a public health concern. In addition to the Healthy US-Style Eating Pattern, the USDA has developed the Healthy Mediterranean-Style and Healthy Vegetarian Eating Patterns. The USDA Food Patterns are notably versatile, because they demonstrate healthy eating patterns that can be applied across the board to many cultures, many personal preferences, and varying dietary requirements. They are a

**TABLE 3.19** Cup and ounce equivalents: USDA's Healthy US-Style Eating Pattern

| | Vegetables | Fruits | Grains | Dairy | Protein |
|---|---|---|---|---|---|
| 0.5 cup equivalent | 0.5 cup green beans | 0.5 cup strawberries | — | — | — |
| | 1 cup raw spinach | 0.25 cup raisins | — | — | — |
| 0.75 cup equivalent | — | 0.75 cup 100% OJ | — | 6 oz. fat-free yogurt | |
| 1 oz. equivalent | — | — | 1 slice bread | — | 1 large egg |
| | — | — | 0.5 cup cooked brown rice | — | — |
| 1 cup equivalent | — | — | — | 1.5 oz. cheddar cheese | — |
| 2 oz. equivalents | — | — | — | — | 2 Tbsp peanut butter |
| | — | — | — | — | 0.5 cup black beans |
| 4 oz. equivalents | — | — | — | — | 4 oz. pork |

Modified from U.S. Department of Health and Human Services and U.S. Department of Agriculture (2015). 2015–2020 *Dietary Guidelines For Americans* 8th Edition. Figure 1-1 Cup-& Ounce-Equivalents. Page 19. https://health.gov/dietaryguidelines/2015/guidelines. Accessed July 27, 2016.

useful tool for planning and serving meals for home, school, work, and other everyday environments.[10]

**Recap** The MyPlate food guide was created as an interpretation of the *Dietary Guidelines* to help Americans apply the central ideas to their individual diets. The USDA Food Patterns summarize ways to meet these nutrient needs without consuming excessive calories.

## ▶ Chapter Summary

The US Department of Agriculture, the Department of Health and Human Services, and other federal government agencies constantly assess the composition of foods and the quality of dietary intake among Americans in an effort to support consumption that meets recommended needs and reduces the risk of chronic disease. The *Dietary Guidelines for Americans* represent the ideal eating behaviors for optimal nutritional status. The *Dietary Guidelines* is the standard against which researchers compare population intake patterns and data collected through the use of dietary quality-assessment tools such as the Healthy Eating Index.

The USDA supplements the *Dietary Guidelines* with consumer education materials and infographics, the most current of which is MyPlate, the result of a 25-year evolution of the Food Guide Pyramid to accurately reflect the messages communicated by the latest *Dietary Guidelines*; its format is most likely to resonate with the American population. The concern of adequately communicating messages to consumers is also demonstrated in the newly revised Nutrition Facts Label. Changes were made to highlight key nutrients contributing to health status, with aesthetics designed to attract customer focus to the important components. Given the progressive change in our country's health status and eating behaviors, nutrition research, legislature, education, and recommendations will continue to adapt to keep up with current trends, knowledge, and needs.

## CASE STUDY

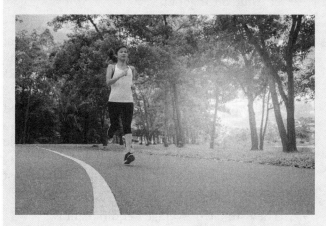

© CrispyPork/Shutterstock.

Providing dietary recommendations to an individual is a complex and involved process, as was discussed in this chapter. Although these recommendations can be made for the broader population, it is often necessary to tailor them to a specific person's needs. Consider Joanne, for example.

Joanne is a 23-year-old woman who is 5' 7" and weighs 135 lbs. She currently works as a teaching assistant at a university, and spends 30 to 60 minutes a day walking around campus. She also jogs 60 minutes a day, six days a week. She has read on the Internet that in order to stay thin, she should limit her carbohydrate intake, and she is, therefore, currently consuming about 150 g of carbohydrate per day. Her daily energy intake is between 1,900 and 2,000 calories. She has been losing weight quite rapidly and is extremely fatigued, not only during her runs but also throughout the rest of the day.

### Questions:

1. Calculate Joanne's estimated energy requirement (EER) using an equation from Table 3.9 and physical-activity coefficient from Table 3.10.
2. Is Joanne currently meeting her caloric requirements for the day?
3. Using the total energy expenditure (TEE) value that you calculate for Joanne, determine how many grams of carbohydrate, protein, and fat she should be consuming each day.
4. Assess Joanne's current carbohydrate intake compared to intake recommended for her. If she is not consuming enough carbohydrate, provide examples of healthy carbohydrate-containing foods that she can incorporate into her diet.
5. Using your calculations and Joanne's current diet and exercise regimen, provide possible reasons why Joanne is feeling fatigued and losing weight.

# Learning Portfolio

## Key Terms

Adequate intake (AI)
Acceptable macronutrient distribution range (AMDR)
Basal Energy Expenditure (BEE)
Dietary Reference Intakes (DRIs)
Energy density
Estimated Average Requirement (EAR)
Estimated Energy Requirement (EER)

Healthy Eating Index (HEI)
Nutrient density
Recommended Dietary Allowance (RDA)
Resting Energy Expenditure (REE)
Thermic effect of activity (TEA)
Thermic effect of food (TEF)
Tolerable upper intake level (UL)

## Study Questions

1. What year were the first *Dietary Guidelines* released?
   a. 1985
   b. 1977
   c. 1980
   d. 1990

2. Who is responsible for issuing the *Dietary Guidelines*?
   a. USDA and HHS
   b. DHS and HHS
   c. USDA and FDA
   d. HHS and FDA

3. What year were the first USDA food guides issued?
   a. 1916
   b. 1956
   d. 1992
   d. 2011

4. Which food guide includes a visual representation for physical activity?
   a. MyPlate
   b. Food Guide Pyramid
   c. MyPyramid
   d. *Food for Fitness*

5. Which of the following is not one of the Dietary Reference Intakes?
   a. Recommended Dietary Allowance
   b. Adequate intake
   c. Acceptable macronutrient distribution range
   d. Estimated Average Requirement

6. The primary uses of the DRIs include all except:
   a. Assessing the intakes of individuals.
   b. Rating the intakes of individuals.
   c. Planning diets for individuals.
   d. Planning diets for groups.

7. The DRI committees have been established by governments of the United States and
   a. Australia.
   b. France.
   c. United Kingdom.
   d. Canada.

8. Which of the following pertains to *relevant* data:
   a. Study results are generalizable to the North American population and to DRI development.
   b. Study results are generalizable to the United States population and to DRI development.
   c. Research was unlikely to have been available to the previous DRI expert panel.
   d. Research has been conducted within the last two years.

9. The Estimated Average Requirement is:
   a. The average daily nutrient intake estimated to meet the needs of half of the healthy individuals in a group.
   b. The average daily nutrient intake level sufficient to meet the nutrient requirement of almost all healthy individuals in a group.
   c. The recommended average daily intake based on observed or experimentally determined approximations or estimations of nutrient intake by a group.
   d. A set of nutrient-based reference values that are quantitative estimates of nutrient intakes used for planning and assessing diets for healthy people.

10. The EAR has not been established for:
    a. Vitamin E
    b. Molybdenum
    c. Phosphorus
    d. Vitamin D

11. The EAR serves as the basis for calculating which other DRI standard?
    a. UL
    b. AI
    c. RDA
    d. EER

12. The main purpose of the EAR is to:
    a. Assess the adequacy of population intakes.
    b. Assess the adequacy of individual intakes.
    c. Be the goal for daily intake by individuals.
    d. Be the goal for daily intake by populations.

13. When the RDA cannot be determined, which other standard of nutrient intake is used?
    a. DRI
    b. EAR
    c. AMDR
    d. AI

14. The RDA is established based on which other standard of nutrient intake?
    a. AI
    b. EAR
    c. DRI
    d. UL

15. Which of the following is not true about the RDA?
    a. It is used to assess the intake of groups.
    b. It is used to assess the intake of individuals.
    c. It is determined from the EAR.
    d. It is sufficient to meet the requirements of 97% to 98% of healthy individuals in a group.

16. RDA is defined as:
    a. The average daily nutrient intake level sufficient to meet the nutrient requirement of half the individuals in a group.
    b. The average daily nutrient intake level sufficient to meet all of the individuals in a group.
    c. The average daily dietary nutrient intake level sufficient to meet the nutrient requirement of nearly all individuals in a group.
    d. The mean intake of a nutrient for individuals in a group.

17. Tolerable upper intake level is defined as:
    a. The recommended average daily intake based on observed or experimentally determined approximations or estimations of nutrient intake by a group.
    b. The highest average daily nutrient intake level likely to pose no risk of adverse health effects to almost all individuals in a group.
    c. A set of nutrient-based reference values that are quantitative estimates of nutrient intakes used for planning and assessing diets for healthy people.
    d. The average daily nutrient intake level sufficient to meet the nutrient requirement of almost all healthy individuals in a group.

18. Tolerable upper intake level has been established for:
    a. All micronutrients.
    b. All macronutrients.
    c. Some micronutrients.
    d. Some macronutrients.

19. Which of the following is true?
    a. As intake increases above the UL, the risk for potential adverse events decreases.
    b. As intake decreases below the UL, the risk for potential adverse events decreases.
    c. As intake decreases below the UL, the risk for potential adverse events increases.
    d. As intake increases above the UL, the risk for potential adverse events increases.

20. The UL was established in response to:
    a. Pressure by the federal government.
    b. The increase in fortified foods and dietary supplementation usage.
    c. The growing number of individuals with toxic levels of nutrients.
    d. The establishment of UL in Canada.

21. Energy requirement is most precisely measured from:
    a. Energy expenditure.
    b. Energy intake.
    c. Energy expenditure and energy intake.
    d. Energy intake and physical activity.

22. All of the following are methods used to measure energy expenditure in humans except:
    a. Indirect calorimetry.
    b. Direct calorimetry.
    c. Doubly labeled water.
    d. Double-blind water studies.

23. Which of the following is not a component of total energy expenditure?
    a. Resting Energy Expenditure
    b. Basal Energy Expenditure
    c. Exercise activity thermogenesis
    d. Resting activity thermogenesis

24. The total number of calories a person needs per day depends on which factors?
    - i. Age
    - ii. Sex
    - iii. Physical activity level
    - iv. Maximal oxygen consumption ($VO_2max$)
    - v. Height
    - vi. Weight
    - vii. Medical condition
    a. i, ii, iii, v, vi
    b. i, ii, iii, iv, v, vi
    c. i, ii, v, vi
    d. i, ii, iii, v, vi, vii

25. The RDA for carbohydrates for adults and children is:
    a. 120 g/day.
    b. 100 g/day.
    c. 130 g/day.
    d. 140 g/day.

26. The EAR for carbohydrates is established based on:
    a. Amount of fat absorbed and stored as adipose tissue.
    b. Amount of protein able to be used by the body.
    c. Average amount of protein needed for physical activity.
    d. Average amount of glucose used by the brain.

27. Insufficient data exists for which standard of nutrient intake to establish any specific recommendations for macronutrients?
    a. EAR
    b. UL
    c. RDA
    d. AMDR

28. The AMDR was established in the interest of the risk for:
    a. Chronic disease.
    b. Obesity.
    c. Malnutrition.
    d. Fat overconsumption.

29. Nutrient-dense foods:
    a. Have a high concentration of nutrients per amount of food.
    b. Have a high concentration of fats and added sugars per amount of food.
    c. Contain a high number of individual vitamins and minerals.
    d. Contain a high number of vitamins, minerals, fats, and sugars.

30. All of the following are nutrient-density profiling tools except:
    a. The nutrient-dense foods index.
    b. The nutrient-rich foods index.
    c. The affordable nutrition index.
    d. The Guiding Stars program.

31. The most widely used front-of-packaging labeling tool is:
    a. Guiding Stars.
    b. Powerhouse Fruits and Vegetables.
    c. Healthy eating systems.
    d. Nutrient Density Climate Index.

32. Energy density is:
    a. The weight of a food or a beverage.
    b. The amount of calories in a food item.
    c. The amount of energy per weight of food or beverage.
    d. The amount of exercise required to burn off a food item.

33. The Healthy Eating Index (HEI) assesses conformance to:
    a. The *Dietary Guidelines for Americans.*
    b. Estimated Energy Requirement.
    c. Recommended Dietary Allowances.
    d. Macronutrient recommendations.

34. Which organization established the HEI?
    a. World Health Organization
    b. Centers for Disease Control and Prevention
    c. Center for Nutrition Policy and Promotion
    d. US Food and Drug Administration

35. Uses of the HEI include all except:
    a. Determining the relationship between diet cost and diet quality.
    b. Evaluating food environments.
    c. Evaluating personal food choices versus the food choices of others.
    d. Examining relationships between diet and outcomes of public health concern.

36. The components of the Alternative Healthy Eating Index (AHEI) include:
    a. Vegetables, fruit, nuts and soy, wheat, polyunsaturated and saturated fatty acids, red and white meat.
    b. Vegetables, fruit, nuts and soy, cereal fiber, monounsaturated fatty acids, red and white meat.
    c. Vegetables, fruit, nuts and soy, cereal fiber, saturated fatty acids, red and white meat.
    d. Vegetables, fruit, nuts and soy, cereal fiber, polyunsaturated and saturated fatty acids, red and white meat.

37. How often are the *Dietary Guidelines* published?
    a. Every 10 years
    b. Every five years
    c. Every year
    d. On an as-needed basis

38. The recommendations in the *Dietary Guidelines* are provided for the purpose of all of the following except:
    a. To promote health.
    b. To prevent chronic disease.
    c. To help people reach and maintain healthy weight.
    d. To help people maintain appropriate weight and manage their chronic diseases.

39. The process for developing the *Dietary Guidelines* includes all of the following except:
    a. Conducting the research.
    b. Reviewing the science.
    c. Developing the *Dietary Guidelines*.
    d. Implementing the *Dietary Guidelines*.

40. The *Dietary Guidelines 2015* recommend Americans:
    a. Consume <20% of their daily calories from added sugars.
    b. Consume <20% of their daily calories from total fat.
    c. Consume >2300 mg sodium per day.
    d. Consume <10% of their daily calories from saturated fats.

41. The size of print has been increased in the new Nutrition Facts Label for which three nutrition factors?
    a. Calories, servings per container, serving size
    b. Calories from fat, servings per container, serving size
    c. Calories, trans fat, serving size
    d. Calories, trans fat, saturated fat

42. Daily values for which three nutrients are being updated?
    a. Sodium, calcium, vitamin D
    b. Saturated fat, vitamin D, dietary fiber
    c. Sodium, dietary fiber, vitamin D
    d. Saturated fat, vitamin D, vitamin C

43. The % daily value is based on a diet of how many calories per day?
    a. 1500
    b. 2000
    c. 2200
    d. 1800

44. Which parameter has been removed from the new Nutrition Facts Label?
    a. Calories from fat
    b. Total fat
    c. Vitamin C
    d. Dietary fiber

45. The recommended daily amount of fruit intake for men and women ages 19 to 30 years old is:
    a. 1.5 cups
    b. 1–1.5 cups
    c. 2 cups
    d. 1 cup

46. The two subgroups of grains are:
    a. Unrefined and refined.
    b. Whole and refined.
    c. Gluten and gluten-free.
    d. White and whole wheat.

47. The healthy US-Style Eating Pattern was formulated to comply with which nutrient intake standards?
    i. DRI
    ii. RDA
    iii. EAR
    iv. UL
    v. AI
    vi. AMDR
    a. i, v, vi
    b. ii, iii, v, vi
    c. ii, v, vi
    d. ii, iiii, v

48. How many different calorie levels of Food Patterns are provided in the healthy US-Style Eating Pattern?
    a. 5
    b. 12
    c. 15
    d. 3

## Discussion Questions

1. What standards and recommendations do you see being incorporated into future dietary guidelines and the USDA Food Guides?
2. Why might the progression of the USDA Food Guides have been geared toward giving consumers a visual representation of portion sizes, and how might the current MyPlate food guide be improved?
3. What are the main differences or improvements between the DRIs and the previous RDA and RNI standards?

4. Explain the key processes for creating and updating the DRIs. What is the basis for the DRI committees to review a nutrient?

5. Which nutrients do you think should be proposed for establishing an EAR in future reviews?

6. Explain why there is no EAR for saturated fat, monounsaturated fat. and cholesterol.

7. How does the RDA differ from the EAR in the way that it is determined, used, applied?

8. Do you think the UL is a useful or necessary DRI standard? Explain.

9. Compare and contrast indirect and direct calorimetry.

10. Consider a way in which an individual might increase total energy expenditure for the day without increasing amount of exercise (i.e. no change in the thermic effect of activity).

11. Discuss some of the ways in which variables such as age, gender, physical activity level, weight, and height contribute to the variation in estimated calorie needs per day (see Table 3.8) among different people.

12. What are some instances in which the AMDR would be useful?

13. What recommendation would you give someone about her daily allowance of saturated fat and cholesterol? Explain why there are no RDAs for these nutrients.

14. Provide examples of foods that are not nutrient dense and suggest preferred options.

15. Think of an example of a common energy-dense meal that is simultaneously low in nutrients. Consider how you might make substitutions to make it less energy dense while being *more* nutrient dense.

16. What initiatives or legislation would you suggest to improve the diet quality of the American population?

17. Describe a diet that would receive a Healthy Eating Index Score of 100. Refer to the *Dietary Guidelines for Americans.*

18. Do you think the *Dietary Guidelines* have been effective in influencing the eating habits of Americans?

19. Describe how new *Dietary Guidelines* would be developed, including the federal departments involved.

20. What other changes to the food label beyond those being implemented do you think would be beneficial and why?

21. Explain the reasoning behind the updates to the Nutrition Facts Label, including added sugars, calories from fat being removed, and daily values for sodium, dietary fiber, and Vitamin D.

22. Does the MyPlate visual adequately represent the food group recommendations specified in the literature?

23. Explain the four main focuses of MyPlate as well as examples of acceptable foods from each of the five food groups.

## Activities

1. In a group of two or three students, write down what you ate for breakfast, lunch, and dinner yesterday. Distribute your food records among the group so that everyone is reading someone's record other than their own. Now identify which foods from your classmate's food record are nutrient dense and which are energy dense. Include the aspects of those foods that led you to label them as either nutrient or energy dense. Write down a suggestion on your classmate's paper about how they might substitute one or two of the foods they are eating with healthier, nutrient-dense options.

2. Review the *Dietary Guidelines for Americans 2015*, including the criteria for a healthy eating pattern. Then write a sample day of eating that follows the guidelines and consists of four different meals. Include food groups and types but not specific portion sizes.

   **Example Meal**
   One serving whole wheat bread
   Mashed avocado
   Two eggs, fried in olive oil
   One medium apple
   Glass of 2% milk

## Online Resources

**Center for Nutrition Policy and Promotion**
www.cnpp.usda.gov

**Department of Health and Human Services**
www.hhs.gov

**Food and Drug Administration**
FDA.gov

**MyPlate SuperTracker**
supertracker.usda.gov

**Nutrition Evidence Library**
NEL.gov

**Nutrition Facts Label**
www.cfsan.fda.gov/~dms/foodlab.html

**Nutrition Information**
www.nutrition.gov

**Office of Disease Prevention and Health Promotion**
health.gov

**United States Department of Agriculture**
USDA.gov

# References

1. US Department of Agriculture (USDA). 2015 Dietary Guidelines for Advisory Committee. DGAC Meeting 1: Materials and Presentations. https://health.gov/dietaryguide lines/2015-binder/meeting1/historycurrentuse.aspx.

2. Institute of Medicine (US), Committee on Use of Dietary Reference Intakes in Nutrition Labeling. Dietary Reference Intakes: Guiding Principles for Nutrition Labeling and Fortification. Washington, DC: National Academies Press; 2003: 4. https://www.ncbi.nlm.nih.gov/books/NBK208878/.

3. Murphy SP, Yates AA, Atkinson SA, Barr SI, Dwyer J. History of nutrition: The long road leading to the Dietary Reference Intakes for the United States and Canada. *Adv Nutr* 2016; 7:157-168.

4. USDA. Choose MyPlate. A brief history of USDA Food Guides. choosemyplate.gov. https://www.choosemyplate.gov/content /brief-history-usda-food-guides. Accessed September 28, 2016.

5. Institute of Medicine of the National Academies. *Dietary Reference Intakes: The Essential Guide to Nutrient Requirements.* Washington, DC: The National Academy Press; 2006.

6. National Academy of Sciences. *Dietary Reference Intakes for Energy, Carbohydrate, Fiber, Fat, Fatty Acids, Cholesterol, Protein, and Amino Acids (Macronutrients).* Washington, DC: National Academy Press; 2002/2005.

7. Academy of Nutrition and Dietetics. Definitions of energy expenditure. Nutrition Care Manual. https://www .nutritioncaremanual.org/topic.cfm?ncm_category_id=11& lv1=144882&lv2=144895&ncm_toc_id=144895&ncm _heading=&. Accessed July 27, 2016.

8. Academy of Nutrition and Dietetics. Energy metabolism. Nutrition Care Manual. https://www.nutritioncaremanual .org/topic.cfm?ncm_category_id=11&lv1=144882&ncm _toc_id=144882&ncm_heading=&. Accessed July 27, 2016.

9. Academy of Nutrition and Dietetics. Measurement of energy expenditure. Nutrition Care Manual. https://www .nutritioncaremanual.org/topic.cfm?ncm_category_id=11 &lv1=144882&lv2=144900&ncm_toc_id=144900&ncm _heading=&. Accessed July 27, 2016.

10. US Department of Health and Human Services (HHS), USDA. *2015–2020 Dietary Guidelines For Americans.* 8th ed. Washington, DC: US Government Printing Office, 2015.

11. HHS, USDA. *2015–2020 Dietary Guidelines For Americans.* 8th ed. Appendix 2. Estimated calorie needs per day, by age, sex and physical activity level. Washington, DC: US Government Printing Office, 2015.

12. Academy of Nutrition and Dietetics. Predictive equations. Nutrition Care Manual. https://www.nutritioncaremanual.org /topic.cfm?ncm_category_id=11&lv1=144882&lv2=144904&ncm _toc_id=144905&ncm_heading=&.

13. Dietary Guidelines Advisory Committee. *Report of the Dietary Guidelines Advisory Committee on the Dietary Guidelines for Americans, 2010, to the Secretary of Agriculture and the Secretary of Health and Human Services.* Appendix E-4: History of the dietary guidelines for Americans. Washington, DC: USDA, Agricultural Research Service, 2010.

14. Hingle MD, Kandiah J, Maggi A. Practice paper of the Academy of Nutrition and Dietetics: Selecting nutrient-dense foods for good health. *J Acad Nutr Diet.* 2016; 116(9):1473-1479.

15. USDA Center for Nutrition Policy and Promotion. Healthy Eating Index (HEI). https://www.cnpp.usda.gov/healthyeating index. Accessed September 28, 2016.

16. Snetselaar L. Are Americans following US dietary guidelines? Elsevier.com. March 2, 2015. https://www.elsevier.com/connect /are-americans-following-us-dietary-guidelines-check-the -healthy-eating-index.

17. Scientific Report of the 2015 Dietary Guidelines Advisory Committee. Appendix E-3.1. Adequacy of USDA Food Patterns. https://health.gov/dietaryguidelines/2015-scientific-report /PDFs/Appendix-E-3.1.pdf. Accessed September 28, 2016.

18. USDA. *A Series of Systematic Reviews on the Relationship Between Dietary Patterns and Health Outcomes.* Alexandria, VA: USDA; 2014. http://www.nel.gov/vault/2440/web/files/Dietary Patterns/DPRptFullFinal.pdf.

19. Office of Disease Prevention and Health Promotion (ODPHP). Dietary Guidelines Purpose. health.gov. https://health.gov/die taryguidelines/purpose.asp. Accessed July 27, 2016.

20. ODPHP. Dietary Guidelines Process. health.gov. https:// health.gov/dietaryguidelines/process.asp. Accessed July 27, 2016.

21. ODPHP. Dietary Guidelines Evolution. health.gov. https:// health.gov/dietaryguidelines/evolution.asp. Accessed July 27, 2016.

22. US Food and Drug Administration (FDA). How to understand and use the Nutrition Facts Label. fda.gov. http://www.fda .gov/Food/IngredientsPackagingLabeling/LabelingNutrition /ucm274593.htm. Accessed September 6, 2016.

23. FDA. Changes to the Nutrition Facts Label. fda.gov. http:// www.fda.gov/Food/GuidanceRegulation/Guidance DocumentsRegulatoryInformation/LabelingNutrition /ucm385663.htm. Accessed September 6, 2016.

24. USDA Choose MyPlate. Choose MyPlate. choosemyplate. gov. https://www.choosemyplate.gov. Accessed September 28, 2016.

25. USDA Choose MyPlate. Fruit. ChooseMyPlate.gov. https:// www.choosemyplate.gov/fruit. Accessed September 28, 2016.

26. USDA Choose MyPlate. Vegetables. ChooseMyPlate.gov. https ://www.choosemyplate.gov/vegetables. Accessed September 28, 2016.

27. USDA Choose MyPlate. Grains. ChooseMyPlate.gov. https:// www.choosemyplate.gov/grains. Accessed September 28, 2016.

28. USDA Choose MyPlate. Protein. ChooseMyPlate.gov. https:// www.choosemyplate.gov/protein-foods. Accessed September 28, 2016.

29. USDA Choose MyPlate. Dairy. ChooseMyPlate.gov. https:// www.choosemyplate.gov/dairy. Accessed September 28, 2016.

30. USDA Choose MyPlate. Oils. ChooseMyPlate.gov. https:// www.choosemyplate.gov/oils. Accessed September 28, 2016.

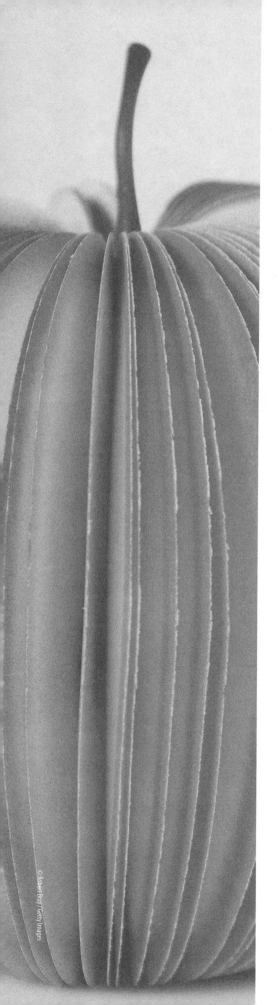

# Methods of Evaluation: Dietary Methods

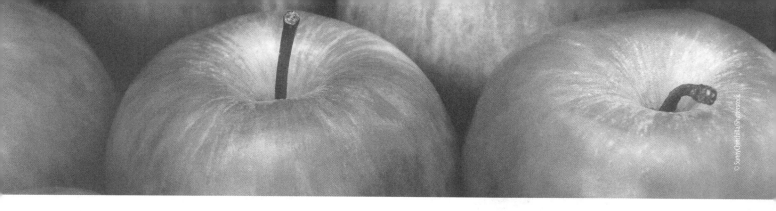

# CHAPTER 4

# Measuring Nutrient Intake

**Crystal L. Wynn**, PhD, MPH, RD
**Nava Livne**, PhD, MS

## CHAPTER OUTLINE

- Introduction
- Relationship between Diet and Health
- Methods for Measuring Usual Dietary Intake
- Methods Designed to Measure Food and Nutrient Intake
- Challenges in Food and Nutrient Intake Measurement Methods
- Chapter Summary

## LEARNING OBJECTIVES

After completing this chapter, the reader should be able to:
1. Discuss the relationship between diet and health.
2. List the methods for measuring usual diet intake.
3. Describe the methods for measuring food and nutrient intake.
4. Explain the various challenges encountered with diet assessment methods.
5. Explain methods for measuring and estimating portion sizes.

## ▶ Introduction

Nutrient intake is a major factor in health and nutritional status. Measuring an individual's nutrient and dietary intake can be extremely difficult and labor intensive. Many factors can affect the reliability of dietary assessment methods. One factor that influences the reliability of data used in nutrition-assessment methods is that nutrition professionals frequently rely on information provided by individuals other than actual patients or clients. Aside from that, self-reported intake has a tendency to differ from actual intake. Memory recall and portion-size errors may create systematic errors in intake measurement.[1]

In this chapter, we will discuss the relationship between diet and disease, as well as the various methods for measuring nutrient intake, their strengths, and their limitations. Challenges involving measuring nutrient intake such as reliability or reproducibility and validity will be reviewed.

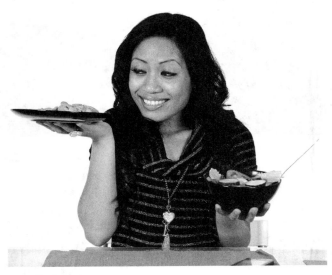

© Mehmet Dilsiz/Shutterstock.

Data collected from dietary intake records are vital in determining relationships between diet and health as well as relationships between diet and disease. For instance, data on food intake and the use of supplements before and during pregnancy helped define the association between low intake of folic acid and neural tube defects in offspring; this was later determined to be a causal relationship.[1,4]

In addition, dietary data are important to assist researchers in identifying populations at risk for inadequate nutrient intake, whether deficiency or excess. Information gathered from research studies can be used to develop interventions, programs, and policies that can aid in health education and promotion.[5]

> **Recap**   Collecting dietary intake data is an important component of monitoring individuals and community health.

# ▶ Relationship Between Diet and Health

> **Preview**   Researchers seek to measure nutrient intake for various reasons. Food and nutrition are important components of health at both the individual and population levels. Monitoring and evaluating eating patterns is important when assessing the effectiveness of public-health interventions to improve diet and health.

## Nutritional Epidemiology

**Nutritional epidemiology** is a sub-discipline of epidemiology that provides data about the relationship between diet and disease. The data collected is used to define diet–disease associations that are converted into the practice of prevention by public-health nutrition practitioners.[2] Nutritional epidemiology is the study of the nutritional factors that contribute to disease in human populations.

Dietary intake normally includes all foods and beverages consumed via the oral cavity. Clinicians such as registered dietitian nutritionists (RDNs) and public-health practitioners measure dietary intake in efforts to acquire quantitative data on the quantities of energy and nutrients accessible for metabolism. Measuring dietary intake is a way of describing the actual food intake of both individuals and groups.[3]

# ▶ Methods for Measuring Usual Dietary Intake

> **Preview**   Researchers, RDNs, nurses, and other healthcare professionals use various methods to measure food intake. Each method has its own advantages and disadvantages. Study design and characteristics of study participants are also presented.

## Research Design

Research falls into two major categories of design type: observational and experimental.[6] Observational studies include cohort, cross-sectional, and case-control. Experimental studies include randomized controlled trials (RCTs). Observational study designs are widely used in studies measuring nutrient intake. **Cohort** studies are generally used to identify factors that may cause a disease to develop in a certain group over time—that is, the natural history of disease development.[6]

Studies can be either prospective or retrospective. A prospective analysis involves observing a group of subjects over an extended period of time to predict an outcome. A retrospective study—also known as a *historic cohort study*—is a study design in which a cohort of individuals is categorized as either having some outcome (case) or not (control). The outcome of interest might be a disease and the medical history associated with that outcome.[7] These research designs are used to collect dietary data. Tools such as **24-hour recall** record, a **food-frequency questionnaire (FFQ)**, or a **food record** are often used to collect nutrient-related data.

In a **longitudinal study**, data are repeatedly gathered for the same subjects over a determined period of time. Longitudinal research projects can extend over many years or decades. For example, the Framingham study is the first longitudinal study that followed a large cohort of subjects to study the etiology of cardiovascular diseases in the United States.[8,9]

The origin of the Framingham study is closely linked to the cardiovascular health of President Franklin D. Roosevelt, who died prematurely from hypertensive heart disease and stroke in 1945.[8] In the year 1948, 5,209 men and women from Framingham, Massachusetts formed the original cohort to identify heritability of cardiovascular diseases and related risk factors.[9] The cohort has contributed to the current understanding of cardiovascular disease and its risk factors.[8]

In healthcare research, a cross-sectional study (also referred to as a *cross-sectional, transversal,* or *prevalence study*) is a category of observational study that examines data collected from a population or from a representative subset at a specific point in time.[6] It typically represent a "snapshot" of the group of interest, including exposure to a specific risk factor, disease outcome, and distribution patterns. Dietary data collected on cross-sectional samples provide information that can be applied to the health and dietary habits of general segments of the population. The diet assessment tool of choice for cross-sectional studies is the 24-hour recall. The National Health and Nutrition Examination Survey (NHANES) is a cross-sectional study in which a sample of the population ages 1 to 74 years was examined in the early 1970s to look at the health and habits of Americans.[10] Subsequent cross-sectional NHANES surveys have been carried out periodically, and the data have been used to examine associations among variables such as dietary intake and prevalence of risk factors for chronic diseases. Health planners depend on disease-prevalence information to allocate sufficient resources to ensure adequate population care.

Cohort studies are used to estimate the incidence of a condition—that is, the proportion of the population susceptible to developing a disease over time. Cross-sectional studies provide information about the prevalence of a specific outcome to describe the proportion of the population that have a disease or demonstrate a specific outcome at one point in time.

Studies done for **case control** retrospectively compare subjects that have an illness or an outcome of interest (cases) to individuals who do not have the condition or the desired outcome (controls). This type of study compares how the frequency of exposure to a risk factor present in the case and control groups determines the relationship between the risk factor and the disease.

Case-control studies are observational because no intervention is tried and no effort is made to modify the development or progression of the disease. These studies are intended to estimate odds.[6]

In both the cohort and case-control studies, the groups are matched or correlated to disease causes. These studies help outline how factors in the past contribute to an existing disease. Nutrition assessment tools used to measure nutrient intake in these types of studies include FFQs. A study by Jansen et al. examined the relationship between fruit and vegetable consumption and pancreatic cancer[11] using a case-control design. The study matched 1,648 patients to 1,514 control subjects from an overall 2,473 patients from a database of patients with pancreatic adenocarcinoma cases. Both groups completed food-frequency questionnaires (FFQs) defining intakes of fruits and vegetables. The results pointed to a statistically significant inverse association between vegetables, fruits, and dietary fiber consumption and pancreatic cancer occurrence.[11]

## Characteristics of Study Participants

Dietary assessment methods are used to measure nutrient intake in a variety of populations, including children, adults, and the elderly. Segments of research populations have different learning needs and concerns that may impact measuring intake in these groups. Factors that should be considered when determining the best research method to use for collecting data with each group include communication, literacy level, and memory. These constraints dictate the most appropriate dietary assessment method for data collection. For individuals who have difficulty communicating or who may experience memory loss, dietary data may need to be collected from another person, such as a parent, a child, or a spouse.[12]

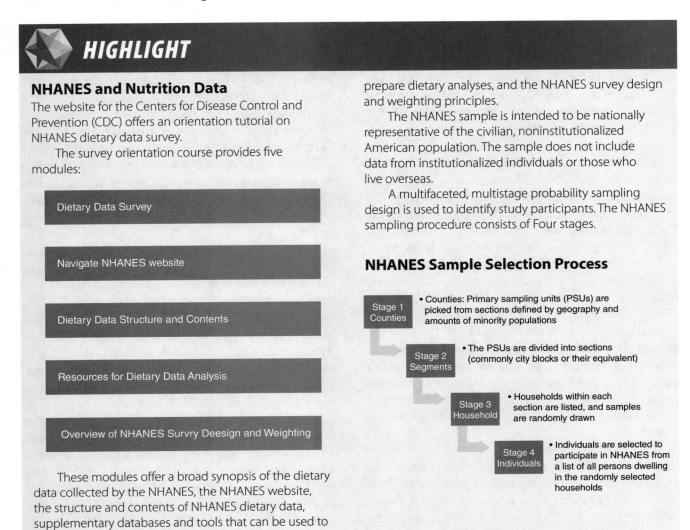

## NHANES and Nutrition Data

The website for the Centers for Disease Control and Prevention (CDC) offers an orientation tutorial on NHANES dietary data survey.

The survey orientation course provides five modules:

Dietary Data Survey

Navigate NHANES website

Dietary Data Structure and Contents

Resources for Dietary Data Analysis

Overview of NHANES Survry Deesign and Weighting

These modules offer a broad synopsis of the dietary data collected by the NHANES, the NHANES website, the structure and contents of NHANES dietary data, supplementary databases and tools that can be used to prepare dietary analyses, and the NHANES survey design and weighting principles.

The NHANES sample is intended to be nationally representative of the civilian, noninstitutionalized American population. The sample does not include data from institutionalized individuals or those who live overseas.

A multifaceted, multistage probability sampling design is used to identify study participants. The NHANES sampling procedure consists of Four stages.

### NHANES Sample Selection Process

**Stage 1 Counties** • Counties: Primary sampling units (PSUs) are picked from sections defined by geography and amounts of minority populations

**Stage 2 Segments** • The PSUs are divided into sections (commonly city blocks or their equivalent)

**Stage 3 Household** • Households within each section are listed, and samples are randomly drawn

**Stage 4 Individuals** • Individuals are selected to participate in NHANES from a list of all persons dwelling in the randomly selected households

Modified from Center for Disease Control and Prevention. Dietary Data Survey Orientation. https://www.cdc.gov/nchs/tutorials/dietary/SurveyOrientation/intro.htm Accessed July 25, 2017.

In some cases, meal observations may be required, as in the case of extremely young children or older adult populations. The 24-hour recall, FFQs, and food records have been used in research studies involving children. For individuals who have literacy challenges, the 24-hour recall or the administered FFQ has been the most effective.[12]

## Factors Affecting Method Selection

Measuring nutrient intake in research studies can be an expensive process from both a monetary and human resource standpoint. The 24-hour recall method requires a trained research interviewer to conduct the recall. This method is labor intensive, and the training for the interviewer can be expensive. In addition, there is daily variation in the reported food intakes, so repeated 24-hour recalls need to be used to control for systematic error measurement.[6] The use of food records requires that research study subjects be trained to complete their intake in the food-record tool. Both the 24-hour recall and food records are demanding because individuals must enter data into a computer for nutrient analysis. Some researchers have found that multiple food records may need to be considered as replacements for multiple or repeated 24-hour recalls because of the reduced respondent burden of memory recall.[13] Another method, the FFQ, can be self-administered, depending on the skill level of the study participants. This questionnaire is least labor intensive because the responses are recorded on a form and then scanned into a computer for analysis.

Overall, for studies requiring a smaller number of subjects, either the 24-hour recall or food record is the preferred method. For large-scale research studies, the FFQ serves as the most appropriate method commonly used.[14]

# VIEWPOINT

## Social Determinants of Health and Their Impact on Obesity

*Diane R. Bridges, PhD, MSN, RN, CCM*

Obesity in the United States can be considered an elusive epidemic. The prevalence of obesity for both adults (those age 20 years and older) and children has been shown to be high in the United States.[1] More than one-third of the adult population is obese, along with one in six children considered obese.[2,3]

Obesity is a condition that crosses many demographics such as ethnicity, gender, and age. Middle-aged and older persons have a higher prevalence (40.2%); 38.8% of women between ages 40 and 59 years were found to be obese.[1] Non-Hispanic black and Mexican American women were found to have a risk of obesity that is twice that of non-Hispanic white women.[4]

Vaccinations are available to treat many viral illnesses, but there is no vaccination to prevent or erase obesity.[5] It can affect the development of chronic diseases from pure physical stress to inflammatory processes, diabetes, arthritis, cardiovascular disease, and other chronic conditions.[4] In addition, the medical costs to treat obesity were shown to be $147 billion annually.[6]

What causes obesity? Many people think obesity can be attributed solely to poor nutrition; typically, the consumption of processed packaged foods high in fructose is to blame. Others contend, however, that a lack of activity and a sedentary lifestyle lead to obesity.[7]

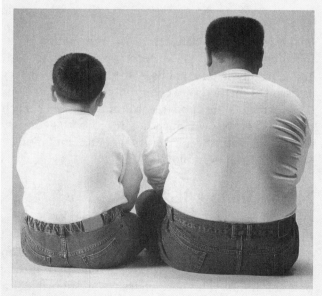

© Topic Images/Getty Images.

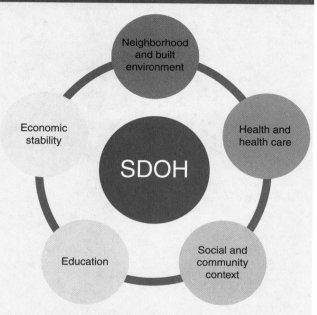

**FIGURE A** Social determinants of health (SDOH) impact one's risk of obesity

Reproduced from Healthy People 2020. U.S. Department of Health and Human Services. https://www.healthypeople.gov/2020/topics-objectives/topic/social-determinants-of-health.

Still others say genetics, race, and ethnicity may all contribute to obesity.[5]

But these are not the only things that affect the rise of obesity. It is the social determinant of health of an individual impact one's risk to obesity as well (see **FIGURE A**). Social determinants of health are "the structural determinants and conditions in which people are born, grow, live, work and age."[8] Income, education, employment, support, stress, food accessibility, transportation, age, race, and ethnicity are all in some way social determinants of health.

Efforts to manage obesity have included education, placing nutritional labels on food packaging, posting nutritional information in restaurants, improving urban development, improving accessibility to food choices, taxing sugared drinks, and policy development.[5] These efforts appear to have had little impact on the prevalence of obesity and adults continue to self-report as obese even in light of their knowledge about the risk of obesity.[5] We need to take on strategies to lower rates of childhood obesity through improved nutritional choices in school, increased physical activity, and allocating more resources to address this important issue.[9]

We need to continue to raise awareness of obesity and other issues in the communities we serve. Students need to be educated in the social determinants of health so they can then become part of the solution.

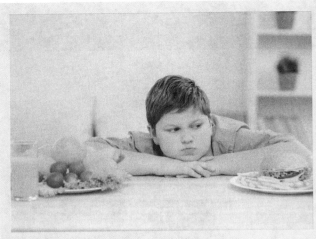

One must become involved in helping to improve the lives of our population by addressing issues that can be prevented.

### References

1. Ogden C, Carroll M, Fryar C, Flegal K. Prevalence of obesity among adults and youth: United States, 2011-2014. US Department of Health and Human Services, Centers for Disease Control and Prevention. *National Center Health Statistic Brief.* 2015; November; 219. Available at http://www .cdc.gov/nchs/products/databriefs.htm. Accessed November 14, 2016.
2. Centers for Disease Control and Prevention. *Adult obesity facts.* Available at https://www.cdc.gov /obesity/data/adult.html. Accessed November 14, 2016.
3. Centers for Disease Control and Prevention. *Childhood overweight and obesity.* Available at https://www.cdc.gov/obesity/childhood/. Accessed November 14, 2016.
4. Graves B. The obesity epidemic: Scope of the problem and management strategies. *J Midwifery Women's Health.* 2010; November–December; 55(6):568–578.
5. Callahan D. Obesity: Chasing an elusive epidemic. *Hastings Center Report.* 2013; 43(1):34–40.
6. Hammond R., Levine R. The economic impact of obesity in the United States. *Diabetes, Metabolic Syndrome and Obesity: Targets and Therapy.* 2010:3:285–295.
7. Radford D, Jones R, Winterstein J. The obesity epidemic. *ACA News (American Chiropractic Association)* [serial online]. 2015; March;11(2):12–17. Available from CINAHL Complete, Ipswich, MA. Accessed November 14, 2016.
8. Heiman H, Artiga S. Beyond health care: The role of social determinants in promoting health and health equity. 2015; November. Available at http:// kff.org/disparities-policy//issue-brief/beyond-health -care-the-role-of-social-determinents-inpromoting -health-and-heal-equity. Accessed November 15, 2016.
9. The role of schools in preventing childhood obesity. The State Education Standard. 2004. Available at: https://www.cdc.gov/healthyyouth/physicalactivity /pdf/roleofschools_obesity.pdf. Accessed November 14, 2016.

**Recap** Researchers use a variety of diet-assessment methods to collect, measure, and analyze nutrient intake. The selection of the assessment tool is primarily determined by the study goal.

## ▶ Methods Designed to Measure Food and Nutrient Intake

**Preview** Measuring nutrient intake can help researchers and care providers across the healthcare spectrum explore the association between diet and disease, determining whether a causal relationship exists between diet and disease, and whether past factors have contributed to current diseases.

Dietary assessment data can reveal information about the long-term past, short-term or immediate past, and current dietary habits. Three types of dietary assessment methods are commonly used: the 24-hour dietary recall, the food record, and the FFQ. Each method has its own purposes in collecting dietary data, along with several advantages and limitations.[14] **FIGURE 4.1** is an example of a FFQ.

### 24-Hour Dietary Recall

One common method for assessing dietary intake is the 24-hour dietary recall. This dietary recall is based on verbal self-reports concerning everything a person ate and drank during a specified time period—the past 24 hours. The interviewer is responsible for recording the dietary data for analysis. Based on this information, generalized assumptions about the individual's eating habits are made. During the interview,

Date:

Name:

| Instructions:  In the past three (3) months did you consume the foods listed below? | | | | | | |
|---|---|---|---|---|---|---|
| **Food Group** | **Frequency** | | | | | |
| | Never | Less than one time per week | 1-6 times per week | 1-3 times per day | 4 or more times per day | Serving size |
| **Dairy:** milk, cheese, yogurt | | | | | | |
| **Chicken:** grilled chicken, baked chicken, fired chicken, etc. | | | | | | |
| **Turkey:** turkey sandwich, soup, breast, roasted, etc. | | | | | | |
| **Beef:** meatballs, steak, etc. | | | | | | |
| **Pork:** cured ham, fresh ham, ribs, pork chops, pulled pork, etc. | | | | | | |
| **Fish and seafood:** shrimp, scallops, fish, shellfish | | | | | | |
| **Other Meat:** lamb, duck, etc. | | | | | | |
| **Nuts:** walnuts, cashews, peanuts, etc. | | | | | | |
| **Beans:** red beans, chick peas, chili, etc. | | | | | | |
| **Egg:** omelet, hard-boiled egg, etc. | | | | | | |
| **Vegetables:** broccoli, cauliflower, green beans, etc. | | | | | | |
| **Fruit:** banana, strawberry, apple, pear, melon, etc. | | | | | | |
| **Grains:** rice, bread, cereal, etc. | | | | | | |
| **Sweets:** cakes, cookies, pies, etc. | | | | | | |
| **Beverages:** coffee, tea, sodas, juices, etc. | | | | | | |

**FIGURE 4.1** Example of a food-frequency questionnaire

Data from Poulain JP, Smith W, Laporte C, Tibere L, Ismail MN, Mognard E., Aloysius M, Neethiahnanthan AR, & Shamsul AM. Studying the consequences of modernization on ethnic food patters: Development of the Malaysian Food Barometer (MFB). Anthropol food. 21 April 2015. Accessed online 26 February 2017 https://aof.revues.org/7735.

the interviewer assists the subject in recalling everything that was consumed during the specified time period. In addition, the interviewer helps the subject estimate the portion sizes of all consumed food items and beverages. The interviewer typically prompts subjects to recall everything they ate in a 24 hour period usually beginning at midnight. During the interview, the subjects are often asked about their activities during the day to facilitate their ability to remember everything they ate or drank during the previous 24 hours. Typically, the researcher reviews the information collected with the subject to ensure that all of the required information has been recorded and to identify errors. Once the data are collected, they can be analyzed using a diet-analysis computer software program.[14]

The 24-hour recall tool can be used in clinical, research, and community settings. It is frequently used in the clinical setting because it has been found to help improve the accuracy of the data reported.

With the advent of digital technology, the use of this tool reduces the burden on the respondent.[15–17]

## Advantages

Regardless of the care setting, the 24-hour recall method has a number of advantages. First, the 24-hour recall is relatively quick and convenient.[18] It is typically inexpensive and places little burden on the subject, who is more willing to respond. Refusals to answer requests for data in this format are less likely. One of the main strengths of the 24-hour recall is that it facilitates comparisons among population groups while describing their unique dietary intakes.[18,19] For example, the NHANES 24-hour recalls have been used to collect data on two consecutive days for describing populations' nutrient intake and group comparisons for identifying relationships between food and diseases between and within groups.[19]

Because this method relies on short-term memory, usual diet and eating habits are less likely to be altered.[18] The 24-hour recall is considered more objective and the preferred method among diet assessment methods.[20,21]

## Limitations

Several limitations have been identified using the 24-hour recall method. These methods are not specific to the clinical setting. An individual's diet intake may vary from day to day, and a 24-hour period may not represent daily variation, which is why collecting data on two nonconsecutive recalls is a best practice when using the 24-hour recall to estimate usual daily dietary intake.[22] To manage limitations, multiple 24-hour recalls on nonconsecutive days be conducted before applying the results to the individual's regular eating habits.[23]

Inaccurate reporting has been identified as another limitation of the 24-hour recall method. Both overreporting and underreporting of actual food intake is common and may occur for various reasons, including inaccurate memory recall, distorted perceptions of portion sizes, and deliberate misreporting to avoid social stigma.

Evidence shows there are gender differences related to the inaccuracies seen in reporting intake on 24-hour recalls.[24] Females have a higher rate of underreporting food intake than males. Among overweight and obese adults, more 24-hour recalls are needed for women than men to reflect an accurate estimate of food intake. As previously mentioned, to control for underreporting systematic biases, collecting data with multiple-pass 24-hour recalls is recommended.[24,25]

The 24-hour recall requires the interviewer and respondent to evoke the previous day's intake several times to obtain accurate information.[25] Depending on the research question, the interviewer might explore facts such as food-preparation methods and the composition of mixed dishes. The quantities of each food consumed are appraised in reference to a commonly used size container such as cups and glasses, standard measuring utensils such as cups and spoons, three-dimensional food models, or visual aids such as food pictures. One advantage of the 24-hour recall is that little burden is placed on the subject. Conversely, one limitation is that data collection depends on the subject's memory and the proficiencies of a well-trained interviewer to diminish recall bias.[14] To reduce limitations and ensure the accuracy of the data collected, adequate, intensive, and thorough training of interviewers is recommended.[26] **TABLE 4.1** shows the advantages and limitations of the 24-hour recall method.

**TABLE 4.1** Advantages and limitations of the 24-hour recall method

| Advantages | Limitations |
|---|---|
| Quick | Diet variation |
| Convenient | Inaccurate reporting |
| Inexpensive | Misreporting |
| Relies on short-term memory | |
| Does not alter the diet | |

Modified from Shim J-S, Oh K, Kim HC. Dietary assessment methods in epidemiologic studies. Epidemiology and Health. 2014;36(e2014009). https://www.ncbi.nlm.nih.gov/pmc/articles/PMC4154347/. Accessed May, 1, 2017.

## Food Record: Diary

The food record or food diary is a subjective dietary intake collection method that relies on the use of open-ended, self-administered questionnaires (see **FIGURE 4.2**). This tool is used to attain detailed information about all foods and beverages consumed over a specified period of time, which can be one or more days.

This open-ended tool offers clinicians and researchers few limitations as to how many items can be inquired about. Normally, subjects are asked to record foods and beverages as they are consumed throughout the day. This is a real-time accounting of their intake. Data collected can include the consumption of dietary supplements. Multiple administrations of a specified number of days are frequently used.

Usually, study participants are provided with a form to record their intake. Oral or written directions (or both) are provided to help participants record pertinent details for all foods and beverages they consume (such as brand name, preparation method, and where consumed). Portion size is either estimated using food models, pictures, or other visual aids; or it is measured using weight scales or volume measures.

The use of food records is widely used not only in research but also in the clinical setting. The information recorded is used to develop nutrition care plans.

Food records or diaries can take different forms. The most simple and cheapest form includes a blank notebook that is small enough to be carried around throughout the day. Typically, when filling out a food diary, the individual estimates meal portion sizes using household measuring utensils such as cups and spoons or measurement scales.[18]

# Food Diary

Use this chart to track the foods you eat over the week. Write in the foods you eat and mark the corresponding check boxes for each serving from a food group to track whether you are meeting recommended servings. Don't forget to include beverages.

| | SUNDAY | MONDAY | TUESDAY | WEDNESDAY | THURSDAY | FRIDAY | SATURDAY |
|---|---|---|---|---|---|---|---|
| Milk & Milk Products<br>Vegetables<br>Fruits<br>Grains<br>Meat & Beans | OOO<br>OOO<br>OO<br>OOOOOO<br>OO | OOO<br>OOO<br>OO<br>OOOOOO<br>OO | OOO<br>OOO<br>OO<br>OOOOOO<br>OO | OOO<br>OOO<br>OO<br>OOOOOO<br>OO | OOO<br>OOO<br>OO<br>OOOOOO<br>OO | OOO<br>OOO<br>OO<br>OOOOOO<br>OO | OOO<br>OOO<br>OO<br>OOOOOO<br>OO |
| Breakfast | | | | | | | |
| Snack | | | | | | | |
| Lunch | | | | | | | |
| Snack | | | | | | | |
| Dinner | | | | | | | |
| Evening Snack | | | | | | | |

**FIGURE 4.2** Example of a food diary

Reproduced from: National Council of California. http://www.healthyeating.org/Healthy-Eating/Healthy-Living/Weight-Management/Article-Viewer/Article/230/Food-Diary.aspx. 2012. Accessed 27 February 2017.

The record includes measures of dietary intake and fluids consumed at breakfast, lunch, and dinner; as well as snacks.

Innovative approaches for evaluating dietary intake are vital in effort to decrease subjects' strain in completing dietary surveys, increase participation rates and thus improve the sample size. It is also important to decrease the effect of quantifying dietary intake on a subject's food choices during the recording period. One method of decreasing the burden placed on those logging dietary intake is to substitute the weighing of foods with approximations of portion size by using tools such as food photographs.

An additional form of food diary that is increasingly popular uses technology-based programs, many of which offer online websites and phone applications (apps) that make logging food intake easy and convenient. Among these programs are MyFitness-Pal, Fitbit, MyPlate, and Lose It! Typically, the apps are downloaded to a smartphone where individuals track their food intake. Some programs allow users to digitally scan barcodes on food packaging for quick item entry. Other apps allow users to take pictures of their meals and have the app estimate portion sizes. Technology-based records also allow users to save a favorite or frequently consumed food to minimize the search time when entering items in the food database.

## Advantages

There are several advantages of food records. For one, they do not rely on an individual's memory, because the data are recorded at the time of consumption.

Young adults prefer technology-based food diaries because they are more accessible and convenient. Kerr et al. found that digital and image-based diet food records could lead to improved cooperation and motivate participants to engage in behavior change such as losing weight, suggesting that digital food diaries may be a useful tool for future health interventions.[11]

## Limitations

Using a food record or diary also has several limitations, regardless of care setting. First, the timing of collecting and recording dietary intakes may be atypical for a participant's regular food intake.[18] Second, subjects who agree to complete a food record may not be representative of the study's target population. Third, completing a food record requires a high literacy level, perhaps excluding those who are not proficient in English. Lack of language proficiency can be an important limitation to consider, because the participant's ability to understand instructions on recording food intake will influence the quality of record keeping.[31] Fourth, this method requires detailed documentation, which may cause individuals to either not fully complete the record for the entire specified time period or cause them to reduce the number of foods eaten. Likewise, the method requires a high level of cooperation, commitment, and compliance.[32] Fifth, the method may alter an individual's diet; participants may decide to eat simpler meals to make record keeping easier, thus eliminating snacks or sugar-sweetened beverages.[32] Sixth, food records provide data on current diet, whereas food intake in the past may be dissimilar. Finally, the method is labor intensive and expensive because of the high cost of training interviewers, administering the tool, and data analysis. **TABLE 4.2** shows the advantages and limitations of food diaries.

## Food-Frequency Questionnaire

FFQs consist of an extensive list of foods and beverages with a range of consumption frequencies that participants can select from for each food. Serving sizes may or may not be present.[18] To evaluate the actual true diet, the number of foods and beverages probed usually ranges from 80 to 120. FFQs are normally created for each study group and research question to ensure that specific characteristics such as ethnicity, culture, an individual's preferences, economic status, and so on are identified. Depending on the interests of the investigator, FFQs can emphasize the collection of data for a specific nutrient and nutritional exposures linked to a disease process, or they can comprehensively assess various nutrients.[22] Through their responses, respondents state how many times a day, week, month, or year they usually consume the foods in question. Although some FFQs include portion sizes, most use a standard portion size based on an amount per serving for a specific age and gender group.[33,34]

There are three basic types of FFQs: the nonquantitative, the semiquantitative, and the quantitative FFQs.[18] The simple or **nonquantitative FFQ** asks respondents how frequently they consume a certain food item per day, week, month, or year; portion sizes are disregarded.[34]

The **semiquantitative FFQ** includes a list of food items, each accompanied with predefined portion sizes, and asks respondents how many times a day, week, month, or year they eat a certain food item (**FIGURE 4.3**).[35]

An FFQ can be used in both clinical and community settings because of its low administration cost and respondent burden. Also, it can be used to measure long-term intake as well as usual intake.[36]

The **quantitative FFQ** asks respondents to describe the daily frequency of food consumption and record the portion size of their serving according to their usual habits.[18] In some instances, respondents are asked to define the portion serving size as small, medium, or large.[37] The usefulness of questions in FFQs related to portion size has been controversial. Some researchers support that between-person deviations in portion size are not significant, because the variation seems to be smaller than the variation in frequency of eating the item.[38] FFQs are normally self-administered. Interviewer administration is done sporadically, usually in cases of low literacy.[18] Once the form is completed, it can be scanned and responses can be downloaded into a computer for analysis.

Three FFQs are widely used in nutrition epidemiological studies: the Harvard Willett Questionnaire, the Block Questionnaire, and the Diet History Questionnaire. The 131-item Harvard Willett includes items such as major sources of nutrients and

| **TABLE 4.2** Advantages and limitations of a food diaries | |
|---|---|
| **Advantages** | **Limitations** |
| Does not rely on memory | Timing of data collection may not be feasible |
| Provides detailed dietary intake data | High literacy level required |
| Can provide personalized dietary feedback | High response burden on participants |
| | Labor intensive |

Modified from Johnson RK, Yon BA, Hankin JH. Dietary assessment and validation. In: Monsen ER, VanHorn L, eds. Research Successful Approaches. 3rd ed. Chicago IL: Diana Faulhaber; 2008:187–204.

| How often, in the past 3 months, did you eat the following? | never | Less than 1 time per week | 1-6 times per week | 1-3 times per day | 4 or more times per day |
|---|---|---|---|---|---|
| **Dairy** (cheese, milk, yogurt, etc.) | | | | | |
| **Chicken** (fried chicken, in soup, grilled chicken, etc.) | | | | | |
| **Turkey** (turkey dinner, turkey sandwich, in soup, etc.) | | | | | |
| **Fish and Seafood** (tuna, shrimp, crab, etc.) | | | | | |
| **Pork** (ham, pork chops, ribs, etc.) | | | | | |
| **Beef** (steak, meatballs, in tacos, etc.) | | | | | |
| **Other Meat** (duck, lamb, venison, etc.) | | | | | |
| **Eggs** (omelet, in salad, in baked goods, etc.) | | | | | |

**FIGURE 4.3** Example of a food-frequency questionnaire

Reproduced from: National Council of California. http://www.healthyeating.org/Healthy-Eating/Healthy-Living/Weight-Management/Article-Viewer/Article/230/Food-Diary.aspx. 2012. Accessed 27 February 2017.

foods of interest.[39] Open-ended questions are used to identify brands of margarine, cooking oils, vitamin or mineral supplements, ready-to-eat cereals, and other foods consumed one time a week. The Harvard Willett questionnaire has one standard portion size for each food item, and respondents are asked to indicate the relative frequency of consumption from nine different response alternatives ranging from less than one time per month to six or more times per day.[39] The self-administered questionnaire is best used in circumstances where intake of simple sugars, sweet foods, and fructose is of major concern.[18]

The 60-item, semiquantitative Block Questionnaire was originally developed by the National Cancer Institute. As a self-administered tool, it can be used in two ways: pen and paper and web based.[39] Several versions to address the needs of many subpopulations such as children, adolescents, adults, and dialysis patients have been developed, as has a Spanish version. Food screeners for adults address nutrients such as sodium, fiber, sugar, and folic acid as well as food groups such as fruits and vegetables.[40] Respondents are asked to estimate their consumption frequencies—daily, weekly, monthly, yearly, rarely, or never—by indicating the exact number of times each food was eaten.[39] Participants also must indicate whether their usual portion size is small, medium, or large compared with a standard.[18,39] For children and adolescents, the Block Kids Food Screener has been used for ages 10 to 17 years. It assesses the intake by food group.[41] Other FFQs used in children and adolescents are Block Questionnaires for ages 2–7 years and 8–17 years, English and Spanish versions, and Block Food Screeners for ages two to 17 years.[42]

To assist participants in estimating the portion sizes, the questionnaire may be accompanied by different sample portion sizes of each food item, geometric models, or food photographs in three portion sizes.[18] Completed questionnaires are checked for accuracy and completeness. Daily intakes of energy and nutrients are estimated by multiplying frequency responses with the specified portion sizes and the nutrient values assigned to each food item in the nutrient database. No information on dietary supplements is usually collected.

A comparison between the Block and Willett questionnaires showed that the Block instrument yielded an overall underestimation bias. The comparison also showed that the Block questionnaire was more accurate in calculating the participants' percent intake of energy from fat and carbohydrate. The Willett questionnaire, in turn, showed no overall underestimation bias and was accurate in determining the intake of vitamin A and calcium.[39]

The Diet History Questionnaire is another self-administered instrument and includes 124 questions about such items as portion sizes and nutrition supplement intake.[43] The questionnaire was developed by the US National Cancer Institute's Risk Factor Monitoring and Methods Branch. This tool is also available in print and web forms.

**TABLE 4.3** shows the advantages and limitations of FFQs.

## Advantages

Regardless of the setting, the FFQ method can be self-administered, takes little time to complete (30–60 minutes), and places minimal burdens on study participants.[44] Administrating this tool to large population groups is inexpensive and can assess current or past diet. The short versions can focus on precise nutrients with few food

**TABLE 4.3** Advantages and limitations of a food-frequency questionnaire

| Advantages | Limitations |
|---|---|
| Self-administered Inexpensive Representative of usual intake | Relies on memory recall Consumption is not quantifiable Lack of homogeneity in food choices |

Modified from Adamson AJ, Collerton J, Davies K, et al. Nutrition in advanced age: dietary assessment in the Newcastle 85+ study. *Eur J Clin Nutr.* 2009;63(S1):S6-S18.

sources. Data received from this method are representative of usual intake and capture habitual food intake. The advantages listed make the FFQ the preferred method for evaluating diet–disease relationships in epidemiologic studies.[45]

## Limitations

Data collected through the use of FFQ have non-negligible limitations and are not unique to one particular care setting. Facts generated are subjective because of reliance on participant memory recall.[44] Unlike the 24-hour recall and food record methods, that are completed soon after the food is eaten, FFQs describe average consumption and are not as quantifiably precise. Information such as food preparation, specific food and beverages consumed, and brand names for products is not recorded. Because FFQs consist of a prespecified food list, no one single FFQ could

reflect the eating patterns of a given population. The use of a FFQ in one group of participants is not transferable to a different population.[46] Moreover, FFQs are limited to 150 items that may not represent the usual foods of respondents or provide meal-pattern information.[44] Another major limitation in interpreting data from FFQs is the absence of consistency in food-composition tables.[46]

**FIGURE 4.4** shows different ways to estimate portion sizes.

## Measuring and Estimating Portion Sizes
### Why Do Portion Sizes Matter?

Portion size can be defined as the total amount of food one chooses to eat at a single eating occasion regardless of the location and meal (home, restaurant, lunch meal, or snack).[47] The inclusion of portion sizes in 24-hour recalls, food records, or FFQs is important because it may lead to greater consumption of certain foods and explain within- and between-person variations.[14] Figure 4.4 shows an example of methods used to measure portion sizes. Considerable evidence indicates that portion sizes have increased incrementally over the last three decades, contributing to the rising incidence obesity and chronic diseases.[14,47–49] Rolls et al. showed that excess energy intake is portion-size dependent in that larger portions of food led to greater food consumption across adult men and women.[48] In this study, participants consumed 30% more energy when offered larger portion sizes of an entrée on one day compared to smaller portion sizes offered on another day. Portion sizes also influenced the energy intake of children three to five

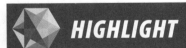

**HIGHLIGHT**

### Technological Advances in Diet-Assessment Methods

Nutrition-assessment methods have been used in the United States since the early 1900s. These methods have evolved from traditional paper-and-pencil ways to computer and digital methods. The National Institutes of Health has sponsored several projects that focus on improving food records using mobile phone apps.

One project, the Technology Assisted Dietary Assessment (TADA), has developed algorithms to allow the use of a single image (picture) in estimating food

volume. TADA uses a standard or point of reference within the image to fragment the different food components on the plate. When the location and identification of each food item is recognized, the volume of food is identified. The volume-assessment procedure used by TADA involves categorizing each picture section into a geometric class such as a sphere, cube, or mound and then developing measurements from the image and employing a formula to calculate volume. These calculations can be conducted using a handheld device. TADA have been used to determine the accuracy of food-volume estimation.

Data from Stumbo PJ. New technology in dietary assessment: a review of digital methods in improving food record accuracy. *Proc Nutr Soc.* 2013;72(1):70–76.

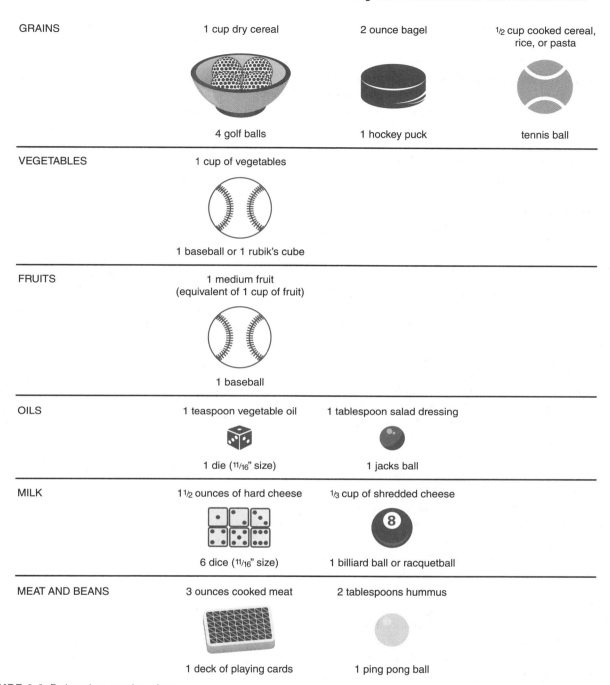

**FIGURE 4.4** Estimating portion sizes

years old, making parent-focused, portion-education interventions imperative.[48] Portion sizes also determined the extent of energy self-regulation for the dietary intakes of young children from 4 to 24 months of age.[50] Fox et al. found that portion sizes were negatively associated with energy consumption.[50] Children who eat more often during the day consume smaller-than-average portion sizes compared with those who eat less often during the day and consume larger-than-average portion sizes.[51]

Accounting for the quantity of food consumed is an important part in assessing the dietary intakes of populations and individuals. Individuals who consume foods based on expected satiation formed by pleasure foods have a tendency to underestimate the portion sizes they consume when compared to actual food intake. Conversely, healthy adults who ate based on hunger accurately estimated the portion sizes they consumed compared with their actual food intake.[51] These findings reinforce the significance of measuring portion sizes as part of the dietary assessment routine.

Food models are the most common and simplest method to measure portion sizes in a clinic or research setting. Portion sizes can also be measured using household artifacts (such as measuring cups and spoons), premeasured portion sizes, or food photographs. Measurements can be from two-dimensional and three-dimensional food forms. Familiar household items such as cups and spoons or bowls and plates are commonly used by study participants for estimating portion sizes. The use of food photographs of various food-portion sizes has increased in the research setting.

### Food Artifacts

Household artifacts are portion-size estimation objects intended to help people estimate food-portion sizes.[52] Household measures are widely used because they resemble real-life, authentic objects and serve as tangible, visual objects.[53] People with varying literacy levels can best recall and estimate food-portion sizes using visualization and comparison aids. They often estimate portion sizes based on the size or shape of the container while using their hands to indicate the equivalent portions.[52]

Chaudhry et al. found that people associate estimates of liquids with the household containers they usually use—for instance, estimating the portion size of coffee with a drinking cup.[52] The association with the containers is made without the necessarily knowing the actual volume. People also tend to estimate portion sizes of solid food container based on the similarity to the shape of the actual container.[52]

In a recent study, Gibson et al. compared the accuracy of "the width of the fingers," fist and fingertips for estimating portion sizes with that of household measures (cups and spoons).[54] Estimated weights were compared with true weights, using a percentage difference to compare the precision between the hand and household measures. University of Sydney staff and students estimated the portion sizes of multiple foods and beverages. Surprisingly, the hand method, which yielded a rough estimation of portion sizes, was more accurate than the household method. The hand estimation was 80% within the ±25% of the true weight of foods, and 13% were within the ±10% of accuracy. Conversely, the household estimation accuracy produced only 29% within the ±25% of the true weight of foods, and 8% were within the ±10%. The researchers concluded that the finger-width method for portion-size estimation was superior to using the household measures, particularly for geometrically shaped foods.[54]

Research supports that household measures and other food models produce poor accuracy in estimating portion sizes when used by children.[55] Children ages 4 to 16 years of age who used food photographs or an interactive portion-size assessment were more accurate in their portion-size estimation of foods served at school. Using household measures and other food models, the participants' estimation was least accurate.[55] Overall, these findings showed that household measures are not always the best option for estimating food-portion size.

### Unit Measurement

Food intake can be measured by different units of portion sizes—for example, grams versus servings.[56] Note that the two units are not interchangeable because they represent different entities. Although a portion is the amount an individual consumes, a serving relates to a standardized amount of food listed on a food label or the information about a food within a food group such as in dietary guidance.[57,58] Moreover, different foods are associated with different serving sizes, such as measured cups, ounces, grams, slices, or numbers (three crackers), which indicates that a portion size may not match a serving size.[57] Nöthlings et al. examined whether the portion-size unit—for example, grams versus servings—may have different impacts on food consumption.[56] Using a cohort study of more than 200,000 participants, the authors found that the two measures could be interchangeable in predicting disease risk. Inversely, Herman and Policy[59] affirmed that norms related to portion sizes were determined by the amount of food served versus the number of food items provided. For example, when served pizzas were cut into different sizes, more food was eaten when portion sizes were larger because of a cognitive bias.[47,59] Geier et al. further confirmed that there is a unit bias—that is, larger portion sizes subconsciously encourage people to consume more food.[60] Likewise, the normal amount of food that should be eaten will determine the amount served. Could larger portion sizes of food also encourage the consumption of large portion sizes of fruit and vegetables that are not energy dense? Unfortunately, evidence showed that larger servings of vegetables and fruit did not result in their greater intake. Together, these findings point to the limitations of using subjective unit measures to determine their impact on food intake.[49]

### Food Photographs

Food photographs have been used as alternative methods to estimate food-portion sizes.[56,61] Foster et al.

found that both food photographs and an interactive portion-size assessment resulted in good accuracy of portion-size estimates in relation to the true food intake.[55] When compared to using household measures and food models, children using food photographs and an interactive method were more effective in improving accuracy in estimating portion sizes. Food photographs and the interactive portion-size assessment produced more accurate estimation of the amount of food served rather than that consumed.[55] Steyn et al. confirmed that two-dimensional real-life drawings and as well as three-dimensional food models produce a high degree of portion sizes' accuracy that closely resembled the real food portion presented to children.[61] Two-dimensional food drawings provided better estimates of total energy intake for fats and carbohydrates than did three-dimensional food models. The study found significant ethnic differences in using one tool over the other. Overall, black children selected the use of drawings and models more often than white children. As a result, both aids probably could be used in dietary interviews using urban black children as subjects. With adolescents, using food models will increase accuracy.[61]

The effectiveness of accuracy when using digital portion-size photographs was investigated using adult subjects.[62] Participants viewed different computerized portion sizes and selected the most-appropriate portion size of food served at a buffet the previous day. The results indicated that no one image produced the most-accurate estimation of food served. However, the number of images presented at one time influenced accuracy in estimating portion size. Accuracy outcomes were not statistically significant, indicating that one image form was not more accurate than another. Accuracy results showed that the use of eight images rather than four yielded greater accuracy. Results also confirmed that showing simultaneous images was preferred to showing sequential images.[62] Food photographs also yielded a high agreement between estimated energy intake and actual weight of food when rated by trained researchers.[63] Trained raters estimated the weight of food served in two schools, and found that food photographs resulted in high precision of meals served by staff rather than self-serving portion sizes. The bias of the method was more pronounced with bigger portion sizes. Overall, food photographs can constitute acceptable estimates of energy intake but were limited in their validity and generalization.[63]

> **Recap** The use of 24-hour recall, food-record diaries, and FFQ methods for assessing dietary intake has both advantages and limitations. The introduction of other measures such as portion sizes increases accuracy in estimating dietary intake. Including portion sizes in dietary assessment methods may lead to greater accuracy for measuring actual food intake.

# ▶ Challenges in Food and Nutrient Intake Measurement Methods

> **Preview** There is no gold standard for measuring food and nutrient intake. Various diet-assessment methods have been developed; each method has its own set of challenges or limitations. Underreporting seems to be the major and most common challenge among diet-assessment methods.

## Reliability

**Reliability**, also known as *reproducibility*, represents the internal consistency of an instrument to provide repeated results with the same group of participants. A reliability study links intake results from two administrations of a tool in the same group of participants. In a reliable instrument, the mean of the measurements (for instance, the mean intake of a nutrient) should not vary significantly between the two administrations. Furthermore, correlation coefficients for the outcomes of interest (i.e., intake of a specific nutrient) assessed from the two administrations of the research instrument in the same group of subjects should be high and usually in the matching range of 0.6–0.7. Reliability is an easy measure and provides a level of certainty as to the accuracy of a research tool.[64] Overall, reliability values range from 0.00 to 1.00, where a value of $r \geq 0.7$ is considered sufficiently reliable for dietary assessments.[65]

In general, reliability is instrument specific and reflects errors because of the use of a specific dietary assessment instrument. Therefore, ideally, the reliability of each new food questionnaire should be determined for each new population being assessed.[66]

Reliability can take different forms under different situations. The interrater reliability indicates the extent of agreement of dietary assessment among judges.[66] The internal consistency reliability, commonly expressed by Cronbach's α, reflects the extent to which all the items within a single instrument measure the same concept and yield similar results.[65,67] Equivalent form reliability describes how two different forms of the same instrument yield the same results. Test–retest reliability designates the extent to which a single instrument produces the same results for the same individuals on two different occasions.[66] Of the four reliability forms, the test–retest reliability is closely related to reproducibility.[68] *Reproducibility* refers to the variation in measurements made on a single assessment instrument for the same respondents under changing conditions.[68] In dietary-intake assessments, the changing conditions are prone to error measurement over some time period. A dietary assessment is reliable or reproducible if the same instrument yields similar results for repeated measures of the same respondents under different passages of time between administrations.[66] For example, respondents may complete a dietary assessment twice within a two-week period or on the first day of the month and again on the first day of the following month.

There are fundamental challenges relating to the reliability of dietary assessment reports. Dietary assessments of respondents' records are subjected to memory bias.[69] Cardoso et al. found a low to moderate reliability of the FFQ (0.52–0.75) within one-month intervals of three 24-hour dietary recalls among 93 low-income women.[69] In addition, the long-term reliability (one-year interval) of the same instrument was lower (0.30–0.56), reflecting memory bias. Andersen et al. administered a dietary assessment with both 24-hour recall and food-frequency questionnaire portions within two weeks of the initial assessment to sixth-grade students.[70] The results indicated no significant differences in responses between the two time periods. The authors attributed the high reliability to short time periods between the assessment as students remember their responses to the initial asse\ssment, and record them on the subsequent assessment.[70]

Although longer periods between testing minimize the risk of participants replicating previous answers, they introduce a new challenge. If periods are too long between assessments, seasons may change during that time, which can affect the types of foods eaten or the food-frequency consumption. Marchioni et al. administered FFQs to high school sophomores in Brazil three times each, one month apart.[71] Although the test–retest reliability was reasonable for most of the nutrients assessed, the FFQ internal consistency of the second assessment was lower than that of the initial assessment, as reflected by the corresponding intraclass correlation coefficient values of the two FFQs. Researchers suggested the students consumed different seasonal foods during the study duration because they came from low-income populations for which seasonal changes could affect food availability.[71]

To control the time interval variable, four to eight weeks are suggested as an acceptable time duration between dietary assessments.[33] Hebden et al. established that a one-month period was appropriate for investigating the FFQ reliability.[72] In this study, two FFQs were administered to Australian male and female students four weeks apart. The results indicated good reliability for all nutrients of interest and for fruit and vegetable servings. Researchers declared that one month was enough to easily administer FFQs and obtain good reliability for assessing diet in young adults.[72] Fallaize et al. also administered two FFQs to students at the University of Reading in the United Kingdom four weeks apart.[73] This study found insignificant differences of macronutrient and micronutrient dietary intakes between the first and second FFQs. Based on their results, researchers maintained that four weeks was the best time interval between repeated measures of FFQs to obtain reproducibility or test–retest reliability because it could minimize changes and error measurement in reporting dietary intake.[73] In a similar study, Filippi et al. administered two online FFQs to 185 Italian adolescents ages 14 to 17 four weeks apart.[74] Analysis of the results showed that differences in dietary intake estimates were not statistically significant for all food groups, indicating that the FFQ was a reliable instrument for estimating food groups, energy, and nutrient intakes for this population.[74]

Dietary assessment self-reports could also be dependent on individual characteristics, thus reducing their reliability. Neuhouser et al.[75] found that individuals also tended to report dietary data quite differently, depending on their age, body mass index, and ethnicity. Specifically, their findings indicated that participant characteristics correlated with energy and protein intake misreporting, confirming the existence of systematic bias in dietary self-reports and reducing the reliability of dietary assessment self-reports.[75] Together, these findings help to define the importance of obtaining good reliability for dietary assessment instruments.[66]

## Validity

Reliability concerns the internal consistency of dietary assessment items, but **validity** refers to the extent to which an instrument measures what it purports to measure.[66,76-79] Validity is important in the development of a tool and vital in evaluating the performance of the developed tool. Validity necessitates that an instrument be reliable, but an instrument can be reliable without being valid. This means an assessment tool can consistently deliver similar outcomes but not that the results are necessarily accurate.[80] Most dietary assessments aim to measure the participants' usual food intake over a defined time period.[77]

Accuracy is defined as a measurement of the degree of closeness of measurements of a quality to that quantity's true value.[81] This trait is particularly relevant to dietary assessment because of the large variability in people's eating habits.[18]

Validity evidence is fostered over time, with validations taking place in different populations. Validity can take four forms.[66] **Face validity** is the extent to which the instrument is assumed to measure a characteristic based on the participants' judgment.[66,67] **Relative validity** compares a new measurement method with at least one established method that is believed to have a greater degree of demonstrated face validity. **Content validity** explores the relevance and comprehensiveness of a tool's content (tool construction). It is usually evaluated by a group of experts who consider the appropriateness of the tool in relation to its planned purpose and use. **Construct validity** emphasizes the extent to which an assessment parameter performs in agreement with theoretical expectations.[82] In other words, if the tool's performance is consistent with expectations, then construct validity is established in relation to the variables tested. This type of validity is a conclusion based on gathering evidence from several studies using a specific measuring instrument. All confirmation of validity, including content- and criterion-related validity, adds to the evidence of construct validity.[77] **Criterion validity**, in turn, is the extent to which an instrument correlates with an external reference tool that has already been validated, signifying the most accurate estimates of food intake.[66,67] For example, the doubly labeled water (DLW) method is a reference standard in energy metabolism that measures free-living **energy expenditure** in humans. It can be used to independently validate self-reported energy intake and detect true reporting bias.[77,83] Measuring food and nutrient intake may require the comparison of multiple valid instruments to determine the best tool for the project.

Studies validating tools to evaluate nutritional intake have been limited.[18] Most have been traditionally conducted by comparing dietary data collected from an FFQ with data obtained from food records or 24-hour recalls to determine which tool provides greater accuracy.[18,34,84,85] For instance, Vioque et al. developed and evaluated the reliability and validity of a modified FFQ compared with the average of three 24-hour recalls in 169 young Spanish children.[45] The findings demonstrated low to moderate reliability, ranging from 0.3 to 0.7, while the validity was lower across nutrients (average $r = 0.30$). Liese et al. also developed a modified SEARCH FFQ for collecting nutrient intake from youth with type 1 diabetes and examined its validity against three 24-hour recalls within one month.[86] Participants were given two FFQ forms to complete one month apart; in between they also completed the three 24-hour recalls. The results indicated that the SEARCH FFQ demonstrated lower relative validity compared to that of the 24-hour recalls.[86] The 24-hour recalls reported higher nutrient intakes in all food groups when compared to the SEARCH FFQ for all food items except meat, nuts, seeds, fats, and oils.[45] Overall, the SEARCH FFQ demonstrated low to moderate reliability, highlighting the importance of demonstrating both reliability and validity in dietary assessments.

Wong et al. further investigated the test–retest reliability and relative validity of the New Zealand Adolescent FFQ (NZAFFQ) to assess food-group intake in 52 adolescents ages 14 to 18 years.[87] The NZAFFQ was administered twice within two weeks to measure reliability, whereas four food records were used to assess the instrument's validity. Results showed that the new FFQ has good to excellent reliability, ranging from 0.54 to 0.89 across nutrients, whereas the validity was poor to reasonable, ranging from 0.32 to 0.70. Estimates of some of the vegetable intakes was particularly inaccurate.[87]

Christian et al. validated their 24-hour Child and Diet Evaluation Tool (CADET) recall against a one-day weighed food record in the United Kingdom intended for children 8 to 11 years old.[88] The CADET exhibited good validity compared against weighed food records, especially for fruits, vegetables, and their combination ($r = 0.7$). The CADET also recorded higher amounts of macronutrient intakes when compared to the weighed food record.[88]

Some researchers question the use of FFQs in nutrition epidemiological research because it limits the interpretability studies' results.[89] In some studies, the FFQ significantly underestimated fat and protein intakes and overestimated carbohydrate intake with the high-fat diet compared with a food record.[90] Others doubt the use of food records and 24-hour recalls as the criterion method.[90,91]

Determining the reliability and validity of dietary intake assessments can be an arduous task. As a rule, the traditional dietary intake methods (24-hour recalls, food records, and FFQs) rely on subjective participants' self-reports. To reduce error rate in the data collected, objective measures should be defined.[18] Also, to control for errors in measurement, the validity and reliability of the instrument should be considered when selecting the assessment tool.[66] Instruments with a low validity contribute to errors related to measuring the wrong characteristics, whereas an instrument with low reliability lacks precision. To address these issues, biomarkers and energy-expenditure tests can be added to dietary assessment because they reflect a more objective, accurate measurement of dietary intake.[18]

## Sensitivity and Specificity

Sensitivity and specificity are statistical measures for evaluating the results of diagnostics and screening tests. *Sensitivity* measures the amount of the actual positives, and *specificity* accounts for the proportion of the negatives. Sensitivity measures the number of positive results that are correctly identified as such. This is also called a *true positive rate*—that is, the ratio of sick people who are correctly recognized as having the illness.[92] Specificity is defined as the number of individuals without disease who are properly identified by a screening test.[93]

A highly sensitive test shows few false-negative results—that is, few actual cases are missed, and therefore it has a strong value for screening.[92] A negatively sensitive test means that the proportion of persons who have a disease are diagnosed with negative test results—that is, as not having the condition.[94]

Specificity is the test's ability to correctly diagnose an individual without the disease as negative.[92] A highly specific test means there are few false-positive results, making it valuable because of low false-positive errors. In contrast, a negatively specific test erroneously diagnoses many individuals without the disease as having the condition. A negatively specificity test can potentially lead to providing unnecessary treatment such as invasive, risky, or expensive follow-up diagnostics.[92] DeVellis noticed that the higher the specificity of a test, the stronger the test indicators correlate with one another.[95]

The goal is to use tools with high sensitivity and specificity and thereby minimizing the misclassifications. To that end, sensitivity and specificity are used to establish reference intervals against which nutrition-assessment instruments can be compared to determine their effectiveness.[94]

## Use of Biological Markers

All of the traditional dietary assessments—the 24-hour recall, food records, and FFQs—rely on subjective self-reports that involve systemic bias and error in measurement.[66,96-98]

The National Academy of Medicine (formerly the Institute of Medicine) has debated whether **biological markers** could predict functional outcomes and chronic diseases. They should thus be used as external, independent criteria to validate overall diet quality measured as total energy intake or the intake of selected nutrients.[18,97]

Sources of biological markers include DLW for energy expenditure, urine, blood, and tissue for specific nutrients.[18,75,97,101] These markers are generally readily accessible and can objectively assess food and nutrient intake without bias and self-reported dietary intake.[96]

Urinary nitrogen, sodium, potassium, vitamin E, vitamin C, carotenoids, and fatty acids in adipose tissue are among the most commonly used biomarkers in research. Although numerous studies have used biomarkers as tools for validation, few studies translate their results in terms of the validity coefficient.[102-105]

## Doubly Labeled Water: The Gold Standard for Energy Expenditure

Doubly labeled water is an established biomarker that is considered the gold standard for validating total energy intake or energy-expenditure measurement.[18,75] The DLW method is considered the most relevant, although costly, technique for calculating energy expenditure in animals and humans. It is based on the exponential disappearance from the body of the stable isotopes deuterium ($^2$H) and oxygen ($^{18}$O) after a bolus dose of water labeled with both isotopes. The $^2$H is lost as water and the $^{18}$O as both water and carbon dioxide ($CO_2$). After correction for isotopic fractionation, the excess disappearance rate of $^{18}$O relative to $^2$H is a measure of the $CO_2$ production rate.[106] Urine or saliva samples are collected and analyzed to measure the disappearance of the isotopes.[101] This rate can be transformed to an approximation of total energy expenditure by using a known or estimated respiratory quotient and the principle of indirect calorimetry.[107] When weight conditions are stable, energy intake equals energy expenditure.[108]

The doubly labeled water biomarker provides a more objective method of assessing energy intake and is often used to assess underreporting in dietary assessments.[75,101] A study by Neuhouser et al. found that women who participated in the Women's Health Initiative Dietary Modification Trial underreported energy intake by 32% as measured by a DLW protocol.[75] African Americans and Hispanic women underreported energy intake more than Caucasians.[75] Participants in the Observing Protein and Energy Nutrition Study underreported total energy intake as measured by the 24-hour recalls as FFQs as compared with the DLW protocol.[101] Men underreported energy intake by 12%–14% on the 24-hour recalls and 31%–36% on FFQs, whereas women underreported energy intake by 16%–20% on 24-hour recall and 27%–32% on FFQs.

The use of the DLW technique has both advantages and limitations. Advantages include the fact that it has been deemed an accurate, objective measurement of energy expenditure. Other advantages include ease of administration, participants' ability to engage in daily activities, and restriction-free settings.[18]

Limitations to using the DLW technique include the assumption of a constant rate of $CO_2$ and a consistent water pool throughout the measurement period. Aside from this, there is variability in the process researchers process to calculate the isotope pool spaces, the constant elimination rate, the fractionation factors, and the mode of $CO_2$ transformation into energy.[83] Other challenges with using DLW in dietary assessments include the high cost of stable isotopes and the expertise required to activate a sophisticated spectrometer.[18]

One important aspect to consider is that the DLW is time restricted because it is held by the body for only 14 days. Some researchers have tried to compensate for this time restriction by distributing surveys. In doing so, the DLW technique is no longer objective.

## Nutritional Biomarkers

When compared to using self-reported nutrition intake instruments, the use of nutritional biomarkers has been deemed more accurate in assessing nutritional intake or status. Nutritional biomarkers have been used to validate self-reported intake, assess intake of food items when food-composition databases are inadequate, and more accurately link eating patterns with disease risk and nutritional status.

Nutritional biomarkers can be classified into short-term, medium-term, and long-term markers or indicators. Short-term indicators suggest intake for the past few hours or days. Medium-term markers reflect intakes for the past few weeks or months. Long-term nutritional markers show the individual's intake for the past months or years. The type of sample used is the main determinant of time (blood, hair, adipose tissue).[109] The use of hair and nail samples are easily obtained and can be used to address trace elements. The validity of using these samples has not been established.[110] Venipuncture blood samples are the preferred biologic specimen for large-scale studies. Blood samples are simple to obtain add negligible burdens on the subjects, and can be easily managed for large-scale studies. Spot blood samples are used for nutrients such as vitamin A and folate.[111,112] Samples of fatty acids may not be truly reflective of the amount of fatty acid consumed via the diet.[113] Blood fatty acids from phospholipids have also been used to validate the traditional dietary measurement because of their relationship with chronic diseases.[114]

Intake of dietary essential fatty acids (eicosapentaenoic acid and docosahexaenoic acid) found in fish were related to blood fatty acids.[18] Fatty acids from adipose tissues showed comparable results for odd numbers of fatty acids but were not valid biomarkers for saturated and monounsaturated fatty acids.[115] Apparently, dietary essential fatty acids were better biomarkers for validation. Plasma concentration of carotenoids, tocopherols, retinol, folic acid, vitamin C, vitamin $B_{12}$, and flavonoids also performed well as biomarkers and reflected accurately their corresponding ingested foods.[18,114,116]

Serum concentrations of carotenoids and ascorbic acid (vitamin C) were indicative of fruit and vegetable consumption.[18] For example, moderate correlations between fruit and vegetable intake and changes in plasma concentration of vitamin C and specific carotenoids ($r = 0.39$ and $0.37$, respectively) have been found among women in the Netherlands.[117] Similarly, Scott et al. showed that the dietary intakes of lutein, lycopene, and beta-carotene found in fruits and vegetables correlated with changes in plasma concentrations of lutein, lycopene, and beta-carotene ($r = 0.64$, $0.47$, and $0.45$, respectively).[118] Serum concentration of folate, vitamin $B_{12}$, and α-tocopherol (vitamin E) were strongly linked to fruits and vegetables, whole and fortified grains, and enriched breakfast cereals.[97,100] Note that biomarkers do not always perform better than other assessments of dietary intake because of their limitations.[115]

Biomarkers are subject to individual variability and may be influenced by confounding factors other than the nutrient of interests.[119] Moreover, rapid turnout of nutrient concentrations in the blood because of half-life (e.g., carotenoids) or to preserve homeostasis limits their sensitivity as biomarkers in the long run.[115,119] Some enzyme activities may serve as functional biomarkers that mirror long-term status but are influenced by confounding factors or several micronutrients that limit their generalizability.[66,119] Likewise, biomarkers' effectiveness depends on the existence of reference values and cutoff points for populations of interest.[119]

Although nutritional biomarkers usually offer a more accurate reflection of the subjects' dietary intake, influences that may not be present in traditional dietary assessment methods could distort biomarker measures of dietary intake. Factors that can distort biomarker measures involve genetic inconsistency, lifestyle habits (such as high consumption of alcohol), dietary factors such as nutrient–nutrient interactions, and analytical procedures.[120] More research is needed in this area. As a result, when using nutritional biomarkers, it is vital to evaluate a biomarker's validity, reproducibility, aptitude to distinguish changes over time, and generalizability across various populations. Strengths and limitations for the different biomarkers needs to be assessed.

In summary, nutritional biomarkers are objective and valid measures of dietary estimates but should complement other subjective estimates, such as 24-hour recalls, food records, or FFQs because of their limitations.[14]

**Recap**   Accurately assessing the intake of food and beverages is essential to nutrition and health research, including surveillance, epidemiology, and intervention studies. Dietary intake and the process for consuming food and beverages is dynamic and complex. Dietary intake habits change over time and through the different stages of the life cycle. The area of evaluating food intake is filled with challenges.

## ▶ Chapter Summary

Nutrient intake determines an individual's health and nutritional status. Dietary intake plays a crucial role in assessing nutrient deficiencies intended to regulate disease prevention or develop management strategies for chronic diseases among target populations. Current assessment methods include subjective and objectives measures. The three most common subjective methods of dietary measurement are 24-hour recalls, food records, and food-frequency questionnaires. Each method has its advantages and limitations as supported by evidence-based research, unveiling problems in reliability and validity that restrict the ability to predict true dietary intake. Limitations of the dietary-intake tools underscore the need to also include biological biomarkers because they are objective, independent measures that can improve the estimates of dietary consumption. Specific biomarkers mirror the status of selected nutrients or dietary components, either as recovery-based markers that indicate a direct relationship to nutrient intake, as in the case of a 24-hour urinary nitrogen for protein intake or urinary excretion of potassium; or concentration-based markers of a specific nutrient such as plasma or serum concentration of carotenoids or ascorbic acid signifying fruit and vegetable intake. Because nutritional biomarkers have several limitations, current recommendations include the use of both subjective dietary measures and objective nutritional biomarkers as a way to improve the accuracy and precision of dietary intake measurement.

 **CASE STUDY**

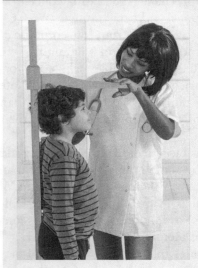
© BSIP SA / Alamy Stock Photo.

Childhood obesity continues to remain a nationwide epidemic. Since the late 1990s, rates have significantly increased among ethnic minorities.

You have been assigned a research project in an urban school district. As part of the project, you need to research all of the factors that can contribute to unhealthy diet intake and physical inactivity among children and adolescents.

**Questions:**

1. What type of nutrient-assessment methods will be used in your methodology?
2. What validation or reproducibility issues may arise in your selected nutrient-assessment methods?
3. In addition to nutrient assessment, will you need to use biomarkers?

# Learning Portfolio

## Key Terms

24-hour recall
Biological marker
Case control
Cohort
Construct validity
Content validity
Criterion validity
Energy expenditure
Face validity
Food-frequency questionnaire (FFQ)

Food record
Longitudinal study
Nonquantitative FFQ
Nutritional epidemiology
Quantitative FFQ
Relative validity
Reliability
Semiquantitative FFQ
Validity

## Study Questions

1. Observational studies include all of the following except:
   a. cohort.
   b. cross-sectional.
   c. randomized controlled trial.
   d. case control.

2. What is the purpose of cohort studies?
   a. To collect data in one point in time
   b. To investigate two groups at a time
   c. To investigate factors that may cause a disease to develop in a particular group over time
   d. To compare and contrast disease prevalence in multiple groups

3. What is the Framingham study?
   a. A case-control study investigating diabetes
   b. A correlational study investigating fiber and colon cancer
   c. A cohort study investigating obesity in children
   d. A longitudinal study investigating cardiovascular disease

4. What does NHANES stand for?
   a. Nutrition Health Assessment and Nutrition Education System
   b. National Health Assessment Nutrition Education Surveillance
   c. Nutrition Health and National Examination System
   d. National Health and Nutrition Examination Survey

5. Cross-sectional studies are also known as
   a. incidence studies.
   b. large approach studies.
   c. small-scale studies.
   d. prevalence studies.

6. Case-control studies are used to investigate two groups known as
   a. case and control.
   b. case and exposure.
   c. case and placebo.
   d. subject and control.

7. What is incidence?
   a. The proportion of the population that is not susceptible to develop a disease immediately
   b. The proportion of the population that has the disease at one point in time
   c. The proportion of the population that is susceptible to develop a disease over time
   d. The proportion of the population that is more susceptible to develop a disease at one point in time

8. What is prevalence?
   a. The proportion of the population that does not develop a disease over time
   b. The proportion of the population that has the disease at one point in time
   c. The proportion of the population that is susceptible to develop a disease over time
   d. The proportion of the population that develops the disease over time.

9.  For individuals who have literacy issues, what is the most effective diet-assessment method?
    a.  Food-frequency questionnaire
    b.  Food record
    c.  Diet History Questionnaire
    d.  24-hour recall

10. For large-scale studies, what is the most effective diet-assessment method?
    a.  Food Record
    b.  24-hour recall
    c.  Food-frequency Questionnaire
    d.  Weighed Food Record

11. The 24-hour dietary recall is defined as:
    a.  a self-report of everything an individual eats and drinks during a specified time period.
    b.  the record of everything an individual eats and drinks over a consecutive three days.
    c.  an extensive list of all foods and beverages an individual has consumed over the past month.
    d.  an extensive questionnaire of foods frequently consumed by individuals over the past week.

12. Advantages of 24-hour dietary recall includes all of the following except
    a.  Quick
    b.  Convenient
    c.  Inexpensive
    d.  Captures usual dietary intake

13. What are the limitations to a 24-hour dietary recall?
    a.  It does not account for diet variation.
    b.  It is expensive.
    c.  It is quick.
    d.  It captures usual dietary intake.

14. A food diary requires participants to track all foods and beverages over what time period?
    a.  During the previous time period
    b.  Over the past month
    c.  During a specified time period
    d.  Over the past week

15. What is an advantage to the food diary method?
    a.  It relies on information in the past.
    b.  It relies on memory.
    c.  It is labor intensive for the subject.
    d.  It does not rely on memory.

16. All of the following are limitations to the food diary method except:
    a.  timing of data collection may not be convenient for subject.
    b.  a high literacy level is needed.

c.  a method may alter an individual's diet.
d.  it is quick.

17. Which of the following data are collected through the use of a food-frequency questionnaire?
    a.  Frequency of consumption of specific foods and nutrients
    b.  Intake within the past 24 hours
    c.  Current intake
    d.  Historical intake

18. What are advantages of the FFQ?
    a.  It quantifies intake.
    b.  No standard method exists.
    c.  It is self-administered.
    d.  It is not culturally tailored.

19. Limitations of the FFQ include all of the following except:
    a.  it relies on memory.
    b.  items may not represent usual intake.
    c.  data may not be quantifiable.
    d.  it reduces participants' burden.

20. What is the Harvard Willet Questionnaire?
    a.  a 131-item questionnaire
    b.  a 150-item questionnaire
    c.  a 300-item questionnaire
    d.  a 250-item questionnaire

21. What is the reliability value range?
    a.  0 to 1
    b.  1.5 to 2.5
    c.  3 to 4
    d.  0.5 to 1.5

22. All of the following are forms of validity, except:
    a.  face.
    b.  criterion.
    c.  content.
    d.  structure.

23. What are not sources of biological markers?
    a.  Urine
    b.  Blood
    c.  Carbohydrates
    d.  Vitamin E

24. What is the gold standard for validating total energy intake?
    a.  Mineral water
    b.  Doubly labeled water
    c.  Plasma levels
    d.  24-hour recall

25. What is an example of a recovery-based marker?
    a.  Plasma levels of carotenoids
    b.  Adipose tissue
    c.  24-hour urinary nitrogen
    d.  Tocopherols

26. All of the following are forms of reliability except:
    a. internal consistency.
    b. test–retest.
    c. reproducibility.
    d. equivalence.

27. All of the following are examples of food models except:
    a. household artifacts.
    b. food photographs.
    c. premeasured portion sizes.
    d. food demonstrations.

28. Food artifacts are most widely used for the following reasons:
    a. They resemble authentic objects.
    b. They have historical value.
    c. They are edible.
    d. They are accessible.

29. Food intake can be measured in which of the following units?
    a. Weights
    b. Kilometers
    c. Grams
    d. Scales

30. Food photographs are most useful during which of the following nutrient-assessment methods?
    a. Food-frequency questionnaire
    b. Food record
    c. Biomarkers
    d. 24-hour recall

31. Food photographs are most useful during which of the following nutrient-assessment methods?
    a. Food-frequency questionnaire
    b. Food record
    c. Biomarkers
    d. 24-hour recall

## Discussion Questions

1. Reflect on the impact of nutrition epidemiology studies. Many of these studies investigate a specific nutrient and disease. Data on intake of foods and supplements before and during pregnancy revealed the association between low folic acid intake and neural tube defects in offspring; this was later determined to be a causal relationship. Design a research study focused on a particular nutrient and disease. What specific nutrient-assessment methods could be used? Why? Write your research proposal.

2. You have been assigned the role of a research assistant to collaborate in a research study investigating the relationship between fiber and gastrointestinal diseases. Your target population is 60 years of age and older. What nutrient-assessment methods would be most appropriate for the study? Why?

3. You are conducting a literature review focused on the dietary intake of children younger than 10 years. You are planning to replicate one of the research studies. What steps should you take to ensure your results are reliable and valid?

## Activities

### Individual Activities

1. Evaluation of various diet-assessment tools:
   a. Work with a partner. You are trying to determine if your subject consumes sufficient fruits and vegetables in a day. Which of the tools listed below will you have your subject complete? Why?
      i.   a 24-hour dietary recall
      ii.  a three-day food record
      iii. the National Cancer Institute's Diet History Questionnaire
   b. Discuss the advantages and disadvantages of each tool.

2. Nutrient analysis of diet-assessment tools:
   a. Using the data from the diet-assessment tool used in Activity 1, complete a nutrient analysis using a nutrient-analysis software such as MyDietAnalysis, iProfile, or MyPlate.
      i.  After completing the nutrient analysis of the tools, discuss the nutrient deficiencies and excesses, as well as nutrients that were met for each analysis.
      ii. Include recommendations and suggestion for how individuals can improve or maintain their nutrient status.

## Group Activities

1. Diet assessment and diet-related diseases:
   a. Identify five diet-related diseases.
   b. Assign each member of the group one diet-related disease.
   c. For each disease, identify a research design that can be used to investigate the diet and disease relationship.
   d. Identify a diet-assessment tool.
   e. Identify a validation method.

## Online Resources

### Diet History Questionnaire II (DHQ II) and Canadian Diet History Questionnaire II (C-DHQ II)

This website provides access to two web-based food-frequency questionnaires. Both can be used by researchers, clinicians, and teachers without permission. The DHQ II has a food list that consists of 134 food items and eight dietary-supplement questions. The C-DHQ II has a food list of 153 food items and 10 supplement questions that reflects the diet of Canadians. The website includes a nutrient database, paper-based forms, web-based questionnaire, and the Diet*Calc Analysis Software. The questionnaire is sponsored by the National Cancer Institute. Go to https://epi.grants.cancer.gov/dhq2/

### National Health and Nutrition Examination Survey

This website provides information about the NHANES survey and the key research studies that have used the survey. In addition, it provides information for participants in research studies, information for health professionals regarding the benefits of the data, questionnaires, dataset, and proposal guidelines for the survey. See https://www.cdc.gov/nchs/nhanes/

### What's in the Foods You Eat Search Tool

This website provides nutrient profiles for commonly eaten foods in the United States. Go to https://www.ars.usda.gov/northeast-area/beltsville-md/beltsville-human-nutrition-research-center/food-surveys-research-group/docs/whats-in-the-foods-you-eat-emsearch-toolem/

### Automated Multiple Pass Method—USDA

This website provides a computerized method for collecting interviewer-administered 24-hour dietary recalls either in person or on the telephone. The method is research based and uses five steps to ensure accurate recall and reduce response burden. See https://www.ars.usda.gov/northeast-area/beltsville-md/beltsville-human-nutrition-research-center/food-surveys-research-group/docs/ampm-usda-automated-multiple-pass-method/

### Short Dietary Assessment Instruments

This website provides a list of tools that have been evaluated and have been used in large population studies. These tools assess the intake of fruit and vegetables and the percentage energy from fat, fiber, added sugars, whole grains, calcium, dairy products, and red and processed meats. See https://epi.grants.cancer.gov/diet/screeners/index.html#screeners

### Healthy Eating Index

This website provides information about the USDA's Healthy Eating Index. This is a measure of diet quality that assesses conformance to the *Dietary Guidelines for Americans*. This can be used to evaluate 24-hour recall. See https://www.cnpp.usda.gov/healthyeatingindex

## References

1. Subar AF, Freedman LS, Tooze JA, et al. Addressing current criticism regarding the value of self-reports dietary data. *J Nutr*. 2015; 145(12):2639-2645. doi: 10.3945/jn.115.219634.
2. Boeing H. Nutritional epidemiology: New perspectives for understanding the diet-disease relationship? *Eur J Clin Nutr*. 2013; 67;424-429. doi:10.1038/ejcn.2013.47.
3. Rutishauser I. Dietary intake measurements. *Public Health Nutr*. 2005;8(7A):1100–1107. https://www.cambridge.org/core/services/aop-cambridgecore/content/view/S136898000 5001369. Accessed February 13, 2017.
4. Lumley J, Watson L, Watson M, Bower C. Periconceptional supplementation with folate and/or multivitamins for preventing neural tube defects. *Cochrane Database Sys Rev*. 2001; (3):CD001056. https://www-ncbi-nlm-nih-gov.ezproxy.rosalindfranklin.edu/pubmed/11686974. Accessed on February 7, 2017.
5. Buzzard I. Rationale for an international conference series on dietary assessment methods. *Am J Clin Nutr*. 1994;59(1):143S–145S.
6. Yamamoto ME. Analytic nutrition epidemiology. In: Monsen ER, VanHorn L, eds. *Research Successful Approaches*. 3rd ed. Chicago IL: Diana Faulhaber; 2008: 89–116.
7. Jacobsen K. *Health Research Methods: A Practical Guide*. Fairfax, VA: Jones and Bartlett Learning; 2012.
8. Mahmood SS, Levy D, Vasan RS, Wang TJ. The Framingham heart study and the epidemiology of cardiovascular diseases: A historical perspective. *Lancet*. 2014; 383(9921):999-1008. doi: 10.1016/S0140-6736(13)61752-3. https://www.ncbi.nlm.nih.gov/pmc/articles/PMC4159698/. Accessed February 7, 2017.

9. Tsao CW, Vasan RS. Cohort profile: The Farmington Heart Study (FHS): Overview of milestones in cardiovascular epidemiology. *Int J Epidemiol*. 2015; 4(6):1800-1813. doi: https://doi.org/10.1093/ije/dyv337. https://academic.oup.com/ije/article/44/6/1800/2572656/Cohort-Profile-The-Framingham-Heart-Study-FHS. Accessed February 7, 2017.

10. Hulley SB, Cummings SR, Browner SB, et al. *Designing Clinical Research*. 4th ed. New York, NY: Wolters Kluwer-Lippinncott, William and Wilkins; 2013.

11. Jansen RJ, Robinson DP, Stozenberg-Solomon RZ, et al. Fruit and vegetable consumption is inversely associated with having pancreatic cancer. *Cancer Causes Control*. 2001; 22(12):1613–1625. doi: 10.1007/s10552-011-9838-0. Accessed February 7, 2017.

12. Liu K. Statistical issues related to the design of dietary survey methodology for NHANES III. In National Center for Health Statistics. Dietary methodology workshop for the Third National Health and Nutrition Examination Survey. Hyattsville, MD. US Department of Health and Human Services, Public Health Service Centers for Disease Control. 1992.

13. Carroll RJ, Midthune D, Subar AF, et al. Taking Advantage of the Strengths of 2 Different Dietary Assessment Instruments to Improve Intake Estimates for Nutritional Epidemiology. *Am J Epidemiol*. 2012;175(4):340-347. doi:10.1093/aje/kwr317.

14. Shim JE, Oh K, Kim HC. Dietary assessment methods in epidemiologic studies. *Epidemiol Health*. 2014;36: e2014009. doi: 10.4178/epih/e2014009CID. https://www.ncbi.nlm.nih.gov/pmc/articles/PMC4154347/. Accessed February 13, 2017.

15. Illner AK, Freisling H, Boeing H, Huybrechts I, Crispim SP, Slimani N. Review and evaluation of innovative technologies for measuring diet in nutritional epidemiology. *Int J Epidemiol*. 2012; 41:1187–1203.

16. Shriver BJ, Roman-Shriver CR, Long JD. Technology-based methods of dietary assessment: recent developments and considerations for clinical practice. *Curr Opin Clin Nutr Metab Care*. 2010;13:548–551.

17. Stumbo PJ. New technology in dietary assessment: a review of digital methods in improving food record accuracy. *Proc Nutr Soc*. 2013;72:70–76. https://www.ncbi.nlm.nih.gov/pubmed/23336561. Accessed February 12, 2017.

18. Johnson RK, Yon BA, Hankin JH. Dietary assessment and validation. In: Monsen ER, VanHorn L, eds. *Research Successful Approaches*. 3rd ed. Chicago, IL: Diana Faulhaber; 2008; 187–204.

19. Ahluwalia N, Dwyer J, Terry A, Moshfegh A, Johnnson C. Update on NHANES dietary data: Focus on collection, release, analytical considerations, and uses to inform public policy. *Adv Nutr*. 2016; 7:121-34. doi: 10.3945/an.115.009258. http://advances.nutrition.org/content/7/1/121.full. Accessed February 9, 2017.

20. Briefel R. Assessment of the US diet in national nutrition surveys: National collaborative efforts and NHANES. *Am J Clin Nutr*. 1994; 59(suppl):164S–167S.

21. Guenther P. Research needs for dietary assessment and monitoring in the United States. *Am J Clin Nutr*. 1994; 59(suppl):168S–170S.

22. National Cancer Institute. National Cancer Institute: Dietary Assessment Primer. 24-hour Dietary Recall (24HR) at a Glance. 2017. https://dietassessmentprimer.cancer.gov/profiles/recall/. Accessed February 9, 2017.

23. Stote KS, Radecki SV, Moshfegh AJ, Ingwersen LA, Baer DJ. The number of 24 h dietary recalls using the US Department of Agriculture's automated multiple-pass method required to estimate nutrient intake in overweight and obese adults. *Public Health Nutr*. 2011; 14(10):1736.

24. Schoch AH, Raynor HA. Social desirability, not dietary restraint, is related to accuracy of reported dietary intake of a laboratory meal in females during a 24-hour recall. *Eat Behav*. 2012; 13(1):78-81. doi: 10.1016/j.eatbeh.2011.11.010.

25. McNutt S, Hall J, Cranston B, Soto P, Hults S. Quality control procedures implemented for the dietary assessment component of the 1999-2000 National Health and Nutrition Examination Survey. *FASEB J*. 2000; 14:A759.

26. McNutt S, Hall J, Cranston B, Soto P, Hults S. The 24-hour dietary recall data collection and coding methodology implemented for the 1999-2000 National Health and Nutrition Examination Survey. *FASEB J*. 2000; 14:A759.

27. National Institutes of Health, National Cancer Institute. National Institutes of Health National Cancer Institute. Dietary Assessment Primer, Evaluating the effect of an intervention on diet. 2017. https://dietassessmentprimer.cancer.gov/approach/intervention.html) Accessed July 27, 2017).

28. Bartkowiak L, Jones J, Bannerman E. Evaluation of food record charts used within the hospital setting to estimate energy and protein intakes. *Clin Nutr ESPEN*. 2015; 10(5):e184–e185.

29. Foster E, Hawkins A, Simpson E, Adamson AJ. Developing an interactive portion size assessment system (IPSAS) for use with children. *J Hum Nutr Diet*. 2014; 27(1):1-18. doi: 10.1111/jhn.12127. https://www.ncbi.nlm.nih.gov/pubmed/23682796. Accessed February 9, 2017.

30. Hankin JH, Wilkens LR, Kolonel LN, Yoshizawa CN. Validation of a quantitative diet history method in Hawaii. *Am J Epidemiol*. 1991; 33;616–628. https://www.ncbi.nlm.nih.gov/pubmed/2006649. Accessed February 9, 2017.

31. Kerr DA, Harray AJ, Pollard CM, et al. The connecting health and technology study: A 6-month randomized controlled trial to improve nutrition behaviors using a mobile food record and text messaging support in young adults. *Int J Behav NutrPhys Act*. 2016; 13:52. doi: 10.1186/s12966-016-0376-8. https://www.ncbi.nlm.nih.gov/pmc/articles/PMC4839101/. 2016. Accessed February 9, 2017.

32. O'Connor LM, Lentjes MA, Luben RN, Khaw KT, Wareham NJ, Forouhi NG. Dietary dairy product intake and incident type 2 diabetes: A prospective study using dietary data from a 7-day food diary. *Diabetologia*. 2014; 57(5):909–917.

33. Block G, Hartman AM. Issues in reproducibility and validity of dietary studies. *Am J Clin Nutr*. 1989; 50:(5 Suppl):1133-1138; discussion 1231-1235. https://www.ncbi.nlm.nih.gov/pubmed/2683721. Accessed February 11, 2017.

34. Feskanich D, Rimm E, Giovannucci E, et al. Reproducibility and validity of food intake measurements from a semi-quantitative food frequency questionnaire. *J Am Diet Assoc*. 1993; 93(7):790–796. https://www.ncbi.nlm.nih.gov/pubmed/8320406. Accessed February 12, 2017.

35. Dehghan M, del Cerro S, Zhang X, et al. Validation of a semi-quantitative food frequency questionnaire for Argentinean adults. *PLoS One*. 2012; 7(5):e37958. http://journals.plos.org/plosone/article?id=10.1371/journal.pone.0037958. Accessed February 10, 2017.

36. Pritchard JM, Seechurn T, Atkinson SA. A food frequency questionnaire for the assessment of calcium, vitamin D and vitamin K: A pilot validation study. *Nutrients*; 2010; 2(8):805–819. doi:10.3390/nu2080805.

37. Sarmento RA, Riboldi BP, Rodrigues DC, Jobim de Azevedo M, Carnevale de Almeida J. Development of a quantitative food frequency questionnaire for Brazilian patients with type 2 diabetes. *BMC Public Health*. 2013; 13:740.

https://www.ncbi.nlm.nih.gov/pmc/articles/PMC3751547/. Accessed February 10, 2017.

38. Samet JM, Humble CG, Skipper BE. Alternatives in the collection and analysis of food frequency interview data. *Am J Epidemiol*, 1984; 120:572–581.

39. Wirfält AK, Jeffery RW, Elmer PJ. Comparison of food frequency questionnaires: the reduced Block and Willett questionnaires differ in ranking on nutrient intakes. *Am J Epidemiol*. 1998; 8(12):1148–1156. https://www.ncbi.nlm.nih.gov/pubmed/9867258. Accessed on February 10, 2017.

40. Block G, Wakimoto P, Block T. A revision of the Block Dietary Questionnaire and database, based on NHANES III data Feb [online]. 2009; at http://www.nutritionquest.com/B98_Dev.pdf. Accessed February 6, 2017.

41. Hunsberger M, O'Malley J, Block T, Norris JC. Relative validation of Block Kids Food Screener for dietary assessment in children and adolescents. *Matern Child Nutr*. 2015; 11(2):260-70; doi: 10.1111/j.1740-8709.2012.00446.x.

42. Nutrition Quest. Assessment and Analysis Service, Questionnaires and Screeners. 2017; http://nutritionquest.com/assessment/list-of-questionnaires-and-screeners/. Accessed July 22, 2017.

43. Thompson F, Suba A, Brown C, et al. Cognitive research enhances accuracy of food frequency questionnaire reports: Results of an experimental validation study. *J Am Diet Assoc*. 2002; 102:212–225.

44. Thompson FE, Byers T. Dietary assessment resource manual. *J Nutr*. 1994; 24(11 Suppl): 2245S-22317S. http://www.ucdenver.edu/research/CCTSI/programs-services/ctrc/Nutrition/Documents/Dietary-Assessment-Methods.pdf. Accessed February 10, 2017.

45. Vioque J, Gimenez D, Navarrete-Muñoz EM, et al. Reproducibility and validity of a food frequency questionnaire designed to assess diet in children aged 4-5 years. *PLoS One*. 2016; 11(11):e0167338. doi: 10.1371/journal.pone.0167338. https://www.ncbi.nlm.nih.gov/pmc/articles/PMC5127574/. Accessed February 10, 2017.

46. Liu L, Wang PP, Roebothan B, et al. Assessing the validity of a self-administered food-frequency questionnaire (FFQ) in the adult population of Newfoundland and Labrador, Canada. *J Nutr*. 2013; 12:49. doi: 10.1186/1475-2891-12-49. https://nutritionj.biomedcentral.com/articles/10.1186/1475-2891-12-49/. Accessed February 10, 2017.

47. Benton D. Portion size: What we know and what we need to know. *Crit Rev Food Sci Nutr*. 2015; 55(7):988–1004. doi: 10.1080/10408398.2012.679980. https://www.ncbi.nlm.nih.gov/pmc/articles/PMC4337741/. Accessed February 14, 2017.

48. Rolls BJ, Morris EL, Roe LS. Portion size of food affects energy intake in normal-weight and overweight men and women *Am J Clin Nutr*. 2002; 76(6):1207–1213. doi: 10.1017/S000711450779390X. http://ajcn.nutrition.org/content/76/6/1207.long. Accessed February 13, 2017.

49. Small L, Lane H, Vaughan L, Melnyk B, McBurnett D. A systematic review of the evidence: The effects of portion size manipulation with children and portion education/training interventions on dietary intake with adults. *Worldviews on Evid Based Nurs*. 2013; 10(2):69–81. https://www.ncbi.nlm.nih.gov/pubmed/22703240. Accessed February 14, 2017.

50. Fox MK, Devaney B, Reidy K, Razafindrakoto C, Ziegler P. Relationship between portion size and energy intake among infants and toddlers: evidence of self-regulation. *J Am Diet Assoc*. 2006; 106(1):S77-83. https://www.ncbi.nlm.nih.gov/pubmed/16376632. Accessed February 14, 2017.

51. Nguyen A, Chern C, Tan SY. Estimated portion size versus actual intake of eight commonly consumed foods by healthy adults. *Nutr Diet*. 2016; 73:490-7. http://onlinelibrary.wiley.com/doi/10.1111/1747-0080.12292/abstract. Accessed February 14, 2017.

52. Chaudry BM, Connelly K, Siek KA, Welch JL. Formative evaluation of a mobile liquid portion size estimation interface for people with varying literacy skills. *J Ambient Intell Humaniz Comput*. 2013; 4(6):779–89. doi: 10.1007/s12652-012-0152-9. http://europepmc.org/articles/pmc3891775-R28. Accessed on February 14, 2017.

53. Chamber E IV, Godwin SL, Vecchio FA. Cognitive strategies for reporting portion sizes using dietary recall procedures. *J Am Diet Assoc* 2000; 100(8);891–897. doi: http://dx.doi.org/10.1016/S0002-8223(00)00259-5. http://www.andjrnl.org/article/S0002-8223(00)00259-5/abstract. Accessed February 14, 2017.

54. Gibson AA, Hsu MS, Rangan AM, et al. Accuracy of hands v. household measures as portion size estimation aids. *J Nutr* Sci. 2016;5:e29. doi: 10.1017/jns.2016.22. https://www.ncbi.nlm.nih.gov/pmc/articles/PMC4976119/. Accessed February 14, 2017.

55. Foster E, Matthews JN, Lloyd J, et al. Children's estimates of food portion size: The development and evaluation of three portion size assessment tools for use with children. *Br J Nutr*. 2008; 99(1):175-184. doi: 10.1017/S000711450779390X. https://www.ncbi.nlm.nih.gov/pubmed/17697426/. Accessed February 14, 2017.

56. Nöthlings U, Murphy SP, Sharma S, Hankin JH, Kolonel LN. A comparison of two methods of measuring food group intake: grams vs servings. *J Am Diet Assoc*. 2006; 106(5):737–739. https://www.ncbi.nlm.nih.gov/pubmed/16647334. Accessed February 14, 2017.

57. National Institute of Health, National Institute of Diabetes Digestive and Kidney Diseases. Just enough for you: About food portions. 2016; https://www.niddk.nih.gov/health-information/health-topics/weight-control/just-enough/Pages/just-enough-for-you.aspx. Accessed February 21, 2017.

58. United States Department of Agriculture. Dietary Guidelines for Americans 2015-2020. 2016; https://health.gov/dietary guidelines/2015/resources/2015-2020_Dietary_Guidelines.pdf. Accessed February 21, 2017.

59. Herman PC, Polivy J. Normative influences on food intake. *Physiol Behav*. 2005; 86(5):762–772. doi: 10.1016/j.physbeh.2005.08.064. https://www.ncbi.nlm.nih.gov/pubmed/16243366. Accessed on February 21, 2017.

60. Geier AB, Rozin P, Doros G. Unit bias. A new heuristic that helps explain the effect of portion size on food intake. *Psychol Sci*. 2006; 17(6):521–5. doi: 10.1111/j.1467-9280.2006.01738.x. https://www.ncbi.nlm.nih.gov/pubmed/16771803. Accessed February 21, 2017.

61. Steyn NP, Senekal M, Norris S, et al. How well do adolescents determine portion sizes of foods and beverages? *Asia Pac J Clin Nutr*. 2006;15(1):35–42. https://www.ncbi.nlm.nih.gov/pmc/articles/PMC2684582/. Accessed February 13, 2017.

62. Subar AF, Crafts J, Zimmerman TP, et al. Assessment of the accuracy of portion size reports using computer-based food photographs aids in the development of an automated self-administered 24-hour recall. *J Am Diet Assoc*. 2010; 110(1):55–64. doi: 10.1016/j.jada.2009.10.007. https://www.ncbi.nlm.nih.gov/pmc/articles/PMC3773715/. Accessed February 13, 2017.

63. Olafsdottir AS, Hornell A, Hedelin M, et al. Development and validation of a photographic method to use for dietary assessment in school settings. *PLoS One.* 2016; Oct. doi:10.1371/journal.pone.0163970. http://journals.plos.org/plosone/article?id=10.1371/journal.pone.0163970. Accessed February 14, 2017.

64. White E, Armstrong BK, Saracci R. *Principles of Exposure Measurement in Epidemiology.* New York: Oxford University Press; 2008.

65. Deniz MS, Alsaffar AA. Assessing the validity and reliability of a questionnaire on dietary fiber-related knowledge in a Turkish student population. *J Health Popul Nutr.* 2013; 31(4):497–503. https://www.ncbi.nlm.nih.gov/pmc/articles/PMC3905644/. Accessed February 11, 2017.

66. Leedy PD, Ormrod JE. *Practical Research: Planning and Design.* 3rd ed. Saddle River, NJ: Pearson Education; 2010.

67. Nunnally JC, Bernstein IH. *Psychometric Theory.* 3rd ed. New York, NY: McGraw-Hill; 1994; 736. http://psychology.concordia.ca/fac/kline/library/k99.pdf. Accessed February 10, 2017.

68. Bartlett JW, Frost C. Reliability, repeatability, and reproducibility: Analysis of measurement errors in continuous variables. *Ultrasound Obstet Gynecol.* 2008; 31(4):466–475. https://www.ncbi.nlm.nih.gov/pubmed/18306169. Accessed February 10, 2017.

69. Cardoso MA, Tomita LY, Laguna EC. Assessing the validity of a food frequency questionnaire among low-income women in São Paulo, southeastern Brazil. *Cad. Saúde Pública, Rio de Janeiro.* 2010; 26(11):2059-2067. http://www.scielo.br/pdf/csp/v26n11/07.pdf. Accessed February 11, 2017.

70. Andersen LF, Bere E, Kolbjornsen N, Klepp KI. Validity and reproducibility of self-reported intake of fruit and vegetable among 6th graders. *Eur J Clin Nutr.* 2004; 58(5):771–777. https://www.ncbi.nlm.nih.gov/pubmed/15116080. Accessed February 11, 2017.

71. Marchioni D, Voci S, Lima F, Fisberg R, Slater B. Reproducibility of a food frequency questionnaire for adolescents. *Cad. Saude Publica, Rio de Janeiro.* 2007; 23(9):2187–2196. http://www.scielo.br/scielo.php?script=sci_arttext&pid=S0102-311X2007000900026. Accessed February 11, 2017.

72. Hebden L, Kostan E, O'Leary F, Hodge A, Allman-Farinelli M. Validity and reproducibility of a food frequency questionnaire as a measure of recent dietary intake in young adults. *PLoS One.* 2013; 8(9):e75156. https://www.ncbi.nlm.nih.gov/pmc/articles/PMC3776736/. Accessed February 11, 2017.

73. Fallaize R, Forster H, Macready AL, et al. Online dietary intake estimation: reproducibility and validity of the Food4Me food frequency questionnaire against a 4-day weighed food record. *J Med Internet Res.* 2014; 11:16(8):e190. doi: 10.2196/jmir.3355. https://www.ncbi.nlm.nih.gov/pmc/articles/PMC4147714/. Accessed February 11, 2017.

74. Filippi AR, Amodio E, Napoli G, et al. The web-based ASSO-food frequency questionnaire for adolescents: relative and absolute reproducibility assessment. *J Nutr.* 2014; 13(1):119. doi: 10.1186/1475-2891-13-119. https://nutritionj.biomedcentral.com/articles/10.1186/1475-2891-13-119. Accessed February 11, 2017.

75. Neuhouser ML, Tinker L, Shaw PA, et al. Use of recovery biomarkers to calibrate nutrient consumption self-reports in the Women's Health Initiative. *Am J Epidemiol.* 2008; 167(10):1247-59. doi: 10.1093/aje/kwn026. https://www.ncbi.nlm.nih.gov/pubmed/18344516. Accessed February 10, 2017.

76. Mohsen T, Reg D. Making sense of Cronbach's alpha. *Int J Med Edu.* 2011;2:53–55. doi: 10.5116/ijme.4dfb.8dfd 53. https://www.ijme.net/archive/2/cronbachs-alpha.pdf. Accessed February 10, 2017.

77. Institute of Health, National Cancer Institute. Methodology—NCS dietary assessment literature review. 2016; https://epi.grants.cancer.gov/past-initiatives/assess_wc/review/about/methodology.html. Updated September 30, 2016. Accessed February 11, 2017.

78. Lennernas M. Dietary assessment and validity: To measure what is meant to measure. *Scand J Food Nutr Naringsforskning.* 1998; 42(1):63-65. http://www.polarresearch.net/index.php/fnr/article/viewFile/1765/1672. Accessed February 11, 2017.

79. Cameron M, Van Staveren W. *Manual on Methodology for Food Consumption Studies.* New York, NY: Oxford University Press; 1988.

80. Jones JM. Validity of nutritional screening and assessment tools. *Nutrition.* 2004;20(3):312–317.

81. Working Group 2 of Joint Committee for Guides in Metrology. *International Vocabulary of Meteorology—Basic and General Concepts and Associated Terms (VIM).* JCGM/WG 2 Document N318. 2006. https://www.nist.gov/sites/default/files/documents/pml/div688/grp40/International-Vocabulary-of-Metrology.pdf. Accessed May 6, 2017.

82. Carmines EG, Zeller RA. Reliability and validity assessment. In: M.S Lewis-Beck ed., *Basic Measurement.* Newbury Park, CA: Sage Publications; 1994; 19.

83. Buchowsi MS. Doubly labeled water is a validated and verified reference standard in nutrition research. *J Nutr.* 2014; 144(5):573-574. doi: 10.3945/jn.114.191361. https://www.ncbi.nlm.nih.gov/pmc/articles/PMC3985818/. Accessed February 12, 2017.

84. Rimm E, Giovannucci E, Stampfer M, Colditz G, Litin L, Willet W. Reproducibility and validity of an expanded self-administered semi-quantitative food frequency questionnaire among male health professionals. *Am J Epidemiol.* 1992; 135(10):1114–1126. https://www.ncbi.nlm.nih.gov/pubmed/1632423. Accessed February 12, 2017.

85. Munger R, Folsom A, Kushi L, Kaye S, Sellers T. Dietary assessment of older Iowa women with a food frequency questionnaire: Nutrient intake, reproducibility, and comparison with 24-hour dietary recall interviews. *Am J Epidemiol.* 1992; 136(2):192-200. https://www.ncbi.nlm.nih.gov/pubmed/01415141. Accessed February 12, 2017.

86. Liese AD, Crandell JL, Tooze JA, et al. Relative validity and reliability of an FFQ in youth with type 1 diabetes. *Public Health Nutr.* 2015; 18(3):428–437. doi: 10.1017/S1368980014000408. https://www.ncbi.nlm.nih.gov/pmc/articles/PMC4353637/. Accessed February 12, 2017.

87. Wong WW, Roberts SB, Racette SB, et al. The doubly labeled water method produces highly reproducible longitudinal results in nutrition studies. *J Nutr.* 2014; 144(5):777–783. doi: 10.3945/jn.113.187823. https://www.ncbi.nlm.nih.gov/pmc/articles/PMC3985832/. Accessed February 26, 2017.

88. Christian MS, Evans CEL, Nykjaer C, Hancock N, Cade JE. Measuring diet in primary school children aged 8-11 years: Validation of the Child and Diet Evaluation Tool (CADET) with an emphasis on fruit and vegetable intake. *Eur J Clin Nutr.* 2015; 69(2):234–241. doi:10.1038/ejcn.2014.160. https://www.ncbi.nlm.nih.gov/pubmed/25139558. Accessed February 13, 2017.

89. Briefel R, Flegal K, Winn D, et al. Assessing the nation's diet: Limitations of the food frequency questionnaire. *J Am Diet Assoc.* 1992; 92(8):959–962.

90. Schaefer E, Augustin J, Schaefer M, et al. Lack of efficacy of a food-frequency questionnaire in assessing dietary macronutrient intakes in subjects consuming diets of known composition. *Am J Clin Nutr.* 2000; 71(3):746–751. http://ajcn.nutrition.org/content/71/3/746.abstract. Accessed February 13, 2017.

91. Kowalkowska J, Slowinska MA, Slowinski D, et al. Comparison of a full food-frequency questionnaire with the three-day unweighted food records in young polish adult women: Implications for dietary assessment. *Nutrients*; 2013; 5(7): 2747–2776. doi: 10.3390/nu5072747. https://www.ncbi.nlm.nih.gov/pmc/articles/PMC3738998/. Accessed February 9, 2017.

92. Maxi LD, Niebo R, Utell MJ. Screening test: A review with examples. *Inhal Toxicol.* 2014; 26(13):811–828. doi: 10.3109/08958378.2014.955932. https://www.ncbi.nlm.nih.gov/pubmed/25264934.

93. Miller-Keane Encyclopedia. Specificity. *Miller-Keane Encyclopedia and Dictionary of Medicine, Nursing, and Allied Health*, 7th ed. Philadelphia, PA: Saunders; 2003. http://medical-dictionary.thefreedictionary.com/specificity. Accessed July 28, 2017.

94. Moran MB, Archer S, Van Horn L. Descriptive epidemiologic research. In: Monsen ER, VanHorn L, eds. *Research Successful Approaches.* 3rd ed. Chicago IL: Diana Faulhaber; 2008:57–64

95. DeVellis RF. *Scale Development: Theory and Application.* 3rd ed. Newbury Park, CA: Sage; 2012:74–75.

96. Hedrick VE, Dietrich AM, Estabrooks PA, et al. Dietary biomarkers: Advances, limitations, and future directions. *Nutr J.* 2012; 11:109–122. doi: 10.1186/1475-2891-11-109. https://nutritionj.biomedcentral.com/articles/10.1186/1475-2891-11-109. Accessed February 22, 2017.

97. Lampe JW, Huang Y, Neuhouser ML. Dietary biomarker evaluation in a controlled feeding study in women from the Women's Health Initiative cohort. *Am J Clin Nutr.* 2017; 105(2):466–475. http://ajcn.nutrition.org/content/early/2016/12/27/ajcn.116.144840.abstract. Accessed February 22, 2017.

98. Mossavar-Rahmani Y, Sotres-Alvarez D, Wong WW, et al. Applying recovery biomarkers to calibrate self-report measures of sodium and potassium in the Hispanic community health study/study of Latinos. *J Hum Hypertens.* 2017; Feb;8(4):1–4. doi: 10.1038/jhh.2016.98. https://www.ncbi.nlm.nih.gov/pubmed/28205551. Accessed February 23, 2017.

99. Institute of Medicine of the National Academies. Dietary reference intakes: Research synthesis workshop summary. Washington, DC: National Academies Press; 2007. http://70.89.103.33/bota/USDA/11767.pdf. Accessed February 23, 2017.

100. Playdon MC, Moore SC, Derkach A, et al. Identify biomarkers of dietary patterns by metabolomics. *Am J Clin Nutr.* 2017; 105(2):450-465. doi: 10.3945/ajcn.116.144501. https://www.ncbi.nlm.nih.gov/pubmed/28031192. Accessed February 23, 2017.

101. Subar AF, Kipnis V, Troiano RP, et al. Using intake biomarkers to evaluate the extent of dietary misreporting in a large sample of adults: The OPEN Study. *Am J Epidemiol.* 2003; 158(1): 1–13. https://www.ncbi.nlm.nih.gov/pubmed/12835280.

102. Willet W. Future directions in the development of food-frequency questionnaires. *Am J Clin Nutr.* 1994; 59(1):171S-174S. http://ajcn.nutrition.org/content/59/1/171S.abstract. Accessed February 13, 2017.

103. Willet W. *Nutritional Epidemiology.* 2nd ed. New York, NY: Oxford University Press; 1998.

104. McNaughton S, Marks G, Gaffney P, Williams G, Green A. Validation of a food frequency questionnaire of carotenoid and vitamin E intake using weighed food records and plasma biomarkers: The method of triads model. *Eur J Clin Nutr.* 2005; 59(2):211-218. https://www.ncbi.nlm.nih.gov/pubmed/15483635. Accessed February 25, 2017.

105. Day N, McKeown Y, Welch A, Bingham S. Epidemiological assessment of diet: A comparison of a 7-day diary with a food frequency questionnaire using urinary markers of nitrogen, potassium, and sodium. *Int J Epidemiol.* 2001; 30:309–317. https://www.ncbi.nlm.nih.gov/pubmed/11369735. Accessed February 25, 2017.

106. Schoeller DA. Insights into energy balance from doubly labeled water. *Int J Obes* (Lond). 2008; 2:S72-S75.

107. Schoeller DA, Hnilicka JM. Reliability of the doubly labeled water method for the measurement of total daily energy expenditure in free-living subjects. *J Nutr.* 1996;126 (Suppl):348S–54S.

108. Livingston M, Black A. Markers of the validity of reported energy intake. *J Nutr.* 2003; 133(3):895S-920S. http://jn.nutrition.org/content/133/3/895S.long. Accessed on February 25, 2017.

109. Potischman N. Biologic and methodologic issues for nutritional biomarkers. *J Nutr.* 2003; 133: 875S-880S.

110. Bates CJ, Thurnham DL, Bingham SA, Margetts BM, Nelson M. Biochemical markers of nutrient intake. In: Margetts BM, Nelson M, eds. *Design Concepts in Nutritional Epidemiology.* New York, NY: Oxford University Press; 1981; 192–265.

111. Craft NE, Bulux JV, Valdez C, Li Y, Solomons NW. Retinol concentrations in capillary dried blood spots from healthy volunteers: method validation. *Am J Clin Nutr.* 2000; 72: 450–454.

112. O'Broin SD, Gunter EW. Screening of folate status with use of dried blood spots on filter paper. *Am J Clin Nutr.* 1999; 70: 359–367.

113. Linscheer WG, Vergroesen AJ. Lipids. In: Shils ME, Olson JA, Shike M, eds. *Modern Nutrition in Health and Disease*, 8th ed. Philadelphia, PA: Lea and Febiger; 1994: 47–88.

114. McNaughton SA, Hughes MC, Marks GC. Validation of a FFQ to estimate the intake of PUFA using plasma phospholipid fatty acids and weighed food records. *Br J Nutr.* 2007; 97:561-568.

115. Yokota RT, Miyazaki ES, Ito MK. Applying the triads method in the validation of dietary intake using biomarkers. *Cad Saúde Pública.* 2010; 26(11):2027-2037. http://dx.doi.org/10.1590/S0102-311X2010001100004. Accessed February 22, 2017.

116. Tasevska N, Runswick SA, McTaggart A, Bingham SA. Urinary sucrose and fructose as biomarkers for sugar consumption. *Cancer Epidemiol Biomarkers Prev.* 2005; 14(5); 1287–1294. doi: 10.1158/1055–9965. http://cebp.aacrjournals.org/content/14/5/1287.long. Accessed February 26, 2017.

117. Bogers RP, Van Assema P, Kester AD, Westerterp KR, Dagnelie PC. Reproducibility, validity, and responsiveness to change of a short questionnaire for measuring fruit and vegetable intake. *Am J Epidemiol.* 2004; 159(9):900-909. doi: https://doi.org/10.1093/aje/kwh123.

118. Scott KJ, Thurnham DI, Hart DJ, Bingham SA, Day K. The correlation between the intake of lutein, lycopene, and beta carotenoid from vegetables and fruits and, and blood plasma concentrations in a group of women aged 50–65 years in UK. *Br J Nutr*. 1996; 75(3);409–418. https://www.ncbi.nlm.nih .gov/pubmed/8785214. Accessed February 26, 2017.

119. Elmadfa I, Meyer AL. Developing suitable methods of nutritional status assessment: A continuous challenge. *Adv Nutr*. 2014; Sep;5:590S-598S. http://advances.nutrition.org/content/5/5/590S.abstract. Accessed February 22, 2017.

120. Jenab M, Slimani N, Bictash M, Ferrari P, Bingham S. Biomarkers in nutritional epidemiology: Applications, needs, and new horizons. *Hum Genet*. 2009; 125: 507–525. doi: 10.1007/s00439-009-0662-5.

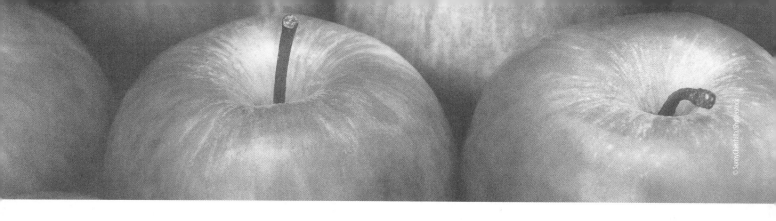

# CHAPTER 5

# National Food and Nutrition Surveys

**Elizabeth F. Eilender**, MS, RD, CDN

## CHAPTER OUTLINE

- Introduction
- Food-Consumption Surveys: Background
- Creation of the National Health and Nutrition Examination Survey
- Creation of a National Nutrition-Monitoring System
- Monitoring Versus Surveillance
- Dietary Assessment Methods
- Defining the Elements of a Healthy Diet
- How Well Do Americans Eat: The Healthy Eating Index
- Chapter Summary

## LEARNING OBJECTIVES

After reading this chapter, the learner will be able to:

1. Describe the early history and development of health and food-consumption surveys, and how they created the groundwork for the monitoring and surveillance instruments used today.
2. Explain how the National Health and Nutrition Examination Survey (NHANES) developed into its current form, and its relevance to research and national nutrition-monitoring activities.
3. Discuss the significance of the National Nutrition Monitoring and Related Research Act to the coordinated and effective collection and use of nationwide diet and health data.
4. Differentiate between nutrition monitoring and nutrition surveillance, and cite examples of each.
5. Identify the most commonly used dietary assessment methods, and the strengths and weaknesses of each one.
6. Recommend healthy eating patterns that align with the *Dietary Guidelines for Americans*.
7. Explain the key principles of the *Dietary Guidelines for Americans*.
8. State the significance of the Healthy Eating Index in evaluating diet quality among Americans.

# ▶ Introduction

How do nutrition experts and researchers determine the extent to which people adhere to evidence-based dietary guidelines, and whether or not the nutrient intake among subsections of the population is adequate? There are many data-collection methods used for diet and nutrition monitoring and surveillance, both nationwide and for select populations, that gather accurate and time information. The data can then be useful for creating effective health policies, designing nutrition-education programs, and making informed decisions related to federal food and nutrition-assistance programs, population-based nutrition interventions, nutrient adequacy of the American food supply, and food safety. This chapter covers the evolution of diet and health surveys in the United States, from the early food-consumption studies of the 1930s to the establishment of nutrition and health examination surveys performed today.

In one form or another, health surveys have been around for a a couple of centuries. Their precursors began in 18th-century Europe when German physician and public-health pioneer Johann Peter Frank (1745–1821) used a rudimentary form of surveying during part of his life in Italy as sanitary inspector general. In this role, he surveyed the health and social conditions in several Italian provinces as he studied the relationship between socioeconomic status, poverty, and the presence of disease.[1] Later, in the 19th century, other health officials performed similar "poverty studies" in cities throughout Great Britain to ascertain the connection between impoverishment and poor health. Eventually, these surveys were done in the United States in certain cities such as Buffalo, New York (1887), New York City (1905), and Baltimore, Maryland (1916–1917).[1]

During the early 20th century, government and health authorities were concerned about the rise in infectious-disease epidemics in rapidly expanding American cities. In 1912, the US Public Health Service conducted "sanitary surveys" to understand the link between human disease and unsound public-sanitation practices. These early surveys showed the importance of having some organized method of observation in the study of health and socioenvironmental conditions.[1]

At that time, the country's major health threats were typhoid, cholera, and yellow fever—contagious diseases associated with poor hygiene and sanitation. But many observers were also aware of the health problems resulting from poor nutrition, such as goiter and pellagra.[2]

As medical discoveries and scientific advancement gave way to increased life expectancy later in the 20th century, scientists and researchers became more interested in how to develop methods for assessing a population's **morbidity rate**, or how frequently diseases appear in a population. Consequently, public-health research and programs shifted from a focus on infectious diseases to the effects of chronic conditions on population health, such as cardiovascular problems and cancer.[1,2]

During the winter of 1935–1936, the US Public Health Service implemented the country's first major government-supported National Health Survey (NHS). This enormous endeavor showed the potential and feasibility of gathering huge amounts of data from a large sample of households relatively quickly.[1] At the time, the NHS was the largest morbidity survey ever done, and it was the first one to focus on chronic disease and disability in the United States.[3] It reached 2.8 million people throughout 19 states and showed on a grand scale that the health of the nation could be evaluated based on the level of disease occurrence rather than **mortality rate**, or the number of deaths in a population per unit of time. The NHS also illuminated the fact that that the poor suffered disproportionately from illnesses because of inadequate health care compared to those of higher economic status.[3]

Over the next 20 years, the findings from this historic survey became the primary source of data on the health status of the American public and the health services they used.[1] Among its many conclusions, the NHS revealed that one person in six in the United States suffered from a chronic disease, a bone-related impairment, or problems with hearing or vision. Consequently, the survey brought widespread national attention to the idea that chronic disease was a major public-health problem linked to pervasive issues such as unsanitary conditions, overcrowding, and poor nutrition.[3]

By 1956, a congressional health bill—the National Health Survey Act—created a permanent version of the NHS, now known as the National Health Interview Survey (NHIS), and established a data-collection agency to be used by those responsible for the country's health policies. The act authorized a continuing survey of disease, injury, impairment, and disability in the United States as overweight, smoking, exposure to air pollution, and other environmental factors entered the realm of epidemiological research.[4]

Today, the NHIS is the principle source of information on the health of the American civilian, noninstitutionalized population and is one of the country's major data-collection programs. Information from the NHIS is used widely throughout the US Department of Health and Human Services (HHS) to monitor trends in illness and disability and track progress in achieving national health objectives. The NHIS is a cross-sectional survey that gathers information through a personal household interview of family members on topics related to health status and limitations, injuries, and healthcare access. Although the survey has been conducted continuously since 1957, its content and questions have been updated every 10 to 15 years.[5]

In addition to the NHIS, the 1956 act also provided the legislative authority for a more comprehensive National Health Examination Survey (NHES), for which data were collected from three major sources:[6]

1. Direct interview of individuals
2. Physical examination, measurements, and clinical tests
3. Places where people receive medical care such as hospitals, clinics, and doctors' offices

The first three such surveys were conducted in the 1960s, and each had a sample size of approximately 7,500 people (see **FIGURE 5.1**).

Although this string of surveys provided vital data for shaping governmental health policies with respect to chronic disease, many researchers agreed that national health-monitoring efforts needed to pay closer attention to the roles that food consumption and nutritional intake had on the health of the nation's population, as well as the extent to which hunger and food insecurity existed throughout the country.

NHES I: 1960 to 1962
Focus: selected chronic diseases of adults ages
   18 to 79

NHES II: 1963 to 1965
Focus: growth and development of children ages
   6 to 11

NHES III: 1966 to 1970
Focus: growth and development of children ages
   12 to 17

**FIGURE 5.1** List of US National Health Examination Surveys conducted between 1960 and 1970

Modified from Centers for Disease Control and Prevention. National Center for Health Statistics. History. https://www.cdc.gov /nchs/nhanes/history.htm. Accessed August 6, 2017.

# ▶ Food-Consumption Surveys: Background

**Preview** Emerging concern about the quality of American diets prompted the initiation of the nation's first major consumer-purchases study, to be followed later by other surveys in the 1940s and 1950s, and eventually by more-expanded surveys over the past 50 years that explored the population's food consumption habits.

Early studies that specifically focused on food and nutrition in the United States began in the 1890s with the work of W.O. Atwater, a renowned food and nutrition scientist who invented the respiratory calorimeter (a device that measures the exchange of oxygen and carbon dioxide in order to calculate the heat energy released after consuming food). His food-consumption studies focused on working-class men who volunteered to provide information on the weight and cost of the foods they ate from a written inventory of items they brought into their household for the duration of the study.[7]

During the Great Depression of the 1930s, concern grew about the quality of American diets. Although not fully representative of the American population, the US Department of Agriculture (USDA) began small and periodic nationwide surveys to examine food consumption and nutritional adequacy.[7] By the middle of the decade, a milestone survey known as the 1935–1936 Consumer Purchases Study provided a more detailed picture of household food consumption. At the time, researchers examining American dietary habits increasingly recognized that malnutrition, in addition to chronic disease, was a central area of public-health concern. The Consumer Purchases Study was the first large-scale, federally funded *dietary* survey in the United States, and it revealed that one-third of American families had diets that were deemed nutritionally poor. These findings were instrumental in spearheading government efforts to enrich flour and bread products with iron and the B vitamins; thiamin, niacin, and riboflavin, as well as bring about the establishment of the federal school-lunch program.[7,8]

A few years later, the 1942 Spending and Saving in Wartime Survey measured the early effects of World War II on food consumption among urban, rural, and farm families at different income levels. Although the survey found significant improvement in American diets overall compared with the 1930s, many families had an inadequate intake of several nutrients in comparison with the Recommended Dietary Allowances (RDAs) that were issued in 1941 by the federal government's Food and Nutrition Board.[7]

More than a decade afterward, the USDA conducted an even larger and more nationally representative study known as the 1955 Household Food Consumption Survey (HFCS), which showed that the adequacy of American diets was improving.[7] Up until this point, many of these food surveys focused on eating patterns within a household, but by the mid-1960s researchers recognized the value in examining the diets of individuals. In 1965, the USDA started to gather data on individual food intakes of household members as part of the nationwide 1965–1966 Household Food Consumption Survey.[8] This more recent HFCS was useful in showing the positive impact of **food fortification** on different age groups, and its success as a survey led to a greater expansion of the next one of its kind, which was renamed the 1977–1978 Nationwide Food Consumption Survey (NFCS). This study was the largest of all the USDA surveys until that time and collected information from 14,000 households as well as dietary-intake data from some 36,000 individuals. It also included data on food-use estimates based on income, season, and region, in addition to food costs at home and away from home.[7]

Ten years later, the 1987–1988 NFCS was the last of this survey type to include both household food use and individual intake components. The collection of both kinds of information in the same survey was burdensome for the respondents and consequently resulted in low response rates during the previous study. Therefore, the USDA did not include a household food-use component in subsequent surveys. Moreover, because of the necessity to assess the nutrient adequacy of diets, analyzing the diet quality of individuals rather than households in comparison with RDA standards made more sense.[7]

## Continuing Survey of Food Intakes by Individuals

In the early 1980s, several committees of the National Academy of Sciences recommended that American food-consumption surveys should be conducted more frequently than every 10 years to accurately assess year-to-year changes in food choices and dietary status. Consequently, the USDA devised the Continuing Survey of Food Intakes by Individuals (CSFII).[8] Introduced in 1985, this survey represented a major change in the frequency of USDA monitoring efforts because it was the first nationwide dietary survey to be conducted yearly in the United States. The purpose was to measure the food and nutrient content of American diets over time, indicate changes in food and nutrient intake, and collect data frequently enough to provide timely information on the adequacy of the diets of selected population groups and therefore enable better planning of government food-assistance and educational programs.[7,9]

In addition, the CSFII was intended to complement the NFCS (conducted every 10 years) by providing continuous data on the dietary status of selected population subgroups, especially those who might be at nutritional risk. The first CSFII, for example, focused on women ages 19 to 50 years and their children ages one to five years in nationally representative samples of all income groups, including those with lower income status. The study gathered six days of dietary data from each participant, including how the meals were prepared and the kinds and amounts of ingredients.[9]

The second CSFII focused on women of childbearing age and young children, with an emphasis on what dietary habits most often failed to provide recommended amounts of nutrients. There was also a collection of one-day dietary data on a nationally representative sample of men ages 19 to 50 years.[9]

The ability to observe trends and anticipate potential problems based on CSFII results have helped policy makers formulate better health regulations and programs related to agriculture, food assistance, nutrition education, and food fortification.[9] Researchers have used data from the CFSII to improve their understanding of factors that affect food choices, as well as to learn how extensively people comprehend and follow federal dietary guidelines. In this way, the survey links individual knowledge and attitudes about nutritional recommendations to practiced dietary behavior.[8]

## Diet and Health Knowledge Survey

Given the assumption that an individual's knowledge and attitudes about food and dietary behavior influences his or her food choices, in 1989 the USDA came out with the Diet and Health Knowledge Survey (DHKS).[7] This survey provided questions to men, women, and children of all ages and included a 24-hour recall and a two-day food diary. It also consisted of a telephone follow-up interview with the CSFII. In so doing, it documented individual attitudes and knowledge about healthy eating and how these perspectives connect with reported food choices and nutrient intakes.[10] Because many nutrition education initiatives are often designed to target the pre-behavioral determinants of dietary choices, obtaining some form of assessment of knowledge, attitudes, and beliefs is useful for designing and evaluating population-based intervention programs.[11]

## What We Eat in America

In 2002, both the CSFII and the DHKS merged to become the National Food and Nutrition Survey, which is also known as What We Eat in America (WWEIA). The newly integrated survey is conducted as a partnership between the USDA and HHS; the former oversees the maintenance of the databases used to code and process the information as well as data review; the latter is responsible for sample design and data collection.[12,13] WWEIA is one of the most important nationwide nutrition and health surveys in the United States and is the dietary information component of the NHANES—the cornerstone of the country's health and nutrition-monitoring system.

> **Recap** The US Department of Agriculture implemented nationwide food-consumption surveys in the 1930s because malnutrition was a major public-health concern. Findings led to the enrichment of flour and bread products with certain key nutrients. Over several decades, more-expanded food-consumption surveys followed to assess the nutritional adequacy of the American diet, including the Nationwide Food Consumption Survey, the Continuing Survey of Food Intakes by Individuals, and What We Eat in America.

## ▶ Creation of the National Health and Nutrition Examination Survey

> **Preview** The **National Health Examination Survey (NHES)** had been in place since the early 1960s. Health advocates called for a dietary component to the survey as research studies continued to support the observed link between diet and health. As a result, the first National Health and Nutrition Examination Survey (NHANES) began in 1971 and continues today.

During the late 1960s, in response to concerns about hunger and malnutrition in the United States, a federal legislative mandate gave rise to the Ten-State Nutrition Survey. The data collected focused only on low-socioeconomic communities and was therefore not representative of the nation as a whole, but it did include a physical assessment. The Ten-State Nutrition Survey was conducted during from 1968 through 1970, utilizing participants selected from urban and rural families living in New York, Massachusetts, Michigan, California, Washington, Kentucky, West Virginia, Louisiana, Texas, and South Carolina.[14]

Among the 30,000 families identified for the survey, 23,846 of them participated in it and more than 80,000 people provided interview data, out of which 40,847 underwent a clinical assessment.[14] The survey included extensive demographic information on each participating family; information regarding its food utilization; and a 24-hour dietary recall for infants up to 36 months of age, children 10 to 16 years of age, pregnant and lactating women, and individuals 60 years of age and older.[14] The collection of this type of data, which included a physical examination, paved the way for a new phase of health and nutrition monitoring in the United States.

After the third and last National Health Examination Survey (NHES III) was well underway starting in 1966, health advocates called for added emphasis on exploring the dietary habits of the participants. The study of nutrition and its relationship to health status had become increasingly important as researchers began to discover additional links between diet and disease.[6] In response to this growing concern, the federal government instituted a National Nutrition Surveillance System in 1970 to evaluate the nutritional status of the American population and observe subsequent changes. A newly created task force recommended that such a surveillance system should also include physical evaluations as well as the collection of dietary-intake patterns. As a result of these recommendations, the surveillance system was combined with the NHES to form the **National Health and Nutrition Examination Survey (NHANES)**, ultimately administered by the HHS.

Today, the NHANES is the nation's most comprehensive form of nutrition and health monitoring because it is collects a cross-section of population-wide data throughout the country. It is unique in using both household interviews and physical examinations, and it comprises a series of nationally representative health studies of adults and children that are conducted in mobile examination units or

1971–75: National Health and Nutrition Examination Survey I (NHANES I)
1976–80: National Health and Nutrition Examination Survey II (NHANES II)
1982–84: Hispanic Health and Nutrition Examination Survey (HHANES)
1988–94: National Health and Nutrition Examination Survey (NHANES III) and
1999–present: National Health and Nutrition Examination Survey (Continuous NHANES)

NHANES I was based on a national sample of 28,000 persons ages one to 74. The data were collected by interview, physical examination, and a series of clinical measurements and tests from all members of the sample.

NHANES II involved interviewing and examining 28,000 people between six months and 74 years of age. To establish a baseline for assessing changes over time, data collection for NHANES II were made comparable to NHANES I data so that many of the same measurements were taken in the same way on the same age segment of the American population in both surveys.

The NHANES, conducted from 1982 to 1984, aimed at producing estimates of health and nutritional status for the three largest Hispanic subgroups in the United States—Mexican Americans, Cuban Americans, and Puerto Ricans—that were comparable to the estimates available for the general population. The HHANES was similar in design to the previous NHANES studies, interviewing and examining 16,000 people in various regions across the country with large Hispanic populations.

NHANES III included 40,000 people selected from households in 81 counties across the United States in which black Americans and Mexican Americans were selected in large proportions in NHANES III. It was also the first survey to include infants as young as 2 months of age and adults with no upper age limit. For the first time, a home examination was developed for those persons who were unable or unwilling to come into the exam center but would agree to an abbreviated examination in their homes. To obtain reliable estimates, infants and young children (1 to 5 years old) and older persons (60+ years) were sampled at a higher rate. NHANES III also placed an additional emphasis on the effects of the environment on health. Data were gathered to measure the levels of pesticide exposure, the presence of certain trace elements, and the level of carbon monoxide in the blood.

Data collection on the current NHANES began in early 1999 and remains a continuous annual survey. Each year, approximately 7,000 randomly selected residents across the United States participate in the latest NHANES.

**FIGURE 5.2** National Health and Nutrition Examination Surveys 1971 to the present

Modified from Centers for Disease Control and Prevention. National Center for Health Statistics. History. https://www.cdc.gov/nchs/nhanes/history.htm. Accessed August 6, 2017.

clinics. The surveys monitor changes over time by gathering information on dietary intake, biochemical tests, physical measurements (anthropometric data), and clinical assessments for evidence of nutritional deficiencies.[15]

The clinical examinations and laboratory tests follow a specific standard protocol to ensure as much as possible that the data across sites and providers are comparable. The survey results are then used to determine the prevalence of major diseases as well as risk factors for them, as well as assess nutritional status. In addition, the findings serve as the basis for national standards for such measurements as height, weight, and blood pressure.[15]

A total of seven national examination surveys were conducted from 1960 to 1994 in distinct cycles encompassing several years, but the NHANES has become a continuous annual survey since 1999. Data are collected every year from a representative sample of the civilian, noninstitutionalized American population (See **FIGURE 5.2**).[15]

**Recap** Concern about hunger and malnutrition in the United States gave rise to an early nationwide dietary survey in the late 1960s, called the Ten-State Nutrition Survey. At the same time, health advocates observed the growing link between diet and health and urged policy makers to modify the already existing National Health and Examination Survey to include a dietary component. This change led to the establishment of the National Health and Nutrition Examination Survey, which is the nation's most comprehensive form of nutrition and health monitoring.

# ▶ Creation of a National Nutrition-Monitoring System

**Preview** By the 1970s, the US government had a long-established system for monitoring dietary behavior across the country. However, the system had its weaknesses, chief among them a lack of efficient coordination between the two federal agencies responsible for those activities. In response to the problem, the National Nutrition Monitoring System (NNMS) was created.

Since the 1930s, the American government has tracked food usage in the country, starting with the Consumer Purchases Study, which eventually expanded to become the Nationwide Food Consumption Survey of the late 1970s. The consensus was that further development in the breadth and approach of federal nutrition-monitoring activities was needed, along with a revised mechanism for setting priorities. As a result, between 1969 and 1977, a congressional committee investigated not only the pervasiveness of hunger in the United States but also how effectively the federal government was at measuring the nature and extent of the problem.[16] As serious shortcomings of the federal nutrition-monitoring apparatus came to light, such as a lack of timely and effective data collection that hindered drawing scientifically valid conclusions over time, lawmakers saw a need for a more fully coordinated and comprehensive system.[16,17]

In answering this need for legislative action, the two federal agencies most responsible for nutrition monitoring—the USDA and the HHS—aimed to improve the scope and coordination of their national surveys. The central problem was that food availability data from the USDA and dietary-intake data from both the USDA and the HHS were gathered in surveys that used different collection methods from a wide variety of sample populations, which used different kinds of food-composition databases and consequently produced results that could not be compared. These differences made it difficult for researchers to use the data to reach reliable conclusions about dietary changes.[17]

In response to these challenges, the 1977 Food and Agriculture Act instructed the USDA and the DHSS (then called the Department of Health, Education, and Welfare) to submit to Congress a proposal for a comprehensive nutrition-status monitoring system that would integrate the ongoing nutrition survey activities of both departments. The primary objective was that the USDA and HHS should achieve the highest level of coordination between the two largest and most-important components of the system: the USDA's Nationwide Food Consumption Survey (NFCS) and the HHS's NHANES.[9] The act also called for the creation of a reporting system and the delivery of periodic reports to Congress based on survey results and related nutrition-monitoring activities.[18] Together, the two federal departments submitted the Joint Implementation Plan for a Comprehensive National Nutrition Monitoring System to Congress in 1981.[9]

## The Goals of the National Nutrition Monitoring System

The **Nation Nutrition Monitoring System (NNMS)** has the following five goals:

1. Provide the scientific foundation for the maintenance and improvement of the nutritional status of the American population and of the nutritional quality and healthfulness of the national food supply.
2. Collect, analyze, and disseminate timely data on the nutritional and dietary status of the American population, the nutritional quality of the food supply, food-consumption patterns, and consumer knowledge and attitudes concerning nutrition.
3. Identify high-risk groups of individuals and geographic areas, as well as nutrition-related problems and trends, in order to facilitate prompt implementation of nutrition-intervention activities.
4. Establish national baseline data for the NNMS and develop and improve uniform standard methods, criteria, policies, and procedures for nutrition monitoring.
5. Provide data for evaluating changes in agricultural policy related to food production, processing, and distribution that may affect the nutritional quality and healthfulness of the American food supply.

The implementation plan called for the integration of some of the current monitoring system's existing elements such as using the same coding system, coordination of questions and interviewer training, and compatible databases for gender and age categories.[9]

In 1983, a joint USDA and HHS nutrition-monitoring and evaluation committee issued the country's first report providing an in-depth summary of the dietary and nutritional status of the American population. Several recommendations for future survey data collection and nutrition monitoring were suggested, and in 1988 the Interagency Committee on Nutrition Monitoring was formed to enhance planning, coordination, and communication of these activities with the federal government (in 1991 it was replaced by the Interagency Board for Nutrition Monitoring and Related Research).[18]

In 1990 Congress passed the National Nutrition Monitoring and Related Research Act, which established the National Nutrition Monitoring and Related Research Program (NNMRRP) and was the culmination of efforts to create a coordinated collaboration between federal, state, and local government agencies.[18] Today, the data obtained from the NNMRRP are used to direct research initiatives, develop education activities and services, and make policy decisions regarding nutrition programs such as food labeling, food and nutrition assistance, and food safety. Reports of the various efforts are issued every five years or so and provide information on trends, knowledge, attitudes and behavior, food composition, and factors that influence the food supply.[10] **FIGURE 5.3** summarizes some of the important uses of national nutrition-monitoring data.

> **Recap** Although a federal nutrition-monitoring program had been in place for many years, lawmakers saw a need for a more fully coordinated and comprehensive system that allowed the USDA and HHS to better coordinate their activities. The 1977 Food and Agriculture Act paved the way for the creation of the NNMS. Among other objectives, the NNMS is responsible for identifying groups at high risk for nutrition-related problems; collect, analyze, and disseminate timely data on the nutritional and dietary status of the American population; and provide data for evaluating changes in agricultural policy related to food production, processing, and distribution.

## ▶ Monitoring versus Surveillance

> **Preview** Although often used interchangeably, the terms *monitoring* and *surveillance* in their strictest sense do not share the same definition. **Monitoring** refers to quantitatively accurate measures with the goal of observing trends with precision, and **surveillance** refers to a system of collecting less-precise data for use in timely population-based interventions.

- To observe trends in food and nutrient intake (e.g., total fat and saturated fat intake, fruit and vegetable intake).
- To observe trends in the prevalence of disease and related risk factors (e.g., hypertension, overweight, obesity, and diabetes).
- To observe trends in intake and household food security.
- To monitor the current and future safety of the food supply (e.g., exposure of seafood to methyl mercury, pesticide levels in raw agricultural products, and bacterial contamination).
- To evaluate whether nutrient intakes are consistent with the *Dietary Guidelines for Americans*.
- To monitor trends in supplement use and composition.
- To monitor trends in dietary knowledge and behavior.
- To review food fortification policy and labeling.
- To assess food-assistance programs (e.g., SNAP, WIC, and school breakfast and lunch programs).

**FIGURE 5.3** Uses of nutrition-monitoring data

Modified from Dwyer J, Picciano MF, and Raiten DJ. "Future Directions for What We Eat in America -NHANES: The Integrated CSFII-NHANES." *Journal of Nutrition.* February 1, 2003, Volume 133, No. 2; 576S-581S.

Throughout this chapter, we have discussed topics related to food and nutrition monitoring and surveillance in a general sense, with these terms often meaning the same thing. However, in a more narrow and specific context, the two terms are not interchangeable and have subtle differences. The distinction between monitoring and surveillance is related to the goals of these activities rather than to specific methods of implementation. *Monitoring* refers to the collection and analysis of quantitatively accurate measures from representative samples of a population, with the goal of observing trends with precision. *Surveillance* refers to a system of data collection of less-precise measures, but it is intended to elicit prompt interventions when a meaningful trend or problem is detected.[11]

Therefore, nutrition-monitoring systems usually evaluate large, representative samples of the population that are national or regional with direct and accurate measures such as body weight and detailed diet recalls. In contrast, nutrition-surveillance systems usually assess state or local samples that may not be representative of the entire population and use more-superficial and more-rapid measures such as self-reported weight and brief food-frequency questionnaires.[11]

Nutrition-monitoring data tend to be analyzed as direct estimates of nutritional parameters of larger populations over the time span of years, whereas surveillance data tend to be analyzed as indirect indicators of nutritional status of smaller, local populations over the time span of months. Therefore, the differences between the methods are rooted in the quantitative accuracy of the measures, the differences in population size, and the differences in the timelines in question.[11]

Monitoring surveys such as the NHANES produce dietary-intake estimates that are representative of the national population but are not designed to provide measures representing any particular locality. Furthermore, analyses of national-survey monitoring data are often not performed until several years after the information is collected. Therefore, dietary surveillance is necessary to provide a locally representative and timely measure of any behaviors or nutritional determinants that are needed for planning, targeting, and evaluating nutrition-intervention programs.[11] In the United States, nutritional surveillance has traditionally focused on populations served by maternal and child health programs in order to detect trends in undernutrition and iron deficiency. However, a growing number of surveillance initiatives have been searching for trends related to chronic-disease risks such as obesity, dietary fat intake, and inadequate consumption of fruits and vegetables. In this respect, local data are helpful for intervention purposes given that national data can lack timeliness and localized representation of a given audience.[11]

Two examples of past nutrition-surveillance systems that were operated jointly by state departments of health and the Centers for Disease Control and Prevention (CDC) are the Pediatric Nutrition Surveillance System and the **Pregnancy Nutrition Surveillance System (PNSS)**. Data are analyzed locally on a monthly or quarterly basis to identify and track individual cases of nutritional inadequacy such as anemia or low weight for height.[11] State health agencies, in conjunction with the CDC, currently operate the Behavioral Risk Factor Surveillance System designed to measure the major behavioral causes of chronic diseases and injuries in each state. Policy makers use this information to design, target, and evaluate prevention programs.[11]

## Behavioral Risk Factor Surveillance System

Although national estimates of health risk behaviors among American adult populations had been periodically obtained through surveys conducted by the National Center for Health Statistics (NCHS), these data were not available on a state-by-state basis. This situation was viewed as a critical obstacle to efforts by state health agencies to target resources aimed at behavioral-risk reduction. Meanwhile, telephone surveys emerged as an acceptable method for determining the prevalence of many health risk behaviors among populations, and they were more cost-effective than face-to-face interviewing.

In 1984, the CDC established the **Behavioral Risk Factor Surveillance System (BRFSS)**, and 15 states participated in monthly data collection. The CDC developed a standard core questionnaire for states to use to provide data that could be compared across states. Initial topics included smoking, alcohol use, physical inactivity, diet, hypertension, and seatbelt use; in 1988, the agency introduced optional question modules on specific topics. The BRFSS became a nationwide surveillance system in 1993 using a redesigned questionnaire that included rotating core questions. States have used the BRFSS to address urgent and emerging health issues, such as monitoring vaccine shortages during the 2004–2005 flu season, and using questions to ask about influenza-like illness during the 2009 H1N1 flu pandemic.[19]

In 2008, the BRFSS started to include cell phones in the survey to reach segments of the population that were previously inaccessible—those who have cell phones but not landlines—and produce a more representative sample and higher-quality data. More than 450,000 interviews are conducted each year, making the BRFSS the largest telephone survey in the world.[19,20] Currently data are collected monthly in all 50 states, the District of Columbia, American Samoa, Palau, Puerto Rico, the US Virgin Islands, and Guam.[20] For most local health departments, the BRFSS is the only source of state data on health and health risk behavior related to chronic disease. The BRFSS gives communities and states, as well as the CDC and other federal agencies, the necessary information to plan, conduct, and evaluate public-health programs at local, state, and national levels.[19]

Each year, states can choose to add several optional modules to their core surveys, which can include questions related to chronic illnesses, workplace conditions, diet, and prevention behaviors such as disease screenings and immunizations. They can also develop and add questions that they develop to meet their specific needs. All states use the same methods to conduct their surveys, as well as any additional modules and added questions, to yield comparable results between states or local areas.[19]

## Youth Risk Behavior Surveillance System

The **Youth Risk Behavior Surveillance System (YRBSS)** was created in 1990 to monitor priority health-risk behaviors that contribute markedly to the leading causes of death, disability, and social problems among youth and young adults in the United States. These behaviors, which are often established during the childhood years and early adolescence, include:[21]

- Behaviors that contribute to unintentional injuries and violence
- Sexual behaviors related to unintended pregnancy and sexually transmitted infections, including HIV infection
- Alcohol and other drug use
- Tobacco use
- Unhealthy dietary behaviors
- Inadequate physical activity

In addition, the YRBSS monitors the prevalence of obesity and asthma and other priority issues related to health such as sexual identity and behavior.

Conducted every two years, the YRBSS has collected data from more than 3.8 million public and private high-school students (ninth through 12th grade)

from 1991 through 2015 in more than 1,700 separate surveys, which were designed to do the following:[21]

- Determine the prevalence of health behaviors
- Assess whether health behaviors increase, decrease, or stay the same over time
- Examine the co-occurrence of health behaviors
- Provide comparable national, state, territorial, tribal, and local data
- Provide comparable data among subpopulations of youth
- Monitor progress toward achieving the federal government's Healthy People objectives and other program indicators

## Pediatric Nutrition Surveillance System

In 1973, the CDC began working with five American states to develop a system for continuously monitoring the nutritional status of low-income children participating in federally funded maternal and child health and nutrition programs. By 1997, the **Pediatric Nutrition Surveillance System (PedNSS)** had expanded to include 44 states, the District of Columbia, and five tribal governments.[22] The PedNSS was replaced in 2012 by the Special Supplemental Nutrition Program for Women, Infants, and Children Participants and Program Characteristics (WIC PC), which summarizes the characteristics of those receiving services nationwide based on income, nutrition risk, and breastfeeding initiation rates. Data are generated every two years from WIC's state management system.[23,24]

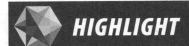

## HIGHLIGHT

### A Closer Look: The Youth Risk Behavior Survey

Among American high-school students, 14% are obese and 48% do not attend physical-education classes in an average week. This data comes from the national 2015 Youth Risk Behavior Survey, a surveillance system set up by the Centers for Disease Control and Prevention in the early 1990s. Since 1991, the Youth Risk Behavior Surveillance System (YRBSS) has collected data from more than 3.8 million high-school students from more than 1,700 separate surveys to monitor priority health risk behaviors. Some of the issues include unhealthy dietary choices, inadequate physical activity, and examining the prevalence of obesity.

The procedure for conducting the YRBSS is designed to protect student privacy by allowing anonymous participation, which is voluntary but requires

parental permission. Students must complete a self-administered questionnaire during one class period and record their responses on a computer-scannable booklet or answer sheet. The survey takes approximately 35 minutes to complete, and no physical exam is involved.

The YRBSS questionnaires are only available in English, but they are in the public domain and may be freely translated and used in any language. The data are available only for large urban school districts or counties. No data are available by zip code, census tract, or school because of sample-size limitations and confidentiality requirements.

National YRBSS data sets and documentation are available at https://www.cdc.gov/healthyyouth/data/yrbs/data.htm for download at no charge, and permission is not required to access or use the information.

# ▶ Dietary Assessment Methods

**Preview**  Dietary assessment methods are used by researchers to obtain the data they need for effective nutrition monitoring or surveillance of targeted populations. Food-consumption records, 24-hour dietary recalls, food records, dietary histories, and food-frequency questionnaires are the methods most commonly used.

Dietary assessment methods are the "tools of the trade" used by researchers to obtain the data they need for effective nutrition monitoring or surveillance of targeted populations. The type, quantity, and nutrient composition of an individual's diet can be challenging to measure with the accuracy needed to render the results scientifically meaningful. Inaccurate dietary assessment may present a significant hindrance to understanding the extent to which diet affects health, so it is important to explore the benefits and limitations of each type of method.[25] This section offers a brief review of the dietary assessment methods most often used in population-based research that are put into practice singularly or in combination with one another (see **TABLE 5.1**). These methods include food-consumption records, the 24-hour dietary recall, the food record, the dietary history, and the food-frequency questionnaire.

A **food-consumption record** involves collecting dietary information on the subject's food-preparation and food-consumption habits in his or her home. It is performed by a skilled fieldworker making objective observations. This approach is especially useful in developing countries with low literacy rates where the subjects may have difficulty filling out questionnaires or reading food checklists; it is not helpful for subjects who frequently eat outside the home. Similarly, a **food record** collects real-time data by having subjects self-record what they consume at the time they eat, which may or may not include weighing the foods consumed, thus reducing their reliance on memory. On the other hand, to collect accurate data, respondents must be trained before participating in the survey. Consequently, there is a relatively large burden imposed on the subjects.[25]

Also commonly used in nutrition survey research is the **dietary recall (24-hour)**, which is an open-ended survey that collects a variety of detailed information about the subject's food consumption over a specific time period. It is used mostly in nutrition-surveillance and nutrition-monitoring studies, which assess a population's intake and helps researchers identify subgroups that may require dietary intervention.[26] The 24-hour recall is typically conducted through an in-depth interview and often requires 20 to 30 minutes to complete for a recall of one day. Depending on the purpose of the research, the interviewer may collect information about the subject's food preparation methods, the ingredients used in mixed dishes, and the brand name of the commercial products that are used. The amounts of each food consumed can be estimated by referencing common sizes of dishware and kitchen implements (such as bowls, cups, drinking glasses, and standard measuring cups and spoons) or by using a three-dimensional food model or photographs. A big advantage of the 24-hour recall is that it places a relatively small burden on respondents. The accuracy of the information, however, depends on the subject's memory as well as the skills of a well-trained interviewer to minimize recall bias.[25]

Both the 24-hour recall and the food records are frequently applied to randomized clinical trials and cohort studies.[25] These methods also have some limitations in that both mainly focus on short-term intake, which is not optimal for studying chronic diseases unless multiple 24-hour recalls and food records are used. Use of such repeated measurements requires a lot of resources and time, and survey repetition may also influence a respondent's diet unintentionally through the process of self-reflection, which in turn may skew the results.

A **dietary history** is used to assess individual long-term dietary intake. It requires that subjects complete a 24-hour recall, a three-day food diary, and a checklist of foods they typically eat. A dietary history requires a highly skilled professional to

**TABLE 5.1** Summary of dietary assessment methods and applications

| Method | Food Records | 24-Hour Recall (Multiple) | 24-Hour Recall (Single) | Food-Frequency Questionnaire | Biomarkers |
|---|---|---|---|---|---|
| Applications | Monitoring compliance of dietary intervention studies Validation of other dietary-intake assessment methods | Monitoring compliance of dietary intervention studies Assessment of trends in dietary intake (i.e., currently used in NHANES) Validation of other dietary-intake assessment methods | National surveillance of dietary intake (mean population) Assessment of trends in dietary intake (i.e., earlier versions of NHANES) | Analysis of dietary and disease associations in large epidemiological studies Assessment of past dietary intake | Analysis of dietary and disease associations in smaller epidemiological studies Monitoring of compliance in intervention trials Validation of other dietary-intake assessment methods |

Modified from Satija A., Yu E., Willett WC, and Hu FB. "Understanding Nutritional Epidemiology and Its Role in Policy." *Advances in Nutrition.* 2015;6:5-18.

collect the information on the subject's usual diet through an in-depth interview, which may take 90 minutes to complete, and is therefore used far less often in epidemiological studies compared with other methods.[25]

The **food-frequency questionnaire (FFQ)** is an advanced form of the checklist used in the dietary history method. It asks respondents how often and how much food they ate over a specific time period. The method is used in a vast majority of nutritional epidemiology studies that assess association between diet and disease.[26] The FFQ often lists about 100 to 150 foods and takes 20 to 30 minutes to complete, but it can be self-administered or conducted through an interview. This method is highly useful for assessing long-term dietary intakes in a relatively simple, cost-effective, and time-efficient manner, and therefore has been widely used since the 1990s.[25]

**Biomarkers** are biological measures that are used to perform a clinical assessment, such as finding out cholesterol level or iron status. Biomarkers help with monitoring and predicting states of health for use in determining appropriate therapeutic interventions. In epidemiological studies, specific biomarkers have been used to measure the dietary intake of selected nutrients or food components. These markers have been found to be highly correlated with dietary intake levels, are not subject to social desirability bias or the

subject's memory failures, and therefore may provide more-accurate measures than do dietary intake estimates. Several biomarkers are influenced by their absorption and metabolism after food consumption and ones that are also affected by disease or homeostatic regulation in such a way that their values cannot be translated into the subject's absolute dietary intake.[25]

Many foods and nutrients lack sensitive or specific biomarkers, or their assessment always includes error from multiple sources. Obtaining and testing for biomarkers is also expensive and burdensome, so their use to investigate the links between nutrients and disease has been mostly limited to case-control studies and small trials.[27]

**Recap** Inaccurate dietary assessment may significantly hinder our understanding the degree to which diet and health are linked. It is therefore important to weigh the benefits and limitations of each type of assessment method. Some have more ease of application compared with others, or require training of the survey interviewer. Other methods may be subject to recall bias or place a relatively large burden on the respondent. These methods can be used singularly or in combination.

# ▶ Defining the Elements of a Healthy Diet

> **Preview** Mounting evidence suggests that certain long-term dietary patterns significantly reduce the risk of many chronic conditions. The 2015 *Dietary Guidelines for Americans* emphasizes the importance of variety in what people eat, rather than a narrow focus on specific nutrients or foods in isolation. Specific healthy eating patterns are recommended.

With almost universal agreement, health experts believe there is no single perfect diet suitable for everyone. However, after decades of data collection and scientific research, there is a preponderance of evidence demonstrating that certain long-term dietary patterns significantly reduce the risk of many chronic conditions.[28]

Today, federal dietary guidelines are based on the belief that what people routinely eat and drink can confer positive cumulative effects on health over time. To encourage not just better choices of particular foods but also improved eating habits overall, the federal government's latest set of **Dietary Guidelines for Americans** (issued in 2015) emphasizes the importance of variety in what people eat rather than a narrow focus on specific nutrients or foods in isolation—the pursuit of **healthy eating patterns**.[28]

Research shows that a healthy eating pattern includes a *high* intake of fruits, vegetables, whole grains, fat-free or low-fat dairy, seafood, legumes, and nuts. A healthy eating pattern also includes a *low* intake of meat, processed meat, sugar-sweetened foods and beverages, and refined grains. To put these recommendations into practice, the *Dietary Guidelines* suggest that people focus on one of three broad eating styles: Healthy US-Style Eating, Healthy Mediterranean-Style Eating, and Healthy Vegetarian Eating.[28]

## The Healthy US-Style Eating Pattern

This eating pattern is based on the types and proportions of foods Americans typically eat but in nutrient-dense and sensible portion sizes. An example of a Healthy US Style Eating Pattern based on a 2,000-calorie daily diet is:

- 2½ cups of vegetables
- 2 cups of fruit
- 6 ounces of grains (half should be whole grains)
- 3 cups of dairy
- 5½ ounces of protein foods (8 ounces of seafood *per week*; 26 ounces of meat, poultry, and eggs *per week*; 5 ounces of nuts, seeds, and soy products *per week*)
- 5 teaspoons of healthy oils per day.

The Dietary Approaches to Stop Hypertension (DASH) is an example of a healthy eating pattern that has many of the same features as the Healthy US-Style Eating Pattern. Studies of DASH have shown that it significantly lowers blood pressure and LDL-cholesterol levels, thereby reducing the risk for cardiovascular disease compared to diets that are similar to a typical American diet. DASH is high in vegetables, fruits, low-fat dairy products, whole grains, poultry, fish, beans, and nuts and is therefore rich in potassium, calcium, magnesium, fiber, and protein. The DASH plan is also low in sweets, sugar-sweetened beverages, and red meats, and therefore low in saturated fats. It is also lower in sodium than the typical American diet.

## The Healthy Mediterranean-Style Eating Pattern

The Healthy Mediterranean-Style Eating Pattern is an eating plan that consists of more fruits and seafood and fewer dairy choices than the Healthy US-Style Eating Pattern. An example of a daily 2,000-calorie diet includes:

- 2½ cups of vegetables
- 2½ cups of fruits
- 6 ounces of grains (half of which are whole grains)
- 2 cups of dairy
- 6½ ounces of protein foods, which include a combination of meat, poultry, and eggs (26 ounces *per week*)
- Seafood (15 ounces *per week*)
- A combination of nuts, seeds, and soy products (5 ounces *per week*)
- 5 teaspoons of healthy oils per day

## The Healthy Vegetarian Eating Pattern

When compared to the Healthy US-Style Eating Pattern, the Healthy Vegetarian Eating Pattern includes more legumes (beans and peas), soy products, nuts and seeds, and whole grains. It contains no meats, poultry, or seafood. An example of a daily 2,000-calorie diet includes:

- 2½ cups of vegetables
- 2 cups of fruit
- 6½ ounces of grains (3½ of which is whole grains)
- 3 cups of dairy substitute
- 3½ ounces of protein foods, including eggs (3 ounces *per week*)
- Legumes (6 ounces *per week*)
- Soy products (8 ounces *per week*)
- Nuts and seeds (7 ounces *per week*)
- 5 teaspoons of healthy oils per day

**Recap** Current federal dietary guidelines call for an emphasis on healthy eating patterns because evidence suggests that what people routinely eat and drink can confer a positive cumulative effect on health over time. Research shows that a healthy eating pattern includes a high intake of fruits, vegetables, whole grains, fat-free or low-fat dairy, seafood, legumes, and nuts; as well as a low intake of meat, processed meat, sugar-sweetened foods and beverages, and refined grains.

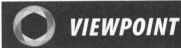

# VIEWPOINT

## Health Literacy

*Charlotte M. Beyer, MSIS, AHIP*

### What Is Health Literacy?

Health literacy is defined as the degree to which individuals have the capacity to obtain, process, and understand basic health information and services needed to make appropriate decisions for their care. According to *Healthy People 2020*, everyone has the right to health information that helps them make informed decisions. In addition, health services should be delivered in ways that are understandable and beneficial to health, longevity, and quality of life.[1]

The modern healthcare system is complex and expects patients to effectively communicate with healthcare providers. This can be greatly affected by barriers such as education, culture, and knowledge of health care. Examples of low health literacy include an inability to identify medications or conditions, read appointment slips, or navigate insurance plans.

### Low-Health-Literacy Nutrition Example

A patient with diabetes is referred to a dietitian. The patient believes he does not eat a lot of sugar and cannot possibly have high blood sugar. He feels it was the candy bar he ate the day before he had his blood drawn that is causing the problem; if his blood were drawn today, the blood-sugar level would be normal. He feels he does not need information on a high-blood-sugar diet.

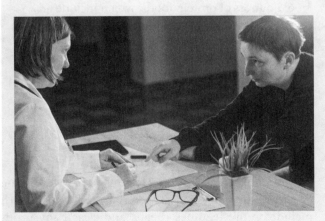

© igorstevanovic/Shutterstock.

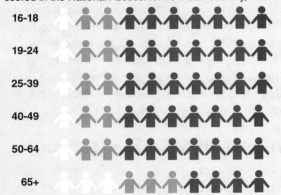

*Health Literacy by Age*

Listed below are the general percentages of how age groups scored in the National Assessment of Adult Literacy, 2003.

16-18
19-24
25-39
40-49
50-64
65+

Below Basic   Basic ▨   Intermediate ▩   Proficient ■

**Note:** data has been rounded.

Modified from U.S. Department of Education, Institute of Education Sciences, National Center for Education Statistics, 2003 National Assessment of Adult Literacy.

### Why Is It Important?

According to the National Assessment for Adult Literacy, six of 10 adults over age 65 years scored in the basic or below basic levels.[2] This means these individuals struggle to perform tasks such as calculating a healthy weight based on a body mass index chart. Note that health literacy is separate from prose literacy, which is being able to read and comprehend continuous text. This is because health care as a whole is unfamiliar to a vast majority of the public, regardless of education. This lack of health literacy proficiency has far-reaching impacts in health care, including the lack of preventive healthcare use as well as increased rates of hospitalization that, in turn, increase healthcare costs.

### What Strategies Might Improve Health Literacy?

Healthcare providers can employ a few strategies to improve the health literacy of their patients. Before a potential intervention, for example, select patient education materials that are easy to understand and use plain language. One great resource for these types of materials is MedlinePlus—https://medlineplus.gov/all_easytoread.html. One of the most important methods to improving health literacy is evaluating users' understanding at every point of the intervention. One tool providers can use is the teach-back method, in which the patient is asked to repeat instructions in their own words. If there is any misunderstanding, the provider adjusts the instructions.[3] Using any of these strategies can greatly help patients understand their health issues and improve their health and well-being.

---

**Strategies for Improving Health Literacy**

✓ Choose easy-to-read materials.

✓ Use the teach-back method to evalute patient understanding.

✓ Revise your approach if there is a lack of understanding.

---

Modified from Quick Guide to Health Literacy: Improve the Usability of Health Information. Office of Disease Prevention and Health Promotion. https://health.gov/communication/literacy/quickguide/healthinfo.htm Created April 26, 2006. Accessed August 1, 2017.

### References

1. Office of Disease Prevention and Health Promotion. Healthy People 2020. National Action Plan to Improve Health Literacy. https://www.healthypeople.gov/2020/tools-resources/evidence-based-resource/national-action-plan-improve-health-literacy.
2. Kutner M, Greenberg E, Jin Y, Paulsen C. *The Health Literacy of America's Adults: Results from the 2003 National Assessment of Adult Literacy (NCES 2006–483)*. Washington, DC: National Center for Education Statistics; 2006.
3. Use the Teach-Back Method: Tool #5. Rockville, MD: Agency for Healthcare Research and Quality. http://www.ahrq.gov/professionals/quality-patient-safety/quality-resources/tools/literacy-toolkit/healthlittoolkit2-tool5.html.

---

## ▶ How Well Do Americans Eat? The Healthy Eating Index

**Preview**   The Healthy Eating Index is a nationwide survey that assesses the extent to which a cross-section of the population adheres to federal dietary guidelines. The survey uses data collected through a 24-hour recall.

Although Americans are encouraged to understand and follow the basic principles of the federal *Dietary Guidelines for Americans*, an important nationwide survey known as the **Healthy Eating Index (HEI)** has been used for more than 20 years as a way to assess the extent to which a cross-section of the population adheres to the *Guidelines*. This diet-quality survey uses data that are collected through a 24-hour dietary recall. The original HEI was created by the Center for Nutrition Policy and Promotion in 1995.[13]

Because of its assessment purposes, the HEI is a diet-quality index of major significance to public health. The original 1995 index had 10 components that measured five major food groups and four nutrients that should be consumed in moderation and variety, with a score of 100 being as close to adherence to the guidelines as possible.[29] The latest available HEI results are from 2010, and they reflect changes in diet quality over time. They also examine the relationship between diet cost and diet quality, evaluate the diets of subpopulations, assess the quality of foods provided through USDA nutrition-assistance programs, and measure the impact of nutrition interventions. The information has also been used in research to better understand relationships between nutrients, foods, dietary patterns, and health-related outcomes.[13] The most recent version of the HEI also uses a score from 0 to 100 and has 12 components:[30]

- Adequacy (higher consumption results in a higher score)
  - Total fruit (5 points)
  - Whole fruit (5 points)
  - Total vegetables (5 points)
  - Greens and beans (5 points)
  - Whole grains (10 points)
  - Dairy (10 points)
  - Total protein (5 points)
  - Seafood and plant proteins (5 points)
  - Fatty acids (10 points)

- Moderation (lower consumption results in a higher score)
  - Refined grains (10 points)
  - Sodium (10 points)
  - Empty calories and added sugar (20 points)

A diet with a score greater than 80 is considered *good*, one with a score of 51 to 80 is considered *fair*, and one with a score of less than 51 is considered *poor*.[31] Based on the 2009 to 2010 NHANES, the average HEI for Americans age two and older was 57.[32] The most-recent HEI-2010 scores for the total American population aged two or older, children 2 to 17 years of age, and older adults 65 years of age or older was based on data from NHANES 2011 to 2012 and are summarized in **TABLE 5.2**. The average score for the total American population is 59—a small increase from the previous result, indicating that Americans had not

**TABLE 5.2** Healthy Eating Index 2010: Total and component scores for the US total population, children and older adults, NHANES 2011–2012

| HEI-2010 Dietary Component (Maximum Score) | Mean Score (Standard Error) | | |
|---|---|---|---|
| | Total Population ≥2 Years (*n* = 7,933) | Children 2–17 Years (*n* = 2,857) | Older Adults ≥65 Years (*n* = 1,032) |
| Total fruit (5) | 3.00 (0.11) | 3.91 (0.18) | 3.84 (0.22) |
| Whole fruit (5) | 4.01 (0.17) | 4.78 (0.22) | 4.99 (0.05) |
| Total vegetables (5) | 3.36 (0.08) | 2.10 (0.09) | 4.16 (0.19) |
| Greens and beans (5) | 2.98 (0.15) | 0.70 (0.09) | 3.58 (0.47) |
| Whole grains (10) | 2.86 (0.13) | 2.50 (0.10) | 4.23 (0.34) |
| Dairy (10) | 6.44 (0.14) | 9.03 (0.22) | 5.99 (0.16) |
| Total protein foods (5) | 5.00 (0.00) | 4.44 (0.13) | 5.00 (0.00) |
| Seafood and plant proteins (5) | 3.74 (0.20) | 3.05 (0.17) | 4.91 (0.18) |
| Fatty acids (10) | 4.66 (0.14) | 3.29 (0.18) | 5.60 (0.36) |
| Refined grains (10) | 6.19 (0.15) | 4.91 (0.16) | 7.34 (0.31) |
| Sodium (10) | 4.15 (0.06) | 4.85 (0.25) | 3.66 (0.26) |
| Empty calories (20) | 12.60 (0.23) | 11.50 (0.28) | 14.99 (0.44) |
| Total HEI score (100) | 59.00 (0.95) | 55.07 (0.72) | 68.29 (1.76) |

Modified from United States Department of Agriculture, Center for Nutrition Policy and Promotion (n.d.).

made much progress in improving the quality of their diets over that time frame. Work still must be done to improve our food choices to promote health and prevent disease.

> **Recap**  For more than 20 years, the Healthy Eating Index has been used to evaluate the extent to which Americans follow federal dietary guidelines. The survey reflects changes in diet quality over time, examines the relationship between diet cost and diet quality, and measures the impact of nutrition interventions. The index contains 12 components made up of food groups and certain nutrients that are each assigned a score based on level of consumption. A total Index score of 80 and above is *good*, 51 to 80 is *fair*, and less than 51 is *poor*.

## ▶ Chapter Summary

From national food-consumption surveys in the early 20th century to the present-day nutrition-monitoring and nutrition-surveillance systems, evidence suggests that the lifestyle and eating habits among Americans have changed dramatically. Chronic diseases such as hypertension, obesity, and diabetes have grown to be the great public-health issues of our time, and government agencies are tasked with determining the best policy approaches to pursue, based on the information and data they can acquire. Nutrition and dietary survey collection methods are far from perfect, but on balance they contribute significantly to our understanding of how diet and health outcomes are linked, and they are critical to the production and maintenance of a nutritionally sound, accessible, and safe food supply.

The challenge health experts and researchers now face is the continued development of surveys that address the evolving food landscape among a larger and more diverse American population, where disparities in diet quality and health continue to widen. Now more than ever, policy makers at all levels of government need access to high-quality data on the nation's dietary habits, health status, and attitudes and knowledge about nutrition to make informed and effective decisions about the nation's food system in the 21st century.

 **CASE STUDY**

In recent years, San Antonio, Texas, has seen a significant rise in maternal and child morbidity rates. For example, there has been a rise in maternal obesity and infant birthweights that are large for gestational age.

As part of a state task force set up to explore diet quality among low-income pregnant women throughout the city, Dr. Ellen Ramirez is collecting data in order to quantify two things: 1) fresh fruit and vegetable consumption; and 2) pregnant women's access to fresh, unprocessed foods during the second and third trimesters.

### Questions:

1. Based on the information addressed in this chapter, identify which method of nutrition assessment would be most appropriate for collecting this type of data, and explain the reasoning behind your answer.

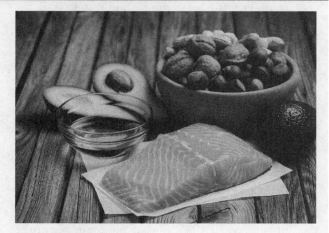
© JulijaDmitrijeva/iStock/Getty Images.

# Learning Portfolio

## Key Terms

Behavioral Risk Factor Surveillance System (BRFSS)
Biomarker
*Dietary Guidelines for Americans*
Dietary history
Dietary recall (24-hour)
Food record
Food-consumption record
Food-frequency questionnaire (FFQ)
Food fortification
Healthy Eating Index (HEI)
Healthy eating patterns

Monitoring
Morbidity rate
Mortality rate
National Health and Nutrition Examination Survey (NHANES)
National Health Examination Survey (NHES)
National Nutrition Monitoring System (NNMS)
Pediatric Nutrition Surveillance System (PedNSS)
Pregnancy Nutrition Surveillance System (PNSS)
Surveillance
Youth Risk Behavior Surveillance System (YRBSS)

## Study Questions

1. The USDA's 1935–1936 Consumer Purchases Study was considered to be a milestone survey because:
   a. It was the first survey to reveal that malnutrition existed in the United States.
   b. The survey was the first to measure the impact World War II had on food consumption among Americans.
   c. More than 14,000 households participated in the study.
   d. It was the first large-scale, federally funded dietary survey in the United States.

2. The USDA's 1965–1966 Household Food Consumption Survey was different from its predecessors because it:
   a. Was the largest of the USDA surveys until that time.
   b. Included data on individual food intake for the first time in addition to household intake.
   c. Spearheaded the enrichment of flour and bread products with key essential vitamins.
   d. Examined the diets of rural farm families at different income levels.

3. Introduced in 1985, one of the main purposes of the Continuing Survey of Food Intakes by Individuals was to:
   a. Measure the food and nutrient content frequently enough to provide timely information on dietary adequacy.
   b. Collect clinical data based on a physical exam.
   c. Assess the frequency with which select foods are eaten among the general population.
   d. Evaluate individual perceptions and attitudes about food and dietary behavior.

4. The importance of the Diet and Health Knowledge Survey is based on the premise that:
   a. Dietary choices are always made spontaneously.
   b. Many nutrition education programs are designed to address overeating.
   c. Many nutrition-education programs are designed to address the prebehavioral determinants of dietary choices.
   d. Knowledge exclusively determines dietary choices.

5. The Ten-State Nutrition Survey collected data on communities in low socioeconomic areas in response to:
   a. Concerns about hunger and malnutrition in the United States.
   b. Chronic disease and disability in the United States.
   c. Issues related to the cost of food in the United States.
   d. Problems with food distribution in the United States.

6. One primary reason why health advocates recommended that a dietary component be added to the National Health Examination Survey (NHES) in the 1960s was that:
   a. Hunger and malnutrition had reached the highest levels ever.
   b. Infant mortality was rising.
   c. Rates of acute illness had been declining for decades.
   d. Researchers continued to discover links between dietary habits and chronic disease.

7. The National Health and Nutrition Examination Survey (NHANES) is the nation's most comprehensive system for nutrition and health monitoring and is unique because it:
   a. Is conducted every 10 years.
   b. Includes children as well as adults.
   c. Examines a cross-section of the American population.
   d. Includes both household interview and physical examination methods.

8. The Hispanic Health and Nutrition Examination Survey (HHANES) was conducted from 1982 to 1984 to evaluate the three largest Hispanic subgroups in the United States, including:
   a. Costa Ricans, Mexican Americans, and Puerto Ricans.
   b. Mexican Americans, Ecuadorians, and Costa Ricans.
   c. Mexican Americans, Cuban Americans, and Puerto Ricans.
   d. Cuban Americans, Ecuadorians, and Mexican Americans.

9. NHANES III was the first survey to include:
   a. Hispanic Americans.
   b. Adults older than 70 years.
   c. Women.
   d. Infants as young as 2 months of age.

10. One of the shortcomings of the federal nutrition-monitoring system during the 1970s included:
    a. Invalid survey questions.
    b. A lack of timely and effective data collection.
    c. Inadequate numbers of survey interviews.
    d. Poor response rates.

11. The two American federal departments that are most involved with coordinating and implementing the nation's largest health and nutrition surveys are the:
    a. Department of Commerce and the Department of Agriculture.
    b. Department of Health and Human Services and Department of Agriculture.
    c. Department of Health and Human Services and the Department of Education.
    d. Department of Veterans Affairs and the Department of Agriculture.

12. Which one of the statements below is true? One goal of the National Nutrition Monitoring System (NNMS) is to:
    a. Provide data for evaluating changes in American agricultural policy related to food production, processing, and distribution.
    b. Identify high-risk groups of individuals in a highly limited number of geographic areas.
    c. Develop uniform standard methods but not criteria or policies for nutrition monitoring.
    d. Collect data on the nutritional and dietary status of the American population but not consumer knowledge of nutrition.

13. The data collected by the National Nutrition Monitoring and Related Research Program (NNMRRP) are used for the following purposes except:
    a. Directing research activities.
    b. Developing education initiatives.
    c. Providing direct funding for clinical research.
    d. Making policy decisions.

14. Which of the following statements is not true? Nutrition monitoring:
    a. Refers to a system of data collection of state or local population samples.
    b. Involves the collection and analysis of quantitatively accurate measures.
    c. Evaluates large and representative samples of the population.
    d. Requires the analysis of data several years after the information is collected.

15. Which of the following is an example of a nutrition-monitoring survey?
    a. BRFSS.
    b. CDC.
    c. WIC PC.
    d. NHANES

16. For most state health departments in the United States, which of the following is the only source of data and health risk behavior related to chronic disease?
    a. NHANES.
    b. HHS.
    c. PedNSS.
    d. BRFSS.

17. The YRBSS is designed to do the following except:
    a. Determine the prevalence of health behaviors.
    b. Provide comparable data among subpopulations of youth.
    c. Collect anthropometric data.
    d. Monitor progress toward reaching Healthy People objectives.

18. Dietary assessment methods can potentially hinder understanding the extent to which diet impacts health because:
    a. The type, quantity, and nutrient composition of an individual's diet can be difficult to accurately measure.

b. Few if any dietary assessment methods have been validated for scientific research.

c. There are insufficient numbers of skilled survey interviewers and fieldworkers.

d. It is challenging to recruit enough study participants.

19. The creation of food-consumption records whereby a trained surveyor observes food preparation and intake in the home is especially useful for research in developing countries because of:
a. The low cost of designing surveys.
b. Low literacy rates.
c. Use of brief checklists.
d. The utilization of in-depth interviews.

20. A key feature of the food record used in nutrition-research studies is the:
a. Need for a trained interviewer.
b. Opportunity for respondents to self-record the foods and beverages they consume.
c. Requirement that respondents fill out a checklist of commonly eaten foods.
d. Involvement of a trained outside observer to provide documentation.

21. A drawback to using biomarkers in dietary assessment includes all of the following except:
a. Many foods and nutrients lack sensitive or specific biomarkers.
b. Metabolism influences certain biomarkers after food consumption.
c. Certain biomarkers are affected by disease.
d. They are not useful or cost-effective in small case-controlled studies.

22. The broad eating styles recommended by the *Dietary Guidelines for Americans* reflects the basic idea that:
a. Individual nutrients matter more than dietary habits to achieve good health.
b. Certain food groups are more important than others to reduce chronic disease risk.
c. Dietary intake should consist of variety in the form of a healthy eating pattern.
d. Only two or three eating patterns are suitable for everyone.

23. Which of the following statements is false? A healthy eating pattern:
a. Can include 8 to 15 ounces of seafood per week.
b. Can include 5 teaspoons of healthy oils per day.
c. Should not include eggs.
d. Should consist of a low intake of red and processed meat.

24. A key feature of the DASH diet is that it includes an abundance all of the following except:
a. Fruits and vegetables.
b. Lean beef and pork.
c. Low-fat dairy.
d. Poultry and fish.

25. According to the *Dietary Guidelines*, processed meat and poultry can be included in a balanced diet as long as they fall within recommended limits for all of the following except:
a. Protein
b. Sodium.
c. Saturated fats.
d. Total calories.

26. Certain oils such as coconut oil, palm kernel oil, and palm oil are not included in the *Dietary Guidelines* list of healthy oils because they contain significantly higher amounts of:
a. *Trans* fats.
b. Saturated fats.
c. Hydrogenated fats.
d. Cholesterol.

27. Replacing total fat or saturated fats with which of the following is not associated with a reduced risk of cardiovascular disease?
a. Carbohydrates.
b. Polyunsaturated fatty acids.
c. Monounsaturated fatty acids.
d. Omega-3 fatty acids.

28. According to the *Dietary Guidelines*, moderate coffee consumption consists of a daily intake of:
a. One eight-ounce cup.
b. One to two eight-oz. cups.
c. Two eight-oz. cups.
d. Three to five eight-oz. cups.

29. The Healthy Eating Index is used to assess the extent to which a cross-section of the American population adheres to:
a. The *Healthy People 2020* objectives.
b. The American Heart Association recommendations.
c. The Agency for Healthcare Research and Quality parameters.
d. The *Dietary Guidelines for Americans*.

30. The most recent score of the Healthy Eating Index indicates that the quality of the American diet can be characterized as:
a. Significantly improved in the last 25 years.
b. Good.
c. Fair.
d. Poor.

## Discussion Questions

1. Explain why data collected from a 24-hour dietary recall is different from an attitudes and knowledge survey, and describe how each can be useful in understanding the population sample's dietary habits.

2. Discuss why it is important for government nutrition-monitoring and nutrition-surveillance efforts to collect food-consumption data that are representative of the national population as a whole, but also target individual state or local dietary habits and health information.

## Activities

1. Locate a health or news article that reports on the results of a specific diet and health survey. Identify the specific survey used, the target population, and the significance of the results. How might the results be used to develop local, state, or national policies related to healthy eating?

2. Create a food-frequency checklist aimed at a specific population such as high-school students at a particular school or older adults in an assisted-living facility. Think about how long or short the questionnaire should be. What food and beverage items would you include for this population, and why? How might you use the results?

3. Team up with a classmate and conduct a 24-hour dietary recall on one another. Then summarize how closely the results of the recalls adhere to the key principles of the *Dietary Guidelines for Americans*.

## Online Resources

### Behavioral Risk Factor Surveillance System (BRFSS): State-by-State Listing of How Data are Used

This page contains examples of how BRFSS data support ongoing projects and what states have already accomplished by using this information, and it lists the name and contact information for each state BRFSS coordinator. https://www.cdc.gov/brfss/state_info /brfss_use_examples.htm

### National Collaborative on Childhood Obesity Research: Catalog of Surveillance Systems

This resource provides one-stop access to more than 100 publicly available data sets relevant to childhood obesity research. Searches can be filtered by age group, racial/ethnic group, study design, scope of geographic area, and other parameters. https://tools.nccor .org/css

### NHANES Analysis Course

These five modules demonstrate how to analyze NHANES data with a selected number of statistical techniques. The course begins with a module on descriptive statistics, which introduces how to generate means, geometric means, and proportions for NHANES data. The module on hypothesis testing highlights the use of *t*-test and chi-square statistics to test statistical hypotheses about population parameters in NHANES data analysis. Age standardization and population estimate analyses are united in one module because they both use census data either to perform age adjustment or generate population totals. Another module introduces simple and multiple linear-regression models, showing how to examine the association between covariate(s) and a health outcome. The last module is on logistic regression, which demonstrates how to assess the probability of a disease or health condition as a function of one or multiple risk factors. https://www.cdc.gov/nchs/tutorials /nhanes/nhanesanalyses/nhanes_analyses_intro.htm

### What We Eat in America: Dietary Data Web Tutorial

The National Cancer Institute, National Center for Health Statistics, and US Department of Agriculture developed this tutorial to meet the growing needs of NHANES dietary data users. The tutorial offers step-by-step guidance for conducting an analytical project from beginning to end with examples of many common analytic procedures. https://www.cdc.gov/nchs /tutorials/Dietary/index.htm

### Youth Risk Behavior Surveillance System (YRBSS): 2015 YRBS Data User's Guide

This 102-page manual provides information on data edits, calculated variables, data analysis variables, technical notes on analysis software, and 2015 survey questions. https://www.cdc.gov/healthyyouth/data/yrbs /pdf/2015/2015_yrbs-data-users_guide_smy _combined.pdf

# References

1. Johnson TP. Origins and development of health survey methods. Chapter 1 in: Johnson TP, ed. *Handbook of Health Survey Methods*. New York, NY: John Wiley & Sons; 2015. www.britannica.com/biography/johann-peter-frank.

2. Achievement in public health 1900-199: Changes in the public health system. *Morb Mortal Wkly Rep*. 1990; December 24; 48(50);1141-1147.

3. Weisz G. Epidemiology and health care reform: The National Health Survey 1935-1936. *Am J Public Health*. 2011; 101: 438-447.

4. US Public Health Service. The National Health Survey Act. *Public Health Rep*. 1957; 72(1):1-4. https://www.ncbi.nlm .nih.gov/pmc/articles/PMC2031124/pdf/pubhealthreporig 00133-0005.pdf .

5. Pennington J. Nutrition monitoring in the United States. In: Berdanier CD, Dwyer JT, Feldman EB, eds. *Handbook of Nutrition and Food*. 2nd ed. New York, NY: Taylor & Francis Group; 2007.

6. Centers for Disease Control and Prevention (CDC). Nutrition Health and Nutrition Examination Survey: History. https:// www.cdc.gov/nchs/nhanes/history.htm.

7. Tippett KS, Enns CW, Moshfegh AJ. Food consumption surveys in the US Department of Agriculture. *Nutrition Today*. 1999; 34(1):33-46.

8. Rizek RL, Pao EM. Dietary intake methodology I. USDA survey and supporting research. *J Nutr*. 1990; 120(Suppl 11):1525-1529.

9. Welsh S. The Joint Nutrition Evaluation Committee. In: National Research Council (US), Food and Nutrition Board. *What Is America Eating? Proceedings of a Symposium*. Washington, DC: National Academies Press; 1986. https://www .ncbi.nlm.nih.gov/books/NBK217499/.

10. Mahan LK, Raymond JL. Behavioral-environmental: The individual in the community. Chapter 9. In: Mahan LK, Raymond JL, eds. *Krause's Food & the Nutrition Care Process*. 14th ed. New York, NY: Elsevier; 2017.

11. Willett W. Nutritional epidemiology. In: Byers T, ed. *Nutrition Monitoring and Surveillance*. 2nd ed. New York, NY: Oxford University Press; 1998.

12. Dwyer J, Picciano MF, Raiten DJ. Future directions for what we eat in America—NHANES: The Integrated CSFII-NHANES. *J Nutr*. 2003; 133(2):576S-581S.

13. US Department of Agriculture, Center for Nutrition Policy and Promotion. *Healthy Eating Index*; n.d. www.cnpp.usda .gov/healthyeatingindex.

14. Lowe CU, Forbes GB, Garn S, et al. The Ten-State Nutrition Survey: A pediatric perspective. *Pediatrics* 1973; 51(6): 1095–1099.

15. National Center for Health Statistics. National Health and Nutrition Examination Survey (NHANES); n.d. https://www .cdc.gov/nchs/nhanes/about_nhanes.htm.

16. Kuczmarski MF, Kuczmarski RJ. Nutrition Monitoring in the United States. In: Shils ME, Shike M, Ross AC, Caballero B, Cousins RJ, eds. *Modern Nutrition in Health and Disease*. 10th ed. Philadelphia, PA: Lippincott Williams and Wilkins; 2006.

17. Nestle M. National nutrition monitoring policy: The continuing need for legislative intervention. *J Nutr Ed*. 1990; 22(3):141-144.

18. McDowell MA. Nutrition monitoring in the United States. Chapter 29. In: Berdanier CD, Dwyer JT, Heber D, eds. *Handbook of Nutrition and Food*. 3rd ed. Boca Raton, FL: CRC Press; 2013.

19. CDC. Monitoring Health Risks and Behaviors Among Adults ataGlance2016.https://www.cdc.gov/chronicdisease/resources /publications/aag/brfss.htm.

20. CDC. Division of Population Health. https://www.cdc.gov /nccdphp/dph/index.html#.

21. CDC. Youth Risk Behavior Surveillance System (YRBSS) Overview. https://www.cdc.gov/healthyyouth/data/yrbs/over view.htm.

22. CDC. *Pediatric Nutrition Surveillance, 1997: Full Report*. Atlanta, GA: US Department of Health and Human Services; 1998. https://www.cdc.gov/nccdphp/dnpa/pdf/pednss.pdf.

23. CDC. Surveillance Systems; 2016. https://www.cdc.gov /obesity/data/surveillance.html.

24. Women, Infants, and Children (WIC) Participant and Program Characteristics: Summary. https://www.fns.usda.gov /wic/women-infants-and-children-wic-participant-and -program-characteristics-2012.

25. Shim J-S, Oh K, Kim HC. Dietary assessment methods in epidemiologic studies. *Epidemiol Health*. 2014; 36:e2014009. doi: 10.4178/epih/e2014009.

26. Naska A, Lagiou A, Lagiou P. Dietary Assessment methods in epidemiological research: Current state of the art and future prospects. *F1000Research*; 2017;6:926. doi: 10.12688 /f1000research.10703.1.

27. Satija A, Yu E, Willett WC, Hu FB. Understanding nutritional epidemiology and its role in policy. *Adv Nutr*. 2015; 6:5-18.

28. US Department of Health and Human Services, US Department of Agriculture. *Dietary Guidelines for Americans 2015–2020*. 8th ed. December 2015. http://health.gov /dietaryguidelines/2015/guidelines/.

29. Guenther PM, Casavale KO, Kirkpatrick SI, et al. Update of the Healthy Eating Index: HEI-2010. *J Acad Nutr Dietet*. 2013; 113(4):569-580.

30. National Collaborative on Childhood Obesity Research. The Healthy Eating Index 2010: Fact Sheet; n.d. http://nccor.org /downloads/NCCOR_HEI-factsheet_v8.pdf

31. Snetselaar L. Are Americans following the US Dietary Guidelines?ChecktheHealthyEatingIndex.2015;March2.www .elsevier.com/connect/are-americans-following-us-dietary -guidelines-check-the-healthy-eating-index.

32. US Department of Health and Human Services, Office of Disease Prevention and Health Promotion; n.d. "Scientific Report of the 2015 Dietary Guidelines Advisory Committee. Appendix E-2.25: Average Healthy Eating Index-2010 Scores for Americans ages 2 years and older (NHANES 2009-2010)." https://health.gov/dietaryguidelines/2015-scientific-report /data-table-23.asp.

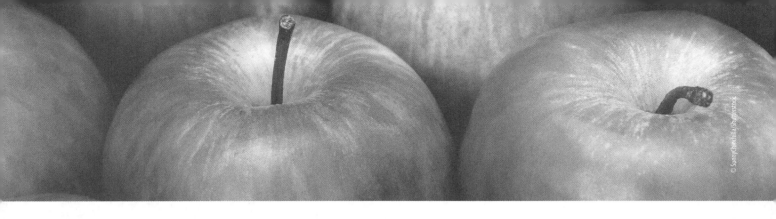

# CHAPTER 6

# Computerized Food and Nutrition Analysis Systems

**Lona Sandon**, PhD, MEd, RDN

## LEARNING OBJECTIVES

After reading this chapter, the learner will be able to:

1. Discuss the advantages and disadvantages of dietary assessment methods commonly used in nutrition research and clinical practice, including food records, 24-hour dietary recall, food-frequency questionnaires, and screeners.
2. Describe three types of innovative technologies that can be used to enhance the collection of dietary data for more-accurate and objective nutrient analysis.
3. Evaluate the appropriateness of a computerized diet analysis, based on factors to consider in selecting a computerized diet-analysis application for nutrition research.
4. Choose a computer-based diet-analysis application to meet clinical or research needs.
5. Select an Internet-based diet-analysis application to meet clinical or research needs.

## ▶ Introduction

Researchers and clinicians in the United States and Great Britain have been interested in determining dietary intake since the 1930s, when the first reports of dietary records appeared in the literature.[1] These early records revealed discrepancies in results coming from the method used to capture the dietary intake and determine the amount of food eaten. In addition to the challenge of accurately recording the actual foods and amount of foods consumed, accurately determining the actual food composition is another concern in dietary-intake assessment.[1] Until the advent of the computer, clinicians and researchers analyzed and calculated dietary intake by hand. As computers became more widely available in the 1980s and 1990s, the need for calculating nutrient intake manually was nearly eliminated, although many clinicians still use quick methods such as the exchange system to quickly assess an individual's dietary intake. Nonetheless, the difficulty of determining the nutrient composition of the total diet and foods available for consumption persists.

As technology continues to advance, so has the number of foods and beverages available for consumption. Early database systems for dietary-intake analysis may have only included a few hundred food items and limited nutrient data to select nutrients. Today's databases are capable of searching hundreds of thousands of food items and are much more robust, with a wider array of nutrient-composition data for individual food items. Nutrient-composition databases can contain information from multiple sources, including the US Department of Agriculture (USDA), research databases, food manufacturers, and restaurant menus and webpages.

Although early computerized nutrient-analysis systems sped up calculating nutrient intake, they did not address the inherent problems and bias in methods used to collect dietary-intake data that truly represents the usual diet. Clinicians and researchers are well aware that one day's record of food intake is not sufficient to determine an individual's usual nutrient intake; multiple days or weeks are required. In addition, bias influences the validity of records of dietary intake.

Current technology can introduce new methods and enhance traditional methods of collecting dietary-intake data to improve accuracy and reduce bias in the data-collection process. Technology may also reduce researcher, clinician, and participant burden associated with dietary-intake data collection, data entry, analysis, and reporting. This chapter discusses traditional dietary-intake assessment methods, evolving technologies for capturing dietary-intake data, existing **computer-based diet-assessment applications**, **Internet-based diet-assessment applications**, and factors to consider in choosing an assessment tool to meet the needs of the researcher or clinician.

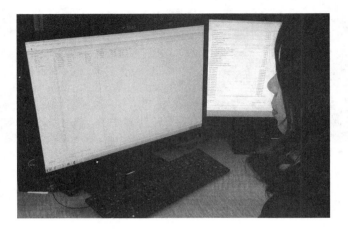

# ▶ Dietary-Intake Assessment Methods

**Preview** Dietary-intake assessment relies on self-reported data in both clinical and research settings. Traditional tools used to capture dietary-intake data include dietary-history questionnaires, food records, 24-hour dietary recalls (24-hour recall), **food-frequency questionnaires (FFQs)**, and **screeners**. Each method mentioned comes with its own set of potential errors, benefits, and drawbacks to gathering valid and reliable dietary data. The ease and ability of managing and analyzing data differs with each method.

## Food Records

A **food record**, also sometimes referred to as a *food diary* (**FIGURE 6.1**), may be useful for evaluating associations between health outcomes and dietary intake. Food records intend to provide a complete record of all foods and beverages consumed over a designated period, typically including several days of dietary intake. Clients or research participants are instructed to document all food or beverage items consumed during the designated time period; weigh, measure, or estimate portion sizes of items eaten using standard household measurements; provide descriptions of food items and methods of food preparation; state specific brands if applicable; and record the time and place where food items are consumed. The clinician or researcher may review the food record with the client or participant to clarify recorded items and portion sizes, thereby improving the quality of dietary data collected. In the food-record

**Food Diary**

| Date/Time | Meal | Food item | Serving size | Calories | Notes |
|---|---|---|---|---|---|
| | Breakfast | | | | |
| | | | | | |
| | | | | | |
| | | | | | |
| | | | | | |
| | Lunch | | | | |
| | | | | | |
| | | | | | |
| | | | | | |
| | Dinner | | | | |
| | | | | | |
| | | | | | |
| | | | | | |
| | Snack | | | | |
| | | | | | |
| | | | | | |
| | | | | | |

**FIGURE 6.1** Food diary sample

method, participants are supposed to record all foods and beverages at the time they are consumed. Recording at the time of intake reduces reliance on memory, which leads to better-quality intake data. This is one strength of the food-record method over other intake-assessment methods.[2,3] Weighed or measured food records that account for plate waste or unconsumed portions of food also improve the accuracy of the dietary data. Food records may benefit dietary-intervention studies in which the intent of the intervention is to improve eating behavior. Recording dietary intake can motivate some participants to make better food and beverage choices.[4] However, this is not an advantage if the researcher or clinician is trying to measure participants' usual intake. The food record is the most thorough method of collecting dietary intake.[2,3]

The process of obtaining dietary data through food records has several limitations. First, participants must be literate enough and have the language skills to record their own dietary intake. Second, participants must be willing and motivated to complete food records, and they may not represent the general population.[4] Third, because of the burdensome

nature of food records, participants may not record data in real time and instead rely on memory to record data at a more convenient time. This introduces **recall bias** into the method.[2] Participants also may alter their eating habits to make recording intake easier or to be more acceptable to the researcher or clinician; this introduces **reactivity bias** and **social**-**approval bias** and affects the ability to assess usual intake.[2,3] Also, food records may also not represent usual intake because they are typically limited to a narrow period that represents current intake but does not provide information about past intake.[4] Multiple days are needed to capture variability in daily dietary intake. The more days required, the more respondent burden, which may affect data quality. Traditional food records have been recorded using pen and paper, an arduous process for clients and participants.[3] Food records sometimes underestimate nutrient intake, including energy and protein intake, when compared to biochemical measures of nutrient intake.[2] Furthermore, food records are also labor intensive for researchers. This limits the use of food records in large population studies.[4] Data entry and management for analyzing food records is time-consuming for researchers or clinicians and prevents them from providing immediate feedback to participants. Current technologies including the Internet and smartphones may offer quicker ways to document dietary intake in real time and directly into databases that may lead to both better-quality data and faster analysis.

## 24-Hour Dietary Recall

A **24-hour recall** uses a structured interview process typically conducted by a trained clinician or interviewer who asks participants to list the foods consumed in the previous 24 hours or a recent 24-hour period. See **FIGURE 6.2**. The interviewer asks questions to prompt the participant to recall intake details, including portion sizes, brand names, how foods were prepared, condiments added, timing of meals or snacks, and missed items. Use of pictures, food models, and measuring cups or spoons aid memory and improve the estimates of portions consumed. The process is relatively quick, does not require literacy on behalf of the participant, and has no influence on intake as it collects information; there is also little burden put on participants.[3,4] A structured and standardized interview process will likely lead to better data collection and coding of items consumed.[2,3] As Thompson et al.[2] state,

| 24-Hour Recall | Instructions: Record the time, the amount and food item consumed. Describe the food preparation method and document where were you when the food item was consumed. The location can be places such as: home in the kitchen, in front of the TV, at work, in my desk, etc. | | | |
|---|---|---|---|---|
| **Time** | **Amount consumed** | **Food and/or beverage consumed** | **Method of preparation** | **Where consumed (location)** |
| | | | | |
| | | | | |
| | | | | |
| | | | | |
| | | | | |
| | | | | |
| | | | | |
| | | | | |
| | | | | |
| | | | | |
| | | | | |
| | | | | |
| | | | | |
| | | | | |
| | | | | |
| | | | | |
| | | | | |
| | | | | |

**FIGURE 6.2** 24-hour dietary recall form

"Twenty-four-hour recalls can be used to describe dietary intake, examine associations between diet and other variables such as health, and evaluate the effectiveness of an intervention study to change diet."[2] Data from 24-hour recalls better represent the usual mean intake of a group as opposed to an individual, given the high variability in day-to-day intake and the need for multiple 24-hour recalls from individuals to determine usual intake. This makes the 24-hour recall a good tool for comparing dietary intake between different groups.[3,4]

One drawback of the 24-hour recall is that it relies on the participant's memory. This introduces recall bias and random error and thereby influences data reliability and validity. Underestimation or underreporting of intake is a common problem of 24-hour recalls. In addition, variation in intake from day to day introduces random error. Collecting multiple 24-hour recalls can reduce the potential for error.[2,3] Between eight and 32 days of 24-hour recalls may be needed to reach 80% reliability for energy intake and fruit intake, respectively.[5] Similar to food records, data entry of 24-hour recalls is time-consuming. Existing computer-based technologies help standardize the interview process and allow direct data entry at the time of interview, thereby reducing

time and effort for data collection and entry. Current technology also allows for self-administered 24-hour recalls using standardized questions and algorithms to guide the self-administered interview process. However, these self-administered applications may limit the ability to capture complete descriptions of food items sought by a trained interviewer.[4]

## Food-Frequency Questionnaires

Food-frequency questionnaires (FFQ) are commonly used in large epidemiological studies because they are less costly than other assessment methods and easier for researchers to administer. See **FIGURE 6.3**. It is the most objective method for assessing intake because it uses a specific list of foods.[2,4] An FFQ asks questions about the usual frequency of a finite list of foods and beverages consumed over a defined time such as a year, month, or week. An FFQ commonly includes portion-size choices on the questionnaire. The number of items may vary, depending on food and beverage items of interest among the study population, nutrients of interest, and customization for items commonly eaten among specific populations. Generally, an FFQ is self-administered and does not require an interviewer. An FFQ is beneficial for assessing food

Date:

Name:

| Instructions: In the past three (3) months did you consume the foods listed below? | | | | | | |
|---|---|---|---|---|---|---|
| **Food Group** | **Frequency** | | | | | |
| | Never | Less than one time per week | 1-6 times per week | 1-3 times per day | 4 or more times per day | Serving size |
| **Dairy:** milk, cheese, yogurt | | | | | | |
| **Chicken:** grilled chicken, baked chicken, fired chicken, etc. | | | | | | |
| **Turkey:** turkey sandwich, soup, breast, roasted, etc. | | | | | | |
| **Beef:** meatballs, steak, etc. | | | | | | |
| **Pork:** cured ham, fresh ham, ribs, pork chops, pulled pork, etc. | | | | | | |
| **Fish and seafood:** shrimp, scallops, fish, shellfish | | | | | | |
| **Other Meat:** lamb, duck, etc. | | | | | | |
| **Nuts:** walnuts, cashews, peanuts, etc. | | | | | | |
| **Beans:** red beans, chick peas, chili, etc. | | | | | | |
| **Egg:** omelet, hard-boiled egg, etc. | | | | | | |
| **Vegetables:** broccoli, cauliflower, green beans, etc. | | | | | | |
| **Fruit:** banana, strawberry, apple, pear, melon, etc. | | | | | | |
| **Grains:** rice, bread, cereal, etc. | | | | | | |
| **Sweets:** cakes, cookies, pies, etc. | | | | | | |
| **Beverages:** coffee, tea, sodas, juices, etc. | | | | | | |

**FIGURE 6.3** Food frequency questionnaire

groups and dietary patterns of certain foods and beverages and their relationships to disease outcomes. Variability in daily intake does not influence an FFQ, which also takes into account seasonal variation in intake.[2,3] Moreover, an FFQ is the preferred instrument for use in retrospective case-controlled studies. It is the only instrument that asks about long-term past dietary intake.[2]

As with other methods, the reliability and validity of data from an FFQ may be affected by recall bias and the inability to capture total dietary intake because of missing intake items that might be common to the population of interest. The inability to assess the total diet makes the FFQ a poor instrument for clinical settings or settings in which adequacy of nutrient intake is important for assessing individual intake. It is less precise than other methods.[4] In a study comparing an FFQ to a seven-day diet record, the FFQ underestimated sodium and overestimated macronutrient and energy intake. Only weak correlations were found

between the FFQ and 24-hour recalls before adjusting for within-person variation, which improved correlations slightly.[6] This calls into question the validity and reliability of FFQ dietary data. Similar to 24-hour recalls, FFQs are subject to social-approval bias—that is, expected norms for behavior influence participants' reported intakes. Miller et al. demonstrated in a randomized blinded study that intervention participants who received prompts related to recommended intake and the benefits of consuming fruits and vegetables were more likely to report higher intakes of fruit and vegetables on an FFQ and 24-hour recall.[7] Underreporting of intake can also be a limitation when using FFQs, which underestimate energy and protein intake when compared to biochemical markers to determine the validity of self-reporting of intake.[2] Underreporting or overreporting of intake can occur if portions listed on the questionnaire are different from what the participant usually consumes.[4] Lastly, traditional paper-based FFQs increase researcher time and effort for data entry and analysis. Technology-based FFQs may decrease the time and effort needed to administer, enter data by the researcher or clinician, and analyze data. Technology also enhances the ability to incorporate food images into the questionnaire, which may help respondents better estimate portion sizes and improve validity.

## Screeners

Dietary screeners are more cost-effective and present less burden for participants than previously described intake-assessment methods. Screeners are similar to FFQs but differ by including a shorter list of questions typically related to specific dietary behaviors (**FIGURE 6.4**). This tool is used to convey gross estimates of the intake of specific dietary components such as fruits and vegetables or usual beverage intakes in both adults and children.[8,9,10] When accurate levels of intake are required, avoid using screeners because they do not assess total diet.[8] Self-administered screeners are easy to use and implement in large cross-sectional studies to determine mean intake of certain dietary components, and they are comparable to 24-hour recalls or FFQs in terms of determining frequency of intake.[2,8] England et al. conducted a review of 47 studies describing 35 different brief questionnaires (having fewer than 35 items) that were designed to assess fat intake, Mediterranean-diet compliance, patterns of healthy eating, and intake of fruits and vegetables.[11] They concluded that validated and reliable brief instruments could guide clinical decision-making when carefully selected to match the client population with the sample population.[11] Short questionnaires allow clinicians and researchers to assess dietary intake quickly. Screeners or brief questionnaires have the advantage of quick and easy scoring. Innovative technologies may further improve the ease of scoring screeners and provide immediate feedback to participants, clinicians, and researchers.

## Technology in Nutrition Assessment

Researchers have called for improvements to current methods or the development of new methods of obtaining and analyzing dietary information. Innovative technologies developed in the past decade offer the opportunity to improve on dietary data-collection methods and add objective data. Potential benefits of incorporating the use of technology into dietary-intake data collection include greater ability to standardize the data-collection process: question sequencing, automated and rapid dietary analysis allowing immediate access to results, and improved data management with direct entry and

| Fruits, Vegetables, and Grains | Less than 1/WEEK | Once a WEEK | 2-3 times a WEEK | 4-6 times a WEEK | Once a DAY | 2+ a DAY |
|---|---|---|---|---|---|---|
| Fruit juice, like orange, apple, grape, fresh, frozen or canned. (Not sodas or other drinks) | O | O | O | O | O | O |
| How often do you eat any fruit, fresh or canned (not counting juice?) | O | O | O | O | O | O |
| Vegetable juice, like tomato juice, V-8, carrot | O | O | O | O | O | O |
| Green salad | O | O | O | O | O | O |
| Potatoes, any kind, including baked, mashed or french fried | O | O | O | O | O | O |
| Vegetable soup, or stew with vegetables | O | O | O | O | O | O |
| Any other vegetables, including string beans, peas, corn, broccoli or any other kind | O | O | O | O | O | O |
| Fiber cereals like Raisin Bran, Shredded Wheat or Fruit-n-Fiber | O | O | O | O | O | O |
| Beans such as baked beans, pinto, kidney, or lentils (not green beans) | O | O | O | O | O | O |
| Dark bread such as whole wheat or rye | O | O | O | O | O | O |

**FIGURE 6.4** Fiber screener

ease of data processing and transfer. The use of technology also affects the time costs of interviewer-led 24-hour recalls and increases acceptability among younger populations.[2,12,13,14] Technology also can add more layers of contextual information such as meal timing and location and eating patterns, as well as more food images to improve reporting of portion sizes. This allows multiple databases to increase the specificity of foods consumed and integration this information with biochemical data.[2] Disadvantages of incorporating innovative technologies include participants' technological literacy; older adults may not be familiar with newer technologies or have difficulty using them because of factors associated with aging (difficulty seeing or hearing). Disabilities can also be a limitation if keyboard or mouse skills are required. Access to technology may limit participation for some socioeconomic groups. Lastly, technology can be more expensive to use than survey instruments that use pen and paper.[12,14]

Incorporating technology into nutrient intake assessment has its advantages and disadvantages. See **TABLE 6.1**.

**Recap** Frequent criticism of traditional methods of dietary-intake assessment result from the known systematic errors in data collection, including recall, reactivity, and social-approval bias as well as poor sensitivity to changes in dietary intake.[2,12] Some researchers believe that no dietary data collected from memory recall can be trusted and that only objective data should be used to assess intake. Thompson et al. recommend the use of objective biochemical measures in addition to self-reported data for validation of dietary-intake assessment.[2] In addition, traditional methods that rely on survey tools requiring pen and paper or interviewer-administered instruments limit researchers in their ability to assess larger populations and hard-to-reach populations. They also require more time, money, and effort of researchers and clinicians to obtain, enter, manage, and analyze dietary-intake data. The introduction of technology into nutrition assessment offers the benefits of reaching larger populations; improving data collection, management, and analysis; and potential increased objectivity in data collection.

---

**TABLE 6.1** Advantages and disadvantages of using technology in nutrition assessment

| Advantages | | Disadvantages |
|---|---|---|
| ■ Reduced cost of labor for data collection<br>■ Increased time effectiveness: data can be automatically stored; no data entry is needed<br>■ Higher acceptance among some populations (e.g., adolescents, young adults)<br>■ Able to assess larger populations with minimal extra cost<br>■ Ability to standardize the data-collection process, including question sequencing<br>■ Automated and rapid dietary analysis | ■ Prevent incomplete or implausible data entry<br>■ Immediate access to results<br>■ Improved data management with direct entry and electronic transfer to central database<br>■ Capture of contextual information (meal timing, location, eating patterns)<br>■ Greater number of real food images to improve reporting of portion sizes<br>■ Help features assist users<br>■ Incorporate multiple databases to increase specificity of foods consumed<br>■ Integrate biochemical data | ■ Self-report bias still exists with new technology<br>■ Requires technological literacy of the participants<br>■ May require keyboard or mouse skills<br>■ Older adults may not be familiar with newer technologies or have difficulty using them because of aging factors (e.g., difficulty seeing or hearing, arthritis)<br>■ May not be easily accessible to individuals with physical impairments<br>■ Accessibility of technologies may limit participation of some socioeconomic groups<br>■ Technology can be more expensive to use than survey instruments requiring pen and paper |

Data from Thompson FE, Kirkpatrick SI, Subar AF, et al. The National Cancer Institute's Dietary Assessment Primer: A resource for diet research. *J Acad Nutr Diet.* 2015; 115:1986–1995. Long JD, Littlefield LA, Estep G, et al. Evidence review of technology and dietary assessment. *Worldviews Evid Based Nurs.* 2010;7(4):191–204. Boushey C, Kerr D, Wright J, Lutes K, Ebert D, Delp E. Use of technology in children's dietary assessment. *Eur J Clin Nutr.* 2009;63(Suppl 1): S50–S57. Probst YC, Tapsell LC. Overview of computerized dietary assessment programs for research and practice in nutrition education. *J Nutr Educ Behav.* 2005;37(1):20–26.

# ▶ Innovative Technologies in Nutrition Assessment

**Preview** Broad categories of current technologies in use or development for clinical or research-based dietary-intake assessment includes computer or Internet-based applications. The technology can be utilized in handheld devices, mobile phones with cameras, audio or video recording devices, and other scanner- or sensor-based devices.[2,12]

## Image-Assisted Dietary Assessment

**Image-assisted dietary assessment (IADA)** is a new approach to dietary-intake capture. See **FIGURE 6.5**. It has been described as any "method that uses images/video of eating episodes to enhance self-report of traditional methods or uses images/video as the primary record of dietary intake."[16] New technology in the form of handheld devices with built-in cameras such as smartphones and wearable cameras or sensors have made it easier to objectively capture dietary intake as opposed to relying solely on self-report. Captured images support traditional methods by aiding recall, identifying misreporting, and uncovering unreported food items, and it may increase the validity of energy-intake estimates.[16] Other purported benefits are the reduced burden of recording for the participant, increased engagement in record keeping, and better estimation of food portions.[2] A drawback of this method is that users must remember to capture images of meals before and after eating. The images also must be of adequate quality for assessment. Not

meeting these criteria leads to underestimation of dietary intake and reduces the method's reliability and validity.[16]

Gemming categorized IADA as either an active or a passive approach, depending on the type of technology used. The active approach requires the participant to use a handheld device to capture food and beverage items before and after each eating episode. In most instances, participants must include a reference marker in the image view to assist with either manual or automated analysis. Depending on the software used, the participant may add supplementary text or an audio recording to confirm information about the food items such as type, preparation, and portions. For reliability and validity of the dietary data, it is critical that participants capture the image before food intake at each eating episode.

The passive approach uses wearable cameras that automatically record images of dietary intake and require little or no input from participants. No manual recording is necessary, and recorded images can aid recall. This approach also captures activities unrelated to eating, and no reference marker is included to aid in analysis.[16] The lack of a reference marker may affect the validity and reliability of determining the correct portion sizes of foods.

## Dietitian-Assessed Food Photographs

Handheld devices and mobile phones with integrated cameras offer a means of gathering dietary-intake data with less recording burden on the user. See **FIGURE 6.6**. Methods include recording images of food and beverages before and after eating, along with audio- or text-recorded data about the meal. Images are sent to the researcher or clinician for analysis.

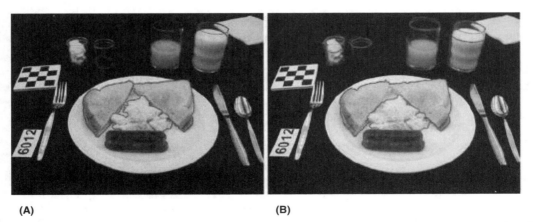

(A)                                    (B)

**FIGURE 6.5** Separation of an image captured by an adolescent during a controlled feeding study. (A) Ground truth segmentation. (B) Results of automated segmentation.

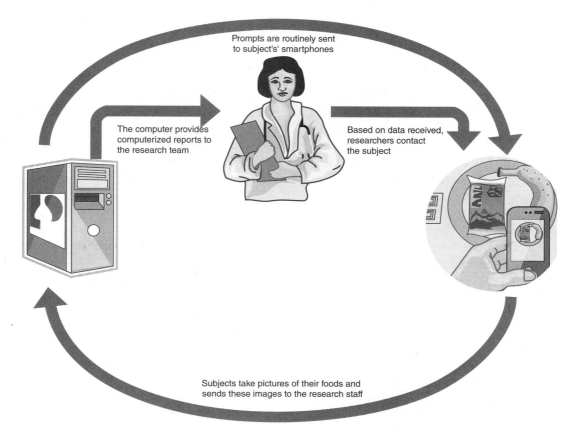

**FIGURE 6.6** Food photographs used in intake assessment

Multiple studies have attempted to validate the IADA method. At least three studies have compared the Wellnavi method to a weighed-food record. The Wellnavi method requires participants to capture food images with a visual reference marker from a 45-degree angle and provide written text describing foods and ingredients. Registered dietitian nutritionists (RDN) then manually analyze images with incorporated text. Two studies found no significant differences between energy or macronutrient intake when comparing the Wellnavi method to a weighed food-record, and the third study (Kikunaga) significantly underestimated macronutrient intake and underestimated energy intake using the Wellnavi method, thereby affecting validity.[17,18,19] Reasons for the results of the later study may have been the lack of text descriptions with the food images. Other studies have documented similar results and noted difficulties with capturing clear images, remembering to capture images before and after eating occasions, and including corresponding text or voice recordings.[16]

Rollo et al. conducted a study comparing energy intake obtained from a 3-day food record using the Nutricam Dietary Assessment Method (NuDAM) to energy expenditure measured by the doubly labeled water (DLW) technique.[20] A weighed food record was used to determine relative validity. Both the NuDAM and weighed food-record methods significantly underestimated energy intake compared to total energy expenditure determined by DLW, indicating the validity of the method is a concern. Moderate correlations were found between the weighed food record and NuDAM for energy, carbohydrate, protein, and alcohol. Interrater reliability was also assessed among three dietitians. Agreement on estimates of nutrients between dietitians was lower than agreement between NuDAM and the weighed food-record.[20] Assessing nutrient intake based on images does not appear to be superior to traditional methods of gathering and assessing dietary data.

## Automated Food-Photograph Analysis

More-advanced technology exists to recognize food and beverages from digital images based on their shapes, colors, or textures. The mobile phone food record (mpFR) captures multiple digital images of foods and beverages before and after a meal or snack. Estimating volume typically requires more than one image and an item of known size, or a reference marker must be included in the image. A server receives and analyzes the digital images based on features such as color and texture to automatically identify the food and estimate the portion size. The reference marker (e.g., ruler, card, or USB stick) helps the software application create a three-dimensional image of the food or beverages to estimate volume. The user confirms that the items identified by the imaging application are correct. Next, a database automatically analyzes nutrient composition for the researcher or clinician based on the analysis of the image and estimate of portion size.[21] When participants forget to capture images during eating episodes, they enter food-record data into an electronic food record built into the mobile phone.[16] In addition to reducing the recording burden, capturing food images may also increase reporting accuracy and reduce or eliminate recall bias in food reporting.

The Technology Assisted Diet Assessment (TADA) tool, developed at Purdue University, uses a single food image with a reference marker—a checkerboard card—to identify and quantify foods. The image-analysis software application automatically separates foods in the image by outlining each item and labeling it by food type. Items must not overlap. The geometric shape of the food is used to determine the volume. The user can confirm the type of food and volume. The food is analyzed for nutrient content by connecting with a database.[1] Researchers validated the TADA tool by comparing it against known portion sizes and nutrient contents of food items. The mean percentage error ranged from 1% to 10%, indicating good validity and accuracy.[22]

Children and adolescents are challenging populations when considering accurate assessment of nutrient intake. The accuracy of dietary-intake reporting and recording among children and adolescents is generally poor. Better methods are needed to assess nutrient intake in these populations. Some researchers hypothesize that mobile technologies are more acceptable and easily adopted by adolescents, although challenges still exist. Six et al. found that adolescents were open to using the mpFR technology but require additional training to improve the accuracy of food-image capturing.[21] A small study of children aged 11 to 14 years asked them to keep an mpFR for three to seven days; fewer than half of those studied were able to correctly follow instructions for capturing food images before and after eating. Participants recorded an average of 3.2 days and an average of 2.2 meals per day. Of the meals captured, many did not include all foods or the required reference marker. The results indicate that children of this age are capable of using an image-based food record. This might

require additional training and prompts for capturing images and reminders to include the reference marker and provide text descriptions of foods to increase the accuracy of analysis.[23] Boushey et al. reported similar findings among adolescents of the same age, in addition to other findings.[13] Girls were more likely to capture food images, and breakfast and lunch were more likely to be reported compared to snacks and dinner. Adolescents also reported they might be more likely to use the mpFR if it incorporated a game or other form of entertainment.[13] An earlier study evaluated usability among both adolescents and adults. Researchers provided participants with instructions on how to capture food and beverage images correctly. Adults were more likely to capture all foods and beverages in the image, required more attempts, and found remembering to capture food images easy. Both groups had difficulty including the reference marker in the images. As with others, results suggest that training and practice are necessary to increase accuracy of capturing images correctly to improve results of dietary analysis using an mpFR.[24] Validation studies using the mpFR are yet to be published.[16] Its correct use is essential for future validity and reliability testing.

### Food Intake and Voice Recorder

The Food Intake and Voice Recorder (FIVR) is another mpFR tool. The FIVR captures food images along with a reference marker to estimate food volume using the three best images. The camera uses a three-dimensional point cloud method to detect the shape and area of the food for volume estimation. Food-recognition software receives the data and calculates the volume. Users also provide a voice recording that includes the name and a description of each food consumed. The food names are compared with color and texture of foods detected in the image and the database of foods available in the software system. The foods are then matched with a nutrient-composition database for analysis.[1,25]

Dietary Data Recorder System is another tool. This tool eliminates the need for a reference marker by using a laser beam to detect the size of the food portion. The laser beam displays a grid over the food item in the image, which the researcher uses to identify the food item, the portion size, and the composition.[1]

## Wearable Image-Capturing Systems
### SenseCam

**SenseCam** is a wearable camera attached to a lanyard worn around the neck. The camera captures and stores images automatically on a continuous cycle for

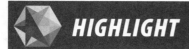

### Bite-Counting Technology

Bite counters are a new technology for monitoring portion intake and estimating the energy intake of foods consumed. Bite counters are worn on the wrist like a watch or embedded in a fork or spoon. Each time the hand with the bite counter is lifted toward the mouth, the device counts a bite based on the movement of an internal gyroscope or accelerometer. Therefore, bite counters may offer an objective and possibly more accurate measure of food intake. Salley et al. conducted a study to evaluate the accuracy of a bite-based estimate of energy intake compared to estimates of energy intake by participants when energy information is available or not available. Researchers measured bite count and energy intake among study participants who consumed a meal in a cafeteria. After the meal, study participants estimated their energy intake with or without a menu containing caloric information. Both age and gender predicted energy per bite, and the number of bites better estimated energy intake compared to participants' estimation of intake with or without the help of caloric information. Bite count may be a suitable objective measure of energy intake in a free-living population.[1]

### References

1. Salley JN, Hoover AW, Wilson ML, Muth ER. Comparison between human and bite-based methods of estimating caloric intake. *J Acad Nutr Diet.* 2016; 116:1568–1577.

---

12 to 16 hours. The researcher downloads the images from the camera to analyze the recorded dietary intake.[16] One study found that reviewing SenseCam data increased estimates of energy intake by 12% to 23% when compared to food record alone, by revealing unreported and misreported food items. Difficulties with the SenseCam included poor quality images in poor lighting and users not wearing the device correctly.[26] When used correctly, this technology offers the opportunity to improve validity of dietary-intake assessment.

## eButton

The **eButton** is a device worn on the chest like a pin. The eButton contains a miniature camera, an accelerometer, a GPS unit, and other sensors that passively capture images of food intake and other health behaviors. The eButton does not require additional self-reporting. Its camera automatically captures images of each eating event every two seconds. Using captured images, the software detects the shapes of plates, bowls, and utensils. It segments food items based on their texture, color, and complexities. The software estimates the volume of food based on the shape of a food-specific model. The food-specific model, which is a virtual wire-mesh frame of known volume sized to the food on the plates. A nutrient database analyzes dietary intake using the software-captured data.[27] Researchers compared the eButton data to manual visual rating of food images and physical measurement of 100 foods to determine the accuracy of its estimated food portions. The error was no more than 30% on 85 food items for the computer analysis. The computer estimates showed less bias and variability than the manual raters did. Irregularly shaped foods or poor-quality images were more likely to cause errors. Overall, the eButton estimates were more accurate for food volume than were visual-rater estimates.[28]

## Crowdsourcing Image-Based Assessment Applications

At least two mobile phone applications, Meal Snap and Platemate, are available and promise to deliver estimated energy intake of a food item based on a single image using crowd sourcing. Crowd sourcing relies on a group of individuals, trained or untrained, who are willing to provide information about the food image. The user simply captures an image of the food item and sends it to a server location for analysis. Analysis is relatively rapid and occurs within a matter of minutes. However, validity and reliability are questionable because it is not known who is providing the information and where the information came from. Informal testing has shown inconsistency in the ability to provide accurate data through crowdsourcing using a single image.[1] At this time, it cannot be recommended for use in research or clinical applications.

**Recap** Adding images to food records and food recalls appears to increase estimates of energy intake and identify unreported or misreported foods. Images may also improve portion-size estimates and better identify types of foods consumed. However, images do not capture ingredients such as added fats and sugar that may increase energy content, so relying only on images as the only source of dietary-intake information will likely lead to inaccuracies in assessing true intake.[16]

# ▶ Selecting a Computerized Diet-Analysis System for the Research Nutritionist

**Preview** Several factors should be considered when choosing a computerized diet-analysis application for nutrition research. First, the researcher must keep in mind the purpose and objectives of the nutrition research and the level of detail of dietary information needed to answer the study questions.[2] Other factors to consider include the cost of the analysis application, ease of use by the researchers or study participants, ability to import or export data for statistical analysis, the source of the nutrient data, reports that can be generated, and the number of food items and nutrients available in the database for analysis.[29]

## Types of Research and Study Questions

Before selecting a diet-analysis application, consider the type of research that will be conducted and the study questions that will need answering. The application you choose must be able to capture the type of data needed to answer your research questions. Therefore, your first step is to define your research objectives and dietary variables of interest. A 24-hour recall will provide details about the total diet and nutrient intake, whereas an FFQ or screener may be limited to only a few components of the diet.

The Dietary Assessment Primer, developed by the National Cancer Institute (NCI), provides guidance on the type of dietary assessment methods deemed most appropriate for differing study designs and research objectives. Common research objectives for dietary assessment include determining usual dietary intake of a group, identifying associations between dietary intake and health outcomes,

identifying associations between group characteristics (age, race, socioeconomics) and dietary intake, and determining the effect(s) of dietary interventions.[2,30] If your research objective were to describe the usual dietary intake of a group, compare usual dietary intake between groups, or determine the prevalence of individuals meeting a specified level of dietary intake, then an application capable of collecting multiple 24-hour recalls from each study participant would be optimal. A computerized FFQ might be useful but would provide less dietary detail and is not useful for determining the proportion of individuals meeting dietary intake criteria. The recommendation is to use multiple 24-hour recalls when evaluating health outcomes related to dietary intake in cross-sectional and prospective studies. Retrospective studies must rely on FFQs to look for relationships between diet and health outcomes. The NCI recommends using multiple 24-hour recalls for prospective and cross-sectional studies evaluating relationships between study-participant characteristics and their influences on dietary-intake variables.

A single 24-hour recall at each observation time point is useful for intervention studies that aim to examine change in intake over a period of time, look for a difference in the change of usual intake between groups, and compare post-intervention intake between groups. To determine change in the prevalence of individuals or differences in prevalence between groups meeting specific dietary criteria, multiple 24-hour recalls at each measurement time point are recommended.[30]

## Required Levels of Dietary Detail

The degree of detail needed for diet analysis is a factor in determining the most appropriate dietary-analysis system. Whether you plan to use the analysis software for clinical nutrient assessment or metabolic diet research will help you determine the level of detail needed. Questions the clinician or researcher must answer before selecting a system include the following:

- Can the application assess dietary patterns?
- Does the application assess total diet nutrient intakes?
- Does the application assess intake by meal, day, and/or multiple days?
- Does the application assess standard nutrients or food components not typically assessed (i.e., oxalates, bioactive food components?

Applications that only include FFQ or screeners capture less detail. The USDA Automated Multiple-Pass Method

(AMPM) and the Automated Self-Administered 24-Hour Dietary Assessment Tool (ASA24) assess both total nutrient intake and dietary patterns. Less commonly assessed nutrients and food components such as oxalates will likely require an application designed specifically for food and nutrition research centers, such as the Nutrient Data System for Research (NDSR) application.

## Accuracy and Quality of the Nutrient Database

Researchers and clinicians must consider how accurately the system captures dietary-intake information. Validity and reliability testing prior to use in a research study is ideal. The ability of users to search for food items consumed, correctly identify them, and correctly estimate portion sizes will influence reliability and validity of data. Nutrient-analysis systems are capable of automatically checking for implausible data entry and providing memory prompts to increase the likelihood of including all foods and beverages consumed. The quality of the database, and quantity of the food items and nutrients found in the database of the computerized system, is a key factor for accuracy in dietary analysis as well. Missing data and missing food items will detrimentally affect validity. For research purposes, food and nutrient databases need to be accurate, complete, up to date, include a large number of food and beverage items, incorporate brand names or restaurant items to help select correct food items, and have the ability to analyze a wide variety of nutrients of interest to the researcher. A system should be in place by the application developer to make regular updates to the food and nutrient database. In addition, the ability of the researcher, clinician, or user to add new foods and recipes to the database improves the ability to assess a participant's dietary intake accurately. The nutrition researcher should be able to determine the source of the food and nutrient database, the frequency of updates to the database, and the nutrients assessable before selecting an application.[29]

Research-quality databases commonly used by computerized dietary assessment applications include the USDA's Food and Nutrient Database for Dietary Studies (FNDDS), the Food Pattern Equivalent Database (FPED), and the NDSR from the Nutrition Coordinating Center of the University of Minnesota. The USDA FNDDS is the nutrient database used for determining nutrient intake of the nutrition-assessment portion of the National Health and Nutrition Examination Survey (NHANES). It is also the main database used for the SuperTracker, the NCI's Dietary History Questionnaire II (DHQ II), and the Automated Self-Administered 24-hour recall (ASA24). The FNDDS includes 8,536 main food descriptions and codes and an additional 12,128 food descriptions related to the main foods, along with 64 nutrients or food components (USDA Agricultural Research Service: https://www.ars.usda.gov).[31] The FPED uses the FNDDS as the source of nutrient values to convert foods and beverages into 37 different USDA food pattern components using portion equivalents to compare to the *Dietary Guidelines for Americans 2015–2020*. For example, the FPED database converts the reported dietary intake of fruits and vegetables into cup equivalents.[31] Lastly, the NDSR boasts more than 18,000 food items, 8,000 brand name items, 23 common restaurant menu items, and 165 nutrients and food components. It also has the capacity to assess food-group equivalents. The main source of nutrient values for the NDSR is the National Nutrient Database for Standard Reference, maintained by the USDA to provide nutrient-composition data. Additional nutrient data are obtained from other databases and published research.[32]

## Technology Requirements

When selecting an application for dietary analysis, determine and consider required network capabilities, Internet connection speed, type of browser, and hardware and software requirements. Some applications may run on a network system instead of individual computer hard drives or vice versa. When installed on individual computers, hardware memory capabilities must be sufficient for storing data and running the application. Operating systems (Microsoft Windows, MAC-OSX, Linux), personal computer (PC) or Macintosh, for example, also must be capable of running the application. Internet connection speed is important for Internet-based applications and the ability to quickly enter, analyze, download, and generate reports based on dietary intake. Note the type of web browser best suited for using Internet-based applications. Ideally, these applications are usable with multiple current versions of web browsers. Whether the Internet-based application can be accessed using mobile phone or tablet devices may also be of interest, because this offers greater flexibility for users. Applications such as the ASA24 is an example of a web-based system that eliminates the need for the researcher to meet specific hardware and software requirements, but requires the researcher and the research participant to access the application from an Internet connection using a web browser anytime, anywhere.

## Cost

Cost is another consideration in choosing a dietary assessment application. Consideration should be given to the cost of equipment needed (i.e., computers, handheld devices, and sensors) and staff and administration costs for data collection and analysis.[15] Handheld devices such as the SenseCam and mobile camera phones cost hundreds of dollars and therefore may be prohibitive for large studies. Image-based food records that do not include automated methods for identifying and analyzing food items will require significant labor costs for expert analysis. Furthermore, most computerized or Internet-based applications require an initial licensing fee that may vary, depending on the number of application users, and they may require an annual renewal fee. The licensing fee may or may not include regular updates to the database or software, and this should be clear before purchasing. In addition, there may be a fee associated with technical support of the system and data storage on a network server or cloud-based system. The amount of data needing storage often determines the fees. Regular updates, technical support, and sufficient data storage are benefits often worth purchasing. Some systems may require payment for analysis of the results, which can be costly. Diet-analysis applications developed with federal grant funds may be free to use but likely come with less support. These include the NCI's DHQ II and the ASA24.

## Data-Management Efficiency

A primary reason for the development of computerized diet-analysis systems is to make collecting and analyzing dietary-intake data more efficient and therefore reduce the burden on researchers, clinicians, and respondents. Applications that allow for self-administration of 24-hour recalls or FFQs and direct entry of food records improve time efficiency by eliminating the need for data entry by the researcher or clinician from traditional paper-based records. This greatly reduces administration time and effort by the researcher and clinician. In addition, systems that use built-in algorithms that allow for skipping unnecessary questions based on previous answers reduces the burden on respondents.[15] This shortens the number of questions that the participant is required to answer and therefore may lead to better-quality data by reducing the fatigue associated with long questionnaires. Internet-based applications that allow data entry anytime, anywhere without requiring the participant to travel to a research center reduces respondent burden as well.

Another important factor regarding data-management efficiency includes coding, transferability, and storage. The efficiency of coding data by automated systems reduces time and effort by the researcher or clinician. The exportability or importability of data to statistical-analysis applications without additional data handling also improves efficiency. Finally, how and where the data will be stored are important considerations. Data should be easily stored on a secure system to prevent loss of confidentiality and easily backed up to prevent loss of data. Internet-based applications typically use a server or cloud-based system to store and retrieve data. This system will generally have in place a method for regularly backing up data.

## Applicability

The researcher or clinician must consider the population for which they intend to collect dietary-intake, and whether or not it is necessary to collect multiple measures of dietary intake. The target population must have the ability to access the technology-based system. Although mobile phones and Internet access are widely available, some target populations such as low-income groups or older adults may not have access to or be comfortable using the technology. The population size also matters. Some systems may limit the number of users or number of data-set entries. In the case of 24-hour recalls in which multiple recalls are beneficial to better estimate usual intake, the computerized system must be capable of handling multiple entries by the same users.

## Usability

In choosing a technology-based dietary assessment method, usability is a factor for researchers, clinicians, and participants. Cognitive effort, time for completion, necessity of training, level of literacy required, and computer skills are all usability items identified by Illner et al. as important to assess.[15] Usability among differing age groups is another consideration because not all age groups will be appropriate for some forms of technology or dietary assessment methods. Different age groups may be more accepting of certain technologies and more comfortable using technology and therefore require less training. One could expect that the lesser the learning curve on using technology in dietary assessment, the better the outcomes. As previously discussed, the user's ability to correctly follow instructions and capture images using a mobile-phone food-recording system influenced the quality and quantity of dietary data collected. How easily the system can be incorporated into a user's lifestyle may also make a difference. Self-administered systems must be easy for the participant to access, navigate, search for food items, and correctly enter information. The researcher should look for applications that are intuitive to users and include help features such as multiple food images in varying portion sizes, avatars, or help wizards. Applications should also allow the user to choose from multiple measurement options (cups, ounces, tablespoons, grams) for ease of portion-size determination and multiple food-preparation methods for food selection, thereby improving quality of data entered. The majority of dietary-analysis applications available on the market allow researchers and clinicians to access a demonstration version of the application to evaluate ease of use prior to purchasing and implementation.

## Reports and Data Analysis

Another factor to consider in selecting a dietary-analysis system is data reporting and analysis. Consider the types of reports you want to generate, such as daily menus for production of metabolic meals, summary of nutrients over multiple days, single-meal or single-day nutrient intake reports, or summary reports of group mean intakes of dietary data. The quality of the report format and layout on the screen or in print is important for easier interpretation of results. The ability to save the reports as a common file type, such as a portable document format (PDF), assists in the ability to share data with other researchers, clinicians, and participants. Other questions to consider include are: What types of analysis will the application provide? Can the raw data be easily exported and imported for statistical analysis by statistical software applications?

## Data Security and HIPAA Compliance

Dietary-analysis systems may allow for the entry and collection of data that includes personal health information and therefore is protected information through the Health Information Portability and Accountability Act (HIPAA). The researcher must consider if the dietary assessment system meets HIPAA compliance standards. Institutional research boards and clinical facilities will most likely require that any computerized systems used to collect participant information and dietary data comply with HIPAA. Any dietary data-collection system should have a means of ensuring data are stored in a secure location to prevent data breaches and maintain confidentiality. Individual researcher, clinician, and

user passwords are means to protecting access to the data.

**TABLE 6.2** provides a summary of factors to consider in choosing a technology for dietary-intake assessment.

**Recap** In summary, many factors must be considered when selecting a computerized dietary assessment application. Start with identifying your research objectives and variables; this will help determine the most appropriate dietary assessment method to choose, thereby narrowing the choice of assessment applications. Quality of the food and nutrient database and the number of foods and nutrients included for analysis are also important factors for accuracy of assessment. Cost, ease of use, technology requirements, and ability to analyze data are other considerations for the nutrition researcher. Finally, data security is of utmost importance to protect confidentiality.

## ▶ Computer-Based Diet-Assessment Applications

**Preview** A computer-based diet-assessment application requires specific hardware and software components for use. They were initially introduced in the last few decades of the 20th century with the advent of the personal computer. Illner et al. contends that their use does not necessarily change the methodology of data collection but enhances it by increasing the potential of increased cost-effectiveness of dietary assessment. It also reduces the time and effort needed for data collection and analysis. For these reasons, it may be a more acceptable means of collecting dietary data. Dietary intake can be collected by a trained interviewer who enters the participant's response directly into the computer application. Otherwise, the dietary interview can be self-administered using standardized, structured prompts and a question sequence in which the participant directly inputs responses.

## Automated Multiple-Pass Method

The USDA developed the Automated Multiple-Pass Method (AMPM) based on the science–based methodology of the 24-hour recall commonly used in surveys to evaluate dietary intake in the American population. The AMPM is used for collecting data during the NHANES dietary interview portion.[33] It is

| **TABLE 6.2** Summary of factors to consider when choosing a technology-based dietary assessment instrument | |
| --- | --- |
| **Selecting a Technology-Based Dietary Assessment Instrument** | |
| Type of Research and Research Question | Define the type of research and research variables<br>Research objective(s) and question(s)<br>Determine the level of dietary detail required |
| Level of Detail Required | Analyze for dietary patterns or individual foods<br>Analysis by meal, day, or multiple days<br>Type and number of nutrients or food components available for analysis |
| Technology Requirements | Network-based or computer-workstation–based<br>Internet-based, web-browser requirements<br>Internet connection speed<br>Hardware and software requirements<br>Handheld or tablet capabilities |
| Accuracy and Quality of the Database | Individual or group validity and reproducibility<br>Food identification<br>Automatic check for implausible data<br>Incorporation of memory prompts<br>Number of foods and beverages included<br>Portion-size estimation<br>Completeness of the database |
| Costs | Equipment and licensing<br>Database or software updates<br>Staff and administration cost<br>Data analysis or storage fees<br>Technical support |
| Data-Management Efficiency | Data-collection duration and entry<br>Transfer of data<br>Data coding<br>Data storage, retrieval, and backup |
| Applicability | Population size<br>Target specific groups<br>Repeated measures |
| Usability | Required training<br>Cognitive effort<br>Time to complete<br>Literacy<br>Computer skills |
| Reports and Analysis | Ease of generating reports<br>Types of reports and analysis<br>Variety of file formats for reporting<br>Format of report |
| Data Security and HIPAA Compliance | Secure data storage and access<br>Meets HIPAA requirements for electronic data |

Data from Thompson FE, Kirkpatrick SI, Subar AF, et al. The National Cancer Institute's Dietary Assessment Primer: A resource for diet research. *J Acad Nutr Diet.* 2015;115:1986–1995. Illner AK, Freisling H, Boeing H, Huybrechts I, Crispim SP, Slimani N. Review and evaluation of innovative technologies for measuring diet in nutritional epidemiology. *Int J Epidemiol.* 2012;41:1187–1203. Vozenilek, G. Choosing the best nutrient analysis software for your needs. *J Amer Diet Assoc.* 1999;99(11):1356–1358.

designed to be interviewer administered in person or by telephone and is respondent driven. Participants are asked to list foods they consumed in a recent past 24-hour period. The interviewer probes for eating events and commonly forgotten foods or additions to foods and then reviews the list of foods. The companion Food Model Booklet is used to help estimate portion sizes during the recall. The AMPM is programmed to adjust questioning based on participant responses. Foods can be added, edited, or deleted at any time during the interview, and automated data checks look for potential errors in data entry. The AMPM links with two other systems that allow for coding and editing of food items, reformatting, review, and nutrient analysis. The Food and Nutrient Database for Dietary Studies serves as the source of nutrient values of foods and beverages.[33,34]

To assess validity, Blanton et al. compared the AMPM to the Block FFQ and the NCI's DHQ using the DLW technique for measuring total energy expenditure and a 14-day food record for nutrient intake.[35] Energy intake assessed by the AMPM and food record was not significantly different from DLW results. The FFQ and DHQ were found to underestimate energy intake. The AMPM most closely estimated absolute nutrient intakes by the food record, whereas the questionnaires significantly underestimated nutrient intake.[35] These results support the validity of the use of the AMPM in dietary assessment.

In another study, the AMPM was evaluated for its accuracy in assessing reported energy intake by comparison to energy expenditure determined by the DLW technique. Study participants were given the DLW technique at the start of the two-week study. Participants completed three 24-hour recalls, one in person and two by telephone. Compared to total energy expenditure as determined by the DLW, energy intake was underreported by 11%. Normal-weight participants were less likely to underreport energy intake compared to those who were overweight. Obese participants were more likely to report low energy intakes. Acceptable energy intake was reported by 78% of men and 74% of women.[36] These results conclude that the AMPM is an acceptable method of evaluating energy intake and that the validity of reporting of energy intake is influenced by body weight and gender. Future studies using biometric measures alongside the AMPM dietary assessment are necessary to validate its use in nutrition research.

## Nutrition Data System for Research

The NDSR, from the Nutrition Coordinating Center (NCC) at the University of Minnesota, is a software application designed for collecting and analyzing dietary-intake information for research purposes. This Microsoft Windows-based software application allows the entry of food records, 24-hour recalls using a guided multipass method, recipes, and development of menus for immediate analysis. Reports of nutrients can be generated for individual ingredients, foods, meals, and days. More than 18,000 foods and brand name items are included in the NCC Food and Nutrient Database, which is updated annually. The USDA's National Nutrient Database serves as a primary source of data for the database. As the researcher enters food items into the software, the database searches for and automatically codes foods for analysis and converts the quantities into grams. The conversion is typically needed for metabolic diet development and production. Data are available for 165 nutrients, food components, and nutrient ratios. An additional module is available for purchase to assess dietary supplement intake.[32] A free demo of the software is available on request from the NCC website (http://www.ncc.umn.edu/). **FIGURE 6.7** shows an example of the report that can be generated through this system.

## ProNutra

ProNutra is another research-quality software application aimed at meal planning for metabolic feeding studies and analyzing dietary intake in research centers. As food items are entered to create a metabolic diet, nutrient data are immediately calculated and can be seen alongside preset nutrient parameters required for the study's diet protocol. This allows for quick comparisons of nutrients and adjustments in food items and portion sizes. Reports can be generated for meal production, menus, labels, and analysis of dietary intake. Furthermore, data can be exported to statistical software for further analysis. The source of nutrient data is the USDA's Nutrient Database for Standard Reference and the Food and Nutrient Database for Dietary Studies[37]. **FIGURE 6.8** shows a sample report for the ProNutra database.

## The Food Processor

The Food Processor nutrition analysis software, from Esha Research, has a large database of 72,000 foods that includes the USDA's Nutrient Database for Standard Reference. It can analyze for 163 nutritional components and includes an exercise database with more than 900 individual activities, according to information provided on the company's website. It is designed primarily for use in a healthcare setting. Clinicians can manage

**NDSR 2015 Nutrient Totals Report**

Project Abbreviation: 961DS027
Participant ID: 961DS027                                    Date of Intake: 03/13/2016

| Primary Energy Sources | |
| --- | --- |
| Energy (kilocalories) | 1129 kcal |
| Total Fat | 31.953 g |
| Total Carbohydrate | 193.581 g |
| Total Protein | 24.709 g |
| Animal Protein | 12.695 g |
| % Calories from Fat | 25.056 % |
| % Calories from Carbohydrate | 66.706 % |
| % Calories from Protein | 8.470 % |
| **Fat and Cholesterol** | |
| Cholesterol | 80 mg |
| Solid Fats | 26.356 g |
| Total Saturated Fatty Acids (SFA) | 16.104 g |
| Total Monounsaturated Fatty Acids (MUFA) | 10.288 g |
| Total Polyunsaturated Fatty Acids (PUFA) | 3.027 g |
| Total Trans-Fatty Acids (TRANS) | 1.572 g |
| Total Conjugated Linoleic Acid (CLA 18:2) | 0.113 g |
| Omega-3 Fatty Acids | 0.501 g |
| % Calories from SFA | 12.676 % |
| % Calories from MUFA | 8.047 % |
| % Calories from PUFA | 2.359 % |
| Polyunsaturated to Saturated Fat Ratio | 0.188 |
| Cholesterol to Saturated Fatty Acid Index | 20.261 |

**FIGURE 6.7** Nutrient data system for research nutrient totals report

Reproduced from NUTRITION DATA SYSTEM FOR RESEARCH (NDSR) Database Version 2017. © 2017 Regents of the University of Minnesota.

unlimited individual client data; analyze intake; analyze and print labels for recipes; and generate reports for clients, diets, and menus. The clinician is able to compare recommended nutrient intake to client intake, customize and track nutrient intake and weight goals, and monitor physical activity. It also has the ability to add the capacity for clients to enter food and activity data via the Internet.[38]

## Nutritionist Pro

The Nutritionist Pro software is also designed for healthcare settings and can be used in research settings.

It is a PC-compatible application that can be used on a standalone computer or network system. The database includes more than 80,000 foods from the United States and other countries, fast-food items, ethnic foods, and medical foods. Foods and recipes can be added to the database. Similar to other applications, an unlimited number of clients can be managed and monitored for nutrient intake, weight goals, and physical activity. Reports can be generated for nutrient-intake summaries, deficiencies, MyPlate analyses, weight-tracking graphs, nutrient-intake graphs, diet plans, menus, food and shopping lists,

## Low Phosphorus 1800

Modified: November 10, 2015; Last Used: May 05, 2014
Description: 700 mg Pho, 1000 mg Ca, 2 gm Na, 3000 mg K

| Food Item | Food Code | Database | Amount | Measure | Weight (g) | Energy (kcal) | Protein (g) | Total lipid (fat) (g) |
|---|---|---|---|---|---|---|---|---|
| **– Breakfast** | | | | | | | | |
| Bread, white, commercial | 18069 | Custom Da | 50.00 | gram | 50.00 | 133.50 | 4.10 | 1.80 |
| Margarine-like spread, tub | 81103080 | FNDDS Ve | 5.00 | gram | 5.00 | 26.55 | 0.03 | 3.00 |
| Egg, whole, raw, fresh | 01123 | Custom Da | 40.00 | gram | 40.00 | 59.60 | 5.00 | 4.01 |
| Salt, table | 02047 | USDA Cust | 0.30 | gram | 0.30 | 0.00 | 0.00 | 0.00 |
| Orange juice, with calcium | 61210250 | FNDDS Ve | 240.00 | gram | 240.00 | 108.00 | 1.63 | 0.14 |
| Applesauce, canned | 09019 | Custom Da | 100.00 | gram | 100.00 | 43.00 | 0.17 | 0.05 |
| **– Lunch** | | | | | | | | |
| Spaghetti, dry, enriched | 20120 | Custom Da | 50.00 | gram | 50.00 | 185.50 | 6.39 | 0.79 |
| Spaghetti sauce, meatless | 74404050 | FNDDS Ve | 100.00 | gram | 100.00 | 109.00 | 1.80 | 4.80 |
| Beef, ground, 80% lean meat | 23572 | USDA Stan | 60.00 | gram | 60.00 | 152.40 | 10.30 | 12.0 |
| Beans, snap, green, frozen | 11060 | Custom Da | 75.00 | gram | 75.00 | 24.75 | 1.35 | 0.16 |
| Bread, white, commercial | 18069 | Custom Da | 25.00 | gram | 25.00 | 66.75 | 2.05 | 0.90 |
| Pineapple, raw | 09266 | Custom Da | 50.00 | gram | 50.00 | 24.50 | 0.20 | 0.22 |
| Margarine-like spread, tub | 81103080 | FNDDS Ve | 10.00 | gram | 10.00 | 53.10 | 0.06 | 6.00 |
| Salt, table | 02047 | USDA Cust | 0.40 | gram | 0.40 | 0.00 | 0.00 | 0.00 |
| **– PM Snack** | | | | | | | | |
| Cookies, chocolate chip | 18164 | Custom Da | 1.00 | 1 medium | 12.00 | 59.04 | 0.59 | 2.71 |
| **– Dinner** | | | | | | | | |
| Pork, fresh, loin, top loin | 10063 | Custom Da | 85.00 | gram | 85.00 | 198.05 | 23.65 | 10.78 |
| Spices, MRS. DASH Original | | USDA Cust | 1.00 | gram | 1.00 | 0.00 | 0.00 | 0.00 |
| Rice, white, long-grain, regular | 20044 | Custom Da | 50.00 | gram | 50.00 | 182.50 | 3.56 | 0.33 |
| Carrots, frozen, unprepared | 11130 | Custom Da | 50.00 | gram | 50.00 | 19.50 | 0.55 | 0.11 |
| Bread, white, commercial | 18069 | Custom Da | 25.00 | gram | 25.00 | 66.75 | 2.05 | 0.90 |
| Margarine, regular, liquid, soy | 04105 | Custom Da | 10.00 | gram | 10.00 | 72.10 | 0.19 | 8.06 |
| Pears, canned, juice pack | 09254 | Custom Da | 90.00 | gram | 90.00 | 45.00 | 0.31 | 0.06 |
| Salt, table | 02047 | USDA Cust | 0.45 | gram | 0.45 | 0.00 | 0.00 | 0.00 |
| **– HS Snack** | | | | | | | | |
| Crackers, saltine | 54325000 | FNDDS Ve | 8.00 | 1 cracker | 24.00 | 104.16 | 2.21 | 2.83 |
| Cheese, cheddar | 01009 | Custom Da | 14.00 | gram | 14.00 | 56.36 | 3.49 | 4.64 |

| | Energy (kcal) | Protein (g) | Total lipid (fat) (g) | Carbohydrate, by difference (g) | Water (g) | Cacium, Ca (mg) |
|---|---|---|---|---|---|---|
| Diet Target | 1800.00 | 67.50 | 60.00 | 247.50 | 3000.00 | 700.00 |
| Diet Actual | 1790.11 | 69.66 | 64.28 | 233.88 | 786.17 | 702.69 |

**FIGURE 6.8** ProNutra metabolic diet development and analysis tool

Reproduced from ProNutra. Viocare. www.viocare.com/pronutra.html. [Accessed September 18, 2016].

and recipe analyses; these can be exported in a variety of formats similar to those offered by other applications. Clinicians can view nutrients of food items as they are added to dietary-intake analysis, recipes, and menus. The client group feature allows tracking of nutrient data among participants in a research study group, and the data-extraction tool quickly pulls data for statistical analysis.[39]

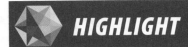

## HIGHLIGHT

### Steps of the Automated Multiple-Pass Method

1. Quick list: List all foods and beverages consumed the previous day.
2. Forgotten foods: Probe for forgotten foods.
3. Time and occasion: Obtain time and eating occasion for each food.
4. Detail cycle: Obtain detailed description and amount for each food and any additions. Review reported items.
5. Final probe: Inquire about any missed items.

### Information Collected by the AMPM

- For each food record:
  - Description of food item
  - Additions to food items (e.g., milk or cream added to coffee)
  - Combination code for foods commonly eaten together (e.g., bread with butter)
  - Quantity of food consumed (e.g., 1 cup, 2 tablespoons, 1 ounce)
  - Time of day eaten
  - Name of eating occasion (breakfast, lunch, dinner, snack)
  - Where food was obtained (grocery store, sit-down restaurant, fast-food restaurant)
  - Was the food eaten at home or away from home?
- Amount of water (bottled or tap) consumed
- Use of salt in food preparation or at the table
- The amount of food consumed on the recall day was usual, more than usual, or less than usual
- Following a diet for weight loss or special diet for health reasons

Modified from U.S. Department of Agriculture.https://www.ars.usda.gov/northeast-area/beltsville-md/beltsville-human-nutrition-research-center/food-surveys-research-group/docs/ampm-usda-automated-multiple-pass-method/.

**Recap**  Computer-based diet-assessment applications described in this chapter are some of the most frequently used in research and clinical settings. These applications are designed for use by nutrition researchers and nutrition professionals. They are not intended for general-public use. The applications mentioned offer similar features but may vary in the number of foods included in the database, number of nutrients available for analysis, ease of use, and cost. The validity and reliability of the dietary-intake data is only as good the data entered and the underlying food composition database.

## ▶ Internet-Based Diet-Analysis Applications

**Preview**  An Internet-based diet-analysis application does many of the same functions as computer-based applications. The main differences are in how the application is accessed and how data are stored and retrieved. For the nutrition researcher, the Internet offers the opportunity to reach a greater number of individuals and to reach groups of individuals previously considered unreachable because of geographical constraints. For the clinician, the Internet makes it possible to collect dietary data for analysis and rapid feedback to improve clinical outcomes.

## Automated Self-Administered 24-Hour Dietary Recall (ASA24)

The Automated Self-Administered 24-hour dietary recall system (ASA24), developed by the National Cancer Institute of the National Institutes of Health, is designed for research studies assessing dietary intake among adults and large-population studies. It is available for free to researchers, teachers, and clinicians without cost.[40] The latest version, ASA24-2016, allows researchers or clinicians to collect both single-day and multiple-day food records. It is currently available in both English and Spanish and in a Canadian version, and it is under development for use in other countries. Researchers or clinicians access the researcher website to set the options available for data collection, manage user accounts, obtain reports to monitor progress of participants, and access analysis files. Analysis for American versions is based on the FNDDS. Users are provided with a website link and login information to access the respondent site for data entry. Guidance through the application is provided through written or audio prompts using the multipass methodology for 24-hour recall. Users enter the eating occasion and the time this meal or snack was eaten; then they search for food and beverage items consumed, including supplements, type of food, and preparation method.[40] Real food images in multiple portion sizes are used to help users accurately estimate the portions consumed. Real food images also act as prompts triggering any missing items or modifying food and drink items. Data on where meals were consumed, sources of foods, whether eaten alone or with company, and if computer or television use occurred during meals can be collected if desired. Multiple recalls or food records can be collected from individual users. The maximum number of recalls is set by the researcher. Lastly, the ASA24 system can be used with computer-screen readers for individuals with disabilities and is accessible with most common web browsers. The ASA24-2016 version is also accessible on mobile devices.[40]

The ASA24 has good potential for use in research or clinical settings for collecting dietary data. When compared to observed intake and plate-waste measurements, the ASA24 performed almost equivalently to dietary recall by AMPM.[41] In addition, Thompson et al. compared the performance of the ASA24 to that of the AMPM with adults across three health systems.[42] There were four groups with each participant completing two recalls: (1) ASA24 and AMPM, (2) AMPM and ASA24, (3) ASA24 and ASA24, and (4) AMPM and AMPM. Study participants preferred the ASA24, and lower attrition was observed among participants who experienced the ASA24 before the AMPM or experienced the ASA24 on both recalls. In addition, energy and nutrient intakes were similar.[42] The greater acceptability, greater retention, and reduced time and cost benefits of using a self-administered system may outweigh the minor differences found between self-administered and interviewer-administered recalls. Note that in a study (in press at the time of writing this chapter) involving this author, adult participants with limited literacy and computer skills had some difficulties using the ASA24 without assistance. Further research is needed to assess the feasibility of use and validity among adult users with limited literacy and computer skills. **FIGURE 6.9** shows an example of the "Add Details" tab indicating portion size for a food item in a 24-hour recall using the ASA24 free demonstration site.

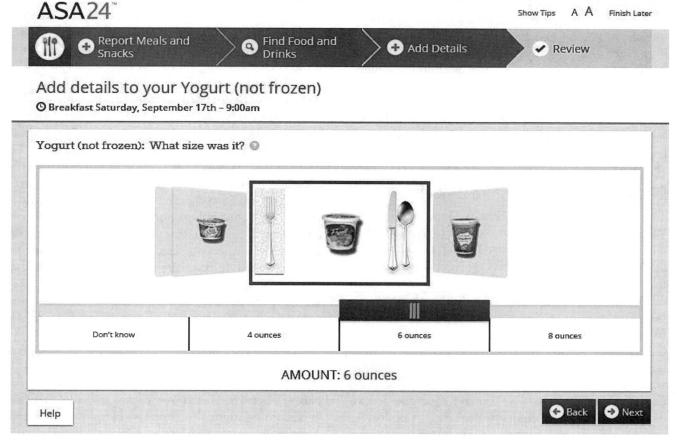

**FIGURE 6.9** ASA24 "Add Details" tab for portion size

## Automated Self-Administered 24-Hour Dietary Recall: ASA24Kids

The ASA24Kids was developed based on the same methodology and features of the ASA24 for use with children 10 years of age and older and is free for use by researchers. Modification for use with children included simplifying wording, removing food and drink items not reported by children in national food and nutrition surveys, removing alcoholic drinks, and removing probing questions that children might not understand or know how to answer. "School" was added as an option for eating location. Obtaining valid and accurate dietary data from children is difficult. In a crossover study, overall matches for reported food intake between the ASA24Kids and an interviewer-led 24-hour recall among children 8 to 13 years old were less than 50%. Younger children had significantly lower matches and were more likely to omit foods and need help with the ASA24Kids.[43] Diep et al. conducted a validation study of the ASA24Kids 2012 version with children ages 9 to 11 years, comparing the web-based self-administered recall to 24-hour recalls conducted by trained interviewers and direct observation of meals consumed.[44] Both modes of obtaining dietary recalls performed inadequately compared to actual observed intakes. Interviewer-administered 24-hour recalls performed only slightly better than the ASA24Kids 2012. Researchers concluded that additional studies are needed to determine at what age children are able to provide dietary data without the assistance of a parent or guardian.[44] Dietary data collected from children must be interpreted cautiously, and automated systems may need to be simplified for children.

## Diet History Questionnaire II–Web

The NCI's web-based Diet History Questionnaire II–Web (DHQII) is simply an electronic version of a paper-based FFQ. However, the DHQII–Web is able to skip unnecessary questions, prevent missed questions and inconsistent responses, allow correction of responses, and allow for completion of the questionnaire over multiple logins as opposed to having to finish within a single session. Four versions of the DHQII–Web are available: (1) past year with portion size, (2) past year without portion size, (3) past month with portion size, and (4) past month without portion size. The DHQII–Web is a free tool, and access can be requested through the website. In addition, researchers can download the PC-based Diet*Calc companion software designed specifically to analyze the DHQII–Web data. The software will provide estimates of nutrient intake and food groups. To date, the

DHQII–Web has not been validated separately from the paper-based version. However, usability studies have been conducted and have demonstrated the ease of use. Results indicate that the web version is less time-consuming than the paper version.[45] **FIGURE 6.10** shows an example of questions relating to the frequency of consumption and portion size consumed of a food item from the DHQII free demonstration site.

## VioScreen

VioScreen is a HIPAA-compliant, web-based, self-administered, graphical FFQ designed for research purposes. VioScreen uses branching logic to avoid unnecessary questions based on user responses, thereby reducing respondent burden, and checks for errors or implausible responses in real time to prevent inaccurate data entry. Users receive memory prompts and are able to choose from food images of differing portion sizes to help them report more accurately. In addition, the FFQ can be completed in English or Spanish. Reports of dietary behavior, estimated nutrient intakes, and food patterns are available instantly. Data can be exported for use in other statistical software applications for further analysis.[46,47] Kristal et al. compared the Graphical Food-Frequency System (GraFFS) to dietary-intake data collected by telephone-administered 24-hour recalls in a validation study.[47] Energy, macronutrients, and 17 micronutrients were estimated using GraFFS and compared to the mean of six 24-hour recalls. The GraFFS was found to underestimate total energy by 9%, carbohydrate by 12%, protein by 5%, and fat by 15%. However, it provided similar results to the 24-hour recalls when comparing macronutrients as a percent of calories. Micronutrients were overestimated in GraFFS compared to 24-hour recalls. Moderate to high correlations were found for the test-retest reliability of GraFFS. Moreover, 100% of participants felt GraFFS was easy to use, 98% would be willing to complete the questionnaire if requested by a doctor, and 80% found the food images to be helpful for estimating portion sizes. In comparing GraFFS to other paper-based FFQs, the authors concluded that GraFFS was equally as good.[47]

## NutraScreen

NutraScreen is a HIPAA-compliant diet-analysis application designed for use in a clinical setting, and it can be incorporated into workplace wellness applications and platforms. It is a web-based application that allows users to enter dietary information using any computer or tablet with an Internet connection.

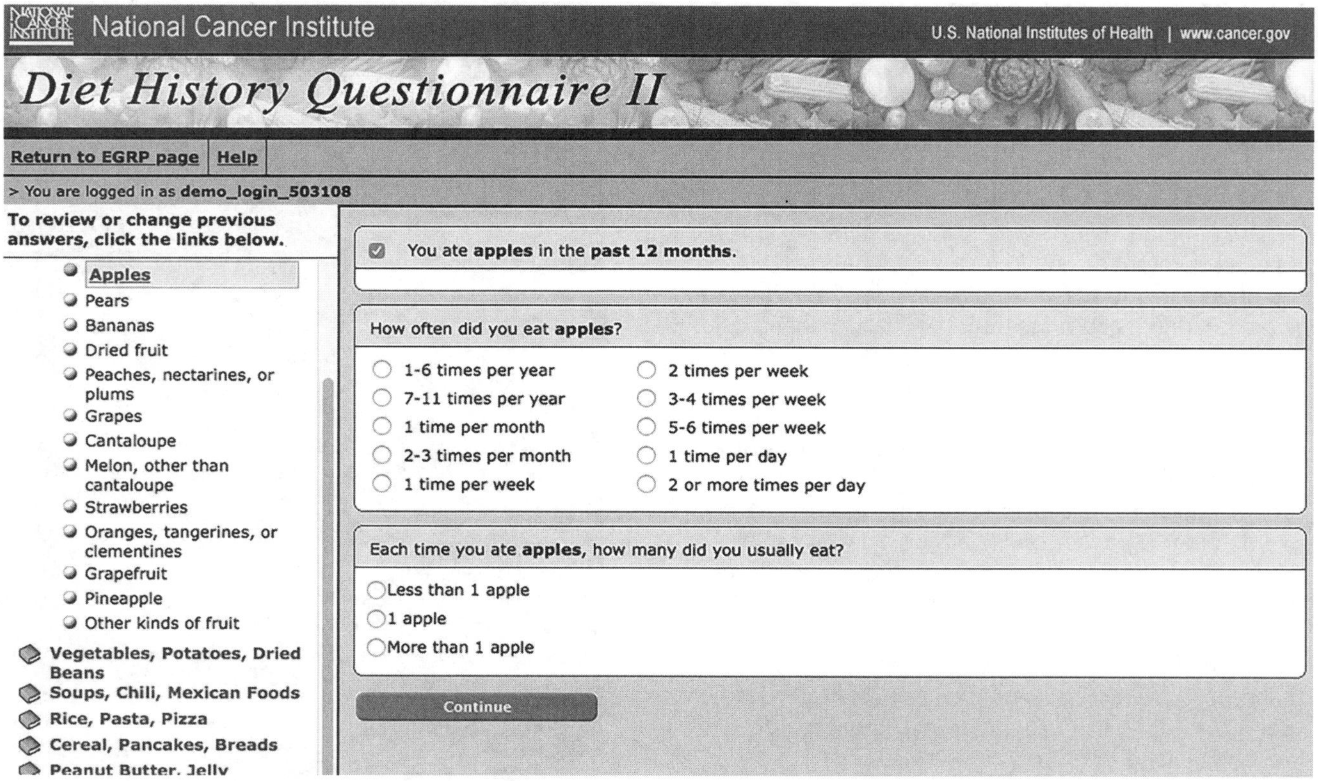

**FIGURE 6.10** DHQII–web questionnaire sample frequency and portion-size questions

Reproduced from Diet History Questionnaire II and Canadian Diet History Questionnaire II: Web-based. National Institutes of Health, National Cancer Institute. epi.grants.cancer.gov/dhq2/. [Accessed October 29. 2016]

Data entry is enhanced by real food photos to assist with portion-size estimates and to allow for quick entry. Results are available immediately for viewing by healthcare providers and users. User data are compared to dietary recommendations, and reports indicate areas needing improvement. A Healthy Eating Index score is also calculated.[48]

## NutritionQuest's Data-on-Demand

Data-on-Demand is a web-based nutrition and physical activity assessment and analysis system developed by NutritionQuest, the source of the well-known and validated Block FFQs. Nutrition researchers may choose any of the Block FFQs or food- or nutrient-specific (e.g., fat, sugar, fruit, vegetable, calcium, sodium) screening questionnaires to deliver on the Data-on-Demand system. Data-on-Demand allows for direct online entry of dietary-intake information for interviewer- or self-administered questionnaires. For the latter, the participant is provided a website address and a login to complete the questionnaire. Researchers may also choose to upload offline data and scanned paper questionnaire data into the system. Data are automatically analyzed when questionnaires are completed, allowing the researcher to see trends

in the data before the study is complete. The data are stored online and backed up daily. The researcher accesses results and manages data through a private, password-protected account. Reports can be printed and data downloaded at any time in batches; for individual subjects, the researcher can track which subjects have completed questionnaires. Automatic transfer of data to a study server is also possible. Like others, the FFQ application uses algorithms to adjust questions based on user responses and skips unnecessary questions, thus reducing time for completion. The Block FFQs, screeners, and physical activity assessment tools have been validated in a variety of studies and groups, as well as used in many research studies assessing dietary intake. A list of validation studies of FFQs and screeners for use with both adults and children is available on the NutritionQuest website.[49]

## Nutribase Cloud Edition

The Nutribase Cloud Edition, by CyberSoft, Inc., is a robust nutrient-analysis application designed for the individual nutrition professional and could be incorporated into methods for collecting dietary intake for research studies. It includes nutrient data on more than 500,000 food items and research-quality databases from

# VIEWPOINT

## Apps

*Randi S. Drasin, MS, RDN*

What's trending in nutrition and fitness? Why, it's "apps," of course! Having an app to track your fitness and nutrition is the newest hot topic and one of the simplest ways to store, analyze, and track your daily routine. So, what is an app?

An app is defined as a self-contained program or piece of software designed to fulfill a particular purpose—an application, especially as downloaded by a user to a mobile device. **FIGURE A** shows the Calorie Counter and Diet Tracker app.

In other words, an app is an application! It can be used on any electronic device, but in today's world we see them being used mostly on smartphones or as wearable units. And these days it seems as if everyone has a smartphone or smart device. Whether it's in your hand, on your wrist (as a watch or a bracelet), in your pocket, in your purse, in your car, in your backpack, on your nightstand, or on your desk, it's usually never far from reach.

And these devices all have the ability to download one or more apps to track your every move, whether it's your steps, your calories burned, the number of floors climbed, your nutrient intake, your health record, your weight, your favorite healthy restaurant down the road, recipes to make the foods you like to eat, or tracking your heart rate, sleep patterns, or blood sugar. There is an app for almost anything you need or want to track.

So where do you start? That is a great question. As nutrition professionals, we want to make sure we are providing our clients with applications that are not only useful to that particular client, but also one that meets them at their literacy level as well as his or her stage of change. We wouldn't want to recommend an app to a client who is not comfortable with advanced technology, nor would we want to provide a client with

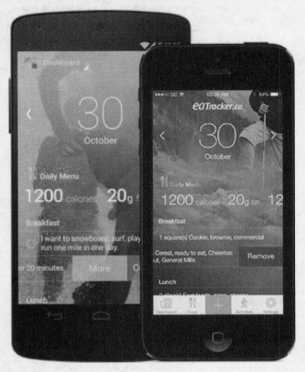

**FIGURE B** EaTracker App

Reproduced with permission from eaTracker.

an app that demands more than they are willing to engage in. **FIGURE B** shows the EaTracker app.

So, what are our best resources? Well, best practice would be to try out several apps yourself to see what you like, what works, and what doesn't. Ask yourself questions: Would my client be able to use this? Is it easy to handle? Confusing? Too detailed? Not detailed enough? Does it have the tracking program that would benefit the client? What is my client trying to accomplish?

Bottom line, is it user-friendly? And what benefit would it be to you as the clinician? Are you actually analyzing the data your clients are tracking? Or is it mainly to encourage self-awareness? Either way, research, research, research and make sure you know the outcome you want to achieve.

Check out the app reviews by three RDNs at the Academy of Nutrition and Dietetics. **TABLE A** shows a few of the top-rated apps with four- and five-star ratings!

### *Resource List*

The Academy of Nutrition and Dietetics: www .eatrightpro.org

The Academy of Nutrition and Dietetics Food and Nutrition Magazine: www.FoodandNutrition.org

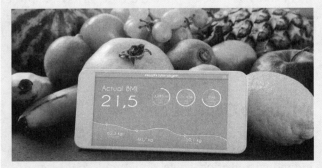

**FIGURE A** Calorie Counter and Diet Tracker app

© Daniel Krason/Shutterstock.

| **TABLE A** | Free Apps available for mobile technology as reviewed by the Academy's spokespeople | |
|---|---|---|
| **App Name** | **Rating** | **Description** |
| EaTipster | 5 stars | Tips to increase healthy eating, fight chronic diseases, and support a healthy weight. Addresses common food and nutrition questions. |
| GluCoMo | 4 stars | An electronic diary to track blood sugar levels, insulin intake, and carbohydrate intake. |
| Calorie Counter & Diet Tracker by MyFitness Pal | 4.5 stars | Tracks weight loss and fitness goals with calorie intake and exercise output. Database of more than 350 exercises with calories burned. |
| Gluten Free Daily | 4.5 stars | Provides resources for following a gluten-free diet. |
| Calorie Counter: Diets & Activities | 4 stars | Tracks calories, water, and fitness along with carbohydrates, protein, fat, cholesterol, saturated fat, and fiber. Offers the ability to create user's own diet and physical-activity plan. |
| Calorie Tracker by Livestrong.com | 4 stars | Food and fitness diary. Tracks calories, fat, cholesterol, sodium, carbohydrates, sugars, fiber, and protein. Is a companion tool for members of The Daily Plate. |

Created by Randi Drasin, from info obtained by the Academy's spokespeople: Marisa Moore, MBA, RD, LD; Jessica Crandall, RD, CDE; Sarah Krieger, MPH, RD, LDN.

both the United States and Canada. It works with multiple smartphone apps for connecting with clients and allows direct entry of dietary intake and physical activity by the client. The cloud-based system makes it easy to synchronize data from any computer. Features of the application include publication-quality food labels, the ability to search food names or brand names, add food items, drag and drop columns of nutrient data and order them according to preference, sort foods from high to low and vice versa based on specific nutrients, send messages to clients, monitor clients' activity at any time, and much more. Data can be backed up and restored on different computers, and backed up to external media such as a flash drive. An extensive list of features and a comparison to other commonly used nutrient-analysis applications is available on the company website at www.nutribase.com.[50] Nutribase may be the most comprehensive application available to date. Previous versions of Nutribase have been used in research studies to analyze self-reported dietary intake. No studies are available assessing its validity and accuracy compared to other methods.

## SuperTracker

Developed by the USDA, the SuperTracker was designed as a consumer-based application for diet tracking and analysis; it also includes a meal-planning tool. The SuperTracker allows for allows for personal goal setting and physical activity and weight tracking encouraging health behavior change through self-monitoring and self-regulation. One of the features of the SuperTracker is the ability for health professionals or nutrition researchers to create private groups with as many as 150 members. Each group member must create a login and is invited to the group by the leader through email or provided an access code for joining the group. The group leader can generate reports of average group intake or individual group members that include age, gender, height, weight and weight history, food intake, physical activity, personal goals, and account activity such as login frequency. Reports can be exported as Excel, Word, or PDF files. Leaders can also send messages and develop healthy eating challenges.[51] This feature allows a new opportunity for nutrition researchers or clinicians to collect and analyze dietary and physical-activity data over time. Incorporating healthy eating challenges or sending messages to the group may serve as an intervention for food and activity behavior changes. The tool could be used with individual or group-based lifestyle interventions and incorporated into analysis to determine the effectiveness of applications for lifestyle changes. Research on feasibility and validity of

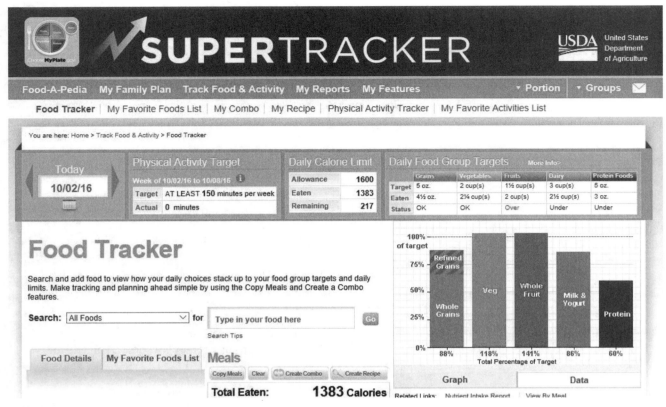

**FIGURE 6.11** SuperTracker food-intake entry page

Reproduced from SuperTracker. United States Department of Agriculture. www.supertracker.usda.gov. [Accessed September 18, 2016].

using SuperTracker in this way is needed. **FIGURE 6.11** shows the food-intake entry page of the SuperTracker along with the bar graph report indicating percent of target for recorded intake of key food groups.

> **Recap** Internet-based dietary assessment applications offer more flexibility for nutrition researchers and professionals. The Internet removes some of the barriers that nutrition researchers face, including reaching certain populations and having greater numbers of participants in nutrition studies. Research participants can provide dietary-intake data without having to travel to the research center, which saves time for both the participants and researchers. The Internet can help remove barriers for clinicians as well, allowing them to connect with patients outside the clinical setting. Clinicians can track food and beverage intake along with weight and exercise goals of clients as they submit information online and provide more immediate feedback to help them meet their nutrition goals. This could lead to improved patient outcomes. Researchers and clinicians may also use these applications to gather data to determine the effectiveness of nutrition interventions.

## ▶ Chapter Summary

Researchers and clinicians have been interested in determining true dietary intake and evaluating its relationship to health outcomes for decades. The ability of traditional methods to collect valid and accurate dietary intake has been criticized because of the known potential for error, primarily recall bias. Traditional methods are also labor intensive and burdensome. There are several advantages with current technologies when it comes to collecting dietary-intake data for analysis. This includes reducing the cost and the time and effort required, providing automatic data storage and rapid analysis, preventing incomplete and implausible data, and incorporating memory prompts and help features. Both computer-based and Internet-based applications improve the dietary interview process by using standardized questions and question sequencing based on the user's response. These applications may also help reduce bias in memory recall and reporting by incorporating multiple real food images and portion sizes, larger databases of food items to correctly identify foods consumed, and reduce the burden of recording dietary intake. Use of computerized technology in nutrition research may increase the objectivity of data collection and allow for larger sample sizes, therefore improving the ability to make stronger conclusions about the relationship of dietary intake to health and disease. Computerized nutrition analysis may also improve assessment in clinical settings and enhance clinical decision making and the provision of care that leads to improved outcomes.

Disadvantages of using technology in dietary assessment include the need for technological literacy on behalf of the participant as well as the research or clinician, keyboard and mouse skills for data entry, a lack of familiarity with or inability to use technology (older adults and the physically impaired may have difficulty using technology), and higher cost than pen-and-paper instruments. In addition, some socioeconomic groups may have limited access to technology. Newer technologies with the capacity to record images of foods consumed can improve the objectivity of reporting intake, aid in memory recall, and reduce

recording burden, and they may be more acceptable to users and thus help correct misreporting. However, there is room for improvement in image-based food records and automated analysis of food items. Image-based food recording also may require more training for the user. Overall, incorporation of technology into dietary assessment has not changed the underlying methodology. Still, in many cases, technology has enhanced the dietary assessment methodology.

Computerized technology is constantly changing and advancing. What is available today will likely change in the near future. Nutrition professionals must be prepared to adopt computerized food and nutrient-analysis systems in any setting and adapt to new technology as it becomes available. This will require acquiring skills in using technology for nutrient intake analysis. In addition, technology-savvy nutrition professionals can lead initiatives to improve systems and work with technology developers to advance systems.

 **CASE STUDY**

You are a postdoctoral fellow working with a prominent senior investigator on a project examining risk factors for dementia.

Nearly one in three Americans are living with hypertension; certain ethnic groups are more affected than others. Lifestyle behaviors, including diet and physical activity, can affect individual risks for developing hypertension, which is itself a risk factor for some leading causes of morbidity and mortality such as cardiovascular disease and stroke. A goal of *Healthy People 2020* is to improve cardiovascular health by controlling risk factors, including hypertension and improving dietary patterns,

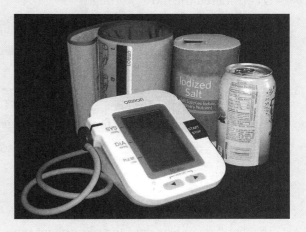

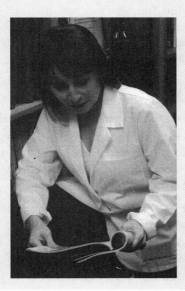

among Americans. Dr. Casas, PhD, RDN, is interested in studying the effects of such dietary components as sodium, phosphorous, and added sugars on hypertension. She wants to know the average intake of these nutrients among a large population of African Americans and Hispanics living in Dallas, Texas. She also plans to conduct a metabolic diet study using diets varying in nutrient composition among a subset of this population.

### Question:

1. Looking back through the information in this chapter, which nutrition assessment method would you recommend for the study procedures, and which tool(s) would be most appropriate, and why?

# Learning Portfolio

## Key Terms

24-hour recall
Computer-based diet-assessment application
eButton
Food-frequency questionnaire (FFQ)
Food record
Image-assisted dietary assessment (IADA)

Internet-based diet-assessment application
Reactivity bias
Recall bias
Screeners
SenseCam
Social-approval bias

## Study Questions

1. Which of the following is an advantage of using a food record to collect dietary-intake information?
   a. Low respondent burden
   b. Quick and easy to analyze
   c. Does not rely on memory
   d. Requires literacy skills

2. Which method of collecting dietary-intake data is considered the most thorough?
   a. Food record
   b. 24-hour recall
   c. Food-frequency questionnaire
   d. Dietary screener questionnaire

3. What is the type of bias in which the respondent changes dietary-intake patterns because of having to record or report food and beverages consumed?
   a. Recall
   b. Reactivity
   c. Social
   d. Recording

4. In what type of bias does the respondent report dietary intake consistent with expected norms or expectations but does not represent true intake?
   a. Recall
   b. Reactivity
   c. Social-approval
   d. Recording

5. Which method of gathering dietary-intake data relies on a structured interview process to obtain information about recently consumed foods?
   a. Food-frequency questionnaire
   b. Food record
   c. Dietary screener questionnaire
   d. 24-hour recall

6. What method of gathering dietary-intake data would be best when working with a population with low literacy levels?
   a. Food-frequency questionnaire
   b. Food record
   c. Dietary screener questionnaire
   d. 24-hour recall

7. Which of the following is a drawback of using the 24-hour recall method for collecting dietary-intake data?
   a. High respondent burden
   b. Introduces recall bias into the data
   c. Requires little time and effort from the researcher
   d. Includes a finite list of foods consumed

8. Which method of obtaining dietary-intake data asks participants to identify how often and sometimes the amount of a specific list of foods they consumed over a period of time, such as a year or month?
   a. Food-frequency questionnaire
   b. Food record
   c. 24-hour recall
   d. Dietary screener questionnaire

9. Which of the following is a benefit of using a food-frequency questionnaire?
   a. It is not affected by variability in daily intake.
   b. It is limited to a specific list of foods.
   c. It can be used to assess the total diet.
   d. It is good for quickly assessing intake of a few food groups.

10. What method of obtaining dietary-intake data is best for retrospective studies?
    a. Food record
    b. Dietary screener questionnaire
    c. Food-frequency questionnaire
    d. 24-hour recall

11. Which method of obtaining dietary-intake data is least burdensome for the participant and provides the least detail?
    a. Food record
    b. Dietary screener questionnaire
    c. Food-frequency questionnaire
    d. 24-hour recall

12. What method would be best to choose for quickly assessing calcium intake among a group of high-school female athletes to determine if an intervention is needed to encourage higher intakes of high-calcium foods?
    a. Food record
    b. 24-hour recall
    c. Food-frequency questionnaire
    d. Dietary screener questionnaire

13. What is a criticism of pen-and-paper methods of gathering dietary-intake data?
    a. It limits the researcher's ability to reach larger populations.
    b. It requires little time and effort for data entry and management.
    c. It is a more objective measure of intake.
    d. Literacy level is not a consideration among study participants.

14. What is a benefit of incorporating technology into dietary assessment methods?
    a. It is easily accessible by all populations.
    b. It is less costly than pen-and-paper methods.
    c. It allows for direct data entry.
    d. It can be easily adapted for people with disabilities.

15. Which of the following is a disadvantage of using technology for gathering dietary assessment data?
    a. Data are automatically analyzed in real time.
    b. A lack of technological literacy among some groups may require more training.
    c. It is more acceptable to use by adolescents.
    d. It limits the amount of data that can be collected because of storage capacity.

16. Image-assisted dietary assessment:
    a. Uses photographs or food models to aid in recall of foods eaten and portions consumed.
    b. Uses images of eating occasions to objectively capture dietary-intake data.
    c. Uses food packaging to estimate portion size of foods consumed.
    d. Requires expensive technology not available to most people.

17. Which of the following is a benefit of using image-assisted dietary assessment for research purposes?
    a. It allows for a more passive approach to collecting dietary data.
    b. It reduces the burden of analysis for the researcher.
    c. It aids in identifying unreported foods.
    d. It it is easier for participants to remember to capture images of foods than to write them down.

18. An example of a passive technology that can be used to capture dietary intake without the participant having to manually record dietary information is:
    a. SenseCam.
    b. A mobile-phone food record.
    c. A mobile voice recorder.
    d. An automated food-photograph analysis.

19. The _____ method requires that participants include (a) a reference marker along with the food in the photograph taken at a 45-degree angle and (b) written text describing the food and ingredients for analysis by an RDN.
    a. SenseCam
    b. NuDAM
    c. Wellnavi
    d. TADA

20. This image-assisted dietary assessment method was found to underestimate energy intakes when compared to the doubly labeled water technique.
    a. SenseCam
    b. NuDAM
    c. Wellnavi
    d. TADA

21. This uses multiple images of foods before and after eating to create a three-dimensional model for estimating nutrient intake.
    a. Dietitian-assessed food photographs
    b. Automated food-photograph analysis
    c. Wearable image-capturing systems
    d. Automated 24-hour recall

22. Which age group likely requires additional training to correctly capture foods and beverages when using the mobile-phone food record for obtaining dietary-intake data?
    a. Adolescents
    b. Adults
    c. Adolescents and adults
    d. No additional training is needed

23. What is a common problem among users of automated food-photograph analysis systems that affects the ability to accurately analyze nutrient-intake data?
    a. Using the wrong reference marker
    b. Forgetting to take images before and after eating
    c. Inability to accurately identify food items
    d. Including too many high-quality food images

24. This tool creates a three-dimensional point cloud and uses recognition software to estimate the volume of food based on three images captured by video recorder.
    a. eButton
    b. Technology Assisted Dietary Assessment
    c. Food Intake and Voice Recorder
    d. Dietary Data Recorder System

25. The _____ eliminates the need to include a reference marker along with food images by displaying a laser-beam grid over the food items in the image.
    a. eButton
    b. Technology Assisted Dietary Assessment
    c. Food Intake and Voice Recorder
    d. Dietary Data Recorder System

26. Users can wear this on the chest to automatically capture food images without additional self-reporting.
    a. eButton
    b. Technology Assisted Dietary Assessment
    c. Food Intake and Voice Recorder
    d. Dietary Data Recorder System

27. Why is it important to consider the type of research and research questions before you choose a dietary assessment method?
    a. The method will determine the cost of data collection.
    b. The method must be able to capture the data needed to answer research questions.
    c. The method will determine the level of detail needed.
    d. The method will determine the accuracy of the data.

28. If your research objective were to evaluate health outcomes related to dietary intake in cross-sectional and prospective studies, what type of dietary assessment method would be most appropriate?
    a. Food-frequency questionnaire
    b. Food record

c. Multiple 24-hour recalls
d. Single 24-hour recall

29. Which of the following can affect the ability to accurately obtain dietary-intake data when using a nutrient-analysis system?
    a. Ability to search for and identify correctly the foods consumed
    b. Cost: Lower-cost systems include fewer food and beverage items.
    c. Efficiency with which data are managed.
    d. The variety and quality of reports available

30. Which of the following is *not* a factor in choosing a computerized nutrient-analysis system?
    a. Cost
    b. Quality of database
    c. Data security
    d. Participant preference

31. Which factor in selecting a computerized diet-analysis system would be most important to evaluate if you have limited time and personnel for data collection, entry, and analysis?
    a. Accuracy and quality of the database
    b. Technical requirements
    c. Data-management efficiency
    d. Usability

32. What is a key difference of computer-based diet-assessment applications versus Internet-based diet-analysis applications?
    a. Computer-based applications are more secure.
    b. Internet-based applications allow access anytime, anywhere.
    c. Computer-based applications require a trained interviewer.
    d. Internet-based applications analyze data in real time.

33. What is the method and system used for gathering dietary-intake data for the National Health and Nutrition Examination Survey?
    a. Diet History Questionnaire II
    b. Nutrient Data System for Research
    c. Automated self-administered 24-hour recall
    d. Automated Multiple-Pass Method

34. Which of the following Internet-based diet-analysis applications are available free of cost for nutrition researchers?
    a. ASA24
    b. ASA24Kids
    c. DHQ II–Web
    d. All of the above

## Discussion Questions

1. Compare and contrast methods of dietary-intake assessment, and give an example of a scenario in which it would be most appropriate to use each method.
2. Describe how you can use technology to improve the collection of dietary-intake data.
3. Choose three computer- or Internet-based diet-analysis applications and create a table comparing the factors to consider in selecting a system.
4. You want to assess dietary intakes of specific nutrients and patterns of food groups among individuals coming to the outpatient cancer center. Which computer-based diet-assessment application(s) would best help gather the data from this population, and why?
5. You are working on a research team across multiple study sites nationwide and are responsible for obtaining data for determining commonly consumed foods and food patterns. Which Internet-based diet-analysis application would best meet your needs, and why?

## Activities

1. Access the ASA24 demonstration site (https://asa24.nci.nih.gov/demo/) and complete at least one 24-hour dietary recall. Note how much time it takes you to complete one 24-hour recall. Reflect on how easy the tool was to use, and provide an example of a research setting in which the tool's use would be appropriate and advantageous.
2. With a group of your peers, brainstorm new ways of using existing technology or ideas for new technology for collecting dietary-intake information. How would your new methods or technology improve the validity and reliability of dietary-intake assessment?

## Online Resources

The ASA24 demonstration site allows clinicians and researchers to experience how user data are entered using the online 24-hour recall system: https://asa24.nci.nih.gov/demo/

The Axxya Systems video "How to use Nutritionist-Pro in a Research Study" can help researchers evaluate whether the application will meet their study needs: https://www.youtube.com/watch?v=GKGoBECue7A

The Dietary History Questionnaire II web demo allows clinicians and researchers to experience entering food-intake data and determine whether the tool is appropriate for their needs: http://epi.grants.cancer.gov/dhq2/webquest/demos.html

This article describes advances made to the eButton health monitor for automatically identifying and quantify food intake: https://www.sciencedaily.com/releases/2013/09/130909131224.htm

This video describes the development and uses for the Microsoft Research Sensecam: https://www.youtube.com/watch?v=g2-FfYCVr_s

This video demonstrates how the SenseCam can be used as a memory aid: https://www.youtube.com/watch?v=gYMQsi7cLqA

## References

1. Stumbo PJ. New technology in dietary assessment: A review of digital methods in improving food record accuracy. *Proc Nutr Soc.* 2013; 72:70–76.
2. Thompson FE, Kirkpatrick SI, Subar AF, et al. The National Cancer Institute's Dietary Assessment Primer: A resource for diet research. *J Acad Nutr Diet.* 2015; 115:1986–1995.
3. Boyle MA. *Community Nutrition in Action: An Entrepreneurial Approach.* 7th ed. Boston, MA: Cengage Learning; 2017.
4. Monsen ER, Van Horn L. *Research: Successful Approaches.* 3rd ed. Chicago, IL: Academy of Nutrition and Dietetics; 2008.
5. St. George SM, Van Horn ML, Lawman HG, Wilson DK. Reliability of 24-hour dietary recalls as a measure of diet in African-American youth. *J Acad Nutr Diet.* 2016; 116:1551–1559.
6. Yuan C, Spiegelman D, Rimm EB, et al. Validity of dietary questionnaire assessed by comparison with multiple weighted dietary records or 24-hour recalls. *Am J Epidemiol.* 2017; 185:570–584.

7. Miller TM, Abdel-Maksoud MF, Crane LA, Marcus AC, Byers TE. Effects of social approval bias on self-reported fruit and vegetable consumption: A randomized controlled trial. *Nutr J.* 2008; 7:18.

8. Yaroch AL, Tooze J, Thompson FE, et al. Evaluation of three short dietary instruments to assess fruit and vegetable intake: The National Cancer Institute's Food Attitudes and Behaviors (FAB) Survey. *J Acad Nutr Diet.* 2012; 112(10):1570–1577.

9. Hedrick VE, Savla J, Comber DL, et al. Development of a brief questionnaire to assess habitual beverage intake (BEVQ-15): Sugar-sweetened beverages and total beverage energy intake. *J Acad Nutr Diet.* 2012; 112(6):840–849.

10. Lora KR, Davy B, Hedrick V, Ferris AM, Anderson MP, Wakefield D. Assessing initial validity and reliability of beverage intake questionnaire in Hispanic preschool-aged children. *J Acad Nutr Diet.* 2016; 116(12):1951–1960. doi: 10.1016/j.jand.2016.06.376.

11. England CY, Andrews RC, Jago R, Thompson JL. A systematic review of brief dietary questionnaires suitable for clinical use in the prevention and management of obesity, cardiovascular disease and type 2 diabetes. *Eur J Clin Nutr.* 2015; 69:977–1003.

12. Long JD, Littlefield LA, Estep G, et al. Evidence review of technology and dietary assessment. *Worldviews Evid Based Nurs.* 2010; 7(4):191–204.

13. Boushey C, Kerr D, Wright J, Lutes K, Ebert D, Delp E. Use of technology in children's dietary assessment. *Eur J Clin Nutr.* 2009; 63(Suppl 1):S50–S57.

14. Probst YC, Tapsell LC. Overview of computerized dietary assessment programs for research and practice in nutrition education. *J Nutr Educ Behav.* 2005; 37(1):20–26.

15. Illner AK, Freisling H, Boeing H, Huybrechts I, Crispim SP, Slimani N. Review and evaluation of innovative technologies for measuring diet in nutritional epidemiology. *Int J Epidemiol.* 2012; 41:1187–1203.

16. Gemming L, Utter J, Mhurchu CN. Image-assisted dietary assessment: A systematic review of the evidence. *J Acad Nutr Diet.* 2015; 115:64–77.

17. Wang DH, Kogashiwa M, Kira S. Development of a new instrument for evaluating individuals' dietary intakes. *J Am Diet Assoc.* 2006; 106(10):1588–1593.

18. Wang DH, Kogashiwa M, Ohta S, Kira S. Validity and reliability of a dietary assessment method: The application of a digital camera with a mobile phone card attachment. *J Nutr Sci Vitaminol.* 2002; 48:498–504.

19. Kikunaga S, Tin T, Ishibashi G, Wang DH, Kira S. The application of a handheld personal digital assistant with camera and mobile phone card (Wellnavi) to the general population in a dietary survey. *J Nutr Sci Vitaminol (Tokyo).* 2007; 53(2):109–116.

20. Rollo ME, Ash S, Lyons-Wall P, Russell AW. Evaluation of a Mobile Phone Image-Based Dietary Assessment Method in Adults with Type 2 Diabetes. *Nutrients.* 2015; 7(6):4897–4910. doi:10.3390/nu7064897.

21. Six BL, Schap TE, Zhu FM, et al. Evidence-based development of a mobile telephone food record. *J Am Diet Assoc.* 2010; 110(1):74–79. doi:10.1016/j.jada.2009.10.010.

22. Zhu F, Bosch M, Boushey CJ, Cel EJ. An image analysis system for dietary assessment and evaluation. *Proceedings/ICIP. International Conference on Image Processing.* 2010; 1853–1856.

23. Casperson SL, Sieling J, Moon J, Johnson L, Roemmich JN, Whigham L. A mobile phone food record app to digitally capture dietary intake for adolescents in a free-living environment: Usability study. Eysenbach G, ed. *JMIR mHealth and uHealth.* 2015; 3(1):e30. doi:10.2196/mhealth.3324.

24. Daugherty BL, Schap TE, Ettienne-Gittens R, et al. Novel technologies for assessing dietary intake: Evaluating the usability of a mobile telephone food record among adults and adolescents. Eysenbach G, ed. *J Med Internet Res.* 2012; 14(2):e58. doi:10.2196/jmir.1967.

25. Weiss R, Stumbo PJ, Divakaran A. Automatic food documentation and volume computation using digital imaging and electronic transmission. *J Amer Diet Assoc.* 2010; 110(1):42–44.

26. O'Loughlin G, Cullen SJ, McGoldrick A, et al. Using a wearable camera to increase the accuracy of dietary analysis. *Am J Prev Med.* 2013; 44(3):297–301.

27. Sun M, Burke LE, Mao Z-H, et al. eButton: A wearable computer for health monitoring and personal assistance. *Proceedings/Design Automation Conference.* 2014; 2014:1–6.

28. Jia W, Chen HC, Yue Y, et al. Accuracy of food portion size estimation from digital pictures acquitted by a chest-worn camera. *Public Health Nutr.* 2014; 17(8):1671–1681.

29. Vozenilek, G. Choosing the best nutrient analysis software for your needs. *J Amer Diet Assoc.* 1999; 99(11):1356–1358.

30. National Institutes of Health, National Cancer Institute. Dietary Assessment Primer. https://dietassessmentprimer.cancer.gov. Accessed September 18, 2016.

31. US Department of Agriculture. Automated Multiple-Pass Method. https://www.ars.usda.gov/northeast-area/beltsville-md/beltsville-human-nutrition-research-center/food-surveys-research-group/docs/ampm-usda-automated-multiple-pass-method/. Accessed September 18, 2016.

32. University of Minnesota, Nutrition Coordinating Center. NDSR. http://www.ncc.umn.edu/products. Accessed September 18, 2016.

33. Falomir Z, Arregui M, Madueno F, Corella D, Coltell O. Automation of food questionnaires in medical studies: A state-of-the-art review and future prospects. *Comput Biol Med.* 2012; 42:964–974.

34. US Department of Agriculture. Food and Nutrient Database for Dietary Studies. https://www.ars.usda.gov/northeast-area/beltsville-md/beltsville-human-nutrition-research-center/food-surveys-research-group/docs/fndds/. Accessed September 18, 2016.

35. Blanton CA, Moshfegh AJ, Baer DJ, Kretsch MJ. The USDA Automated Multi-Pass Method accurately estimates group total energy and nutrient intake. *J Nutr.* 2006; 136:2594–2599.

36. Moshfegh AJ, Rhodes DG, Baer DJ, et al. The US Department of Agriculture Automated Multi-Pass Method reduces bias in the collection of energy intakes. *Am J Clin Nutr.* 2008; 88:324–332.

37. Viocare. ProNutra. http://www.viocare.com/pronutra.html. Accessed September 18, 2016.

38. Esha Research. The Food Processor. www.esha.com. Accessed September 25, 2016.

39. Nutritionist Pro. Nexgen. https://nexgen1.nutritionistpro.com/shop/product-detail/nutritionist-pro-diet-analysis-software-13. Accessed September 25, 2016.

40. National Institutes of Health, National Cancer Institute. Automated Self-Administered 24-Hour Dietary Assessment Tool. http://epi.grants.cancer.gov/asa24/. Accessed September 18, 2016.

41. Kirkpatrick SI, Subar AF, Douglass D, et al. Performance of the Automated Self-Administered 24-hour recall relative to a measure of true intakes and to an interviewer-administered 24-h recall. *Am J Clin Nutr.* 2014; 100:233–240.

42. Thompson FE, Dixit-Joshi S, Potischman N, et al. Comparison of interviewer-administered and Automated Self-Administered 24-hour dietary recalls in 3 diverse integrated health systems. *Am J Epidemiol.* 2015; 181(12):970–978.

43. Baranowski T, Islam N, Baranowski J, et al. Comparison of a web-based versus traditional diet recall among children. *J Acad Nutr Diet.* 2012; 112(4):527–532.

44. Diep CS, Hingle M, Chen T, et al. The automated self-administered 24-hour dietary recall for children, 2012 version, for youth aged 9 to 11 years: A validation study. *J Acad Nutr Diet.* 2015; 115:1591-1598.

45. National Institutes of Health, National Cancer Institute. Diet History Questionnaire II and Canadian Diet History Questionnaire II: Web-based. http://epi.grants.cancer.gov /dhq2/webquest/. Accessed October 29, 2016.

46. Viocare. VioScreen. http://www.viocare.com/vioscreen.html. Accessed September 18, 2016.

47. Kristal AR, Kolar AS, Fisher JL, et al. Evaluation of web-based, self-administered, graphical food frequency questionnaire. *J Acad Nutr Diet.* 2014; 114:613–621.

48. Viocare. NutraScreen. http://www.viocare.com/nutrascreen. html. Accessed September 18, 2016.

49. NutritionQuest. Data-on-Demand. http://nutritionquest. com/assessment/data-on-demand/. Accessed September 18, 2016.

50. Cybersoft. Nutribase Cloud Edition. www.nutribase.com. Accessed September 25, 2016.

51. United States Department of Agriculture. SuperTracker. https://www.supertracker.usda.gov. Accessed September 18, 2016.

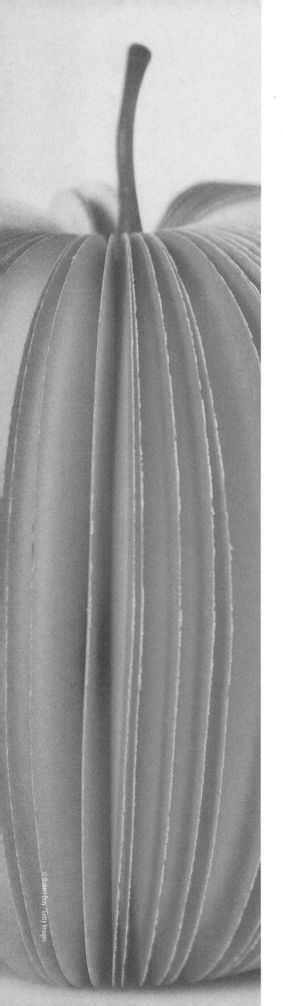

# Method of Evaluation: Anthropometric Methods

CHAPTER 7 Anthropometry

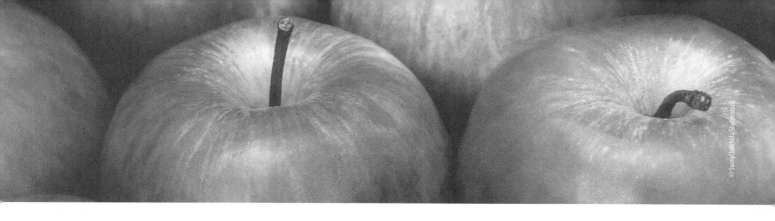

CHAPTER 7

# Anthropometry

**Patricia G. Davidson**, DCN, RDN, CDE, LDN, FAND
**Dwight L. Davidson**, PhD, LMHC

## CHAPTER OUTLINE

- Introduction
- Anthropometric Indicators and Cutoffs
- Plotting and Interpreting Measurements in Children
- Additional Anthropometrics
- Body Composition
- Chapter Summary

## LEARNING OBJECTIVES

After reading this chapter, the learner will be able to:
1. Define anthropometric measures and their use in assessing metabolic disease risk.
2. State and describe age-appropriate anthropometric measurements throughout the life cycle.
3. Demonstrate how to calculate and accurately evaluate body mass index.
4. Evaluate a person's metabolic fitness and nutritional status based on body composition.
5. Compare and contrast methods for assessing body composition.
6. Accurately measure height, weight, and waist circumference.

## ▶ Introduction

Anthropometric measurements are useful in establishing normative data and standards, assessing efficacy of treatments, and determining the impact of disease states. As a tool, it is useful in establishing normative data and standards, assessing efficacy of treatments, and determining the impact of disease states.

## History

The human body has been measured since antiquity because it was essential to the figurative arts of painting and sculpture. Eventually, these systematic measurements were adopted by anthropologists to identify basic "aspects" of human morphology. The term anthropometria dates back to naturalists of the 17th century.[1] The manual *Anthropometria* by Johann Sigismund Elsholtz appears as the earliest recorded effort to investigate and measure the human body for scientific and medical purposes. It brought a quantitative approach to acquiring data concerning variations and changes in the human form, and it described the relationship between the human body and disease.[2]

As a measurement of physiological and developmental human growth, anthropometrics appeared in clinical practices, which used instruments to assess and record individual data and begin establishing norms. The importance of these measurements grew from several intricately linked concepts, including nutrition and infection, psychological and social stress, and food contaminants. Variables linked to socioeconomic conditions indicated that body size was a sign of quality of life. Thus, **anthropometry** became a tool for social welfare. The role of anthropometrics in the pediatric population became the foundation of both research and clinical interventions, with techniques and technologies initially focused on this group. Certain measures were developed, but in practice were limited to the assessment, diagnosis, and intervention of childhood development and disease states.[1]

Accurately assessing a person's nutritional status involves more than just evaluating what a person eats. It also involves determining his or her **body composition** and comparing the person's growth and development to accepted standards. Measuring, monitoring, and accurately evaluating body composition are important skills to define and trend the health status of a person, as well as the population, throughout the life cycle. Overweight and obesity and associated comorbid conditions have been clinical concerns since the 1980s. The health implications associated with these conditions have further stimulated the need for accurate assessment of weight and body composition to determine the risk for such metabolic diseases as diabetes mellitus and cardiovascular disease (CVD), as well as a person's metabolic fitness.

## Definition of Anthropometry

As the science of nutrition has expanded, the need for accurate measures of nutritional status has become essential when performing a nutrition-focused physical assessment. Assessing a person's body composition, protein status, muscle strength, and body fat is crucial for identifying malnutrition and a response to medical nutrition therapy

intervention. Anthropometric assessment is an essential nutrition-evaluation tool. It reveals malnutrition, overweight, and obesity; it also quantifies the loss of muscle mass, increases in fat mass, and redistribution of adipose tissue.

These techniques and methodologies make up the area of **anthropometrics**, which is defined as "the study of human body measurements, especially on a comparative basis."[3] Anthropometrics includes measurements of body weight, stature, composition, and a focus on specific area measurements such as circumference (waist and hip), skinfold (SF), and bone dimensions. Some provide direct measurements (e.g., height and weight), and others are derived (e.g., body composition).[4] The anthropometric measures in common use for adults and children include weight, height, waist circumference (WC), **skinfold thickness** (as measured at different body sites), and a set of weight-for-height indices, such as **body mass index (BMI)**. Often such measures, or a combination of them, are used to determine **body composition (BC)**—for example, percentage of body fat (%BF).

Studies have been conducted to assess the validity of anthropometric measures such as BMI, WC, and skinfold thickness to estimate body fat and using **dual-energy x-ray absorptiometry (DXA)** as the reference. Results indicate modest to excellent agreement. Other studies found that measures of skinfold thickness are better predictors of %BF than other, simpler anthropometric methods such as BMI.[5]

## ▶ Anthropometric Indicators and Cutoffs

**Preview** Anthropometric measurements have two requirements: an anthropometric indicator (measurement) and a cutoff point. By applying statistical analyses to the compiled body measurements of study groups of children, the cutoff points were established.

Anthropometric measurements require: (1) an **anthropometric indicator** and (2) a **cutoff point**. The anthropometric indicator, also known as an *anthropometric index*, is a measurement or measurements (such as height and weight) or a combination of additional data with measurements (e.g., age).

A cutoff point is established below which either individuals or populations will require an intervention or therapy. The application of universal cutoff points has the dual advantage of allowing comparisons between populations and preventing bias on the part of staff when performing an initial assessment or follow-up of patients.[6,7] In addition, cutoff points can be used to characterize changes and trends within a population and identify persons at a higher risk for adverse outcomes.[6,8] The cutoff point of 0.5 has been recommended for waist-to-height ratio (WHtR) to classify central obesity in adults and children and as well as different ethnic groups.[9]

Cutoff thresholds are used to explicate variations in age, gender, ethnicity, and other technical factors that affect anthropometrics alone or in conjunction with social or health causes or outcomes, as well as in policy formulation and advocacy. In growth references, certain Z-scores and percentiles have been chosen for cutoff points to classify problematic growth and nutritional status.[10]

## Body Measurements: Foundations in Pediatrics

The clinical outcomes of alterations in body composition should be a necessary component of any physical assessment, even more so in the care of children. Body measurements are essential in the analysis of the development or progression of disease and for monitoring the efficacy of treatment. Accurate measurement of changes in BC because of interventions is vital in planning nutritional care and the management of developmental and aging processes, disease progression, and rehabilitation efforts. The need for better quantification of what constitutes an excessive deviation from normative standards has sparked a growth in the technologies for measurement of human body composition.[11]

In pediatrics, the essential, static measurements for infants up to age 2 years are length, weight, head circumference (HC), and weight for length. For ages 3 years and older, they are height, weight, and BMI.[7,12]

## Height and Length in Children

To accurately measure a child's height, we must first think in terms of length for those too young to stand. The child should be placed supine on a measuring device or board, and the measurement should be recorded to the nearest 0.1 cm (**FIGURE 7.1**).

For children unable to stand for reasons other than age, alternative methods are used, including

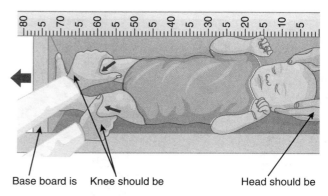

Base board is    Knee should be    Head should be

**FIGURE 7.1** Infant length measured using a standard measuring board

knee height or upper-arm length.[13] The knee height is measured with the specific caliper from the top of the patella to the bottom of the foot, with both knee and foot at a 90-degree angle. The following gender and racial specific formulas are used for calculating the child's height for ages between 6 and 18 years.

White children:

Boys: height = 40.54 + (2.22 × knee height)
Girls: height = 43.21 + (2.15 × knee height)

Black children:

Boys: height = 39.60 + (2.18 × knee height)
Girls: height = 46.59 + (2.02 × knee height)

These values must be compared to specific standard curves designated for knee-height calculations.

To evaluate suspected short or tall stature, accurate measurements of height and weight are plotted on the appropriate age growth chart.[14] Infants and toddlers should have their length, weight, and head circumference plotted on a growth curve at every well or sick visit to the physician. The Centers for Disease Control and Prevention (CDC) and the American Academy of Pediatrics recommend using the World Health Organization (WHO) growth charts for children younger than two years and the CDC growth charts for children older than two years.[15,16]

For patients 2 to 20 years of age, weight, height, and body mass index should also be plotted. Short stature is determined when plotted height is more than two standard deviations below the mean for age, or less than the third percentile. Height in children older than two years should be measured using a wall-mounted stadiometer[14,17,18,19] (**FIGURE 7.2**).

In the United States, use the WHO growth charts to monitor growth for newborn infants and children up to two years of age. Use the CDC growth charts

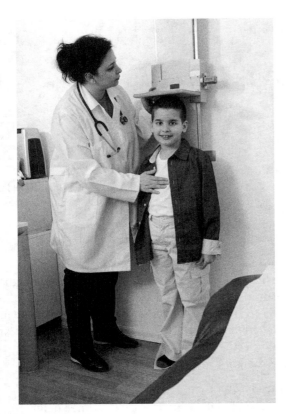

**FIGURE 7.2** Standing-height measurement technique

© Levent Konuk/Shutterstock.

to monitor growth for children ages 2 years and older.[18,19]

## Percentiles and Z-Scores

Widely used in the assessment of children's nutritional status and growth performance are two indicators: percentiles and **Z-scores**. Both are interchangeable, but their respective cutoff points may not be identical.[14,20]

## Percentiles

A **percentile** is defined as the position of an individual on a given reference distribution of 100 points, and it is easier to understand and use in practice by professionals and the public. In addition, a percentile designates the expected percentage of a population that should fall above or below it. Age-specific and sex-specific percentiles are often used to assess growth and nutritional status in children as based on anthropometric measures. There is a growing consensus on using BMI percentiles as cutoffs instead of WHt Z-scores in assessing overweight and obesity in children more than two years old. The most widely used percentiles are the 3rd, 5th, 50th (median), 85th, 95th, 97th, and 99th. The term *percentile* and the related term *percentile rank* are often used in descriptive

statistics and are frequently represented graphically with a normal curve.[21–23]

## Z-Scores

Several considerations support the use of Z-scores. First, they are calculated from the distribution [both mean (μ) and the standard deviation (σ)] of the reference population. Second, Z-scores are standardized measures and comparable across ages, genders, and measures. Third, a group of Z-scores is subject to the measures of statistics such as μ and σ and thus can be studied as a continuous variable. Finally, Z-scores can be used to quantify the growth status of those children falling outside the percentile ranges. In clinical settings, growth references and standards are useful for monitoring populations and research projects.[10]

> **Recap** To address non-normative data obtained from children, whether from malnutrition, disease, or genetic conditions, it is plotted on the growth charts developed by the WHO and the CDC. The resultant percentiles and Z-scores permit the quantification of the measurements in relation to the anticipated parameters.

## ▶ Plotting and Interpreting Measurements In Children

> **Preview** The use of established growth charts facilitates the interpretation of growth data in children. Height and stature can be projected from the height velocity as determined over time.

To plot the growth of a child, first the appropriate growth chart (**FIGURE 7.3**) is selected from either the WHO or CDC. The measurements should be taken at each visit to the physician and recorded by first locating the child's age on the horizontal axis and using a ruler/straight edge to draw a line from the age. Then on the vertical axis locate the particular measurement (weight, height, BMI, and HC) and draw a line across placing a circle where the age and measurement intersect to determine the percentile. The percentile rank is used for assessing nutritional risk base on age/gender/population cutoff value. It is also used as a comparative standard for the child in that it identifies shifts or changes between visits and the need for further evaluation. For example, if the intersect is plotted the 5th percentile, it means that 95 of

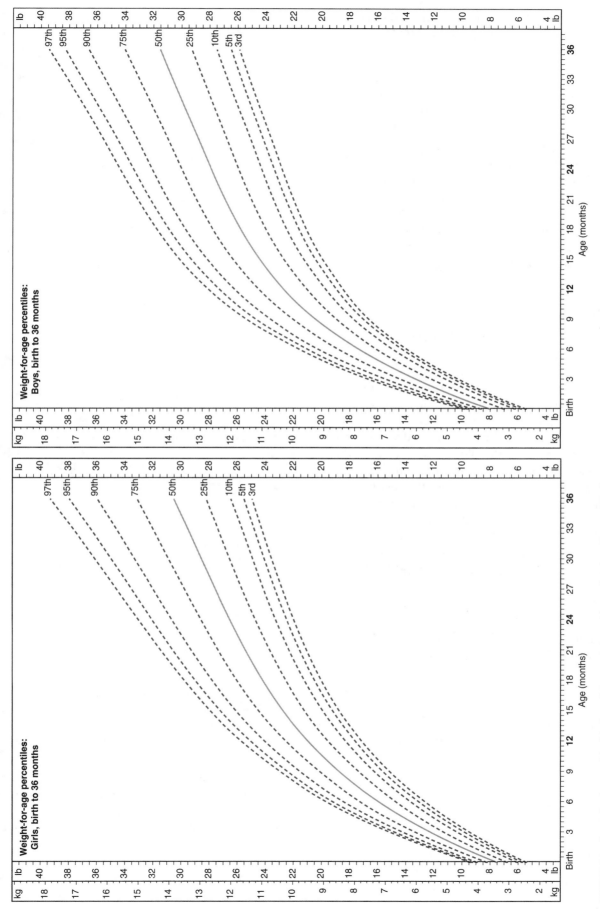

**FIGURE 7.3** Growth charts girls (birth to 36 months) and boys (birth to 36 months)

Data from the National Center for Health Statistics in collaboration with the National Center for Chronic Disease Prevention and Health Promotion (2000).

100 children (95%) of the same age and gender have a lower for-age measurement (Figure 7.3).

## Height Velocity

The most sensitive measurement in detecting growth abnormalities early in the course of all types of chronic illness is **height velocity**.[24] If a child more than two years of age has a height velocity of less than 4 cm/year, he or she should be carefully monitored for nutritional deficits or other causes of short stature, as 95 percent of children have a height velocity more than 4 cm/year.[25] Peak height velocity occurs in puberty, with boys growing 6 to 12 cm/year and girls growing 5 to 10 cm/year; there is a substantial variability in the age of peak height velocity.

## Adult Stature

Height and weight are often used in combination to assess nutritional status, thinness, and fatness. Therefore, height-measurement accuracy is important and should be measured with an accurate stadiometer with a fixed vertical ruler and an adjustable sliding horizontal headpiece. The person being measured, while standing on a hard floor, is requested to stand up straight, look forward with relaxed arms at the sides, straight legs close together, and feet flat with the heels together. The head is positioned by the technician, taking the measurement in the Frankfort horizontal plane in which the lower eye lid or socket is horizontally level with the top of the ear. If a person is unable to stand or is bedridden, then using demispan, knee height (KH), or ulna length (UL) (**FIGURES 7.4, 7.5,** and **7.6**) for estimating a person's height are options.[26,27] The demispan measures from the sternal notch to the web between the middle and ring fingers, and the knee height is measured using a sliding broad-blade caliper while both the knee and ankle are at a

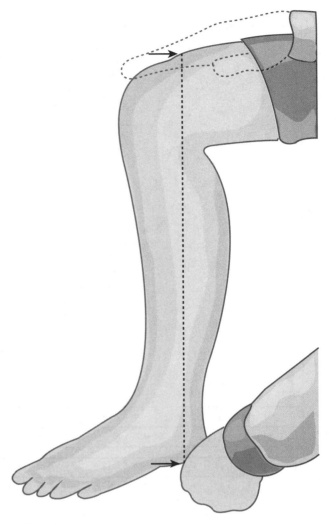

Females
    Height in cm = 84.88 − (0.24 × age)
    + (1.83 × knee height)
Males
    Height in cm = 64.19 − (0.04 × age)
    + (2.02 × knee height)

**FIGURE 7.5** Knee-height calculation

90-degree angle. Using a standard formula for gender, age, and either knee height or demispan, a person's height is calculated.

For ulna-height measurement, the forearm is measured using an anthropometric tape while the person's left arm is bent across the chest with the hand flat on the chest and fingers pointing toward the right shoulder (Figure 7.6).[28] The measurement is taken on a bare arm from the tip of the elbow (olecranon process) to the styloid process (prominent bone of the wrist). It is a useful tool because it is low cost and does not require special equipment, but it has been noted to overestimate height for certain ethnic groups such as healthy Asians and blacks.

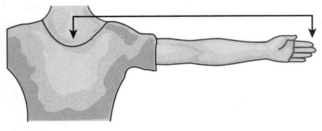

Females
    Height in cm = (1.35 × demispan in cm) + 60.1
Males
    Height in cm = (1.40 × demispan in cm) + 57.8

**FIGURE 7.4** Demispan height calculation

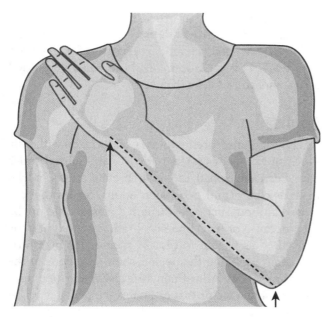

Females
   Height in cm = 95.6 + (2.77 × ulna length in cm)
Males
   Height in cm = 79.2 + (3.60 × ulna length in cm)

**FIGURE 7.6**  Ulna predicted height calculation

## Advantages and Limitations

Like other anthropometric measures, height is influenced by a variety of factors, including racial and ethnic differences, because both of these can affect the actual height measure and interpretation as well as the relationship between them. As people age, height decreases, beginning sometime between ages 30 and 50, and varies by gender, with women's height decreasing more rapidly with age. Factors affecting height measurements include postural changes, decrease in vertebrae height,

and conditions limiting the ability to stand straight (such as **kyphoscoliosis** or disease-related curvature of the spine and arthritis). All of these can limit accurate height assessment and result in poor interpretation of BMI and its associated health risks. Alternative height measures have limited agreement with the exact height because they estimate maximal height, not current height, and are based on a healthy, younger population and do not correlate with hospitalized adults 65 years of age and older.[26] Demispan is considered to be the best alternative height measure because it does not decline like standing height (SH) and is a better measurement to use for calculating BMI for health risk, particularly in the older adults at least 65 years of age.[29] Knee height has limitations, especially for people who are bedridden, preventing appropriate positioning of the leg and requiring specific anthropometric calipers, but KH estimates are closer to SH than to UL. Similar trends are noted when calculating BMI using KH. It is recommended to add 1.8kg/m$^2$ if calculating the BMI with UL, especially if using the BMI to assess for malnutrition.[30]

## Head Circumference

Measurement of head circumference, also known as **frontal-occipital circumference**, is vital in children 3 years old and younger because this corresponds to the period of greatest brain growth. Correct measurement requires a flexible tape measure (usually paper or vinyl) applied at the maximum head diameter, along the supraorbital ridge to the occiput (**FIGURE 7.7**). The value should be recorded to the nearest 0.01 cm and also be plotted on a standardized growth chart. Because children grow in spurts, two measurements at least three to six months apart and preferably 6 to 12 months apart are needed to

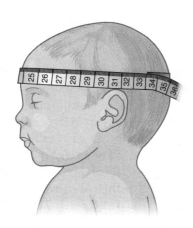
Baby with typical head size

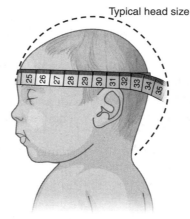
Baby with microcephaly

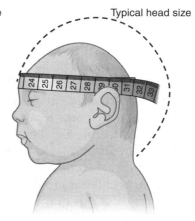
Baby with severe microcephaly

**FIGURE 7.7**  Head-circumference measurement comparison

accurately determine growth velocity. Measurement of head circumference rarely occurs after 16 years of age in a clinical setting.[7,12] Clinically, accurate and ongoing measurement of the HC is important, particularly in tall and short-statured children, because HC has been shown to correlate with both height and weight through adolescence but is particularly strong in the first couple of months of infancy.[31,32]

HC measurement and its strong association with brain development make it an essential component for assessing growth and development in infants and toddlers.[33] Cranial development is influenced not only by age and gender but also by ethnicities; therefore, the measurement needs to be compared to the appropriate HC growth chart.[34] For comparative age, gender, and population, it is considered an abnormal measurement if it is two standard deviations above the mean (macrocephaly) or two standard deviations below the mean (microcephaly). See Figure 7.7. A positive percentile deviation from the comparative age standard is suggestive of hydrocephalus, which is a condition caused by increased pressure on the brain related to excess cerebrospinal fluid in the brain. Craniostenosis is indicated by negative standard deviation, indicating a premature closure of the skull suture(s), thus limiting the growth of the brain and changing the shape of the skull. Rapid changes in cranial growth have also been linked to brain developmental changes and related to the overall growth pattern.[33]

## Weight and Stature: Children and Adults

### Children

Weight and stature are key for assessing growth patterns and determining deviations from the norms for a specified population.[7,22,23] Abnormal growth patterns can signify changes in nutritional status, either because of nutrient malabsorption caused by a disease such as cystic fibrosis and inflammatory bowel or by poor nutritional intake. Malnutrition has variable effects, but clinically these can be noted in changes in anthropometric measures, including height, weight, and changes in lean body mass and adipose tissue. With severe malnutrition, a child's growth is not only stunted but also will appear wasted because of BC changes. In contrast, acute malnutrition will be apparent by BC alterations and wasting, as compared to chronic undernutrition, which will be demonstrated by pattern changes in linear growth.

Measurement of weight in all populations should be taken on a calibrated scale. The infant or toddler should be weighed sans clothing or diaper.

The measurement is recorded to the nearest 0.1 kg. The ratio of **weight-to-length** is used to predict **adiposity** in children under 2 years of age, rather than BMI. This measurement should also be plotted on a standardized growth chart.[7,12]

## Adults

Adult weight measurements are usually taken with only shoes and coats or jackets removed. Specialized scales have been developed to weigh mobile adults, adults in wheelchairs, and bedridden adults. Scales that are moved around, such as bathroom scales, should not be used because of inaccurate calibration. If weight is be monitored as related to disease state or for malnutrition, then weighing the person should be done at the same time of day. Adjustments are also made for amputations using a factor that estimates the percent weight for the amputated limb, using the following formula:

$$(\text{Weight}/100 - \% \text{ amputation}) \times 100$$

Being that weight includes an overall measurement of the body compartments, it is important to include it as a general measure as part of the nutrition assessment. Establishing a reference weight, either by calculating the ideal body weight (IBW) or usual body weight (UBW), is important in assessing a person's nutritional status. In some cases, the 1983 Metropolitan Life Insurance charts have been used as a guide for IBW comparison. These charts are based on weight ranging, incorporating three skeletal frame sizes, and morbidity and mortality. In theory, some use the midrange for determining IBW, but this could potential underestimate IBW and overestimate the excess body weight in a person being evaluated for bariatric surgery.[35] A common formula used for calculating the IBW or reference weight is the Hamwi formula (**FIGURE 7.8**), developed in the 1960s. The main criticism for using IBW is that it does not consider ethnicity, age, or body frame size or the changes in anthropometric trends—that is, increases in both height and weight.[11]

Accurate weight references are important not only for setting weight goals for weight loss but also for assessing nutritional risk or health status. Weight change and current weight compared to either IBW or UBW are indices used clinically. For example, if an adult is <70% of his or her UBW or IBW or has experienced a greater than 5% unintentional weight loss in less than a month, then this adult would be considered at nutritional risk (**TABLES 7.1, 7.2,** and **7.3**). The same would be considered for unintentional weight gain as well.

Males:

106 for 5 feet + 6 lbs per inch over 5 feet

Example: 72" (6 feet) = 12 × 6
= 72 + 106 = 178 lbs

Females:

100 pounds for 5 feet + 5 lbs per inch over 5 feet

Example: 64" (5 feet 4 in) = 4 × 5
= 20 + 100 = 120 lbs

Determine range: Add/subtract (±) 10% to account for body frame size
Adjust for persons less than 5' and >18 yrs
Subtract 1.55 lbs/inch for women
Subtract 1.76 lbs/inch for men

**FIGURE 7.8** Hamwi formula

**TABLE 7.2** Nutritional status and weight change (unintentional)

| Time | Significant (%) | Severe Weight Loss (%) |
|------|-----------------|------------------------|
| 1 week | 1.0–2.0 | > 2.0 |
| 1 month | 5.0 | > 5.0 |
| 3 months | 7.5 | > 7.5 |
| 6 months | 10.0 | > 10.0 |
| 1 year | 20.0 | > 20.0 |

Modified from White JV, Guenter P, Jensen G, et al. Consensus statement of the academy of nutrition and dietetics/American Society for Parenteral and Enteral Nutrition: Characteristics recommended for the identification and documentation of adult malnutrition (undernutrition). *J Acad Nutr Diet*. 2012;112(5):730-738.

**TABLE 7.1** Percent of IBW or UBW

| %IBW = Current weight ÷ IBW × 100% | %UBW = Current weight ÷ UBW × 100% |
|---|---|
| Example: IBW 166#; current wt 142# | Example: UBW 129#; current weight 101# |
| 142# ÷ 166# × 100 = 85.5% | 101# ÷ 129# × 100 = 78.5% |

**TABLE 7.3** UBW and IBW nutritional status

| Index | Mild Deficit (%) | Moderate Deficit (%) | Severe Deficit (%) |
|-------|------------------|----------------------|---------------------|
| IBW | 80–90 | 70–79 | < 70 |
| UBW | 85–95 | 75–84 | < 75 |

Modified from White JV, Guenter P, Jensen G, et al. Consensus statement of the academy of nutrition and dietetics/American Society for Parenteral and Enteral Nutrition: Characteristics recommended for the identification and documentation of adult malnutrition (undernutrition). *J Acad Nutr Diet*. 2012;112(5):730-738.

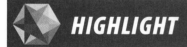 **HIGHLIGHT**

## Estimating Energy Requirements

Indirect calorimetry is considered the gold standard by the Academy of Nutrition and Dietetics for calculating the energy needs of patients in the clinical setting, particularly the critically ill. This method is more accurate than using a predictive equation because it closely estimates actual energy expenditure and accounts for the effects of stress, trauma, and the disease state, thus eliminating the need for adding in a stress factor. If resting energy expenditure cannot be measured by indirect calorimetry, then it may be estimated by a predictive equation, including the Harris-Benedict, Mifflin-St. Jeor, and Ireton-Jones equations. To calculate needs using these equations, an accurate weight in kilograms, height in centimeters, and age in years are needed. Then to determine total energy expenditure or needs, multiply by a stress factor, ranging from 1.3 to 1.5, to indicate additional energy needs associated with activity, fever, trauma, and malnutrition. Both equations consider a decrease in energy needs associated with aging, and separate equations are derived for males and females. A potential source for error in these equations is the lack of distinction between fat and lean mass; in addition, the Harris-Benedict equation is known to overestimate needs by 5% to 15%. The Academy has concluded that the Harris-Benedict equation is not accurate enough to estimate energy expenditure in critically ill patients and does not recommend its use for that purpose.

Mifflin-St. Jeor, the predictive equation, is recommended by the Academy because it demonstrates increased accuracy over Harris-Benedict. This equation calculates total energy expenditure by calculating requirements based on age, weight, height, and stress factor.

### Mifflin-St. Jeor:

Men: EEE = 9.99 × (weight in kg) + 6.25 × (height in cm) − 4.92 × (age in years) + 5

Women: EEE = 9.99 × (weight in kg) + 6.25 × (height in cm) − 4.92 × (age in years) − 161

Example: For a 30-year-old man standing 170 cm tall and weighing 70 kg:

Mifflin-St. Jeor EEE = 9.99 × (70) + 6.25 × (170) − 4.92 × (30) + 5 = 1,619 kcal

### Harris-Benedict:

Men: EEE = 66.5 + 13.8 × (weight in kg) + 5.0 × (height in cm) − 6.8 × (age in years)

Women: EEE = 655.1 + 9.6 × (weight in kg) + 1.9 × (height in cm) − 4.7 × (age in years)

Example: For a 30-year-old man standing 170 cm tall and weighing 70 kg:

Harris-Benedict EEE = 66.5 + 13.8 × (70) + 5.0 × (170) − 6.8 × (30) = 1,679 kcal

### Activity Factors

Based on general activity level
Range: 1.0–1.2 sedentary, 1.3 ambulatory, 1.4 lightly active, 1.5 moderately active, 1.7 very active, 1.9 extra active

### Stress Factors

1.0 fever, 1.2 pneumonia, 1.3 major injury, 1.5 severe sepsis, burns (15% to 30% TBSA), 1.5–2.0 burns (31% to 49% TBSA), 1.8–2.1 burns (> 50% TBSA)

TBSA = total body surface area; EEE= estimated energy expenditure
Modified from Determination of Resting Metabolic Rate: Individual Equations. ADA Evidence Analysis Web site. http://www.adaevidencelibrary.com/topic.cfm?cat=4311. Accessed November 1, 2016.

**Recap** Anthropometric data is only as reliable as the measurements are consistent, both in technique and instrumentation. Whether measuring height, head circumference, weight, or stature, the standardization of the techniques and the plotting of the data necessitate attention to detail.

# ▶ Additional Anthropometrics

**Preview** The anthropometric study of the body now moves from the quantitative (physical measurement) to the qualitative projective (interpolation from specific component measurements).

## Waist-to-Height Ratio

The waist-to-height ratio was developed as an indicator of central obesity and for risk of CVD. However, scant data are available on the utility of WHtR in assessing abdominal obesity and related cardiometabolic risks among children of normal weight or those overweight or obese, as categorized according to BMI values.[36] In theory, this measurement takes into consideration a person's size by dividing the WC by height. There are concerns that this index does not adjust for age, particularly during periods of growth, or for gender. For some ethnicities in which BMI may not identify a person as overweight or obese, WHtR has the potential to identify metabolic abnormalities and risk. WHtR has been studied as a simple anthropometric index in the detection of central obesity and in the assessment of associations between cardiometabolic risk factors and central intra-abdominal obesity.[9] Adult studies have shown that this measure has the ability to identify adverse cardiometabolic risk profiles not only in those with normal weight but also in those with normal metabolic risk profiles in the overweight or obese classifications.[37] The WHtR and obesity risks are listed in **TABLE 7.4**.

## Measures of Adiposity

### Body Mass Index

Central adiposity functions as a complex and active endocrine organ, producing a variety of hormones and cytokines. They play an important role in the dysregulation of inflammatory, metabolic, and hemodynamic processes through various mechanisms, including hepatic lipogenesis and hepatic insulin resistance and release of free fatty acids from adipocytes.[38]

**TABLE 7.4** Waist-to-height ratio and obesity risk

| WHtR Category | Male (%) | Female (%) |
|---|---|---|
| Underweight | <43 | <42 |
| Healthy weight | 43–52 | 42–48 |
| Overweight | 53–62 | 49–57 |
| Obese | >63 | >58 |

Modified from Wildman RP, Muntner P, Reynolds K, McGinn AP, Rajpathak S, WylieRosett J, Sowers MR: The obese without cardiometabolic risk factor clustering and the normal weight with cardiometabolic risk factor clustering: prevalence and correlates of 2 phenotypes among the 8 US population (NHANES 1999-2004). *Arch Intern Med 2008*; 168:1617–1624.

BMI is determined from the measurements of height and weight, calculating the relative proportion between the two. It is a valid predictor of adiposity.[39] BMI will vary based on gender, age, and pubertal stage. The calculation is as follows:

$$BMI = (Weight\ in\ kg) / (Height\ in\ m)^2$$

BMI is recommended in the clinical setting as the most appropriate single indicator of overweight and obesity in the pediatric population. In comparison to other anthropometric measurements, such as waist circumference and **triceps skinfold thickness (TSF)**, BMI is a stronger data point for estimating %BF in children and adolescents.[40,41] The required measurements to calculate BMI are routine, noninvasive, and inexpensive. BMI values are plotted on a BMI reference chart; a child with a BMI above the 85th percentile is overweight, and a child with a BMI above the 95th percentile is obese. A child with a BMI below the 5th percentile is underweight.[7,12] BMI is identified as the best choice among available measures that can be easily assessed at low cost, and it is strongly associated with body fat and health risks. However, as an indirect measure of adiposity, BMI has several limitations, especially when used for children. In children, BMI measures should be expressed as Z-scores or percentiles relative to age and gender because BMI is strongly related to growth and maturation.[36] Children's maturation statuses and growth patterns affect their BC and BMI. BMI is positively associated with height in children. Although there is a correlation between BMI for overweight children and percent fat mass (FM), there is only a weak relationship in thin children, although the data were not analyzed for ethic differences.[41] In contrast, a study evaluating the correlation of BMI strongly correlated with the %BF determined by DXA for a variety of ethnic groups.[42]

In a systematic review of 25 population-based studies, Simmonds et al. found that BMI correctly detected obesity in children (81.9%) compared to reference standards (95% confidence interval [CI], 73–93.8), with a false-positive rate of only 4%, but detected fewer children as overweight (76.3% sensitivity; 95% CI, 70.2–82.4) with a higher false-positive rate of 7.9%. The referenced studies used various methods: five used densitometry, one used deuterium dilution, and the rest used DXA.[5] In comparisons with classification of obesity by comparing %BF to BMI, BMI demonstrated a low sensitivity, although it does have a high specificity. Results also showed that BMI does not always correlate to central obesity.

In adults, BMI has historically been used to assess both risks for obesity-related diseases as well as nutritional risk. As noted, it does not depict BC, but is a good indicator of both ends of the spectrum and the need for further assessment. There are several features for a good measure of body fatness, and BMI possesses a majority of them, including low cost and its value as an easy assessment tool for health risk and body adiposity. However, it does not distinguish the type of fat or account for growth, gender, ethnicity, or athletes, all of which confound the association of BMI to adiposity. It is among several methods used to estimate BC but is not reasonable for daily clinical use.[4]

With a strong association shown between body stores or adiposity and a need for a quick, noninvasive assessment measure, the WHO established classifications to be used for underweight, overweight, and obesity. Adults with a BMI ≤18.5 are classified as underweight and BMI ≥25 as overweight. In general, a BMI between 18 and 25 kg/m² for adults is considered healthy.

Using BMI in a hospital setting can allow for early recognition of malnutrition and thus influence the disease course, decrease the length of stay, and decrease mortality. Established norms for BMI can allow the clinician to estimate morbidity and mortality.

BMI and its association to muscle mass can vary considerably between people of the same height. Bodybuilders and participants in other strength-related sports, are among those who can be incorrectly assessed by BMI typically possessing lower %BF but presenting with a BMI in the overweight or even obese index.[43,44] In contrast, a lower BMI in an adult could be attributed to a loss of **fat-free mass**

(FFM) (lean tissue) caused by **sarcopenia**, increased adipose tissue, or shifts in both. The BMI measure does not distinguish the BC changes and could lead to an incorrect BMI classification or delay in nutrition intervention. If an adult's BMI is determined as nonobese but with unintentional lean body mass weight loss, unintentional loss in lean body mass, the risk for malnutrition could be missed. In contrast, if the weight loss was because of FM, the nutrition risk is less.

BMI is often cited as a correlate of key health indicators of cardiovascular and metabolic disease. However, as BMI cannot differentiate between FFM and adiposity and cannot indicate the distribution of these components in the body, it leads to misclassification on the individual level and has low sensitivity in determining excess adiposity.[45]

The effectiveness of BMI as an assessment tool for adiposity and as a predictor of health complications must be evaluated for cultural and ethnic differences. An analysis of data from some 900,000 participants in 57 prospective studies on four continents confirms that obesity, as measured by BMI, is associated with increased total mortality in both men and women in age classifications ranging from 35 to 89 years.[46] However, even though BMI has been the most widely applied phenotypic technique in measurement of human adiposity, close scrutiny has led to the observation that correlations with adult adiposity are generally modest and that other factors such as age, race, and physical activity levels perplex efforts to correlate BMI and adiposity.[47]

Because BMI does not distinguish between FM and lean (nonfat) mass or FFM, it can vary considerably between individuals of the same height. Data suggest different health effects of FM and FFM. When only BMI is used, these disparate associations cannot be distinguished.[48]

Clearly, the relationship between BMI and FM% differs among ethnic groups and populations. Among Asians of many ethnicities (Chinese, Indians, Indonesians, Malaysians, Japanese), differences in the BMI-FM% relationship have repeatedly been documented when compared with Caucasians.[49] With as much as 5% higher body fat at any BMI value, as well as higher risks of type 2 diabetes and cardiovascular diseases at lower BMIs, Asian Indians consistently demonstrated greatest deviations from Caucasians. These ethnic groups also have their BMIs affected by differences in frame size and relative leg length (relative sitting height).[48,50] To date, the WHO has not redefined the cutoff points in any specific Asian populations.[51]

Research has suggested some ethnic differences in the associations among BMI, %BF, fat distribution, and health risks. Different BMI cutoff points have been recommended for some Asian and Pacific populations. There are biological differences between ethnic groups and populations in BC, the relationships between BMI and %BF, and those between BC and morbidity.[52,53]

There are two sets of international BMI cutoff points in addition to other classifications: one recommended by the WHO and another by the International Obesity Task Force (IOTF). The IOTF values have been used widely worldwide.[54]

The FFM and FM indices (FFMI and FMI) are comparable notions to the BMI (the denominator is the same) and result from the partitioning of BMI into two subcomponents using BC, namely:

$$\text{BMI (kg/m}^2) = \text{FFMI (kg/m}^2) + \text{FMI (kg/m}^2)$$

Thus,

$$\text{FFMI} = (\text{BMI} - \text{FMI}); \text{FMI} = (\text{BMI} - \text{FFMI})$$

Therefore, FFMI, FMI, and BMI use similar ratios for their calculation, the difference being that the numerator is composed of FFM or FM (in kg) rather than body weight. Interpretation of BMI and FM% may fail to allow a clinician to detect the presence of protein-energy malnutrition (PEM). Calculation of FFMI, however, does allow for the identification of an individual as malnourished.[48]

Hull et al. investigated the presence of FFMI differences in 1,339 healthy adults (ages 18–110 years) of different races and ethnicities (Caucasian vs. African American, Hispanic, and Asian). They found that among the four ethnic groups for both genders (males > females), FFMI did differ, with FFMI lowest in Asians and greatest in African Americans. This demonstrated racial disparities in BC and infers that identification by race will show greater susceptibility for disease relative to loss of FFM.[55]

## Waist Circumference

Internationally (WHO and the International Diabetes Federation) and in the United States, WC has been accepted as a valid anthropometric measure for identifying central and visual adiposity as well as an established component of metabolic syndrome, a predictor of risk for cardiovascular disease, and type 2 diabetes.[56] Because of gender, age, and ethnic variations in body fat distribution, consideration for different cutoffs or indices are recommended in assessing health risk. In theory, circumference differences represents FM-to-FFM proportions for any area of

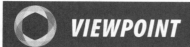

# BMI: The Weight Categories for Older Adults Are Different

*Robin B. Dahm, RDN, LDN*

Eating healthfully and getting adequate physical activity contribute significantly to how well we maintain a healthful weight—one that is neither too high nor too low. A healthful weight is an optimal goal at any age and protects against numerous health problems. Being underweight increases the risk for immediate and acute health challenges such as skin breakdown and chronic diseases. Carrying excess weight also can cause clear and present dangers such as joint and respiratory problems. In addition, overweight adults are statistically likely to develop several diseases associated with aging.[1] Body mass index is a key screening tool for determining weight status and is based on a person's weight-to-height ratio. **Figure A** lists some of the conditions associated with being overweight.

### Older Adults Are Not the Same as Younger Adults

The BMI weight classifications for adults are based specifically on associations between BMI and chronic disease and mortality risk in healthy, *young* adults (20 years and older) populations.[2] What kind of a skew does this create? Consider an older adult whose atherosclerosis (a precursor to cardiovascular disease) began at age 55 years versus a younger adult whose atherosclerosis began at age 20 years. The younger adult is statistically more likely to manifest full-blown cardiovascular disease by age 55 years, whereas the older adult at this age has only the precursor to cardiovascular disease. The 55-year-old is also statistically less likely to develop cardiovascular disease even within her next few years of life because its onset was later in life (which is statistically protective). Yet the BMI population chart treats all adults as a single population, with no distinction between younger adults and older adults and their differing statistics for developing diseases later in life.

A main use of BMI for adults is to determine chronic disease risks associated with higher BMI values. The standard BMI categories are less applicable as age increases; the concept that mortality risk increases as weight increases does not seem to hold as true for older adults.[2]

### Older Adults and Underweight

The BMI weight categories require some adjustment to address health statistics associated with older adults. At a

- High blood pressure (hypertension)
- High levels of LDL cholesterol, low levels of HDL cholesterol, or high levels of triglycerides (dyslipidemia)
- Type 2 diabetes
- Coronary heart disease
- Stroke
- Gallbladder disease
- Osteoarthritis (a breakdown of cartilage and bone within a joint)
- Chronic inflammation and increased oxidative stress
- Some cancers (endometrial, breast, colon, kidney, gallbladder, and liver)

**FIGURE A** Some chronic diseases associated with overweight

Modified from Centers for Disease Control and Prevention. About Adult BMI. https://www.cdc.gov/healthyweight /assessing/bmi/adult_bmi/index.html. Accessed February 2, 2017.

higher BMI, for example, a person at least 65 years of age has a lower mortality risk, whereas the *opposite* is true for younger adults![1,2]

BMI cannot distinguish between lean tissue, fat, and bone mass. Yet as we age, our bodies tend to develop more fat, which increases BMI values. In addition, mortality statistics for older adults show that somewhat higher BMIs are protective.[2] **Figure B** shows how how BMI status for older adults is "more lenient" than for younger adults.

Why is underweight more of a concern for older adults than for their younger counterparts? Underweight older adults might be more susceptible to certain undernutrition-related health problems that often go unrecognized. These include physiologic changes, chronic disease, polypharmacy, and psychosocial changes. Such combinations of underweight and unrecognized conditions may have a stronger effect on older adults than on younger adults.[2,3]

For older adults, carrying "a few extra pounds" can temporarily compensate for unplanned weight loss and hold off the development of secondary conditions that weight loss can trigger such as loss of bone-mineral density.[4]

### Practical Application

Currently, BMI weight classifications do not differentiate between older adults and younger adults. Healthcare practitioners who use the right-shifted BMI weight categories can more appropriately address the health needs of their older adult clients and patients.

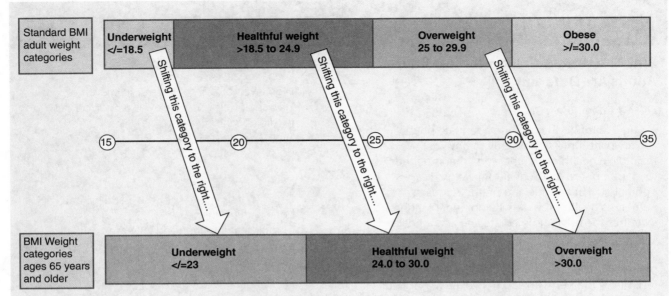

**FIGURE B** Shifting BMI weight categories to the right for adults ages 65 years and older more accurately represents the health statistics associated with this subpopulation.

Modified from Using Body Mass Index. Queensland Government. https://www.health.qld.gov.au/__data/assets/pdf_file/0031/147937/hphe_usingbmi.pdf. Accessed February 2, 2017.

### References

1. Department of Health and Human Services, Centers for Disease Control and Prevention. Body mass index: Considerations for practitioners. https://www.cdc.gov/obesity/downloads/BMIforPactitioners.pdf. Accessed February 2, 2017.
2. Raeburn ED. Higher BMI may be better for older adults. *MedPage Today*. 2014; March 19. http://www.medpagetoday.com/Endocrinology/General Endocrinology/44843. Accessed February 2, 2017.
3. Winter JE, MacInnis RJ, Wattanapenpaiboon N, Nowson CA. BMI and all-cause mortality in older adults: A meta-analysis. *Am J Clin Nutr*. 2014; April; 99(4): 875-890. http://ajcn.nutrition.org /content/99/4/875.long. Accessed February 2, 2017.
4. MedlinePlus. Body mass index. https://medlineplus .gov/ency/article/007196.htm. Accessed February 2, 2017.

the body, with larger measures reflecting a higher percentage of body fat. Circumference measures are taken with a flexible measuring tape and can be performed at the waist, hip, and thigh to assess body fat distribution. Adiposity of the abdomen, as measured by WC, is useful in diagnosing cardiovascular risk factors and metabolic syndrome. Exact location of the WC measurement is necessary. Common WC sites are (1) just beneath the lowest or floating rib, (2) at the midpoint between the iliac crest and the lowest or floating rib, (3) the narrowest point of the abdomen as visualized, and (4) just above the iliac crest. Sites using bony landmarks are preferable (see **FIGURE 7.9**).

In both adults and children, BMI has been the accepted method to identify the overweight and obese; however, visceral fat strongly mediates the association between obesity and weight-related diseases. WC

measurement has emerged as a useful clinical measure in the assessment of those so identified. Specific waist circumference cutoff points have been established to identify overweight and obese adults, but values are not so clearly defined for children, where waist circumference differs between genders and varies with age as well.[57]

WC correctly detected obesity in children (83.8%) compared to reference standards, with a false-positive rate of 3.5%. WC correctly detected overweight in children (73.4%), with a false-positive rate of 5.3%.[3]

WC is particularly useful in adult patients who are categorized as normal or overweight on the BMI scale. Waist circumference has little added predictive power of disease risk at BMIs of at least 35. Therefore, there is no benefit to measuring waist circumference in adults with BMIs of at least 35.[22]

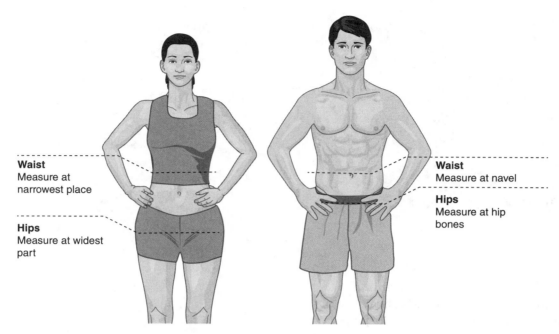

**FIGURE 7.9** Waist circumference measurement female and male

The WHO has identified ethnic groups for which waist circumference may reflect more body fat at a given BMI level. Studies investigating BC and association with health outcomes in Asia have focused on Chinese, Japanese, Korean, or South Asian (or Indian). Some have viewed these ethnic groups as a homogeneous population labeled "Asians" and found a higher %BF in Asians at lower BMIs and an increased prevalence of truncal fat compared to Caucasians.[58]

European men and women display less visceral adipose tissue for a given waist circumference than do Chinese and South Asians (Indians).[59] Correspondingly, an increase %BF across a range of WC values has been recorded in East Asia.[60] Comparisons of indigenous or aboriginal peoples and Caucasians in North America have reported no difference between visceral adipose tissue and BMI, total body fat, or WC.[61] Black women in South Africa, compared to European women, have a slightly lower BMI at a given %BF, but they also have less abdominal adipose tissue as determined by DXA at the same WC.[62] In a few small studies, African women reportedly had less visceral adipose tissue than do white women.[63–65]

One study reported that visceral adipose tissue at a specific WC was not appreciably different in Hispanics than in whites.[66] There have been reports that Pacific Islanders have more muscle mass and less %BF than Europeans have at similar BMIs.[62,67]

Although there is substantial evidence of age and gender variations in WC, there is less evidence for demonstrable ethnic differences. Asian populations have more visceral adipose tissue, and African populations—with possibly Pacific Islanders—have less visceral adipose tissue or %BF at any given waist circumference compared to Europeans. If higher levels of abdominal fat for a WC are reflected in associations with health outcomes, then lower thresholds for these indicators might be needed for the affected ethnicities than for Europeans. Data from Africans and Pacific Islanders are possible indications for more cutoffs than those used for Europeans. Because the objective is to predict disease risk, drawing conclusions about cutoffs based solely on observed risks is not pertinent.[61]

## Skinfold Thickness

One of the earliest techniques used for estimating %BF is skinfold (SF) measurements using specially designed calipers to measure the subcutaneous fat (see **FIGURE 7.10**).[4] Skinfold thickness measurements are based on an assumption that subcutaneous fat is approximately 50% of total body fat. SF measurements are obtained in a minimum of three and as many as nine areas of the body, including subscapular, triceps, biceps, suprailiac, and abdominal; these measurements indirectly predict %BF through population-specific (gender-specific and

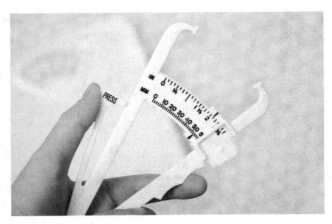

**FIGURE 7.10** Skinfold calipers

© jonathandowney/Getty Images.

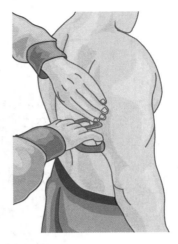

**(a)**

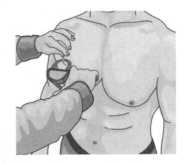

**(b)**

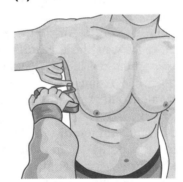

**(c)**

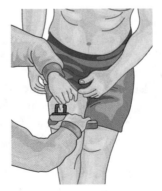

**(d)**

**FIGURE 7.11** Skinfold sites: (a) triceps (b) chest (c) supraillic (d) thigh

age-specific) equations.[68] All measurements for skinfolds are taken using skinfold calipers. To begin, the examiner needs to carefully mark the point for performing the skinfold measurement—either the specified midpoints for the arms and legs or the designated boney points for the trunk of the body. To improve comfort when taking measurements, the procedure should be explained to the child or adult and demonstrated on the patient's hand. Before applying the caliper, a fold of skin along with the **subcutaneous adipose tissue (SAT)** is grasped between the thumb and index finger. Caution should be taken to ensure there is distinction between the fold and the underlying muscle, with the two sides close to parallel. While holding the skinfold, the jaws of the caliper are placed perpendicular to the fold length and measured to the nearest 0.1 mm. the reading is taken within three seconds after the caliper is released. Most calipers can measure up to 44 mm.

The skinfold caliper measurement is prone to interrater error because of difficulty separating the fold of skin from the muscle. The procedure requires that the skinfold include the adipose tissue below and two thicknesses of skin.[7] However, with practice, the interrater error can be as low as 5% if standard protocol is followed and measurements are taken in the same areas.[69,70,71]

### Adults

Measurement recommendations can be gender specific, with only three measurements. For men, measurements include chest, abdomen, and thigh; for women, the measurements include, triceps, suprailiac, and thigh (**FIGURE 7.11**). In addition, site-specific correlations have been established with triceps SF estimating %BF as compared to subscapular skinfolds, with total body fat (TBF) and health risk.[72]

Although SF thickness is inexpensive and easy to measure, it is limited by the training of the of the person performing the assessment, the type of calipers used, and the appropriate selection of the equations to match the population.[68,72] From estimating the TBF percentage, it is possible to calculate lean tissue weight by using the following formula:

$$\text{Lean tissue weight} = \text{Total body weight} - (\text{Total body weight} \times \%BF)$$

Following protocol is essential, particularly the timing for conducting the test. It should be avoided after the person has been swimming, showering, or exercising, all which increase blood flow and skinfold thickness.[8] Other limitations include compression of subcutaneous adipose tissue; variability of the elasticity of the tissues, specifically in elderly and obese individuals; and inaccuracy of site placement, which can alter measurement results by 1 centimeter.[73,74] All of these can decrease the accuracy of measured SAT, with site placement at 39% and site compressibility ranging from 25% to 37%.[74] This emphasizes the importance of training and having the same clinician perform the measurements by following the measurement protocol.

### Children

Skinfold thickness tests correctly detected obesity in children (72.5%) compared to reference tests, with a false-positive rate of 6.3%, and correctly detected overweight in children (78%), with a false-positive rate of 9.7%.[5]

## Mid-Upper-Arm Circumference

Another method to quickly assess for malnutrition, particularly protein and energy reserves, is the mid-upper-arm circumference (MUAC). This is an inexpensive, simple measurement that can be implemented for a variety of populations across the life cycle as well as across ethnicities. MUAC requires minimal equipment and calculations compared to weight and height measurements for calculation of BMI, or other anthropometrics such as skinfold thickness. This measurement can be used from the age of 2 months onward. In children, MUAC is useful for assessing nutritional status, predicting mortality, and in some studies, predicting death in children better than any other anthropometric indicator.[75]

A nonelastic measuring tape is used to measure the posterior surface of the upper left arm, with the person standing, weight even on both feet, and facing away from the examiner. The elbow of the left arm is bent at a 90-degree angle, left palm facing up. The upper-arm length is then measured. The tape is placed at the acromion process (shoulder blade) and extended to the olecranon process (elbow). With the tape in place, the examiner places a mark on the posterior surface as the midpoint of the arm (see **FIGURE 7.12**). The measuring tape is positioned at the midpoint and wrapped flush around the arm, snugly but without causing a compression of the skin, and is measured to the nearest 0.1 cm. An alternative method has the person in a sitting position with the left arm hanging relaxed during the measurements.[76] When the measurement is taken on an infant, a similar procedure is completed with the infant upright, not supine. Numerous studies have shown that MUAC correlates well with BMI in adult populations.[77-79]

In situations when an accurate weight or height is unobtainable, indirect measures are used, leading to poor estimates of the BMI and poor assessment of nutritional status. The MUAC is an anthropometric measurement that correlates with BMI and can be an alternative measure for nutritional status in clinics, the field, and hospitals.[80]

Both the WHO and the United Nations Children's Fund (UNICEF) propose to define nonedematous severe acute malnutrition (SAM) by either an MUAC of <115 mm or by a weight-for-height Z-score (WHtZ) of less than −3.[10] The Academy of Nutrition and Dietetics (the Academy), in conjunction with the American Society for Parenteral and Enteral Nutrition (ASPEN), recommend the MUAC as a measure for detecting and documenting pediatric malnutrition.[81]

Studies with children and adults have documented that MUAC is as good a predictor for mortality as BMI is. Since 2007, because of its specificity for identifying high mortality risks in children, MUAC has been the measurement of choice as the single diagnostic anthropometric measure in the community setting for identifying SAM.[10,61] Briend et al. compared the sensitivity and specificity of using MUAC or WHtZ measurements alone or in combination in 5,751 children; it confirmed that MUAC is a more specific and more sensitive measurement for identifying high-risk children, and that including WhtZ brought no added value.[10] Even though combining the two measures increased specificity, the sensitivity for appropriately identifying children at high risk for SAM decreased. Assessment of nutritional status for children typically uses Z-scores for height and weight for age as well as weight for height. A WHO Mulicentre Growth Reference study not only

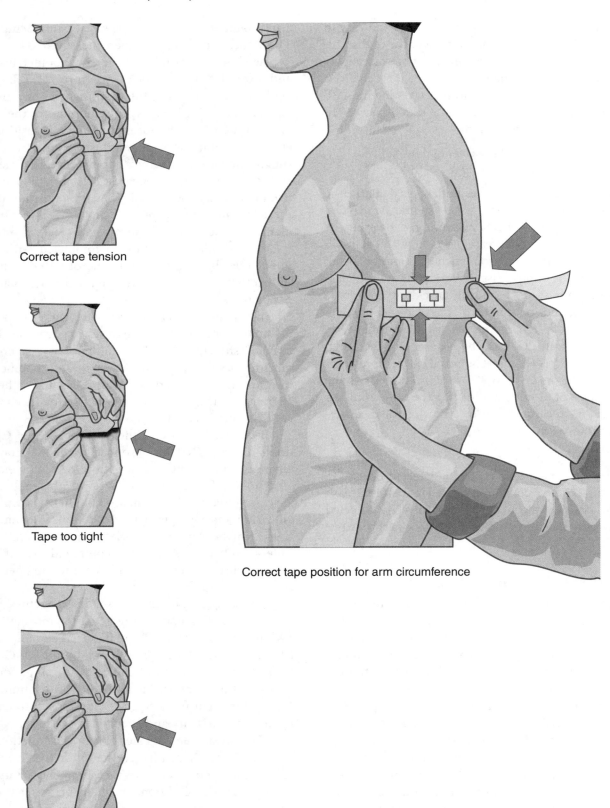

Correct tape tension

Tape too tight

Tape too lose

Correct tape position for arm circumference

**FIGURE 7.12** Appropriate measurement of mid-upper-arm circumference

evaluated height and weight measures, but included multi-age Z-score for MUAC for children, starting at three months of age.[22,23] A comparison between the use of the MUAC and MUAC Z-score in infants (six to 35 months of age) predicted equally short-term mortality risk, with no significant difference in the prevalence of malnutrition or severe malnutrition between the two measures.[82] In lower-income and underdeveloped countries, almost 20 percent of the population are adolescents, underscoring the importance of establishing a cost-effective and rapid anthropometrical measurement for identifying the nutritional status of this population. As an anthropometric measure, MUAC has been shown to have a strong positive correlation with nutritional or protein status with biochemical markers such as serum albumin and serum retinol, confirming its value as a measure of muscle and fat status.[83] Similarly, MUAC, based on its reflecting both muscle and fat stores, is beneficial in obesity screening and determining body fat distribution.[84]

MUAC is beneficial in assessments for weight restoration in children and adolescents being treated for eating disorders. Weight can be of limited value in assessing progress because of time-of-day variability and manipulation by weight loading. Even though peripheral edema caused by fluid restoration following dehydration can affect MUAC, neither rapid water loading nor intense biceps exercising affect the accuracy of this measurement.[85] Research suggests that for children and adolescents being clinically treated for anorexia, MUAC benefits are twofold: First, they confirm the accuracy of weight changes; second, they are better tolerated and produce less anxiety as compared to SF or weight.[86] In adults, MUAC is strongly associated with BMI, but there are no established cutoffs used for identifying malnutrition in the adult population like there is for children. A MUAC at or below 23.5 cm, which indicates an increased risk of low birthweight and poor pregnancy outcomes, has been consistently documented in cross-sectional and longitudinal studies.[84] In healthy, nonpregnant adults and the elderly, a correlation was found between a low BMI (< 18.5) and MUAC (< 24 cm, with women < 22 cm and men < 23 cm) and nutritional risk, with an overall specificity and sensitivity of 70%.

In summary, MUAC has proven to be an accurate, quick method to assess nutritional status and identify acute malnutrition among children and adults, particularly in lower-income environments. It has become one of the main screening indices recommended by the WHO and UNICEF for identifying and starting early treatment for SAM from infancy (three months) to childhood (five years of age).[61] More research is needed for establishing specific MUAC cutoffs to identify not only the risk for malnutrition in adults but also a possible spectrum from moderate to severe, as well as to identify those who will not respond to treatment or are at an increased risk for mortality related to acute malnutrition.

## Mid-Upper-Arm Muscle Area

An indirect measure for estimating midarm muscle (MAMA) and fat (MAMF) combines the TSF and MUAC. These measures, compared to NHANES reference tables, can estimate muscle adequacy and wasting (see **TABLE 7.5**). Estimating MAMA is an evaluation of overall muscle mass and is based on the following assumptions: (1) Arm muscle and bone are circular, and (2) the TSF measurement is twice the thickness of fat and bone. MAMA as a calculated value has historically been overestimated by 15% to 25% but can estimate somatic protein and fat stores.

Midarm muscle or arm muscle area is determined from the MUAC and TSF:

$$\text{MAMA} = [\text{MUAC} - (\text{TSF} \times 0.3122)^2]/12.57$$

The MUAC and MAMA can be easily applied to a subject anywhere and at any time by a trained examiner

**TABLE 7.5** Midarm muscle circumference and muscle status

| Percentage of Standard Measurement | Muscle Status Category |
|---|---|
| 50 | Wasted |
| 60 | Below average—depleted |
| 75 | Average—marginal |
| 100 ± 20 | Adequate |
| > 120 | High muscle |

Reproduced from National Health and Nutrition Examination Surveys I and II;: Anthropometric reference data for children and adults: United States, 2003–2006. Natl Health Stat Report Oct 22 (10): 1–48, 2008.(pgs 24-26.) https://www.cdc.gov/nchs/data/nhsr/nhsr010.pdf

with a flexible tape measure and a caliper. Reference tables for MUAC and MAMA have been published in the United States, the United Kingdom, and Japan (see the resources provided in "Online Resources" section). Two-dimensional MAMA is a better indicator of three-dimensional muscle mass when compared with one-dimensional MUAC.[76]

## Calf and Thigh Circumference

Similar to the MUAC, calf and thigh circumferences can be measured to assess muscle mass. The loss of skeletal muscle and its associated effects on physiological and functional decline occurring with aging has led to the need for quick and accurate noninvasive methods predicting functional capacity, balance issues or risks for falls, and bone-mineral density (BMD).

### Calf Circumference

Because of the complexity and impracticality of using dual-energy x-ray absorptiometry, the National Institute of Aging recommends the use of anthropometric measures such as calf circumference (CC) to assess muscle mass and bone density. Currently, as part of the Mini Nutritional Assessment for Malnutrition and the need for care using either BMI or CC in assessing functional status, the World Health Organization states that CC is a better anthropometric measure and has higher sensitivity than both BMI and MUAC in the older adult.[22] In addition, the CC measurement better depicts body-composition changes, reflecting lower-extremity muscle loss and atrophy contributing to decreased mobility and risk of falling.[87,88] Various cutoffs have been reported in the literature ranging from 29 cm to 33 cm for men and 27 cm to 31 cm for women, with a general cutoff for both of 31 cm as predictive of disability, sarcopenia, and BMD.[89] Higher CC has shown an inverse relationship between CC and frailty and functionality in community-dwelling older adults.[88] Along with the CC as a strong predictor of BMD, particularly for the hip and spine, a higher CC also correlates with structural changes and strength of the hip.

While sitting with feet gently resting on the floor and knee and ankle flexed in a 90-degree angle, the calf circumference is measured using a flexible, nonelastic measuring tape at the bulk area, or the greatest circumference area, of the nondominant leg (i.e., the right leg for a left-handed person); this is most often the midpoint between the patella and the ankle.

To be sure the maximum circumference area is being measured, the examiner should take measurements up and down the calf. For the most accurate measurement and to prevent compressing the subcutaneous fat, the tape measure is pulled snugly but should not constrict the skin; the value is recorded to the nearest 0.1 cm.[7]

### Thigh Circumference

Like CC, thigh circumference (TC) is an alternative marker of muscle mass and a predictor of risk for bone fracture because of its linear correlation with BMD and hip strength.[89] TC alone inconsistently predicts bone strength, and it is speculated that the higher fat content of the thigh may influence the measurement.[90] This higher fat composition limits the TC's strength as a predictor of total lean body mass as compared to CC and MUAC. There is an inverse relationship for TC and risk of cardiovascular disease, with two times the risk in those with a TC <55 cm.[91] The TC is measured to the nearest 0.1 cm using a flexible nonelastic measuring tape at the midpoint of the dominant leg (i.e., the right leg for a right-handed person) while the person stands with the weight shifted onto the nondominant leg.[7]

In summary, there is a strong positive correlation of both CC and TC to muscle mass and its value as a predictor of BMD and disability. However, more studies are needed to validate its use for predicting sarcopenia and BMD that take into consideration the influence of changes in the distribution of fat and skin elasticity occurring with aging, with the potential to affect the accuracy of CC and other anthropometric measures.[92] Assessing for muscle mass by using a simple, quick anthropometric measure such as CC is beneficial in a variety of healthcare settings and community living situations for predicting need for care, early interventions, and improving functionality in the aging adult.[93] Also, consideration for population and gender-specific cutoffs, including ethnicity, race, and age, is recommended.

**TABLE 7.6** provides benefits and limitations associated with the use of anthropometric measurements.

> **Recap** Anthropometrics shift to a predictive milieu. Through standardized techniques, repeated measures provide reliable estimates of the percent of fat in the body. These same methodologies allow for the development of population and cultural norms.

| **TABLE 7.6** Summary of the benefits and limitations of anthropometric measurements ||
|---|---|
| **Benefits** | **Limitations** |
| Low cost: most require only minimal financial investment | Time of day variances: successive measurements in some methods will vary if not conducted at similar time of day |
| Ease of training: no special skill sets are needed nor extensive training required | Variations in location or site of measurement: sites on the body must be marked and recorded to ensure accurate replications |
| Noninvasive: none of the common techniques are invasive | Observational subjectivity: Measurements—especially of length, height, Circumference—can be altered by strength of pull or elasticity of the measuring tape |

Data from McDowell MA, Fryar CD, Ogden CL, Flegal KM. Anthropometric reference data for children and adults: United States, 2003–2006. *Natl Health Stat Rep.* 2008; Oct 22 (10);1–48: 24-26. https://www.cdc.gov/nchs/data/nhsr/nhsr010.pdf.

# ▶ Body Composition

**Preview**  Anthropometrics now shift to qualitative measurements, techniques, and technologies that can provide data on actual body composition.

Assessing changes in BC can augment strategies for the prevention and treatment of disease. BC can be influenced by physical activity, lifestyle choices or interventions, and dietary patterns, as well as by nutritional intake. Accurately assessing and monitoring BC can provide important clinical information for making intervention decisions in disease prevention and in managing and accessing treatment outcomes. As discussed, BMI only assesses a person's weight status or risk for disease and does not portray what proportion or distribution is fat-free mass such as bone and lean mass or adiposity and water.

This section will discuss BC in relation to health and different methods used for assessing BC, including hydrodensity, air-displacement phlethysmography (ADP), **bioelectrical impedance analysis (BIA)**, skinfolds, and densitometry. Depending on the setting, some methods are more applicable for the research, hospital, or community setting. Selecting a technique to use not only depends on the setting but also on its validity, reliability, cost, complexity of what it measures, and practicality.

## Body-Composition Models: Reasons to Measure

To fully realize the nutritional status of a person, a measurement or evaluation of the discrete components of BC, including adiposity (body fat), FFM (bone and lean mass), and water are required. All of these can be influenced by disease status and affects a person's health risks. Both the quantity and distribution of adiposity and FFM vary by age, gender, ethnicity, weight changes (loss and gain), growth, activity level, and disease state(s). They also reflect the impact of nutritional intake and tissue losses and gains over time. Determining a person's BC can lead to the development of comparative standards that are gender-, age-, and disease-specific. An individual's BC can support improved understanding of body changes that are occurring, such as decreasing bone density and increasing adiposity in elderlies, or FFM and adiposity changes from malnutrition, a disease state, exercise, or medications.

Understanding and using BC techniques is important in both research and clinical practice. In research, they are used to assess changes in these components as they relate to age, growth, disease risk, and assessment standards.[94,95] For the clinician, BC comparative standards that are disease, gender, and age specific are used in determining treatment strategies, monitoring the effects of an intervention, and achieving improved outcomes. They are important to consider when selecting the method to use, its reproducibility, its accuracy for the population, and how simple it is to perform. Being able to quantify changes in body weight, particularly FFM and assessing for malnutrition, is critical to improving disease management and decreasing healthcare costs. In contrast to BMI and weight-loss percentage, assessing BC (particularly FFM and FM) is a stronger indicator of clinical outcomes and relationships with mortality.[96,97]

Body fat composition varies throughout the life cycle but begins at 10% to 15% in early infancy and increases to 30% at six months.[98] During adolescence, adiposity increases in females compared to males in which there is a rapid increase in FFM. The difference between genders when comparing body fat to FFM continues into adulthood, with females having a higher percentage of **essential fat** and storage fat (**FIGURE 7.13**).

The rate of increase in body fat slows during early and middle adulthood and is followed by a decline in FFM. It is not clear if there is a true increase in %BF in the elderly or if it just reflects a decrease in FFM caused by sarcopenia or **cachexia**. By definition, sarcopenia is a condition characterized by both a decrease in muscle mass (myopenia) and strength (dynapenia).[92] Depending on the cause, it is classified as either primary (age related) or secondary (related to changes in activity, disease, or nutritional intake).[92] Cachexia differs from sarcopenia because it is a wasting condition occurring concomitantly with a disease state such as cancer, heart

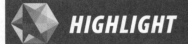
## HIGHLIGHT

### Anthropometrics and Malnutrition: Why Assess?

Malnutrition, or undernutrition, is a problem that occurs not only in the hospital but also in the community. Identifying malnutrition is difficult because it can be the result of inadequate intake or poor nutrient utilization; thus, *malnutrition* and *undernutrition* are synonymous. The prevalence of undernutrition in the hospital setting ranges from 20% to 50% internationally and is a strong factor for extended hospital stays, acute illness, morbidity, mortality, and decreased functionality and quality of life. Since the late 1990s, the Joint Commission—which is an independent, not-for-profit organization, that accredits and certifies nearly 21,000 health care organizations and programs in the United States—has required that institutions assess patients for malnutrition within 24 hours of their admission to a hospital. According to the 10th revision of the *International Classification of Disease*, malnutrition can be identified as a BMI < 18.5 kg/m² or by unintentional weight loss because of an intake of less than estimated needs. Anthropometric data are simple to acquire and are part of the six characteristics—energy intake, weight loss, body fat, muscle mass, fluid accumulation, grip strength—for identifying malnutrition by the

Academy of Nutrition and Dietetics and the American Society for Parenteral and Enteral Nutrition, including weight, grip strength, body-composition fat, and muscle (see **TABLE A**). Accurate measurements of height and weight are essential for estimating energy needs (EENs) and comparing EENs to a person's recent food intake. Consuming less than 75% of EEN is classified as moderate malnutrition if a person is acutely ill for more than seven days or chronically ill for a month or more. Severe malnutrition is consuming less than 50% of energy needs for five or more days in acute illness and one month or more in chronic illness. Whether in a hospital or community setting, weight loss as a percentage of baseline usual body weight over a period of time should be assessed and monitored regularly. Body composition by both physical signs (around the eyes, face, and rib area) and skinfold measurement (triceps, biceps, subscapular, and suprailiac) can identify subcutaneous fat loss, a sign of malnutrition with mild loss being moderate malnutrition in both acute and chronic illness, and moderate loss equaling severe malnutrition in acute illness, and severe loss for severe malnutrition in chronic illness. Why assess? Early identification and intervention leads to better health outcomes and decreased length of stay and overall health costs. Table A shows how to identify malnutrition.

**TABLE A**  Identifying malnutrition

| Criteria | Severe | Moderate/Nonsevere |
|---|---|---|
| Estimated energy needs | ≤50% for ≥5 days | <75% for >7 days |
| Loss of body fat | Moderate | Mild |
| Loss of muscle mass | Moderate | Mild |
| Reduced grip strength | Reduced based on nomogram | Normal |

Modified from White, J. V., Guenter, P., Jensen, G., Malone, A., and Schofield, M. (2012). Consensus statement of the academy of nutrition and dietetics/American Society for Parenteral and Enteral Nutrition: Characteristics recommended for the identification and documentation of adult malnutrition (undernutrition). Journal of the Academy of Nutrition and Dietetics. 112(5). pp. 730–738.

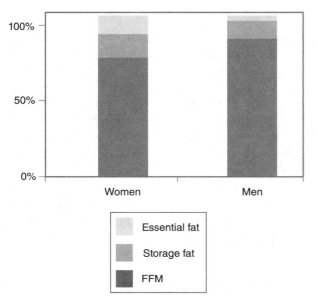

**FIGURE 7.13** Body-composition differences, women and men

Data from Heo M, Faith M, Pietrobelli A, Heymsfield S. Percentage of body fat cutoffs by sex, age, and race-ethnicity in the US adult population from NHANES 1999–2004. *Am J Clin Nutr.* 2012; 95(3):594–602.

failure, or end-stage renal or liver disease. In general, those with cachexia are sarcopenic but not vice versa.[99]

Over the past decade, body fat composition has been considered an important health risk indicator. Body fat composition and distribution appear to be associated with metabolic changes and as a strong predictor for disease risk and not obesity alone.[100] Research demonstrates that the distribution of adipose tissue sets the systemic pathway for increasing the risk for disease development.[100] Body fat is stored in two predominant compartments, **visceral adipose tissue (VAT)** and subcutaneous adipose tissue. VAT makes up 85% of total body adiposity and is located intra-abdominally, surrounding organs. SAT constitutes 10% of total body fat and is found between the muscle and subcutaneous tissue (hypodermis). There are predominantly two body types: **android**, or apple shaped, and **gynoid**, or pear shaped. In the typical android shape, larger fat cells are primarily in the upper part of the body such as the abdomen, which is more common in males and associated with an increased risk for such metabolic diseases as diabetes and cardiovascular disease.[101,102] In the gynoid shape, there are smaller fat cells in the hip and thigh area, which is more common in females. It is not only associated with lower risk for metabolic disease but also may be cardioprotective, especially if located in the thighs, buttocks, and lower abdomen—and is difficult to lose.[103,104] It is possible that the comorbid conditions associated with obesity are related to the visceral fat

opposing the expansion of the protective subcutaneous fat, leading to deposition of fat within the organs such as the liver. Recently, the concept of a VAT:SAT ratio has been studied and found to correlate with increased cardiometabolic risk and as a stronger predictor than BMI or VAT. Thus, evaluating where the fat is stored, along with the ratio, may be more useful in determining a person's health risk.[100]

## Body-Composition Measurements and Models and Techniques

Body composition can be measured both indirectly and directly. Most of the methods used are indirect measures based on assumptions derived from research and cadaver data on expected components for human BC.[4] FFM contains potassium and is as much as 74% water. Potassium content varies between males and females and is expressed in grams/kilogram of FFM.[4,44] Models for determining BC focus on the components measured. The **two-components model** evaluates only body fat mass and FFM, the **three-components model** adds bone, and the **four-components model** adds bone and total body water (**FIGURE 7.14**).

Methods also vary in complexity for what is measured from the whole body (BMI, weight, anthropometry), molecular, cellular, and tissue (blood, bone, adipose tissue, skeletal muscle), or **body cell mass (BCM)**. Models measuring the body tissues are used more in the clinical setting because they are less expensive, noninvasive, and fairly simple to use; these include bioelectrical impedance BIA analysis,

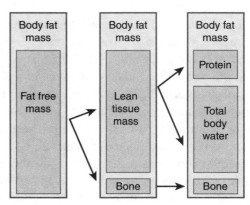

**FIGURE 7.14** Two-, three-, and four-compartment body-composition models

**Courtesy Nancy Munoz**
Reference: Kuriyan R, Thomas T, Ashok S, J J, Kurpad AV. A 4-compartment model based validation of air displacement plethysmography, dual energy X-ray absorptiometry, skinfold technique & bio-electrical impedance for measuring body fat in Indian adults. *The Indian Journal of Medical Research.* 2014;139(5):700–707.

**TABLE 7.7** Body-composition and anthropometric measures for nutritional assessment

| Protein Status | Mid–arm-muscle circumference |
| --- | --- |
| | Grip strength |
| | Plasma proteins |
| Fat Stores | Triceps skinfold |
| | BMI |
| | DXA |
| | BIA |
| | MR or CT |
| | Ultrasound |
| | Waist circumference |
| | Waist to height |
| Body Water | BIA |
| | Weight change |
| | Abdominal girth (waist circumference) |

dual-energy x-ray absorptiometry, and **computerized tomography (CT)** (**TABLE 7.7**).[105]

## Body Cell Mass

Body cell mass (BCM) is a way to assess body composition. This method evaluates the cellular functions of muscles, viscera, blood, and the brain—in other words, the functioning components of the body. Assessing the BCM is considered important clinically because it can demonstrate the effects of disease, medications, and changes in nutritional status or physical activity at an earlier point.[106] The vast majority of the body's potassium (98%) is found in the BCM. Because of the body's tight regulation of potassium and the fact it remains constant in progressive disease states and changes in hydration status, **total body potassium (TBK)** had been historically considered an essential component in assessing nutritional status and BC.[107] Sixty percent of the body's potassium is found in skeletal muscle (SM). An adult model for determining SM using TBK has been established and validated, but its use in children, because of their lower SM, is uncertain. Research has documented a difference of TBK between children and adults, with an SM:TBK ratio in children (0.0071 6 0.0008 kg/mmol) as compared to SM (kg) 0.0082 TBK (mmol) in adults.[107] Using the WBC method for determining TBK is not only safe and noninvasive but also has a lower standard estimated error at 1.5 kg, as compared to other anthropometric and body-composition measures, which range

from 2.2 kg to 2.5 kg. This method also measures BCM and total body protein. Accurately assessing BCM and protein status has an important place in the public-health nutrition arena for evaluating BC changes following nutritional interventions for malnutrition and catch-up growth.[107] BC is often expressed as a percentage of fat and FFM or as a ratio of fat to FFM. Using a two-component model may not be specific enough because the FFM includes bone, water, muscle, and other tissues and thus may not detect significant fluctuations in body protein or loss of lean body mass. TBK is now again being considered as a viable method for assessing protein accretion, particularly in children, because of its potential to more accurately measure protein status rather than FFM or BF percentages.[108]

## Sagittal Abdominal Diameter

In clinical practice, adipose tissue—specifically, abdominal adiposity—correlates with a person's risk for metabolic diseases such as diabetes as well as morbidity and mortality.[103] Gold-standard methods, including computerized tomography, **magnetic resonance imaging (MR)**, and DXA, are expensive and not used as an ongoing assessment method because of radiation exposure.[44,109] For clinical practice and ongoing assessment, waist circumference and sagittal abdominal diameter are more applicable for measuring abdominal obesity.[110,111,112] There are four sites identified for measuring WC and SAD: (1) the narrowest point between the thorax and waist, (2) the midway or slimmest point between the last rib and the iliac crest, (3) the highest point or just above the iliac crest, and (4) the umbilical level. In comparison to SAD, WC is a less reliable measure because the measurement can be influenced by anatomical site used, age, and weight. SAD is measured using a standardized sliding beam abdominal caliper with the subject in the supine position, knees bent. Flaccidity of the abdominal muscles can lead to an overestimation of adipose tissue, and site identification can be masked in those who are have prominent abdominal obesity, thus making it hard to identify the thinnest point for measurement, particularly with WC. Accuracy in SAD measurement is increased by placing the person supine, which effectively redistributes subcutaneous fat along the sides of the abdomen, revealing true abdominal height and allowing accurate assessment of visceral fat.[113]

Measuring SAD midpoint or at the highest point of the iliac crest best predicts AT, particularly VAT, no matter the person's age, gender, level of obesity, or cardiometabolic risk.[110,111] In contrast, WC correlates with SAD. Lack of established population-specific reference ranges and cut points is a primary limiting

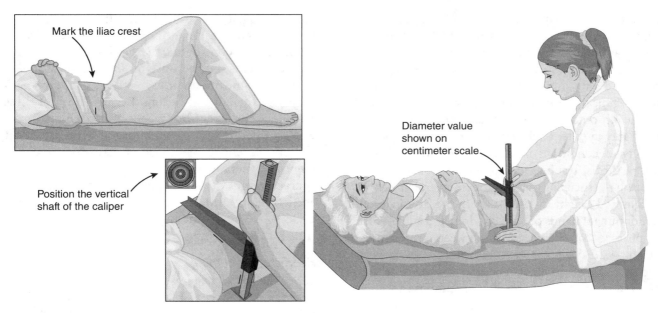

**FIGURE 7.15** Sagittal abdominal diameter measurement

Reproduced from Kahn HS, Gu Q, Bullard KM, Freedman DS, Ahluwalia N, et al. (2014) Population Distribution of the Sagittal Abdominal Diameter (SAD) from a Representative Sample of US Adults: Comparison of SAD, Waist Circumference and Body Mass Index for Identifying Dysglycemia. PLoS ONE 9(10): e108707. doi:10.1371/journal.pone.0108707 Link: https://stacks.cdc.gov/view/cdc/25540/Share

factor to using SAD for nutrition assessment in clinical practice.[4] See **FIGURE 7.15**.

## Handgrip Strength

**Handgrip strength (HGS)** is a quick, quantitative index for assessing upper-body strength and a good predictor of health changes, morbidity, and mortality for adults as well as children. It has become a valid, acceptable measure for muscle strength and a biomarker for identifying sarcopenia.[92] Clinically, HGS is being used to detect a decrease in muscle strength a because low grip strength (GS) strongly suggests pending cognitive decline, physical disability, and morbidity.[114] A **dynamometer** is used to assess GS and can be isokinetic, electrical, digital, or electronic. See **FIGURE 7.16**. Grip strength is a measure of the static force exerted in kilograms and pounds when the hand squeezes the dynamometer. Normative data for comparison are used to assess a person's strength and are stratified by age and gender. Male grip strength is greater than for females, and it peaks between the ages of 30 and 40 years and then declines in a linear direction equally in both genders.[115]

The equipment and procedures used for measuring HGS varies, leading to difficulty in interpreting results and establishing standard protocols and comparative standards. In general, the Jamar dynamometer is the most commonly used device, measuring in kg or pounds in 2-kg (5-lb) increments and rounding to the closest kilogram. There are five positions for the handle; hand size determines where the handle is positioned. The second position is the most used and reliable, with handle positions one and five providing the least reliable measurements. HGS is reduced by fingernail length, that extends from 0.5 cm to 1 cm beyond the fingertip for positions one and two, respectively, because it reduces joint movement. In general, the strength of the dominant hand is 10 percent higher than for the nondominant hand for right-handers but not for left-handers, whose hand strength is equal. Factors affecting the accuracy of the HGS measurement include hand size, posture, joint position and nails, time of day for testing, testing frequency, and hand dominance. Providing encouragement during the testing can influence the results, particularly from the tone and volume of the instructions.

A systematic review shows that HGS predicted mortality, extended length of stay in the hospital, and

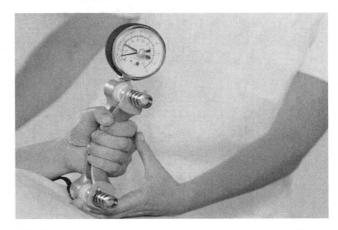

**FIGURE 7.16** Dynamometer

complication risks in older adults better than did other clinical measures such as WHtR, weight loss, and even serum albumin. It is considered to be a strong marker of nutritional status and frailty.[116] Lower HGS is strongly correlated with impaired mobility and is considered a better clinical measure than muscle mass for predicting health outcomes. HGS is used not only in assessing frailty in older adults but also for evaluating a large variety of conditions in children, including rheumatoid arthritis, trauma, and congenital malformations. A strong association has been demonstrated between weight and height in HGS in both the dominant and nondominant hands of both children and adolecents.[117] A positive correlation exists between grip strength, height, and weight. HGS growth curves generate age-specific values, which allows for developmental observation and evaluation of interventions (normative data).[118] Because of its reliability, simplicity, and ease of use in a variety of settings, HGS is considered important as a screening tool for pediatric and adult populations.

## Densitometry

Various **densitometry** methods have been used typically to evaluate body volume (BV) and body density, and extrapolated to predict %BF and FFM.[4] The two most commonly used methods, based on the two-compartment model, are underwater weighing or hydrodensity weighing (HW) and air-displacement phlethysmography (**FIGURE 7.17**).

Both methods assume a consistent body chemical composition, FM density, and FFM density. Variability in bone mineral or water content of the FFM occurring in different conditions or populations inhibits these methods as the reference standard. HW is considered the gold standard for BV measurements, but because of its poor applicability for use in some populations, ADP is used more commonly in the clinical setting. Because both of these assume a consistent body chemical composition of water, minerals, and protein, inaccuracies can occur if there are changes because of disease state, treatment, or therapy and if study population-density characteristics do not apply or are varied (gender, age, ethnicity, athleticism).[109] Each method involves dividing body volume into the body mass and controls for residual lung volume.[7]

### Hydrostatic Weighing

Performing HW requires a large tank of water maintained at 37 degrees Celsius. The person being assessed is lowered into the tank while sitting in a basket or on a platform attached to a scale. While completely underwater, the person being measured expels as much air as possible. Using Archimedes' principle, the volume of displaced water determines the volume of the weight loss by calculating the difference in the body weight (dry weight) before submersion from the weight after submersion. The following formula is used to calculate body density:

$$Wa / [(Wa - Ww) / Dw) - (RV + 100cc)]$$

Note that density of the water (Dw) and residual air volume (RV), as well as air volume can be trapped in the intestine. The %BF is then calculate using the Siri equation:

$$(495 / body\ density) - 450$$

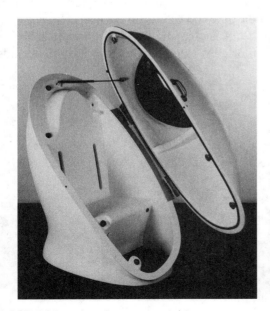
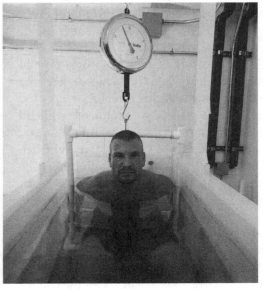

**FIGURE 7.17** BOD POD and underwater weighing

Courtesy of COSMED USA, Inc.

This is the same equation used for skinfold calculations.[7] Even though the body fat estimates are reproducible, this method is not used, because of the test's complexity and problems it presents for some populations, including nonswimmers and those with pulmonary disease, the elderly, and children.[4,109]

*Displacement Plethysmography*

ADP is conducted using similar principles as the HW for determining body density and is an alternative for a wider population. Commercially, for adults between 35 and 200 kg it is known as the BOD POD. For infants up to 8 kg it is known as the PEA POD.[119] This device measures BV by determining air displacement or changes between when the capsule is empty and when the person is sitting inside it. It applies Poisson's law that, at a constant temperature, pressure is inversely related to volume. ADP is a sealed air capsule in which there are two chambers, a test chamber in the front and a reference chamber at the back, connected by a diaphragm that is not only airtight but also flexible. Small volume changes are caused by the vibrating diaphragm in the test chamber, to which both chambers respond. Before entering the capsule, the person is weighed and then sits for two minutes breathing normally in the capsule before performing a breathing exercise. To calculate residual lung volume, the volume of air the person displaces is estimated by the difference between the air pressure when the capsule is occupied and when it is empty. Because of the effects of clothing and hair altering chamber temperature, the person wears minimal clothing such as a bathing suit and a swim cap. In comparison, HW and ADP calculate body density similarly for normal and obese adults and children (10–15 years old).[120,121] Drawbacks to using ADP include its expense, its need for well-trained technicians, and limited size (greater than 35 kg and less than 200 kg for the BOD POD and up to 8 kg for the PEA POD). In general, ADP use for measuring body composition has good within- and between-day measurements. However, ADP has shown some bias in measuring fat mass and has a total error %BF measurement, which can range from 2% to 6%, particularly if there is uncertainty that temperature conditions are met. Variability determining BC has been demonstrated between HW and ADP for athletes and gender, overestimating body fat percent in males by 2% and underestimating it in females by 8%.[44] It is recommended that both of these densitometry methods be combined with other multicompartment methods to confirm the accuracy of body fat estimations.[109,120] As with other BC methods, strict adherence to protocol is essential, including fasting, no exercise within 12 to 24 hours preceding the test, and maintaining normal hydration.

## Dual-Energy X-Ray Absorptiometry

DXA, a three-compartment method, is one of the most versatile methods for assessing body composition in adults and children, providing both regional and whole-body measurements for bone-mineral density, bone-free FFM, and FM. DXA machines transmit low-dose x-rays of different energy peaks. Measuring the amount of x-rays that pass through the bone and bone-free mass, bone density and FFM can be determined by the calculated attenuation ratios (R-values) of the absorption of the two energy frequencies through soft tissue (fat and lean) and bone mineral. The soft-tissue R-value is lower than the bone minerals. A faulty assumption in using DXA is that fat and FFM remain stable, leading to an overestimation of fat in those who are obese and an underestimation in those with lower body fat such as athletes.[122,123] Fluid or hydration status does not seem to affect the DXA BC measurement, but intermachine variability has been documented for both overestimating and underestimating FM.[124] Size and positioning of the person can also lead to errors in body-composition measures.[125,126] Clinical studies have documented limited-effect FM calculations in hemodialysis or in ascites paracentesis but document variations in the measurement in body fat in obese adolescents.[127–129] Also in DXA, comparisons in a four-compartment model indicated good correlations and with no effect of hydration status on body fat measurements.[109,127] Estimating VAT is a recent application of the DXA. This involves measuring SAT width in the abdominal region, along with a geometrically derived formula. The SAT width us subtracted from the total FM to equal the VAT in the abdominal region. There is a concern that DXA overestimates VAT in proportion to increased weight and is not recommended over CT or MRI.

DXA is considered the gold-standard method in determining bone density and for diagnosing osteopenia and osteoporosis.[130] A *T*-score is calculated based on the bone density of a healthy 30-year-old. This reference population is used because this is the age when bones have reached peak development and are at their strongest. The lower the **T-score**, the weaker or thinner the bones, detecting osteoporosis, a condition characterized as porous, fragile bone resulting from the loss of the calcium hydroxyapatite and collagen matrix. Osteoporosis is diagnosed when BMD is 2.5 standard deviations below the reference population. Because of documented differences for gender and ethnicity, a *Z*-score is calculated and represents values derived from a reference population that is age, gender, and ethnicity matched.[130] Often a decreased BMD *T*-score will occur with the *Z*-score remaining stable; thus, the *Z*-score more accurately depicts the BMD changes. BMD is considered to be the most prominent assessment for bone health and fracture risk because the risk for fracture increases with every reduction in standard deviation. Typical DXA focus on the spine and hip because peak bone is reached in these areas by 30 years of age and then declines. Peripheral DXA (P-DXA) scans arms and legs and may not detect changes or risk. The International Society for Clinical Densitometry and the US Preventive Screening Task Force for Osteoporosis recommend the spine and hips (femoral neck or total proximal femur) as the recommended scanning sites.[131,132] Kalkwarf et al. conducted a three-year longitudinal study examining bone-mineral content (BMC) and bone-mineral density (BMD) in children and adolescents.[133] Baseline Z-scores were predictive of the Z-scores at three-year follow-ups, with those at below average scores at baseline continuing with low BMC and BMD at follow-up, indicating screening for BMD earlier using gender- and age-specific Z-scores. These scores, along with clinical risk factors such as smoking, family history, and lifestyle factors, led to the computerized screening algorithm used in the **WHO fracture-risk assessment tool (FRAX)** for men and women.[134]

## Bioelectrical Impedance Analysis

Bioelectrical impedance analysis (BIA) is another method used to determine BC. This method uses measurements of resistance and reactance or impedance of electrical conductivity of the body. In theory, electrical current passes through the low-resistance electrolyte-containing water portion of the body. BIA systems can be single frequency or multi-frequency. Electrodes are placed on the body to transmit a signal that is measuring the opposition of body tissues to the flow of a small (< 1 mA) varying current.[44] The paired placement of electrodes can be arm-leg, leg-leg, or arm-arm (see **FIGURE 7.18**).

The arm-leg pairing is the most commonly used, with four total electrodes, two on the arm and two on the leg, usually on the right side of the body. The leg-leg method concurrently measures weight and impedance and does not estimate FFM as accurately, because

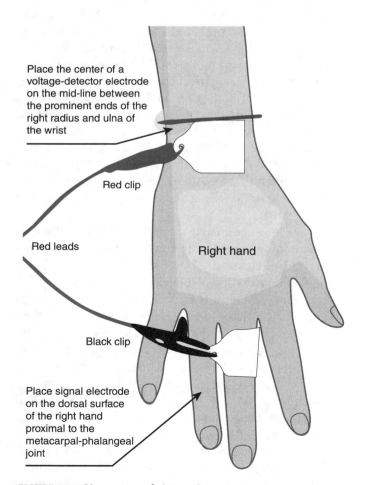

Place the center of a voltage-detector electrode on the mid-line between the prominent ends of the right radius and ulna of the wrist

Red clip

Red leads

Right hand

Black clip

Place signal electrode on the dorsal surface of the right hand proximal to the metacarpal-phalangeal joint

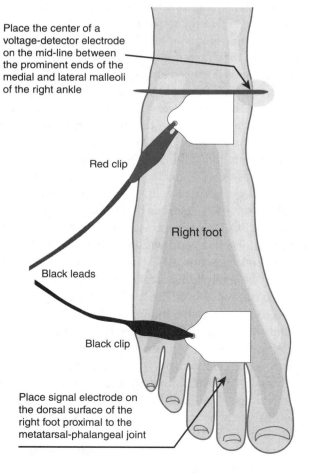

Place the center of a voltage-detector electrode on the mid-line between the prominent ends of the medial and lateral malleoli of the right ankle

Red clip

Right foot

Black leads

Black clip

Place signal electrode on the dorsal surface of the right foot proximal to the metatarsal-phalangeal joint

**FIGURE 7.18** Placement of electrodes

it only measures the legs and part of the abdomen. Similarly, the arm-arm method measures the arms and part of the abdomen. BIA measurements (resistance versus reactance) are calculated based on how resistance correlates with the amount of body water and lean tissue, thus determining the TBW and FFM. The impedance is caused by two vectors: (1) resistance to the tissues, along with (2) the reactance to the strength of the cell membranes, the nonionic tissues, and tissue membrane. Like the other methods described, FFM is calculated with the assumption that hydration status is stable. Total body fat is then determined as the difference between a person's TBW and FFM. In comparison to other methods, BIA is similar, with a margin of error of 3% to 4% for HW, and 2% to 2.5% for ADP.[44,109,120,121] Advantages of using this method include its ease of use in both clinical and research settings, its low expense, and its portability. It also does not require extensive training to operate. Clinically, BIA, particularly multifrequency, is effective in quantifying fluid shifts (extracellular and intracellular) in disease states in patients with renal disease and heart failure.[135] It should not be used if hydration status is not stable—that is, during growth, pregnancy, following exercise, in the morbidly obese, for athletes, and for the undernourished.[44,136,137]

## Total Body Water: Hydration Status

For all BC assessment techniques, understanding hydration status and its effect on accurately determining body fat and FFM is important.[44,138] Errors in the estimation of hydration status from changes in body mass can occur as a result of changes in tissue osmolality due to substrate metabolism and the release of water bound to muscle glycogen.[138] Water is 50% to 70% of total body mass, with lean tissue being predominantly water (70% to 80%) and fat mass (~20%). Alterations in body water can be affected by a disease state, with losses up to 1 liter/hour as in acute diarrhea or in vomiting, and even as much as 3 liters/hour during exercise in hot and humid environments. Disease states that change the metabolism of water, such as malnutrition or edema, can skew hydration calculations. Hydration can be as high as 75% with severe protein malnutrition; similar results are seen with edema. In athletes such as bodybuilders, because of their expanded muscle mass, the hydration constant can increase by 3%.[139] For example, body fat composition estimation can increase by almost 22% with a 10% loss of body water. Both FFM and TBW are both used to determine hydration status, both dehydration and overhydration.[140] Water isotopes such as deuterium oxide used in the deuterium dilution process are the main techniques

used to determine total body water. Bromide is used for extracellular water, and radioactive potassium isotope is used for intracellular water. All of these are expensive and cannot be used to clinically assess short-term fluid shifts. Other less-expensive methods have been used, including urinary tests for color, urine specific gravity and osmolality, plasma osmolarity, and sodium concentration, with urine tests being more reliable in detecting mild to moderate changes in hydration status.

## Imaging

Magnetic resonance imaging and computed tomography are two imaging techniques that provide the most precise and specific tissue-level analyses, including measures of total adipose tissue, subcutaneous adipose tissue, visceral adipose tissue, and intestinal adipose tissue.[44,109] MRI is a noninvasive method that uses strong magnets and radio waves to construct an image; it can provide high-resolution images of vessels as small as 2 mm in diameter, which enables the detection of an occlusion or tumors in difficult-to-access areas. CT is a radiographic technique, with or without intravascular injection of a contrast material, to display a cross-sectional image of targeted areas.

### Magnetic Resonance Imaging

The MRI provides an in-depth view of the chemical composition of body tissue. It is not used to quantify body composition but to form images of organs, structures, and tissues using magnetic fields and radio waves that interact with hydrogen nuclei in the body.[141] To perform this test, a person is placed in a closed system or under a strong magnetic field. The hydrogen nuclei absorb the energy from a radio frequency (RF) pulse and align with the magnetic field. When the energy is released from the nuclei, the nuclei realign and release RF, which are captured to produce an image. In contrast, magnetic resonance spectrometry expands the view to distinguish chemical structures in the area, such as fat from muscle. Both focus on producing images of the body's soft tissues. The MRI is used for a variety of medical purposes, including diagnoses, disease detection, staging, and monitoring treatment. It is used to provide information on something discovered in an ultrasound scan or CT—the causes for bleeding, for example. Segmental MRIs are less expensive and take less time, and research shows they correlate with whole-body tissue measures in cancer and sarcopenic obesity.[109,141]

### Computed Tomography

Complementing both ultrasound and x-ray, computed tomography involves an x-ray tube and a receiver that attenuates the x-rays to produce an image made of pixels, each measuring a unit of attenuation in relation to water and air or Hounsfield unit (HU). The HU value represents the density of the tissue, with adipose tissue equaling −190 to −30 and skeletal muscle 30 HU to 100 HU. The person undergoing the CT scan lays on an examination table that slides in and out of the box- or tunnel-like scanner. Each cross-sectional segment of tissue is calculated. Because of the risk of high radiation exposure, whole-body scans are not done. Similar to the MRI, the CT is a diagnostic test used to detect the presence of a tumor, as well as its size and location, and vascular diseases related to a stroke, pulmonary embolism, or aortic aneurysm.[141,142]

Using an MRI offers several advantages. It is noninvasive, does not use dyes or ionizing radiation, provides good-quality images of soft tissue, and distinguishes the amount and location of body fat, making it a better option than the CT. Also, key minerals can be imaged, including phosphorus, sodium, hydrogen, and potassium. Its biggest disadvantages are cost and that it cannot be used with people who are claustrophobic. The CT has limited use in the assessment of body composition and is not recommended for children, women of childbearing age, and for multiple scans of the same person. For regular everyday use, neither MRI nor CT are recommended for body-composition assessment.

### Ultrasound

Another technique used for assessing body composition is the **ultrasound** transducer, also known as color Doppler imaging (CDI), either A mode or B mode. The A mode scans for the continuity of the area, and CDI involves the use of a brightness-mode ultrasound device (B mode) with a pulsed Doppler flow detector to provide a two-dimensional color image of the of the area being scanned.[143] Often both are used together. The differences in velocity are represented by variations in the colors and their brightnesses. This scanning method allows for isolating and identifying body fat and lean tissue based on sound reflected from ultrasound waves and differences in the acoustic impendence between the tissues, with stronger sound being produced from muscle than from fat. The scanning process uses a bonding gel on the skin or the transducer to improve the sound reflection or decrease sound artifacts. Depending on the reason for the test, the ultrasound technician slides the transducer over the area to be evaluated, ranging from as little as +/−5 mm. To measure body tissue thickness, a two-dimensional picture is produced that shows stronger images or interfaces in white for subcutaneous fat to skin and muscle to

bone but weaker images for the interface between fat and muscle. There are no established protocols for the use of ultrasound for measuring body composition in general. In comparison to other techniques, there is inter-rater variability, similar to but slightly higher than with skinfold measurements, and equal predictive capability of BF% as the DXA, with one-site abdomen measurement for healthy adults and athletes.[73,144] Leahy et al. developed equations, including lower-limb measurements with the abdomen, for men and women, with highly predictive accuracy of body composition.[145]

The advantages of for ultrasound outweigh the limitations, including quick test, non-invasive, portability, low cost, ability to obtain regional and segmental measurements, and to determine muscle and bone tissue thickness. The primary limitation is the interpretation. Results interpretation can be more subjective and difficult because the image that appears contains both continuous, bright, light interfaces (skin-fat, fat-muscle, or muscle-bone) and fascia light streaks which can be confused as body composition interfaces. It is important that the technician be trained to identify the interfaces correctly. There are no standard protocols for ultrasound procedure, but consideration of the site and force of the transducer applied by the technician can vary the subcutaneous adipose tissue by 25% to 37%, and scanning longitudinally is better than scanning vertically.[73]

## Summary of Body Composition Methods

Clinically, DXA or ultrasound appear to be the best measures of sarcopenia, while ultrasound has the added advantage of being able to measure changes in tendons. CT or MRI give excellent measurements of muscles and can delineate fat infiltration, but they are very expensive as capital outlays and in operating and staffing costs. Due to the uncertainty regarding levels of hydration in the subjects, Bioelectrical Impedance BIA measures have questionable value. Both MUAC and calf circumference are inexpensive but inaccurate measures of muscle mass.

**Recap**   These evolving technologies facilitate the non-invasive analysis of body composition. Whether modified from earlier predictive techniques, or innovative adaptations of imaging or applied physics, the barriers to qualitative physical assessment are being removed.

# ▶ Chapter Summary

Since the days of Johann Sigismund Elsholtz and the publication of his *Anthropometria*, there has been a concerted effort to investigate and measure the human body for scientific and medical purposes. Since that time, there has been a quantitative approach to acquiring data concerning variations and changes in the human form, and describing the relationship between the human body and disease. These measurements found a ready application in the assessment of a person's nutritional status, involving more than just evaluating what a person eats, but also in determining his or her body composition and comparing this person's growth and development to accepted standards. Anthropometric assessment rapidly evolved into an essential feature in conducting a nutritional evaluation for determining malnutrition; in defining overweight status and obesity; and in quantifying loss of muscle mass, increase in fat mass, and in the redistribution of adipose tissue.

Anthropometrics includes measurements of body weight, stature or composition; or a focus on specific area measurements, such as circumference (waist and hip), skinfold, and bone dimensions. Some provide direct measurements (i.e., height and weight); others are others derived (i.e., body composition). The application of universal cut-off points has the dual advantage of allowing comparisons between populations and also the prevention of bias on the part of staff when performing initial assessment or follow-up of patients. Additionally, cut-off points can be used to characterize changes and trends within a population and identify persons at a higher risk for adverse outcomes. Body measurements are essential in the analysis of the development and/or progression of disease and also to monitor the efficacy of treatment. Accurate measurement of changes in body composition due to interventions is vital in planning nutritional care and the management of developmental and aging processes, disease progression, and rehabilitation efforts.

In order to evaluate suspected short or tall stature, accurate measurements of height and weight are plotted on a standardized, appropriate-age growth chart. Age-sex-specific percentiles are often utilized to assess growth and nutritional status in children, based on anthropometric measures. Weight and stature are key for assessing growth patterns and determining deviations from the norms for a specified population. Being that weight includes an overall measurement of the body compartments, it is important it be included as a general measure as part of the nutrition assessment.

BMI is determined from the measurements of height and weight; calculating the relative proportion between the two, it is a valid predictor of adiposity. BMI is recommended in the clinical setting as the most appropriate single indicator of overweight and obesity in the pediatric population. Established norms for BMI can allow the clinician to estimate morbidity (chronic-disease risk) and mortality.

Waist circumference has been accepted internationally as a valid anthropometric measurement for identifying central/visual adiposity as well as an established component of metabolic syndrome, a predictor of risk for cardiovascular disease and type 2 diabetes. Skinfold measurement uses specially designed calipers to measure the subcutaneous fat, the original but still useful method for assessing body composition. Additional methods have been developed, including mid-upper-arm circumference, to assess nutritional status, predict mortality, and, in some studies, predict the death of children better than any other anthropometric indicator. MUAC has proven to be an accurate and quick method to assessing nutritional status and identifying acute malnutrition among children and adults, particularly in lower-income environments.

More complex and impractical methods such as DXA have been recommended by various organizations. Ultrasound scanning, another technologically intense method, allows an examiner to isolate and identify body fat and lean tissue based on sound reflected from ultrasound waves and differences in the acoustic impedance between tissues. Even as the technology evolves, the desired outcome remains constant: to best assess the health and growth of the person through accurate, quantifiable, and qualitative measurements.

 **CASE STUDY**

Daniel is a 74-year-old male, of height 5'9" (69"), weight 130 lbs (58.9 kg), and usual body weight 175 lbs (79.37 kg). He is a widower who lives in an apartment of a large continuing-care retirement community (CCRC). Daniel has lived there for many years and gets along quite well. He was diagnosed as having thyroid cancer 1 year ago; in the past 6 months, his weight has gradually decreased to his current 130 lbs. He is seen in the CCRC clinic an average of every three months for regular follow-ups. The facility has a congregate meal program, but lately, he refuses to eat there. Staff members bring him food from the grocery store, and he buys foods that he likes. Much of this goes

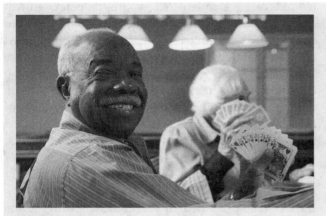

© Monkey Business Images/Shutterstock.

uneaten, however. His labs reveal that his visceral proteins are depleted (low serum albumin). Daniel's triceps skinfold measurement reveals a body fat value that is 50% of the standard. His oral intake ability has decreased gradually; he can only take sips of a high protein supplement (such as Ensure) and occasional bites of food.

### Questions:

1. Daniel's current weight is what percentage of his usual body weight?
2. His current weight is what percentage of his ideal body weight?
3. Calculate the percentage loss of body weight from usual weight.
4. Calculate his BMI at his usual weight. What is his BMI at his current weight? Interpret his current BMI and compare it to his usual weight.
5. Explain what his triceps percentile means as compared to his weight-loss pattern and BMI.
6. What degree of undernutrition is he exhibiting? Explain why you would classify him as exhibiting malnutrition.

### Additional Anthropometrics

Have students perform the triceps skinfold, mid-upper-arm circumference, sagittal abdominal diameter, calf circumference, and waist-circumference measures.

1. Have the students calculate their BMI and WHtR values.
2. Using these measurements, have the students discuss what the numbers mean regarding body composition and health risk.

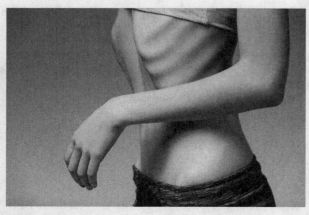

© Vgstockstudio/Shutterstock.

3. Discussion should include outlining the difference between TSF and MUAC. Is one of them better?

### Class Case Study

Barbara is a 30-year-old female, 5'1" (61") tall and weighs 85 lbs (38.5 kg). She has a long history of eating disorders and substance abuse. She calls in sick from her job at the hospital, where she works as a cook. When working, she has the benefit of one free meal on the days she works. She eats most of her other meals out and prepares few meals at home. Because she frequently missed work—this was the third time this month—Barbara's employer insists she bring verification from her doctor that she is cleared to return to work. Her doctor is concerned about her dietary pattern and that she appears undernourished. He calculates the following:

- Ideal weight from the Hamwi equation is 105 lbs. Weight ranges from 94 to 105 lbs.
- BMI: 16.1
- Waist: 20 cm
- Waist-to-height ratio: 33

| Measure | Value | Percentile |
|---------|-------|------------|
| TSF (mm) | 6 | < 5th |
| MAFA (mm²) | 746 | < 5th |
| MUAC (mm) | 258 | 10th to 25th |
| MAMA (mm²) | 4554 | > 75th |

Explain what the percentiles mean for her mid-arm fat area, mid-arm muscle area, and TSF. What conclusions do you have about her body composition from these measurements? What interpretations would you make regarding her body composition and nutritional risk? Would you recommend any other anthropometric measurements? Will the doctor clear her to go back to work?

### Questions:

1. Discuss the innovative adaptations of imaging or applied physics and barriers to qualitative physical assessment.
2. Summarize and discuss the differences between the methods reviewed in the chapter.
3. What is the most accurate method for measuring fat-free mass versus fat mass?
4. Are the techniques appropriate for a hospitalized patient? What about an outpatient in an ambulatory care setting?

### Plotting Case Study

Calculate the percentiles (use growth charts to plot) for a baby boy with the following data, born June 1, 2016.

1. What is the growth velocity at 21/2 months of age? Is it average, below, or above average?
2. What is the growth velocity between 9 and 12 months of age? Is it average, below, or above average?

# Learning Portfolio

## Key Terms

Adiposity
Android
Anthropometric indicator
Anthropometrics
Anthropometry
Bioelectrical impedance analysis (BIA)
Body cell mass (BCM)
Body composition (BC)
Body mass index (BMI)
Cachexia
Computerized tomography (CT)
Cutoff point
Densitometry
Dual-energy x-ray absorptiometry (DXA)
Dynamometer
Essential fat
Fat-free mass (FFM)
Frontal-occipital circumference
Four-components model
Gynoid

Handgrip strength (HGS)
Height velocity
Kyphoscoliosis
Magnetic resonance imaging (MRI)
Percentile
Sarcopenia
Skinfold thickness
Subcutaneous adipose tissue (SAT)
Two-components model
Three-components model
Total body potassium (TBK)
Total body water
Triceps skinfold thickness (TSF)
*T*-score
Visceral adipose tissue (VAT)
Ultrasound
Weight to length
WHO fracture-risk assessment tool (FRAX)
*Z*-score

## Study Questions

1. _____ is a measurement(s) including height and weight assessed in combination with age and gender.
   a. Anthropometric index
   b. Percentile
   c. Cutoff
   d. BMI

2. The purpose of cutoffs is:
   a. To make a change based on the examiner's judgment.
   b. To make comparisons between populations and decrease assessment bias.
   c. Not used for trending data.
   d. Arbitrarily determined by ethnicity and race.

3. A patient has a BMI of 30. This is considered to be:
   a. Obese.
   b. Normal.
   c. Underweight.
   d. Protein energy malnutrition.

4. The IBW range for a female who is 5'7" tall is:
   a. 155 ± 10%.
   b. 135 ± 10%.
   c. 125 ± 10%.
   d. 165 ± 10%.

5. If a patient has a UBW of 200 lbs and now weighs 150 lbs, what is the percentage weight loss?
   a. 25%
   b. 24%
   c. 20%
   d. 15%

6. The patient has experienced an unintentional weight loss of more than 10% in six months. This weight loss is considered:
   a. Moderate.
   b. Severe.
   c. Normal.
   d. Healthy.

7. The TSF:
   a. Measures muscle protein directly.
   b. Represents visceral fat.
   c. Is an index for body fat stores.
   d. Represents visceral protein.

8. Mid-upper-arm circumference:
   a. Measures muscle protein (lean muscle).
   b. Represents visceral fat.
   c. Is an index for body fat stores.
   d. Represents visceral protein.

9. A person who has >85% arm muscle area is considered:
   a. Above average for muscle and excess fat.
   b. Average for muscle and excess fat.
   c. At a deficit for muscle and excess fat.
   d. Below average for muscle and excess fat.

10. A person's basal metabolic rate is directly related to:
    a. Body fat.
    b. Muscle mass.
    c. Total body cell mass.
    d. Fluid mass.

11. Body mass index:
    a. Is synonymous with obesity.
    b. Measures obesity by considering both weight and height.
    c. Measures lean body mass relative to fat mass.
    d. Of 27 corresponds to morbid obesity.

12. A body weight (as a percentage of usual body weight) of 89% is considered to be:
    a. Healthy
    b. Mildly malnourished.
    c. Moderately malnourished.
    d. Severely malnourished.

13. Percent usual body weight is calculated as:
    a. Percent body weight = (current weight/usual weight) × 100.
    b. Percent body weight = (current weight/usual weight) × 50.
    c. Percent body weight = (usual weight/current weight) × 100.
    d. Percent body weight = (ideal body weight/usual weight) × 25.

14. The weight distribution of women who carry most of their weight in the hips is described as:
    a. Android obesity.
    b. Gynoid obesity.
    c. Anthropometry.
    d. A high metabolic health risk.

15. A skinfold assessment is a method for determining total body fat by measuring _____ body fat.
    a. Visceral
    b. Subcutaneous
    c. Essential fat
    d. The ratio of visceral to subcutaneous fat.

16. The most common site used for obtaining skinfold thickness measurements is the:
    a. Biceps skinfold
    b. Fluteal skinfold

    c. Subscapular skinfold
    d. Triceps skinfold

17. _____ fat is the type that is needed by the body to function optimally and protect its organs.
    a. Essential
    b. Storage
    c. Nonessential
    d. Somatic

18. What body-composition measurement technique involves the use of a device that measures the body's resistance to an electrical current?
    a. DXA
    b. BOD POD
    c. PEA POD
    d. BIA

19. In terms of BC measurement, what body tissue is a good conductor of electricity?
    a. Bone
    b. Muscle
    c. Fat
    d. Connective tissue

20. What anthropometric device assesses body composition by displaced air?
    a. DXA
    b. BOD POD
    c. Hydrostatic weighing
    d. BIA

21. What anthropometric device assesses body composition by displaced water?
    a. DXA
    b. BOD POD
    c. Hydrostatic weighing
    d. BIA

22. What anthropometric device assesses body composition by using x-ray technology?
    a. DXA
    b. BOD POD
    c. PEA POD
    d. BIA

23. Which of the following is the most suitable anthropometric measurement for the clinical setting?
    a. BIA
    b. DXA
    c. Air displacement
    d. Underwater weighing

24. _____ fat is considered stored fat.
    a. Subcutaneous
    b. Adipose
    c. Visceral fat
    d. All

25. The fat stored around the organs is known as:
    a. Adipose tissue.
    b. Visceral fat.
    c. Subcutaneous fat.
    d. Topical fat.

26. If a person's weight distribution is characterized by fat stored in the abdominal region and upper body, it is called:
    a. Android.
    b. Gynnoid.
    c. Nonmetabolic.
    d. Protective.

27. Lean mass includes all:
    a. Muscle, bone, and tissue.
    b. Essential fat, tissue, and bone.
    c. Muscle and stored fat.
    d. Stored fat, essential fat, and bone.

28. What is compared when determining body composition?
    a. Muscle to bone
    b. Adipose tissue to muscle

    c. Fat-free mass to muscle
    d. Fat mass to adipose tissue

29. _____ are calculated from the distribution using the mean and standard deviation of the reference population.
    a. Percentiles
    b. *Z*-scores
    c. *T*-scores
    d. Beta scores

30. _____ is a quantitative index for assessing upper-body strength, a good predictor of measure for muscle strength, and a biomarker for identifying sarcopenia
    a. Waist circumference
    b. Handgrip strength
    c. Demispan
    d. Ulna measurement

## Discussion Questions

1. How did the study of anthropometrics transition from the world of art to the world of health?
2. Compare and contrast the differences between anthropometric indicators and cutoff points. Explore NHANE's website (https://www.cdc.gov/nchs/nhanes/) and provide examples of how they are used.
3. Discuss why it is important to use established growth charts. What are the benefits of plotting the data?

## Activities

1. Plotting case study
   At what percentiles (use growth charts to plot) is a baby boy (date of birth June 1, 2016) with the following data:
   a. What is the growth velocity at 2½ months old? Is it average, below average, or above average?
   b. What is the growth velocity between 9 and 12 months? Is it average, below average, or above average?
      (1) At birth: Wt 3.9 kg, Lt 51 cm, HC 35 cm
      (2) At August 15, 2016: Wt 6.18 kg, Lt 60.5 cm, HC 40.5 cm, Wt/Ht:
      (3) At March 1, 2017: Wt 7.9 kg, Lt 71 cm, HC 44.4 cm, Wt/Ht:
      (4) At June 1, 2017: Wt 8.6 kg, Lt 73 cm, HC 45 cm, Wt/Ht:
      (5) At December 1, 2017: Wt 9.0 kg, Lt: 78 cm, HC: 46.1 cm, Wt/Ht:

2. Determining BMI and waist circumference
   Accurately measure your height, weight, and waist circumference. Using the information provided in this chapter, calculate your BMI.
   a. What is your BMI classification?
   b. Based on your BMI classification, what is your health status?
   c. What is your waist circumference classification?
   d. What is your disease-risk classification?

## Online Resources

CDC Growth Charts:
http://www.cdc.gov/growthcharts/who_charts.htm

WHO Growth Standards:
http://www.who.int/childgrowth/en/

Medscape Nutrition and Growth Measurement Technique:
http://emedicine.medscape.com/article/1948024-technique

FRAX® Fracture Risk Assessment Tool:
https://www.shef.ac.uk/FRAX/

Anthropometric Reference Data for US Children and Adults, 2007–2010:
https://www.cdc.gov/nchs/data/series/sr_11/sr11_252.pdf

Nutri Stat—Nutritional Anthropometry Program:
https://nutristat.codeplex.com/

Human Factors and Anthropometric Data:
http://researchguides.library.tufts.edu/humanfactors/anthropometric

FANTA:
https://www.fantaproject.org/sites/default/files/resources/MUAC%20Systematic%20Review%20_Nov%2019.pdf

Anthropometric Procedures:
https://www.youtube.com/watch?v=1ajuqBQOFXg

Arm Circumference:
https://www.youtube.com/watch?v=myaB4eZDBBc

## References

1. Albrizio A. Biometry and anthropometry: From Galton to constitutional medicine. *J Anthro Sci.* 2007; 85:101–123.
2. Ercan I, Ocakoglu G, Sigirli D, Özkaya G. Statistical shape analysis and usage in medical sciences: Review. *Turkiye Klinikleri J Biostat.* 2012; 4(1): 27–35.
3. Merriam-Webster dictionary [online]. http://www.merriam-webster.com/dictionary/anthropometry. Accessed November 8, 2017.
4. Toomey CM, Cremona A, Hughes K, Norton C. A review of body composition measurement in assessment of health. *Top Clin Nutr.* 2015; 30(1):16–32.
5. Simmonds M, Llewellyn A, Owen CG, Woolacott N. Simple test for the diagnosis of childhood obesity: A systematic review and meta-analysis. *Obes Rev.* 2016; 17(12):1301–1315.
6. Woodruff BA, Duffield A. Assessment of nutritional status in emergency-affected populations—Adolescents. UN ACC/Subcommittee on Nutrition. Geneva. UN Statistics Division. 2003. Demographic Yearbook Special Census.
7. ISAK. *International Standards for Anthropometric Assessment* (manual). Marfell-Jones M, Olds T, Stewart A, Lindsay Carter LE, eds. Underdale, South Australia, Australia: International Society for the Advancement of Kinanthropometry; 2012. http://www.ceap.br/material/MAT17032011184632.pdf.
8. FAO. *Uses of Food Consumption and Anthropometric Surveys in the Caribbean.* http://www.fao.org/docrep/008/y5825e/y5825e00.htm. Accessed November 2016.
9. Nambiar S, Hughes I, Davies PS. Developing waist-to-height ratio cut-offs to define overweight and obesity in children and adolescents. *Public Health Nutr.* 2010; 10(10):1566–1574.
10. Briend A, Maier B, Fontaine O, Garenne M. Mid-upper arm circumference and weight-for-height to identify high-risk malnourished under-five children. *Matern Child Nutr.* 2012; 8:130–133.
11. Fryar CD, Gu Q, Ogden CL. Anthropometric reference data for children and adults: United States, 2007–2010. National Center for Health Statistics. *Vital Health Stat.* 2012; 11(252):1-48.
12. Flaherty-Hewitt M, Kline MW, et al. Nutrition and growth measurement technique. *Medscape.* http://emedicine.medscape.com/article/1948024-technique. Accessed November 22, 2016.
13. Bell C, Davies PSW. Prediction of height from knee height in children with cerebral palsy and nondisabled children. *Ann Hum Biol.* 2006; 33(4):493-499. https://www.ncbi.nlm.nih.gov/pubmed/17060071.
14. World Health Organization. *Training Course on Child Growth Assessment.* Geneva: WHO; 2008.
15. Grummer-Strawn LM, Reinold C, Krebs NF. Use of World Health Organization and CDC growth charts for children aged 0–59 months in the United States. Centers for Disease Control and Prevention. [Published correction appears in *MMWR Recomm Rep.* 2010; 59(36):1184.]
16. *MMWR Recomm Rep.* 2010; 59(RR-9):1–15.
17. Barstow C, Rerucha C. Evaluation of short stature and tall stature in children. *Am Fam Physician.* 2015; 91(1):43–50.
18. Centers for Disease Control and Prevention. WHO growth standards are recommended for use in the US for infants and children 0 to 2 years of age. http://www.cdc.gov/growthcharts/who_charts.htm. Accessed November 2016.
19. World Health Organization. The WHO child growth standards. http://www.who.int/childgrowth/en/. Accessed November 2016.
20. World Health Organization. *Physical Status: The Use and Interpretation of Anthropometry.* Report of a WHO Expert Committee. Technical Report. Series No. 454. Geneva: WHO; 1995: 1–452.
21. Wang Y, Moreno LA, Caballero B, Cole TJ. Limitations of the current World Health Organization growth references for children and adolescents. *Food Nutr Bull.* 2006; 27: S175–S188.
22. WHO Multicentre Growth Reference Study Group. WHO child growth standards. Geneva: World Health Organization; 2006.

23. WHO Multicentre Growth Reference Study Group. Assessment of differences in linear growth among populations in he WHO Multicentre Growth Reference Study. *Acta Pediatr.* 2006;450(Suppl.):56–65.

24. Kanof ME, Lake AM, Bayless TM. Decreased height velocity in children and adolescents before the diagnosis of Crohn's disease. *Gastroenterology*; 1988; 95:1523–1527.

25. Tanner JM, Davies PS. Clinical longitudinal standards for height and height velocity for North American children. *J Pediatr.* 1985; 107:317–329.

26. Hirani V, Mindell J. A comparison of measured height and demi-span equivalent height in the assessment of body mass index among people aged 65 years and over in England. *Age Ageing.* 2008; 37: 311–317.

27. Hickson M, Frost G. A comparison of three methods for estimating height in acutely ill elderly population. *J Hum Dietet.* 2003; 16:13–20.

28. Madden AM, Tsikoura T, Stott DJ. The estimation of body height from ulna length in healthy adults from different ethnic groups. *J Hum Nutr Diet.* 2012; 25:121–128.

29. Hirani V, Aresu M. Development of new demi-span equations from a nationally representative sample of older people to estimate adult height. *J Am Geriatri Soc.* 2012; 60:550–554.

30. Lorini C, Collini F, Dastagnoli M, et al. Using alternative or direct anthropometric measurements to assess risk for malnutrition in nursing homes. *Nutrition.* 2014; 30(10): 1171–1176.

31. Geraedts EJ, van Dommelen P, Calibe J, et al. Association between head circumference and body size. *Horm Res Pediatr.* 2011; 75:213–219.

32. Saunders CL, Lejarraga H, del Pino M. Assessment of head size adjusted for height: An anthropometric tool for clinical use based on Argentinian data. *Ann Hum Biol.* 2006; 33: 415–423.

33. Lampl M, Johnson ML. Infant head circumference growth is saltatory and coupled to length growth. *Early Hum Dev.* 2011; 87:361–368.

34. Rollins JD, Collins JS, Holden KR. United States head circumference growth reference charts: Birth to 21 years. *J Pediatr.* 2010; 156:907– 913.

35. Kammerer M, Porter MM, Beekley A, Tichansky DS. Ideal body weight calculation in bariatric surgery population. *J Gastrointest Surg.* 2015; 19: 1758–1762.

36. Mokha JS, Srinivasan SR, Das Mahapatra P, et al. Utility of waist-to-height in assessing central obesity and related cardiometabolic risk profile among normal weight and overweight/obese children: The Bogalusa Heart Study. *BMC Pediatrics.* 2010; 10:73–80.

37. Wildman RP, Muntner P, Reynolds K, et al. The obese without cardiometabolic risk factor clustering and the normal weight with cardiometabolic risk factor clustering: Prevalence and correlates of 2 phenotypes among the 8 US population (NHANES 1999–2004). *Arch Intern Med.* 2008; 168: 1617–1624.

38. Després JP, Lemieux I, Bergeron J, et al. Abdominal obesity and the metabolic syndrome: contribution to global cardiometabolic risk. *Arterioscler Thromb Vasc Biol.* 2008; 28:1039–1049.

39. Malone SK, Zemel BS. Measurement and interpretation of body mass index during childhood and adolescence. *J Sch Nurs.* 2015; 31(4): 261–271.

40. Reilly JJ, Dorosty AR, Ghomizadeh NM, et al. Comparison of waist circumference percentiles versus body mass index percentiles for diagnosis of obesity in a large cohort of children. *Int J Pediatr Obes.* 2010; 5:151–156.

41. Freedman D, Ogden CL, Blanck HM, Borrund LG, Dietz WH. The abilities of body mass index and skinfold thickness to identify children with low or elevated levels of dual energy X-ray absorptiometry-determined body fatness. *J Pediatr.* 2013; 163:160–166.

42. Tuan NT, Wang Y. Adiposity assessments: Agreement between dual-energy x-ray absorptiometry and anthropometric measures in US children. *Obesity*; 2014; 22:1495–1504.

43. Neovius M, Rasmussen F. Evaluation of BMI-based classification of adolescent overweight and obesity: Choice of percentage body fat cutoffs exerts a large influence—The COMPASS study. *Eur J Clin Nutr.* 2008; 62:1201–1207.

44. Ackland TR, Lohaman TG, Sungot-Borgen J, et al. Current status of body composition assessment in sport. Review and position statement on behalf of the ad hoc working group on body composition health and performance, under the auspices of the IOC Medical Commission. *Sports Med.* 2012; 42(3):227–249.

45. Okorodudu DO, Jumean MF, Montori VM, et al. Diagnostic performance of body mass index to identify obesity as defined by body adiposity: A systematic review and meta-analysis. *Int J Obes (Lond).* 2010; 34(5):791–799.

46. Whitlock G, Lewington S, Sherliker P, et al. Body-mass index and cause-specific mortality in 900 000 adults: Collaborative analyses of 57 prospective studies. *Lancet.* 2009; 373:1083–1096.

47. Snijder MB, van Dam RM, Visser M, Seidell JC. What aspects of body fat are particularly hazardous and how do we measure them? *Int J Epidemiol.* 2006; 35:83–92.

48. Dulloo AG, Jacquet J, Solinas G, Montani J-P, Schutz Y. The BMI–FM% relationship may contribute to these racial differences in trunk-to-leg-length ratio, slenderness, and muscularity *Int J Obes.* 2010; 34:S4–S17.

49. Wulan SN, Westerterp KR, Plasqui G. Ethnic differences in body composition and the associated metabolic profile: A comparative study between Asians and Caucasians. *Maturitas.* 2010; 65:315–319.

50. Heymsfield SB, Scherzer R, Pietrobelli A, Lewis CE, Grunfeld C. Body mass index as a phenotypic expression of adiposity: Quantitative contribution of muscularity in a population-based sample. *Int J Obes.* 2009; 33:1363–1373.

51. WHO Expert Consultation. Appropriate body-mass index for Asian populations and its implications for policy and intervention strategies. *Lancet.* 2004; 363:157–163.

52. Yu Z, Han S, Chu J, Xu Z, Zhu C, Guo X. Trends in overweight and obesity among children and adolescents in China from 1981 to 2010: A meta-analysis. *PLoS ONE.* 2012; 7(12):e51949. doi:10.1371/journal.pone.0051949.

53. Davis J, Juarez D, Hodges K. Relationship of ethnicity and body mass index with the development of hypertension and hyperlipidemia. *Ethn Dis.* 2013; 23(1):65–70.

54. Alqahtani N, Scott J. Childhood obesity estimates based on WHO and IOTF reference values. *J Obes Weight Loss Ther.* 2015; 5:249–251.

55. Hull HR, Thornton J, Wang J, et al. Fat-free mass index: Changes and race/ethnic differences in adulthood. *Int J Obes (Lond).* 2011; 35(1):121–127.

56. Bao Y, Lu J, Wang C, et al. Optimal waist circumference cutoffs for abdominal obesity in Chinese. *Atherosclerosis.* 2008; 201(2):378–384.

57. Sabin MA, Wong N, Campbell P, Lee KJ, McCallum Z, Werther GA. Where should we measure waist circumference

in clinically overweight and obese youth? *J Ped Child Health.* 2014; 50:519–524.

58. Wu CH, Heshka S, Wang J, et al. Truncal fat in relation to total body fat: Influences of age, sex, ethnicity and fatness. *Int J Obesity.* 2007; 31(9):1384–1391.

59. Lear SA, Humphries KH, Kohli S, et al. Visceral adipose tissue accumulation differs according to ethnic background: Results of the Multicultural Community Health Assessment Trial (MCHAT). *Am J Clin Nutr.* 2007; 86(2):353–359.

60. Kagawa M, Binns CB, Hills AP. Body composition and anthropometry in Japanese and Australian Caucasian males and Japanese females. *Asia Pac J Clin Nutr.* 2007; 16(Suppl 1): 31–36.

61. Waist Circumference and Waist-Hip Ratio Report of a WHO Expert Consultation GENEVA, 8–11 December 2008.

62. Rush EC, Goedecke JH, Jennings C, et al. BMI, fat, and muscle differences in urban women of five ethnicities from two countries. *Int J Obesity.* 2007; 31(8):1232–1239.

63. Punyadeera C, van der Merwe MT, Crowther NJ, et al. Weight-related differences in glucosemetabolism and free fatty acid production in two South African population groups. *Int J Obes Relat Metabol Disord.* 2001; 25(8):1196–1205.

64. Punyadeera C, van der Merwe MT, Crowther NJ, et al. Ethnic differences in lipid metabolism in two groups of obese South African women. *J Lipid Re.* 2001; 42(5):760–767.

65. van der Merwe MT, Crowther NJ, Schlaphoff GP, et al. Evidence for insulin resistance in black women from South Africa. *Int J Obes Relat Metabol Disord.* 2000; 24(10):1340–1346.

66. Carroll JF, Chiapa AL, Rodriquez M, et al. Visceral fat, waist circumference, and BMI: Impact of race/ethnicity. *Obes (Silver Spring).* 2008; 16(3):600–607.

67. Rush EC, Freitas I, Plank LD. Body size, body composition, and fat distribution: Comparative analysis of European, Maori, Pacific Island and Asian Indian adults. *Brit J Nutr.* 2009; 102(4):632–641.

68. Leahy S, O'Neill C, Sohun R, Toomey C, Jakeman P. Generalized equations for the prediction of percentage of body fat anthropometry in adult men and women aged 18–81 years. *Br J Nutr.* 2013; 109(4):678–658.

69. Fryar CD, Gu Q, Ogden CL. Anthropometric reference data for children and adults: United States, 2007–2010. National Center for Health Statistics. *Vital Health Stat.* 2012; 11(252).

70. Ramírez-Vélez R, López-Cifuentes MF, Correa-Bautista JE, et al. Triceps and subscapular skinfold thickness percentiles and cut-offs for overweight and in a population-based sample of schoolchildren adolescents in Bogota, Colombia. *Nutrients.* 2016; 8:595–610. doi:10.3390/nu8100595.

71. Freeman, DS, Katzmarzyk PT, Dietz WH, Srinivasan SR, Berenson GS. Relation of body mass index and skinfold thicknesses to cardiovascular disease risk factors in children: The Bogalusa Heart Study. *Am J Clin Nutr.* 2009; 90:210–216.

72. NHANES, 2011. Freeman D, Ogden C, Kit BK. Interrelationships between BMI, skinfold thicknesses, percent body fat, and cardiovascular disease risk factors. *BMC Ped.* 2015; 15(1):188–197.

73. Toomey C, McCreesh K, Leahy S, Jakeman P. Technical considerations for accurate measurement of subcutaneous adipose tissue thickness using B-mode ultrasound. *Ultrasound.* 2011; 19(2):91–96. https://doi.org/10.1258/ult.2011.010057.

74. Hume P, and Marfelli-Jones M. The importance of accurate site location for skinfold measurements. *J Sports Sci.* 2008; 26:1333–1340. doi: 1080/02640410802165707.

75. Sachdeva S, Dewan P, Shah D, Malhotra RK, Gupta P. Mid-upper arm circumference v. weight-for-height Z-score for predicting mortality in hospitalized children under 5 years of age. *Public Health Nutr.* 2016; 19(14):2513–2520.

76. Saito R, Ohkawa S, Ichinose S, Nishikino M, Ikegaya N, Kumagai H. Validity of mid-arm muscular area measured by anthropometry in nonobese patients with increased muscle atrophy and variation of subcutaneous fat thickness. *Eur J Clin Nutr.* 2010; 64:899–904.

77. Mazicioglu MM, Yalcin BM, Ozturk A, Ustunbas HB, Kurtoglu S. Anthropometric risk factors for elevated blood pressure in adolescents in Turkey aged 11–17. *Pediatr Nephrol.* 2010; 25:2327–2334.

78. Gueresi P, Miglio R, Cevenini E, Gualdi Russo E. Arm measurements as determinants of further survival in centenarians. *Exp Gerontol.* 2014; 58:230–234.

79. Aparecida Leandro-Merhi V, Luiz Braga de Aquino J, Gonzaga Teixeira de Camargo J. Agreement between body mass index, calf circumference, arm circumference, habitual energy intake and the MNA in hospitalized elderly. *J Nutr Health Aging.* 2012; 16(2):128–132.

80. Kondrup J, Rasmussen HH, Hamberg O, Stanga Z. Nutritional risk screening (NRS 2002): A new method based on an analysis of controlled clinical trials. *Clin Nutr.* 2003; 22(3): 321–336.

81. Becker PJ, Carney LN, Corkins MR, et al. Consensus statement of the Academy of Nutrition and Dietetics/American Society for Parenteral and Enteral Nutrition: Indicators recommended for the identification and documentation of pediatric malnutrition (undernutrition). *J Acad Nutr Diet.* 2014; 114:1988–2000.

82. Rasmussen J, Anderson A, Fisker AB, et al. Mid-upper arm circumference and mid-upper arm circumference z-score: The best predictor of mortality? *Eur J of Clin Nutr.* 2012; 66:998–100.

83. Kulathinal S, Freese R, Korkalo L, Ismael C, Mutanen M. Mid-arm circumference is associated with biochemically determined nutritional status indicators among adolescent girls in Central Mozambique. *Nutr Res.* 2016; 36: 835–844.

84. Tang AM, Dong K, Deitchler M, et al. *Use of Cutoffs for Mid-Upper Arm Circumference (MUAC) as an Indicator or Predictor of Nutritional and Health-Related Outcomes in Adolescents and Adults: A systematic Review.* Washington, DC: FHI 360/ FANTA; 2013.

85. Fernernandez-del-Valle M, Larumbe-Zabala E, Graell-Berna M, Perez-R. Anthropometric changes in adolescents with anorexia nervosa in response to resistance training. *Eating Weight Disord—Stud Anorexia, Bulimia Obes.* 2015; 20(3):311–317.

86. Lam PY, Marshall SK, Harjit GD, Coelho JS, Cairns J. Pinch, or step: Evaluating the effectiveness and acceptability of mid-upper arm circumference measurements in adolescents with eating disorders. *Eat Behav.* 2016; 22:72–75.

87. Portero-McLellan KC, Staudt C, Silva FR, Delbue Bernardi JL, Baston Frenhani P, Leandro Mehri VA. The use of calf circumference measurement as an anthropometric tool to monitor nutritional status in elderly inpatients. *J Nutr Health Aging.* 2010; 14:266–270.

88. Landi F, Onder G, Russo A, et al. Calf circumference, frailty and physical performance among older adults living in the community. *Clin Nutr.* 2014; 33:539–544.

89. Singh R, Gupta S. Relationship of calf circumference with bone mineral density and hip geometry: A hospital-based cross-sectional study. *Arch Osteoporos.* 2015; 10:17–26.

90. Kwon HR, Han KA, Ahn HJ, Lee JH, Park GS, Min KW. The correlations between extremity circumferences with total

and regional amounts of skeletal muscle and muscle strength in obese women with type 2 diabetes. *Diabetes Metab J.* 2011; 35(4):374–383.

91. Min JY, Cho JS, Lee KJ, Park JB, Mi KB. Thigh circumference and low ankle brachial index in US adults: Results from them National Health and Nutrition Examination Survey 1999–2004. *Int J Cardiol.* 2013; 163:40–45.

92. Cruz-Jentoft AJ, Baeyens JP, Bauer JM, et al. Sarcopenia: European consensus on definition and diagnosis; Report of the European Group on Sarcopenia in older people. *Age Ageing.* 2010; 39:412–423.

93. Hsu WC, Tsai AC, Wang JY. Calf circumference is more effective than body mass index in predicting emerging care needs of older adults: Results of a nation cohort study. *Clin Nutr.* 2016; 35:735–740.

94. Chung JY, Kang HT, Lee HR, Lee Y. Body composition and its association with cardiometabolic risk factors in the elderly: A focus on sarcopenic obesity. *Arch Gerontol Geriatr.* 2013; 56:270–278.

95. Christensen HM, Kistorp C, Schou M, et al. Prevalence of cachexia in chronic heart failure and characteristics of body composition and metabolic status. *Endocrine.* 2012; 43:626–634.

96. Thibault R, Le Gallic E, Picard-Kossovsky M, Darmaun D, Chambellan A. Assessment of nutritional status and body composition in patients with COPD: Comparison of several methods. *Rev Mal Respir.* 2010; 27:693–702.

97. Nordén J, Grönberg AM, Bosaeus I, et al. Nutrition impact symptoms and body composition in patients with COPD. *Eur J of Clin Nutr.* 2015; 69:256–269.

98. Carberry AE, Colditz PB, Lingwood BE. Body Composition From Birth to 4.5 Months in Infants Born to Non-Obese Women. *Pediatr Res.* 2010; 68(1):84–88. doi: 10.1203/00006450-201011001-00161.

99. Muscaritoli M, Anker SD, Argiles J, et al. Consensus definition of sarcopenia, cachexia, and pre-cachexia: Joint document elaborated by Special Interest Group (SIG) "cachexia-anorexia in chronic wasting disease" and "nutrition in geriatrics." *Clin Nutr.* 2010; 29:154–159.

100. Booth A, Magnuson A, Foster M. Detrimental and protective fat: Body fat distribution and its relation to metabolic disease. *Horm Mol Biol Clin Invest.* 2014; 17(1):13–17.

101. Koutsari D, Ali AH, Mundi MS, Jensen MD. Storage of circulating free fatty acid in adipose tissue of postabsorptive humans quantitative measures and implications for body fat distribution. *Diabetes.* 2011; 60:2032–2040.

102. Messier V, Karelis AD, Prud'homme D, Primeau V, Brochu M, Rabasa-Lhoret R. Identifying metabolically healthy but obese individuals in sedentary postmenopausal women. *Obesity.* 2010; 18:911–917.

103. Fox CS, Massaro JM, Hoffman U, et al. Abdominal visceral and subcutaneous adipose tissue compartments: Association with metabolic factors in the Framingham Heart Study. *Circulation.* 2007;116:39–48.

104. Porter SA, Massaro JM, Hoffmann U, Vasan RS, O'Donnel CJ, Fox CS. Abdominal subcutaneous adipose tissue: A protective fat depot? *Diabetes Care.* 2009; 32:1068–1075.

105. Thibault R, Genton L, Pichard C. Body composition: Why, when and for who? *Eur Soc Clin Nutr Metabol.* 2012; 31:435–447.

106. Murphy AJ, Ellis KJ, Kurpad AV, Preston T, Slater C. Total body potassium revisited. *Eur J Clin Nutr.* 2014; 68:153–154.

107. Wang A, Heshka S, Pietrobelli A, et al. A new total body potassium method to estimate total body skeletal muscle mass in children. *J Nutr.* 2007; 137: 1988–1991.

108. Murphy AG, Davies PSW. Body cell mass index in children: Interpretation of total body potassium results. *Br J Nutr* 2008; 100:666–668.

109. Fosbol MO, Zerahn B. Contemporary methods of body composition measurement. *Clin Physiol Funct Imaging.* 2015; 35:81–97.

110. Pou KM, Massaro JM, Hoffmann U, Lieb K. Patterns of abdominal fat distribution: The Framingham Heart Study. *Diabetes Care.* 2009; 32:481–485.

111. Yim JY, Kim D, Lim SH, et al. Sagittal abdominal diameter is a strong anthropometric measure of visceral adipose tissue in the Asian general population. *Diabetes Care.* 2010; 33(12): 2665–2670. http://dx.doi.org/10.2337/dc10–0606.

112. de Souza NC, de Oliveira EP. Sagittal abdominal diameter shows better correlation with cardiovascular risk factors than waist circumference and BMI. *J Diabetes Metabol Disord.* 2013; 12:41–46.

113. Dahlén EM, Bjarnegård N, Länne T, Nystrom FH, Östgren CJ. Sagittal abdominal diameter is a more independent measure compared with waist circumference to predict arterial stiffness in subjects with type 2 diabetes: A prospective observational cohort study. *Cardiovasc Diabetol.* 2013; 2:55–63.

114. Leong DP, Teo KK, Rangarajan S, et al. Prognostic value of grip strength: Findings from the Prospective Urban Rural Epidemiology (PURE) study. *Lancet.* 2015; 386: 266–273.

115. Roberts HC, Denison HJ, Martin HJ, et al. A review of the measurement of grip strength in clinical and epidemiological studies: Towards a standardised approach. *Age Ageing.* 2011; 40: 423–429.

116. Bohannon RW. Hand-grip dynamometry predicts future outcomes in aging adults. *J Geriatric Phys Ther.* 2008; 31(1):3–10.

117. Ploegmakers JJ, Hepping AM, Geertzen JH, Bulstra SK, Stevens M. Grip strength is strongly associated with height, weight and gender in childhood: A cross sectional study of 2241 children and adolescents providing reference values. *J Physiother.* 2013; 59:255–261.

118. de Souza MA, de Jesus Alves de Baptista CR, Baranauskas Benedicto MM, Pizzato TM, Mattiello-Sverzut AC. Normative data for hand grip strength in healthy children measured with a bulb dynamometer: A cross-sectional study. *Physiother.* 2014; 100:313–318.

119. Life Measurement Inc., Concord, CA, USA. www.bodpod.com. Accessed December 1, 2016.

120. Fosbol MO, Zerahn B, Noreen EE, Lemon PW. Reliability of air displacement plethysmography in a large, heterogeneous sample. *Med Sci Sports Exerc.* 2006; 38:1505–1509.

121. Hillier SE, Beck L, Petropoulou A, Clegg ME. A comparison of body composition measurement techniques *J Hum Nutr Diet.* 2014; 27: 626–631.

122. Bredella MA, Gill CM, Keating LK, et al. Assessment of abdominal fat compartments using DXA in premenopausal women from anorexia nervosa to morbid obesity. *Obes (Silver Spring).* 2013; 12:2458–2464.

123. Breithaupt P, Colley RC, Adamo KB. Body composition measured by dual-energy X-ray absorptiometry half-body scans in obese children. *Acta Pediatr.* 2011; 100: e260–e266.

124. Malouf J, Digregorio S, Del RL, et al. Fat tissue measurements by dual-energy x-ray absorptiometry: cross-calibration of 3 different fan-beam instruments. *J Clin Densitom.* 2013; 16:212–222.

125. Hangartner TN, Warner S, Braillon P, Jankowski L, Shepherd J. The official positions of the International Society for Clinical Densitometry: Acquisition of dual-energy x-ray absorptiometry body composition and considerations regarding analysis and repeatability of measures. *J Clin Densitom*. 2013; 16: 520–530.

126. Libber J, Binkley N, Krueger D. Clinical observations in total body DXA: Technical aspects of positioning and analysis. *J Clin Densitom*. 2012; 15:282–289.

127. LaForggia J, Dollman J , Dale MJ, Withers RT, Hill AM. Validation of DXA body composition estimates in obese men and women. *Obes (Silver Spring)*. 2009; 17:821–826.

128. Fosbol MO, DuPont A, Alslev L, Zerahn B. The effect of (99m) Tc on dual energy x-ray absorptiometry measurement of body composition and bone mineral density. *J Clin Densitom*. 2012; 16:297–301.

129. Lee S, Kuk JL. Changes in fat and skeletal muscle with exercise training in obese adolescents: Comparison of whole-body MRI and dual energy X-ray absorptiometry. *Obes (Silver Spring)*. 2013; 21:2063–2071.

130. Carey JJ, Delaney MF. T-scores and Z-scores. *Clinic Rev in Bone Min Metab*. 2010; 8(3):113–121.

131. Schoushoe JT, Shepherd JA, Bilezikian JP, Baim S. Executive summary of the 2013 International Society for Clinical Densitometry position development conference on bone densitometry. *J Clin Densitom*. 2013; 16(4):455–466.

132. Nelson HD, Haney EM, Dana T, Bougatsos C, Chou R. Screening for osteoporosis: An update for the US Preventive Services Task Force. *Ann Intern Med*. 2010; 153(2):99–111.

133. Kalkwarf HJ, Gilsanz V, Lappe JM, et al. Tracking of Bone Mass and Density during Childhood and Adolescence. *J Clin Endocrinol Metab*. 2010; 95(4):1690–1698.

134. FRAX® fracture risk assessment tool. https://www.shef.ac.uk/FRAX/. Accessed December 1, 2016.

135. Wabel P, Chamney P, Mossi U, et al. Importance of whole body bioimpedence spectroscopy for the management of fluid balance *Blood Purif*. 2009; 27(1):75–80.

136. Vilaça KH, Paula FJ, Ferriolli E, Lima NK, Marchini JS, Moriguti JC. Body composition assessment of undernourished older subjects by dual energy x-ray absorptiometry and bioelectric impedance analysis. *J Nutr Health Aging*. 2011; 15(6):439–443.

137. Haverkort EB, Reijven PL, Binnekade JM, et al. Bioelectrical impedance analysis to estimate body composition in surgical and oncological patients: A systematic review. *Eur J Clin Nutr*. 2015; 69:3–13.

138. Maughan RJ, Shirreffs SM, Leiper JB. Errors in the estimation of hydration status from changes in body mass. *J Sports Sci*. 2007; 25(7):797–804.

139. Sivapathy S, Chang CY, Chai WJ, Ang YK, Yim HS. Assessment of hydration status and body composition of athlete and non-athlete subjects using bioelectrical impedance analysis. *J Phys Ed Sport*. 2013; 13(2):157–162.

140. Jaffrin MY, Morel H. Body fluid volumes measurement by impedance: A review of bioimpedence spectroscopy (BIS) and bioimpedence analysis (BIA) methods. *Med Eng Phys*. 2008;30(10): 1257–1269.

141. Gray C, MacGillivray TJ, Eeley C, et al. Magnetic resonance imaging with k-means clustering objectively measures whole muscle volume compartments in sarcopenia/cancer cachexia. *Clin Nutr*. 2011; 30:106–111.

142. MacDonald AJ, Greig CA, Baracos V. The advantages and limitations of cross-sectional body composition analysis. *Curr Opin Support Palliat Care*. 2011; 5:342–349.

143. Wagner DR. Ultrasound as a tool to assess body fat. *J Obesity*. 2013; 1–9. http://dx.doi.org/10.1155/2013/280713 Accessed November 21, 2016.

144. O'Neil D, Cronin O, O'Neil S, et al. Application of a sub-set of skinfold sites for ultrasound measurement of subcutaneous adiposity and percentage body fat estimation in athletes. *Int J Sports Med*. 2016; 37(05):359–363.

145. Leahy S, Toomey C, McCreesh K, O'Neill C, Jakeman P. Ultrasound measurement of subcutaneous adipose tissue thickness accurately predicts total and segmental body fat of young adults. *Ultrasound Med Biol*. 2012; 38:28–34.

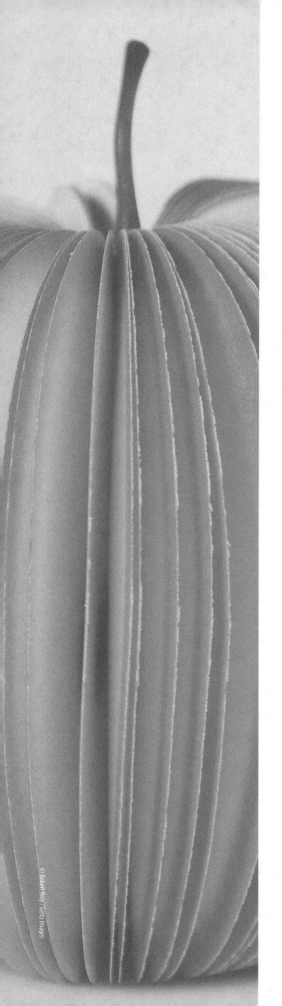

# Method of Evaluation: Biochemical Assessment

CHAPTER 8    Biomarkers in Nutritional Assessment

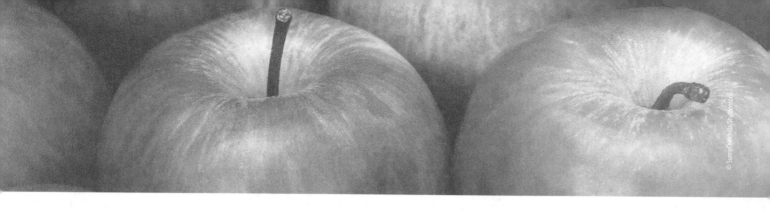

**Dr. Nancy Munoz**, DCN, MHA, RDN, FAND

# CHAPTER 8

# Biomarkers in Nutritional Assessment

## CHAPTER OUTLINE

- Introduction
- Use of Biochemical Measures
- Protein Levels
- Assessing Mineral Levels
- Assessing Vitamin Levels
- Blood Chemistry Studies
- Chapter Summary

## LEARNING OBJECTIVES

After reading this chapter, the learner will be able to:

1. Increase understanding of biochemical markers used in the nutritional assessment of individuals and populations.
2. Define the biochemical markers used in the diagnosis and management of different nutritional deficiencies.
3. Understand the signs and symptoms associated with abnormal biochemical serum-level concentrations.
4. Recognize the laboratory values used in assessing body reserves of vitamin and mineral levels.

## ▶ Introduction

**Biomarker assessment** involves the use of biologically available chemicals inside the body that perform as objective indicators to help clinicians, researchers, and policymakers determine diet and nutrition recommendations to address disease and improve both individual and public health. Biomarker data is one assessment method used by physicians, registered dietitian nutritionists (RDNs), scientists, and those involved in public health assess whether the intake of specific nutrients is inadequate or excessive. Evaluating biomarkers and measuring nutrient intake from foods and dietary supplements are the two main tools used to assess a population's nutritional status.[1] When compared to community and dietary assessments, using biomarker indicators is an objective, more precise approach of measuring nutritional status without the bias of self-reported dietary intake errors, and also without the challenge of intra-individual and diet variability.[2-5]

The National Academies of Science, Engineering, and Medicine's Health and Medicine Division (HMD) has documented the absence of nutrition biochemical markers as a knowledge gap that requires further research. Current knowledge gaps include the need for predictive biomarkers that can forecast functional outcomes and chronic diseases, as well as the need to improve dietary assessment and planning methods.[2] Nutrition biomarkers have their own set of limitations. This includes cost and degree of invasiveness.[6]

A **nutritional biomarker** can be any organic test used as an indicator of nutritional status if it relates to the intake or metabolism of dietary components. This can be a biochemical, functional, or clinical index of the status of an essential nutrient or other dietary component.[7] As an assessment tool, nutrition biomarkers are used to validate self-reported intake methods, assess intake of dietary items when the use of food-composition databases is not possible, and to more accurately link dietary intake with disease risk and nutritional status.[8]

## ▶ Use of Biochemical Measures

> **Preview** The use of biomarkers is common in both research and clinical practice.[9] In nutrition research, a biomarker is a unique biological or biologically derived molecule found in blood, other body fluids, or tissues that is a sign of a process, an event, a condition, or a disease.

The use of biomarkers is common in both clinical research and clinical practice. Some biomarkers have been shown to accurately forecast pertinent clinical outcomes across a range of treatments and populations; for others, the validity is assumed.[10]

### What Is a Biomarker?

In general, HMD defines a biomarker as "a characteristic that is objectively measured and evaluated as an indicator of normal biological processes, pathogenic processes, or pharmacologic responses to a therapeutic intervention."[9] In nutrition-related research, a biomarker is defined as a distinct biological or biologically derived molecule found in blood, other body fluids, or tissues that is a sign of a process, an event, a condition, or a disease.[11] In the nutrition framework, biomarkers are frequently classified as markers of exposure, status, and function or effect.

Biomarkers dealing with exposure can help determine dietary deficiencies as a result of chronic health conditions; intake for specific nutrient(s) for an individual, group, or community; and the needs and risks linked to the consumption level. Status biomarkers describe how a person or a segment of the population (group) relate to accepted standards of nutrition and help determine interventions related to these standards.[11]

Function biomarkers help describe the role of specific nutrients and potential interactions between different nutrients in biological systems, and classify the role of nutrients across the life span and under different physiological states. Effect biomarkers help us understand the direct and indirect results—that is, those affecting cells and those affecting cells and system function—of a nutrient deficiency.[11]

> **Recap** In the nutrition framework, biomarkers are classified as markers of exposure, status, and function or effect.

## ▶ Protein Levels

> **Preview** Several laboratory tests have been used to measure serum protein concentrations. These include albumin, prealbumin, transferrin, and retinol binding protein.

In the clinical setting, the laboratory tests most commonly used in the assessment of individuals are measurements of serum protein concentrations, specifically albumin, prealbumin, and transferrin. Of the three proteins, albumin has been the most extensively researched.

Studies show a strong link between decreased serum albumin levels and high risk of comorbidities and mortality. Jellinge et al. (2014) conducted a prospective and observational cohort study of all patients admitted to a Danish hospital between 2008 and 2009. The study looked at the 30-day mortality rate of all patients with hypoalbuminemia. The researchers reported that mortality for patients with hypoalbuminemia was 16.3% compared to 4.3% for the patients with a normal albumin level.[12]

Serum albumin is not a reliable indicator of nutritional status. Many clinical variables—including hydration status, organ function, infection, and metabolic stress—affect albumin results. For this reason, this protein has been deemed a better marker of severity of illness than of nutritional status.[13]

## Creatinine Excretion and the Creatinine Height Index

### Creatinine

Creatinine has been identified as a potential biomarker for red meat intake. This compound is specific to meat intake and is excreted in the urine.[14]

The creatinine blood test is used to measure kidney function. It is commonly requested as part of a basic metabolic panel (BMP) with other laboratory tests such as blood urea nitrogen (BUN), as well as tests that are obtained to assess the function of the body's major organs. BMP tests are used to screen healthy individuals as part of routine physical exams and to help diagnose acute and chronic illnesses in different care settings. Occasionally, creatinine may be measured as part of a renal panel to estimate kidney function.[15]

Results from a creatinine test are incorporated into calculations that help determine kidney function. When combined with data on age, weight, and gender, blood creatinine levels are used to calculate the **estimated glomerular filtration rate (eGFR)**. It is used as a screening test to assess kidney damage. Blood and urine creatinine levels can be used to estimate a creatinine clearance. This test helps determine how efficiently the kidneys are at cleaning small molecules such as creatinine out of the blood.[15]

Urine creatinine is also used with several other urine tests as a correction factor. Urine concentration varies during the day as a result of fluctuations in the amount of fluid released by the body, in addition to the body's waste products. Because creatinine is produced and removed from the body at a fairly constant rate, the amount of urine creatinine can be used to compare to the amount of other substances. The constant excretion rate is helpful when examining a 24-hour recall

and random urine samples. For instance, the urine's albumin-to-creatinine ratio (ACR) can assess how much albumin is leaking from the kidneys into the urine and be used to determine risk for kidney injury.[14]

Normal levels of blood creatinine are 0.6 to 1.2 milligrams per deciliter (mg/dL) in adult males and 0.5 to 1.1 mg/dL in adult females. A decreased **creatinine clearance** can be an indication of kidney injury, bacterial infection, prostate disease, kidney stones, or other triggers for urinary-tract obstruction.[14]

### Creatinine Height Index

The **creatinine height index (CHI)** is a measurement of a 24-hour urinary excretion collection of creatinine, which is generally related to the individual's muscle mass and an indicator of malnutrition, particularly in young males.[16]

When completing a clinical assessment, an individual's creatinine excretion is compared with the expected excretion rate of a person of similar height and ideal weight. Concrete population standards for this measurement do not exist. Calculated ideal values are applied from the results of the 24-hour excretions of healthy children and adults while on a creatinine or a creatinine-free diet. **TABLE 8.1** shows the formula to calculate CHI values and interpret them.[17]

This test is theoretically beneficial when edema or obesity interferes with obtaining an accurate body weight measurement. Because this measurement relies on the comparison of results to an ideal body weight range as a reference standard, estimates can be inaccurate in individuals above the midrange of the ideal weight-for-height measurement. The test is considered invalid in individuals with reduced urine output, amputations, kidney and liver failure, sepsis, and trauma. Because many factors contribute to decreased creatinine excretion, CHI calculations lead to overestimation of muscle-mass depletion. This makes the CHI an unreliable measurement. Creatinine elimination is

---

**TABLE 8.1** Formula to calculate CHI value

CHI = (actual 24-hour creatinine excretion ÷ ideal 24-hour creatinine excretion) × 100

**Results:**
Above 80% = no protein depletion
60% to 80% = moderate protein depletion
Under 60% = severe protein depletion

Data from Alpers DH, Stenson WF, Taylor BE, Bier DM. Manual of Nutritional Therapeutics. Fifth Edition (2008). Wolters Kluwer/ Lippincott Williams and Wilkins.

higher in individuals engaged in vigorous exercise, who consume red meats, and who are on corticosteroid, testosterone, or antibiotic therapies.[17]

## Nitrogen Balance as a Measurement of Protein Intake

### Dietary Protein

Dietary protein is an essential nutrient for many physiological, metabolic, and structural processes in the human body. Proteins can act as enzymes and have a role in maintaining membrane structures. They transport certain compounds through the blood. Their components, amino acids (AA), serve as precursors for nucleic acids, hormones, vitamins, and other important molecules. The recommended dietary allowance (RDA) is 0.80 grams (g) per kilogram of body weight (kg/BW) of good-quality protein. The RDA for dietary protein was established using the research on nitrogen balance at the time the HMD published the RDA.[18]

Optimal nutrient intake identifies a point in which individual and population nutrient intake meets the cell's metabolic, physiologic, and structural needs without providing too little (contributing to undernutrition) or too much (overnutrition). Optimal nutrient intake contributes to optimal health.[19] As noted above, dietary protein is an essential nutrient contributing to cellular and organ function. To promote optimal health, not only must individuals consume sufficient protein to meet their needs, they must also consume **nonprotein calories** in sufficient amount so that protein is not used to meet energy needs. Likewise, AAs need to be present in the diet in the right balance (in terms of **dispensable amino acids**, **indispensable amino acids**, and **conditionally indispensable amino acids**) in order for ideal protein use to occur.[20]

Worldwide, malnutrition contributes to an estimated one-third of all child deaths.[21] In the United States, protein-energy malnutrition (PEM) is the most common form of nutritional deficiency in hospitalized patients. As many as 50% of all patients admitted to hospitals have some level of malnutrition. A survey conducted in a large children's hospital identified that the prevalence of acute and chronic malnutrition was greater than 50%.[22]

### Nitrogen Balance

**Nitrogen balance** is an assessment parameter that is consistently dependable for measuring protein status in the body. Insufficient protein intake is seen as decreased growth in height and weight in infants and children.[18] Note that the presence of edema and ascites makes the weight–height associations unreliable measurements.[23] Older literature describes low levels of albumin, prealbumin, and other measurements of protein as indicators of malnutrition. We now believe these assessment parameters are an indicator of severity of disease and inflammation and not sensitive indicators of nutritional status.

Nitrogen balance has been deemed the most commonly acceptable process of measuring protein needs. This measurement is defined as the difference between nitrogen intake and nitrogen excretion in the animal body such that a greater intake results in a positive balance and an increased excretion causes a negative balance.[24] See **FIGURE 8.1**. To date, nitrogen balance is the method that has generated the most amount of data in terms of establishing this parameter as a measurement of total protein (nitrogen) requirement. Nitrogen balance shows whether the needs of individuals are met, exceeded, or deficient. Inadequate intake of protein contributes to the development of negative nitrogen balance. To define total protein (nitrogen) needs, high-quality proteins are used as test proteins to measure the negative nitrogen balance that results from inadequate intake of indispensable AAs.[18]

The use of nitrogen balance as a measure of nutritional protein status has its limitations. In adults, the rate of urea turnover is slow. To ensure that a new steady state of nitrogen excretion is being recorded, an adjustment period must be allowed for each level of dietary protein being tested.[25] Measuring nitrogen excretion to determine nitrogen balance is a precise process. Overestimating intake and underestimating excretion are common occurrences that contribute to false-positive results for nitrogen balance.[18] Another limitation of the nitrogen balance method is that because the requirement is demarcated for the individual, and studies seldom specify the precise amount of protein necessary to generate a zero balance, research must include different levels of protein intake in the range being assessed so that estimations of individual requirements can be extrapolated.[18,26] One last limitation is that the dermal and miscellaneous losses must be accounted for. These losses can be influenced by environmental conditions and can be extremely hard to measure. Accounting for dermal and miscellaneous nitrogen losses can have a substantial effect on the final estimates for AA requirements.[27]

## Serum Proteins

As previously mentioned, serum proteins such as albumin, transferrin, and prealbumin (transthyretin) have traditionally been used by clinicians to determine an individual's nutritional status. Recent

**Calculating Nitrogen Balance:**

1. Define nitrogen (N) lost in urine via a 24-hour urinary urea nitrogen (UUN) test.
2. Add 4* to the UUN to account for nonurinary losses of N.
3. Establish nitrogen consumed by dividing the daily protein intake by 6.25.
4. (Value from 2) – (value from 3) = nitrogen balance.

If the nitrogen balance is 0, the person is consuming the correct amount of protein to promote maintenance. If the nitrogen balance is negative (–), increase the protein intake by a factor obtained by multiplying the NB results by 6.25. If the goal is to replete N stores, then increase protein intake over what would result in NB.

**Calculation example:**

Data: Intake: 80 grams of protein. UUN = 15 g

*A factor of 4 is used to appraise the nitrogen losses from nonurine sources such as sweat and feces.

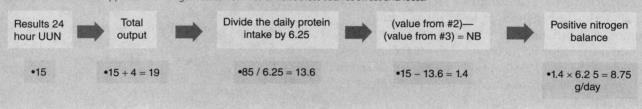

| Results 24 hour UUN | Total output | Divide the daily protein intake by 6.25 | (value from #2)— (value from #3) = NB | Positive nitrogen balance |
|---|---|---|---|---|
| •15 | •15 + 4 = 19 | •85 / 6.25 = 13.6 | •15 – 13.6 = 1.4 | •1.4 × 6.2 5 = 8.75 g/day |

**FIGURE 8.1** Nitrogen balance (NB) calculations.

Data from Nitrogen Balance Caluclator. SurgicalCriticalCare.net: Official website of the Orlando Health Surgical Critical Care Fellowship http://www.surgicalcriticalcare.net/Resources/nitrogen.php. Published 2015. Accessed July 20, 2017.

research contradicts this practice. **TABLE 8.2** shows the significance of abnormal values for these laboratory markers.

## Albumin

Albumin is a serum hepatic protein that functions as a carrier molecule for many minerals, hormones, and fatty acids. It also helps maintain oncotic pressure in the capillaries. Albumin has a half-life of 14–20 days.[28]

Most of the albumin in the body is stored in the extravascular compartment, with only approximately 5% being stored in the liver. This is why an individual's daily protein intake has little influence on his or her albumin level.[29] Albumin is categorized as a negative acute-phase protein. Albumin levels are affected by inflammatory conditions and medications, particularly those that affect liver function such as hepatic failure, burns, sepsis, trauma, postsurgical states, and cancer.[30]

| **TABLE 8.2** Laboratory makers | | |
|---|---|---|
| **Laboratory Marker** | **Reference Range (mg/dL)** | **Significance of Abnormal Values** |
| Albumin | 3.5–5.0 | Increased with dehydration<br>Decreased with edema, hepatic disease, malabsorption, diarrhea, burns, eclampsia, ESRD, stress, overhydration, cancer, inflammation |
| Transferrin | 212–360 | Increased with inadequate iron stores, iron-deficiency anemia, acute hepatitis, polycythemia, oral contraceptive use, pregnancy<br>Decreased with pernicious and sickle-cell anemia, infection, cancer, hepatic disease, nephrotic syndrome, thalassemia |
| Prealbumin | 18–38 | Increased with renal failure, Hodgkin's disease<br>Decreased with acute catabolic state, hepatic disease, stress, infection, surgery |

Data from Pronsky Z, Crowe JP. Food and Medication Interactions. 17th ed. Birchrunville, PA: Food Medication Interactions; 2012.

## Prealbumin

Prealbumin is also a negative acute-phase protein that originates in the liver. As such, levels are affected by inflammatory conditions and liver diseases. Prealbumin has a half-life of two to three days. Prealbumin is degraded in the kidneys, so any kidney injury contributes to increased prealbumin levels. One function of prealbumin is to act as a transport protein for thyroxine, the hormone secreted by the thyroid gland into the bloodstream.

In individuals with hyperthyroidism, prealbumin molecules are used to transport the excessive amount of thyroxine, thus reflecting low levels of measured prealbumin. In instances of hyperthyroidism, prealbumin levels will be high.[29] As seen in Table 8.2, prealbumin levels appear increased with renal failure and Hodgkin's disease. Prealbumin levels are decreased in the presence of hepatic disease, acute catabolic state, stress, infection, and surgery.[31]

## Transferrin

Transferrin is also a negative-phase reactant that has been used to measure the adequacy of nutritional status.[32] The role of transferrin is to transport iron from absorption centers in the duodenum and white-blood-cell macrophages to all tissues. Conditions such as iron-deficiency anemia contribute to increased transferrin levels. Conditions characterized by iron overload contribute to decreased transferrin levels.[33] As with prealbumin, transferrin levels are also increased in the presence of renal failure and with the use of oral contraceptives or estrogen formulas.[29]

## Retinol Binding Protein

Retinol binding protein (RBP) is a component of the retinol circulating complex. Abnormal values of vitamin A and zinc have an impact on RBP serum levels. The retinol circulating complex is degraded in the kidneys. Conditions that trigger renal insufficiency contribute to increased levels of RBP.[34]

Synthesized mostly in the liver, RBP must bind with retinol to activate retinol's secretion.[35] Other sites where RBP synthesis occurs include the kidney, the peritubular and Sertoli cells of the testis, the retinal pigment epithelium, and the choroid plexus of the brain.[36,37,38,39] Formation of RBP in the kidney occurs to return recovered retinol to the body's circulation. Synthesis in the other sites occurs as a way of cells that form the blood-organ barriers of the testis, retina, and brain.[40]

RBP circulates in the blood bound to prealbumin, its carrier protein. This protein-to-protein combination is believed to interact with certain cell receptors to deliver retinol to the target cells. Because of its association with prealbumin, this marker had traditionally been used as a measurement to determine an individual's protein status.[40]

Classified as a negative acute-phase inflammatory reactant, RBP in high concentrations has been associated with insulin resistance in individuals with obesity and type 2 diabetes (T2D).[41] High levels of RBP have also been associated with chronic inflammation, T2D, metabolic syndrome, and cardiovascular disease.[42]

> **Recap**    As a stand-alone assessment tool, biochemical assessments are influenced by non-nutrition aspects related to disease process, physiology, and environmental factors, to name a few. Data obtained from other assessment sources such as diet history and anthropometric references help frame the results obtained from biochemical assessments.

# ▶ Assessing Mineral Levels

> **Preview**    Nutritional mineral deficiencies are well documented and have specific signs and symptoms. Diseases associated with less than desirable mineral biochemical levels include cardiovascular disease, stroke, impaired cognitive function, cancer, eye diseases, poor bone health, and other conditions.

The levels of biochemical markers in the blood and urine can be useful in evaluating the adequacy of intake for individuals and the American population as a whole. These indicators can suggest cumulative intakes from foods, some fortified with micronutrients (such as iron, thiamin, riboflavin, niacin, and folate); and from dietary supplements that contain vitamins, minerals, or both. As previously mentioned, blood or urine concentrations of biochemical indicators can be influenced by factors other than diet, such as diseases.[43]

Nutritional deficiencies are well documented and have specific signs and symptoms. The Centers for Disease Control and Prevention (CDC) report that biochemical concentrations below optimum levels have been linked to adverse health effects. Diseases associated with less-than-desirable biochemical levels include cardiovascular disease, stroke, impaired cognitive function, cancer, eye diseases, and poor bone health. Consuming excessive amount of nutrients can contribute to signs and symptoms of toxicity.[43]

## Iron Levels

Iron functions as a component of proteins and enzymes. Most of the body's iron (approximately two-thirds) is found in hemoglobin (Hg), the protein in red blood cells (RBCs) that transports oxygen to tissues, and some 15% is in the myoglobin of muscle tissue.[44]

The typical American diet offers 10–15 mg of iron per day in the form of heme and nonheme iron.[44] The body absorbs 1–2 mg of iron per day to compensate for body losses (nonmenstruating women).[45] The *2015–2020 Dietary Guidelines for Americans* include iron as an underconsumed nutrient of public-health concern for adolescent adult premenopausal, and pregnant women because of the increased risk of iron deficiency in these groups.[46] Data from the National Health and Nutrition Examination Survey (NHANES) 2003–2006 show that the prevalence of iron deficiency anemia was higher in Mexican American (22%) and non-Hispanic (19%) women 12–49 years of age when compared to non-Hispanic white women (10%).[43]

In the United States, 7% to 9% of toddlers have been classified as iron deficient, and 2% to 3% have been cataloged as having iron-deficiency anemia. iron concentrations decrease in children, and by age 16 years, some 3% of adolescent females develop iron-deficiency anemia. Overall, in the last 40 to 50 years, the prevalence of iron deficiency has not changed much. However, some subgroups have seen great improvements in this condition. For instance, rates of iron deficiency in children up to 2 years of age has decreased from 23% to 11% between the study periods of 1976 to 1980 and 1999 to 2002. The prevalence of iron deficiency is greater in children living at or below the poverty level and in black and Hispanic children.

Iron deficiency is a challenging problem in countries with limited resources.[47] The World Health Organization (WHO) estimates that approximately half the 1.62 billion cases of anemia worldwide are caused by iron deficiency.[48] In most of Africa, Latin America, and Southeast Asia, frequency of anemia ranges from 45% to 65% in children, 20% to 60% in women, and 10% to 35% in men. Most of the anemia occurring in these countries is believed to be related to iron deficiency.[47] See **FIGURE 8.2**.

The RDA for all age groups of men and postmenopausal women is 8 mg/day. The RDA is much higher for premenopausal women, at 18 mg/day. The upper limit (UL) for adults is 45 mg/day. Adverse effects associated with intake over the UL include GI distress.[45]

## Stages of Iron Depletion

Laboratory test levels aid in determining the stages of iron deficiency. During Stage 1, bone-marrow iron stores are low, and hemoglobin and serum iron are within normal levels. During this stage, serum ferritin drops to below 20 ng/mL. The compensatory increase in iron absorption causes an increase in iron-binding capacity that is reflected as an increased transferrin level. Stage 2 is characterized by impaired **erythropoiesis**. In this stage, the transferrin level is

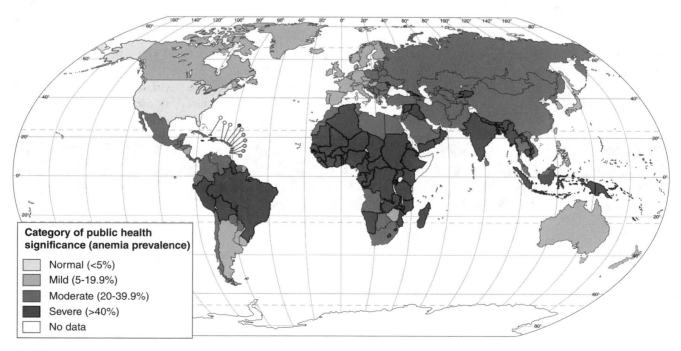

**FIGURE 8.2** Anemia in preschool children by country.

increased (> 8.5 mg/L), and serum iron and transferrin saturation are reduced to (< 50 $\mu$g/dL). Stage 3 is characterized by the presence of anemia with RBCs that appear to be normal. Throughout Stage 4, microcytosis and then hypochromia develop. Stage 5 is fully developed iron deficiency, which affects body tissues; full signs and symptoms are present.[49] See **TABLE 8.3**.

Iron-deficiency anemia is the most severe form of iron deficiency. It is associated with adverse effects such as decreased physical capability and negative pregnancy outcomes.[43,50,51] Even without the signs and symptoms of anemia, iron deficiency has been connected to negative outcomes on cognitive development in infants and adolescents.[43,52,53]

Iron overload is the accrual of excess iron in body tissues. This normally happens as a result of a genetic tendency to absorb above-normal amounts of iron. Increased amounts of iron in the body can also occur because of extreme consumption of iron supplements or numerous blood transfusions.[54] In cases of **hemochromatosis**, the iron collects in the parenchymal cells of several organs, predominantly the liver, followed by the heart and pancreas. This disorder can cause organ dysfunction that can lead to death.[54]

## Serum Ferritin

Serum ferritin is the biochemical indicator used by the NHANES and the CDC to evaluate iron status in the American population. Its main function is to store iron in a soluble, nontoxic form and to shield cells from iron-mediated oxidation–reduction reactions. In circulating blood, it acts as a delivery mechanism. Ferritin is found in the blood in minute amounts.[55] Serum ferritin is in balance with tissue stores. Low ferritin stores are one of the first changes seen in iron-deficiency anemia. Although low serum ferritin concentration is a sensitive indicator of iron deficiency, it does not reflect the severity or progression.[43,56] Ferritin is an acute-phase protein. As such, acute and chronic illnesses, malignancy, and autoimmune conditions may contribute to falsely elevated levels, thus potentially concealing an iron-deficiency diagnosis.[57]

Iron store levels are considered depleted when ferritin levels fall below 15 nanograms per millimeter (ng/mL) for individuals 5 years of age and older and 12 ng/mL for children younger than five years of age.[56] High ferritin levels are measured as values greater than 150 ng/mL for females 12–59 years of age and 200 ng/mL for males over 12 years old.[43]

## Transferring Receptors

Moving iron from one organ to another is done by the reversible binding of iron to the transport protein transferrin, which forms a complex with a highly specific transferrin receptor (TfR) found on cells' plasma membranes. The amount of intracellular transferrin available is controlled through the increased expression of cellular TfR concentration by iron-deficient cells.[43]

Measurement of the soluble transferrin receptor (sTfR), also referred to as *circulating transferrin receptor* or *serum transferrin receptor*, provides a quantifiable measure of total erythropoietic activity. The sTfR concentration in serum is directly proportional to the erythropoietic rate and inversely related to the amount of tissue iron available. In individuals with anemia of chronic disease, sTfR level is normal; it is higher, however, in those with iron-deficiency anemia. In the presence of iron-deficiency anemia, cellular membrane transferrin receptor density rises; as a result, condensed forms of sTfR appear in the serum in higher quantities.[58]

Calculation of the ratio of sTfR (conveyed as mg/L) to ferritin (stated as mcg/L), or the ratio of

**TABLE 8.3** Laboratory tests to determine the progression of iron-deficiency anemia

| Laboratory Test | Iron Storage | Iron Erythropoiesis | Iron-Deficiency Anemia |
|---|---|---|---|
| Hemoglobin | Normal | Normal | Low |
| Transferrin | Normal | Low | Low |
| Erythrocyte protoporphyrin | Normal | High | High |
| Plasma ferritin | Low | Low | Low |

Modified from Braunstein EM. Merck Manual- Iron Deficiency Anemia. 2017. http://www.merckmanuals.com/professional/hematology-and-oncology/anemias-caused-by-deficient-erythropoiesis /iron-deficiency-anemia. Accessed May 14, 2017.

sTfR to the logarithm (to the base 10) of the ferritin concentration, can be useful in determining the presence of anemia of chronic disease versus iron-deficiency anemia. In iron-deficiency anemia, the numerator sTfR is high and normal in the presence of anemia of chronic disease, while the denominator is low in iron-deficiency anemia and normal to high in anemia of chronic disease. A sTfR/log ferritin ratio of less than one is indicative of a diagnosis of anemia of chronic disease. A ratio higher than two implies incidence of iron-deficiency anemia. Individuals with mixed anemia (iron deficiency and chronic-disease anemia) also have a TfR–ferritin index greater than two.[59]

## Transferrin, Serum Iron, and Total Iron-Binding Capacity

Transferrin is a circulating transport protein for iron. It is high in iron-deficiency diagnosis but can be low in those with a diagnosis of anemia of chronic disease. Transferrin can also be reported as total iron-binding capacity (TIBC). The transferrin concentration (mg/dL) can be converted to TIBC (mcg/dL) by multiplying by 1.389.[60]

Transferrin saturation is the ratio of serum iron to TIBC (serum iron ÷ TIBC × 100). In iron deficiency, iron is level is low and TIBC is high, thus reflecting a lower transferrin saturation. Normal values for transferrin saturation range between 25% and 45%.[60] Whereas a level of 16% is typically used to screen for iron deficiency, levels below 10% are common in individuals with iron deficiency.[60]

Iron can be measured in serum or plasma. Serum iron quantifies circulating iron. Decreased serum iron levels are observed in the presence of iron deficiency, as well as in anemia of chronic inflammation and chronic disease. As a rule, serum iron relies on the effectiveness of iron recycling by bone marrow and reticuloendothelial macrophages, which is low in the presence of iron deficiency and anemia of chronic conditions. Serum iron can be influenced by dietary intake. On its own, low serum iron is not sufficient data to assign a diagnosis of anemia. It must be assessed in conjunction with other tests such as transferrin saturation and ferritin.[60]

TIBC is serum test used to measure either iron deficiency or iron overload. Normal TIBC is 250 to 450 $\mu$g/dL. It is used to analyze the transferrin saturation, which is considered a more sensitive indicator of iron status. In healthy individuals, approximately 20% to 40% of the transferrin sites available are used to transport iron.[61]

In iron deficiency, TIBC is high; consequently, transferrin saturation becomes extremely low. In individuals with iron overload, as seen in people with hemochromatosis, TIBC is low to normal, contributing to increased transferrin concentration.[61]

## Erythrocyte Protoporphyrin

Erythrocyte protoporphyrin is a conventional iron indicator, like TIBC and serum iron. It is calculated in $\mu$g/dL. When iron levels are low in the bone marrow, to sustain the assimilation of iron into newly created globin and porphyrin protein, erythrocyte protoporphyrin levels are high. However, erythrocyte protoporphyrin is also elevated with episodes of infection and lead poisoning. This makes erythrocyte protoporphyrin a useful measurement in situations where iron-deficiency levels are common and infections, lead poisoning, and other forms of anemia are rare. Normal level is 80 $\mu$g/dL RBCs for individuals five years and older and 70 $\mu$g/dL RBCs for children under five years of age.[56]

Overall, the erythrocyte protoporphyrin measurement has not been thoroughly studied in the majority of sideroblastic anemia types, thus limiting its value in diagnosis. A high level in total erythrocyte protoporphyrin is a broad result that can be related to several diseases, including iron deficiency, lead poisoning, anemia of chronic disease, and hemolytic conditions.[62]

## Hemoglobin

Hemoglobin is essential for maintaining appropriate oxygen levels in the body tissues. Its presence in erythrocytes can be quite high, influencing RBC shape and viscosity. Disorders that can affect the structure, function, and production of hemoglobin are called *hemoglobinopathies*. These disorders are normally inherited, and their gravity can vary from asymptomatic to death. Some of these conditions include hemolytic anemia, erythrocytosis, cyanosis, and vasoocclusive stigmata.[63]

**Hemolysis** is the rupture or destruction of RBCs. Hemolytic anemia can occur as a result of hereditary or acquired disorders. Conditions such as intrinsic membrane defects, abnormal hemoglobin, erythrocyte enzymatic defects, immune destruction of erythrocytes, mechanical injury, and hypersplenism can contribute to the premature destruction of RBCs.[64]

Hemolytic anemia accounts for about 5% of all anemias. Acute autoimmune hemolytic anemia (AIHA) is fairly rare, with a frequency of 1 to 3 cases per 100,000 population per year.[65] Although not specific to any race, hemolytic anemias are common in Africans, African Americans, some Arabic people, and Aborigines in southern India. Hemolytic anemia does not seem to be gender or age specific. Nonetheless, AIHA seems to be more prevalent in females than in males, and hereditary conditions manifest early in life. AIHA is more common in middle-aged and older adults.[66] See **TABLE 8.4** for a list of different types of anemia. The mortality rate for this condition seems to be low. The risk for mortality is higher in older adults and individuals with cardiovascular disease. Morbidity is influenced by the underlying conditions such as sickle-cell anemia and malaria.[66]

Erythrocytosis is a relative or absolute surge in the number of circulating RBCs, resulting in an increased above the standard range packed cell volume (PCV). The WHO defines erythrocytosis as a hemoglobin level above 18.5 g/dL in men and 16.5 g/dL in women.[67] *Relative erythrocytosis* refers to an increase in RBC numbers derived from an increase in total RBC mass. *Absolute erythrocytosis* is defined as increased RBC numbers as a result of increased RBC mass. This is a rare condition with an unknown prevalence.[68]

Decreased manufacture of hemoglobin as a result of mutation or loss of the globin chain results in thalassemia. iron-deficiency anemia and thalassemia are classified as *hypochromic microcytic anemias*. Thalassemia differs from iron-deficiency anemia in that the decrease of hemoglobin is out of proportion to the decreased mean corpuscular value (MCV).[69]

## Hematocrit

Hematocrit (HCT), also referred to as PCV, is the packed spun volume of blood that contains intact RBCs, calculated as a percentage. HCT can be measured directly following centrifugation of a blood sample, or it can be calculated. Calculating HCT involves direct measurements of the erythrocyte count and the MCV:

$$HCT\ [\mu L/100\ \mu L] = RBC\ [\times 10^{-6}/\mu L] \times MCV\ [fl]/10$$

Any factor that affects the accurate measurement of RBC and MCV will also affect the calculation of HCT.[70] The HCT can also be measured by applying sufficient centrifugal force to pack the cells while diminishing trapped extracellular fluid. Before standardized techniques were developed to quantify hemoglobin, HCT was deemed a simple and accurate method for defining the fractional volume of RBCs and, by extrapolation, the hemoglobin. This process is affected by the different amounts of plasma trapped between the RBCs and the packed cells (approximately 2% to 3%).[71,72] The hematocrit from blood that has abnormal erythrocytes, as in the case of individuals

with sickle cell, thalassemia, and iron deficiency, is high because of the higher plasma level trapped as a result of increased cell rigidity.[72] Hemoglobin level is considered the preferred method to determine the oxygen-carrying capacity of the blood.[70]

## Mean Corpuscular Hemoglobin

Mean corpuscular hemoglobin (MCH) is the average amount of hemoglobin by weight in the RBCs of a blood sample. MCH is measured in picograms. Normal levels of MCH range from 27.5 to 33.2 picograms of hemoglobin per RBC. Individuals with iron deficiency and thalassemia have low MCH values, while those with macrocytosis have levels above the standard range. MCH is calculated as:[73]

$$MCH = \frac{Hemoglobin\ g/l}{RBC\ 10^6/\mu L}$$

Cells with decreased MCH are pale in color and denoted as *hypochromic*. Cells with high MCH are described as *hyperchromic*, and cells with normal volumes of hemoglobin are *normochromic*.[73,74]

## Mean Corpuscular Volume

The MCV measures the average size of RBCs. The size of RBCs helps define the type of anemia present. Large RBCs cells can indicate pernicious anemia caused by vitamin $B_{12}$ or folate deficiency. MCV levels greater than 115 femtoliters (fL) are normally an indication of vitamin $B_{12}$ or folate deficit.

The presence of smaller-than-normal RBCs can be indicative of iron-deficiency anemia or thalassemia. The normal range for MCV is 80 to 100 fL.[75] Even greater values can be seen in the presence of cold agglutinins. This makes the RBCs pass two or three at a time through the count-taking aperture in automated measuring devices.[76] To correct this, the specimen and chemicals should be warmed to body temperature.[77]

Computerized or automated systems are routinely used to determine and report MCV. These assessment tools provide assessments measured in femtoliters ($10^{-15}$ L). Testing measurement involves cells passing through a small aperture (one by one). Light scattering, refraction, or diffraction is used to estimate the size.[77] The MCV can also be calculated by means of the measured RBC count (in standard units of million million cells/microL, equivalent to 106/microL) and the Percent of hematocrit.

## Assessing Iron Status

The CDC has established guidelines for screening different patient groups for iron deficiency. The purpose

**TABLE 8.4** Types of anemia

| Type of Anemia | Cause |
|---|---|
| Iron-deficiency anemia | Iron-deficiency anemia can develop as a result of the body's inability to meet its demands because of decreased iron intake, poor iron absorption, or blood loss. |
| Pernicious anemia | The body cannot make enough healthy RBCs because of the body's inability to absorb sufficient vitamin $B_{12}$ from food. |
| Aplastic anemia | The bone marrow is damaged. As a result, the stem cells are destroyed or do not develop normally. |
| Hemolytic anemia | In acquired hemolytic anemia, the body receives a signal that something is wrong with its RBCs when they are actually normal.<br>Inherited hemolytic anemia is related to problems with the genes that control how the RBCs are made. |
| Immune hemolytic anemia | *Autoimmune hemolytic anemia* is the main cause of hemolytic anemia. The immune system makes antibodies that attack the RBCs.<br>*Alloimmune hemolytic anemia*: A person's immune system makes antibodies against blood that is a different type than his or her own blood.<br>*Drug-induced hemolytic anemia*: Some medications (e.g., penicillin, acetaminophen, antimalaria medicines, and levodopa) may cause an immune reaction that destroys RBCs. |
| Mechanical hemolytic anemia | Hemolytic anemia develops because RBCs are physically damaged. |
| Paroxysmal nocturnal hemoglobinuria | Abnormal stem cells in the bone marrow make blood cells with a defective outer membrane. This causes the body to destroy its RBCs and make too few WBCs and platelets. |
| Other causes of acquired hemolytic anemia | Infections and toxic substances can damage or destroy RBCs, leading to hemolytic anemia. Examples include malaria, blackwater fever, tick-borne diseases, snake venom, and toxic chemicals. |
| Sickle-cell anemia | The body makes abnormal hemoglobin that causes RBCs to take on a sickle or "C" shape. These sickle cells stick together and do not travel easily through blood vessels. |
| Thalassemia | The body does not make sufficient amount of certain types of hemoglobin. This prevent the formation of sufficient healthy RBCs. |
| Hereditary spherocytosis | A defect in the outer membranes of RBCs creates a spherical or ball-like shape. |
| Hereditary elliptocytosis (ovalocytosis) | The RBCs are missing the G6PD enzyme, which makes them fragile. |
| Pyruvate kinase deficiency | RBCs are missing pyruvate kinase (an enzyme). This causes them to break down easily. |

Modified from Department of Health and Human Services. National Institute of Health. National Heart Lung and Blood Institute. Anemia Healthy Lifestyle Changes. NIH Publication No. 11-7629 2011.

of the screening guidelines is to identify insufficiency as early as possible in efforts to curtail severe complications in at-risk populations, and also to develop dietary recommendations to decrease the risk of iron deficiency.[78,79] Screening suggestions involve the following:

- Adolescent and adult females of childbearing age are screened every five to 10 years with a hemoglobin or hematocrit, with more-frequent screening (possibly yearly) if there is substantial menstrual blood loss, decreased iron intake, or a history of iron deficiency. Abnormal results are repeated, and once the presence of anemia is identified, a course of iron therapy is provided. Additional evaluation using RBC indices and serum ferritin is conducted if the trial of iron is unsuccessful. Notation identifying the possibility of sickle-cell disease or thalassemia is made, particularly in high-risk ethnic groups.
- Pregnant women are screened during their first prenatal visit. The criteria for anemia is applied according to the pregnancy stage. If the anemia falls below a predetermined threshold, a therapeutic trial of iron is given.

These guidelines also diverge from a 2015 U.S. Preventive Services Task Force (USPSTF) conclusion that "the current evidence is insufficient to assess the balance of benefits and harms of screening for iron-deficiency anemia in pregnant women to prevent adverse maternal health and birth outcomes."[80] The 2015 document supersedes the 2013 document, which did support screening pregnant women.[80] The latest evidence finds no support for the assertion that conducting regular population screening of men and postmenopausal women for iron deficit is beneficial.[78]

## Zinc Levels

Zinc was first recognized as a distinctive element in 1509 and identified as a vital mineral in the 1900s. A specific association between zinc deficiency, endemic hypogonadism, and dwarfism was recognized in rural Iran in 1961.[81]

Zinc is an important mineral that occurs naturally in some foods, is added to others, and is accessible as a dietary supplement. Zinc is an added ingredient in several over-the-counter cold medications.

Zinc is involved in numerous aspects of cellular metabolism. It is essential for the catalytic activity of nearly 100 enzymes.[82] It also plays a task in immune function, protein synthesis, wound healing, DNA synthesis, and cell division.[83,84] Zinc is important for normal growth and development during pregnancy, childhood, and adolescence, and it is needed to maintain adequate sense of taste and smell.[85–87] Zinc

requirements must be met on a daily basis because the body has no dedicated zinc storage system.[88]

The 1988–1991 National Health and Nutrition Examination Survey (NHANES III) and the 1994 Continuing Survey of Food Intakes of Individuals analysis report that most infants, children, and adults in the United States consume adequate amounts of zinc.[89–91] Conversely, NHANES III data reveal that 35% to 45% of older adults (60 years and older) had decreased zinc levels below the estimated average requirement of 6.8 mg/day for elderly females and 9.4 mg/day for elderly males. Looking at intake data from both diet consumption and dietary supplements, the survey reports that 20%–25% of older adults had insufficient zinc intake.[89,92]

## Plasma Concentration

Plasma zinc level is not considered a sensitive indicator of zinc deficiency, because the measurement does not reflect a true correlation with tissue concentrations. Plasma zinc levels are influenced by the inflammatory process associated with most diseases.[93] Zinc is bound to albumin. Individuals with a low albumin level will also have low zinc levels. Zinc supplementation is recommended for such individuals irrespective of their albumin levels.[94]

Several functional indices are also used to indirectly evaluate zinc status. Some proposed indirect measures of zinc levels include serum superoxide dismutase and erythrocyte alkaline phosphatase. These measures, however, are not widely used.[94]

## Metallothionein and Zinc Status

Several zinc metalloenzymes have been examined as probable biomarkers of zinc status in plasma, RBCs, red-blood membranes (the plasma membrane of the RBC), and in particular cell categories. These involve alkaline phosphatase, d-amino-levulinic acid dehydratase, angiotensin-1-converting enzyme, a-D-mannosidase, extracellular superoxide-dismutase, nucleoside phosphorylase, and ecto purine 50-nucleotidase. Overall, the activity of alkaline phosphatase in serum, RBCs, and red-blood membranes have been studied the most. Results of this said research has yielded inconsistent results, particularly in studies involving community-dwelling individuals, possibly compromised partly by the modest specificity of this enzyme. The proficiency of alkaline phosphatase reflects decreased levels in the presence of severe zinc deficiency, but not in moderate zinc deficit.[95–97]

## Hair Zinc

The use of hair zinc concentrations as a marker of zinc status has been debatable.[98] Evidence indicates that decreased hair zinc concentrations in children, in the absence of malnutrition, suggest chronic suboptimal zinc status. Low hair zinc levels in children have been linked to other indicators of suboptimal zinc status to include impaired taste acuity, low growth percentiles, and high dietary phytate–zinc molar ratios.[99] Hair zinc concentration differs by age, gender, season, hair growth rate, severity of malnutrition, and possibly hair color and hair products. All these factors must be considered when using hair to assess zinc levels. Consistent methods for collecting, washing, and analyzing hair samples need to be followed. A certified reference material to measure the accuracy of the analytical method must also be used. In Belgium, the Institute for Reference Materials and Measurements provides standard reference tools for human hair.[99] More research is needed to determine the validity of hair in determining suboptimal zinc levels.

## Urinary Zinc

Zinc is predominantly eliminated via feces. Renal excretion is a secondary pathway. On a daily basis, the average healthy individual will eliminate approximately 20 to 967 mcg/24 hour. High levels of zinc excreted via the urine, in the presence of decreased zinc levels, may be linked to hepatic cirrhosis, neoplastic disorder, and catabolism.[89]

High levels of zinc in the urine of individuals with normal or elevated serum zinc is indicative of high zinc intake, usually in the form of dietary supplements. Decreased zinc in both the urine and serum levels can be reflective of nutrition deficiency or excessive losses seen in burn patients and gastrointestinal losses.[89]

## Calcium Levels

Calcium is one of the most abundant minerals in the body. It is involved in vascular contraction and vasodilation, muscle function, nerve transmission, intracellular signaling, and hormonal secretion. Approximately 1% of total body calcium is used to support these metabolic functions. Serum calcium levels are closely controlled in the body and do not vary with changes in dietary ingestion. Instead, the body uses bone tissue as a source of calcium to preserve consistent concentrations of calcium in blood, muscle, and intercellular fluids.[100,101]

The bones and teeth store 99% of the body's calcium. The Health and Medicine Division of the National Academies of Sciences, Engineering, Medicine (formerly the Institute of Medicine) defined RDAs for the amounts of calcium as the essential amount needed for bone health and to preserve adequate rates of calcium in healthy individuals. Calcium requirements vary by age and sex.[100] See **TABLE 8.5**.

**TABLE 8.5** RDAs for calcium

| Age | Male (mg) | Female (mg) | Pregnant (mg) | Lactating (mg) |
|---|---|---|---|---|
| 0–6 months* | 200 | 200 | | |
| 7–12 months* | 260 | 260 | | |
| 1–3 years | 700 | 700 | | |
| 4–8 years | 1,000 | 1,000 | | |
| 9–13 years | 1,300 | 1,300 | | |
| 14–18 years | 1,300 | 1,300 | 1,300 | 1,300 |
| 19–50 years | 1,000 | 1,000 | 1,000 | 1,000 |
| 51–70 years | 1,000 | 1,200 | | |
| 71+ years | 1,200 | 1,200 | | |

Modified from Committee to Review Dietary Reference Intakes for Vitamin D and Calcium, Food and Nutrition Board, Institute of Medicine. Dietary Reference Intakes for Calcium and Vitamin D. Washington, DC: National Academy Press, 2010.

The body obtains its calcium through diet intake and nutritional supplements. Calcium is typically associated with the consumption of dairy products such as milk, yogurt, and cheese. Dairy products are the major sources of calcium in the United States[102] and Canada. In the United States, approximately 72% of the calcium consumed comes from these sources or from foods that use dairy products in their preparation[102] such as pizza and lasagna. The rest of the calcium is obtained from other foods such as vegetables, grains, fruits, eggs, and meats.[103]

Calcium carbonate and calcium citrate are the main forms of calcium supplementation. Calcium carbonate is absorbed more efficiently when taken with food. A dose provides 40% elemental calcium. Calcium citrate is well absorbed when taken both with and without food, and a dose provides 21% elemental calcium. Additional forms of calcium supplement include gluconate, lactate, and phosphate.[104] Total amount of calcium absorbed depends on the amount of elemental calcium consumed at one time. As the amount of calcium consumed at one time increases, absorption decreases. Calcium absorption is most efficient at ≤500 mg.[103]

Short-term insufficient calcium intake does not produce any specific signs and symptoms. Circulating blood calcium levels are tightly controlled. Low serum blood levels occur as a result of medical syndromes or treatments such as renal failure, surgical removal of the stomach, and use of medications like diuretics. Signs and symptoms of hypocalcemia include numbness and tingling in the fingers, muscle cramps, convulsions, lethargy, anorexia, and arrhythmia.[105] Untreated calcium deficiency can result in death.

Although more commonly linked with vitamin D deficiency, calcium deficit can increase the risk for the development of rickets.[100] Long-term calcium deficiency results in osteopenia, which is a precursor for osteoporosis. Osteoporosis contributes to increased risk of bone fractures from falls, particularly in older adults.[100]

## Serum Calcium Function

The use of serum-intact parathyroid hormone (PTH) is recommended as the most useful measurement in evaluating hypocalcemia.[106,107]

Other biochemical measurements that can be of value in assessing hypocalcemia include serum magnesium, creatinine, phosphate, the vitamin D metabolites calcidiol and calcitriol, alkaline phosphatase, amylase, and urinary calcium and magnesium elimination.[106–108] Not all of these tests should be performed in every case. The patient's medical history and results of the medical examination should help determine which biochemical assessment parameters to use.[109] See **TABLE 8.6**.

PTH biochemical level is an important element in the assessment of hypocalcemia. However, to ensure accurate interpretation of data, it must be evaluated along with serum calcium concentrations. Decreased calcium levels stimulates PTH production. Individuals with decreased or normal PTH in conjunction with hypocalcemia should be evaluated for **hypoparathyroidism**.[109]

Low serum magnesium induces hypocalcemia by stimulating PTH deficit. In individuals with decreased serum calcium, without a clear etiology, serum

| **TABLE 8.6** Biochemical evaluation of hypocalcemia | | | | | | | |
|---|---|---|---|---|---|---|---|
| **Condition** | **PTH** | **Corrected Serum Calcium** | **Phosphorus** | **Magnesium** | **Calcidiol 25(OH) Vitamin D** | **Calcitriol 1,25(OH) 2 Vitamin D** | **Creatinine** |
| Hypoparathyroidism | Low | Low | High | Normal | Normal | Normal or low | Normal |
| Vitamin D deficit | High | Low or normal | Low or normal | Normal | Low | Normal or high | Normal |
| Chronic kidney disease | High | Low | High | High | Normal or low | Low | High |

Modified from Goltzman D. Diagnostic approach to hypocalcemia. UpToDate. 2016. https://www.uptodate.com/contents/diagnostic-approach-to-hypocalcemia?source=search_result&search=serum%20calcium&selectedTitle=2~150#H4. Accessed May 24, 2017.

magnesium levels should be obtained. When magnesium is the main contributor to an episode of hypocalcemia, calcium levels should be normal immediately after correcting the hypomagnesemia.[109]

Some individuals who suffer from magnesium-responsive hypocalcemia can have normal serum magnesium levels. In this case, the individuals are believed to be tissue magnesium deficient. This is why the use of magnesium supplements might be indicated in people with inexplicable hypocalcemia who trigger a risk for hypomagnesemia as in the case of alcoholic patients.[109]

In individuals with hypocalcemia, phosphate levels might be high, low, or normal, contingent on the condition producing the hypocalcemia. Hypocalcemia that does not respond to treatment in the presence of high phosphate levels with no diagnosis of kidney injury or catabolism can be an indication of PTH deficiency or PTH resistance. Low serum-phosphate levels are usually linked to excessive excretion of PTH. In a hypocalcemia framework, the low phosphate level can be associated with hyperparathyroidism or decreased intake of phosphate, which is a rare occurrence. With episodes of hypocalcemia and normal levels of phosphate, low magnesium or mild vitamin D deficiency can be the reason for the low calcium levels.[109]

Serum levels of calcidiol [25(OH)D] is a more sensitive measurement of vitamin D deficiency than calcitriol (1,25-dihydroxyvitamin D). Decreased calcium levels increase PTH secretion, which stimulates calcitriol production. In individuals with vitamin D deficiencies, the serum level of calcidiol is low and calcitriol is normal or high. Hyperparathyroidism presents with normal calcidiol and decreased calcitriol levels. Examining an individual's dietary intake and adequacy of sunlight exposure is a quick way to screen for vitamin D deficiency.[109]

## Urinary Calcium

Calcium is excreted from the body via feces and urine, as well as by other tissues and fluids such as sweat. The amount of calcium excreted is influenced by several factors. A high intake of sodium increases urinary calcium excretion. Increased protein ingestion also raises calcium elimination and was thought to adversely impact calcium levels.[110,111] Research published in 2005 debunks this idea and suggests that higher protein intake also increases intestinal calcium absorption, essentially counterbalancing its effect on calcium elimination; in this way, body achieves calcium maintenance.[112] The caffeine found in tea and coffee contributes to a minimal increase in calcium excretion and diminishes absorption.[113]

PTH can be a chief factor in urinary calcium elimination; in states of decreased calcium intake, secondary rises in PTH levels result in low urinary calcium elimination. Reduced renal function related to aging illogically decreases calcium loss because of reduced filtration, along with a secondary surge in PTH levels as a result of decreased phosphate clearance. The impaired renal function often seen in older adults can result in decreased renal 1α-hydroxylase activity, which results in a net calcium loss through the kidneys and decreased transport of calcium from the intestine.[100]

## Iodine Levels

Iodine is a trace element found in soil. It is a vital component of the thyroid hormone, which is involved in controlling the body's metabolic processes connected to normal growth and development. Worldwide, iodized salt and seafood are the main dietary sources of iodine. In the United States, where adding iodine to salt is not legally required, dairy products and grains are the main sources of this mineral.[114] Salt is iodized with potassium iodide at 100 parts per million of iodine per kilogram. Approximately 50% to 60% of Americans use iodized salt, although most of the salt consumed by Americans is noniodized salt consumed as an ingredient in processed foods.[45] See **TABLE 8.7** for iodine recommendations.

## Assessing Iodine Status

Iodine deficiency develops when iodide intake falls below 20 $\mu$g/day.[115] Because most dietary iodine is eliminated through the urine, urinary iodine excretion is the measurement of choice for evaluating recent dietary iodine consumption.[116] The WHO classifications for average urinary iodine levels in school-age children are commonly used as the measurement of nutrition status for populations.[116] A supplementary adequacy measurement is that 20% or fewer of the samples collected from children and nonpregnant women be below 50 nanograms per milliliter (ng/mL) of iodine. This is a useful measure for determining population risk. The added criterion is not a useful parameter in determining individual risk status for poor health outcomes. The large variations in urine iodine elimination is counterbalanced by the large samples used in population studies.[117]

For pregnant females, median urinary iodine levels of 150–249 ng/mL represent sufficient iodine

**TABLE 8.7** Iodine recommendations

| Age | Organization | |
| --- | National Academies of Science, Engineering, and Medicine | World Health Organization |
| --- | --- | --- |
| Children 1–8 years | 90 g | |
| Preschool children 0–59 months | | 90 μg |
| Children 9–13 years | 120 μg | |
| Children 6–12 | | 120 μg |
| Adolescents (12–18 years) and nonpregnant adults | 150 μg | 150 μg |
| Pregnant women | 220 μg | 250 μg |
| Lactating women | 290 μg | 250 μg |

Reprinted from World Health Organization, Assessment of iodine deficiency disorders and monitoring their elimination: a guide for programme managers. 3rd ed. Geneva (Switzerland), © 2007.

intake. Median urinary iodine concentrations of <150 ng/mL implies inadequate consumption, 250–499 ng/mL characterizes intake greater than the required amount, and ≥500 ng/mL denotes excessive intake.[116,117]

## Iodine Deficiency

Iodine deficit conditions include mental retardation, hypothyroidism, goiter, cretinism, and variable levels of other growth and developmental irregularities.

According to the WHO, iodine deficiency is the most preventable reason of mental retardation in the world.[116] Thyroid enlargement (goiter) is typically the first clinical sign of iodine deficiency. Thyroid hormone is important in the development of the central nervous system during the fetal and early postnatal periods. In parts of the world where iodized salt is widely used, iodine deficiency is rare.

The most important period for iodine sufficiency is *in utero* through the first two years of life, when thyroid hormones are required for normal brain development.[116] Excess iodine intake contributes to the development of goiters, hyperthyroidism, and hypothyroidism. High iodine consumption has also been linked with higher possibilities of thyroid papillary cancer.[100]

Data from NHANES studies show that urine iodine levels were lowest in young women, and the highest levels were observed in children. Overall iodine levels have been rather steady since the late 980s.[45]

**Recap**   Understanding the effects of mineral concentrations on human health is a challenge. Consuming amounts of minerals in amounts that are too high or too low.

# ▶ Assessing Vitamin Levels

**Preview**   Vitamins are organic compounds that are needed by the body in small amounts. Worldwide, billions of people have vitamin deficiencies.

Vitamins are chemical organic compounds that are essential, in small amounts, for normal body functioning, disease prevention, and well-being. Vitamins must be ingested through diet because they cannot be synthesized by the body, with the exception of vitamin D.

Worldwide, billions of people have vitamin deficiencies. For example, approximately one-third of the developing world's children five years of age and younger have vitamin A deficiencies, thus decreasing their chances for survival.[118]

There are many contributors to vitamin deficiencies. In its basic form, vitamin deficiency is linked to diet. In many countries around the world, individuals with scarce resources do not eat adequate amounts of nutrient-rich foods such as meat, eggs, fish, milk, legumes, fruits, and vegetables. The problem compounds without adequate health care and sanitation and with disease and limited or nonexistent education in infant care and childcare.

## Vitamin A Levels

Vitamin A is the name of a group of fat-soluble retinoids, including retinol, retinal, and retinyl esters.

This vitamin plays a role in immune function, vision, reproduction, and cellular communication.[119]

Vitamin A is critical for adequate vision as an important component of rhodopsin, a protein that absorbs light in the retinal receptors. It also supports the normal differentiation and functioning of the conjunctival membranes and the cornea. Vitamin A is involved in cell growth and differentiation, thus contributing to the full development, function, and maintenance of the heart, lungs, kidneys, and other organs.[120] Inadequate consumption of vitamin A can lead to several disorders. Common signs and symptoms of vitamin A deficiency include night blindness, corneal thinning, and abnormal tissue formation in the conjunctiva. Vitamin A deficiency is the leading cause of blindness in countries with low incomes.[121] This is a rare condition in the United States.[43] Overconsumption of vitamin A can result in nausea, vomiting, headache, vertigo, blurred vision, increased cerebrospinal fluid pressure, and lack of muscular coordination. **Hypervitaminosis** of vitamin A results in dysfunction of the central nervous system such as ataxia, bone and muscle pain, and birth defects that occur *in utero*.[43] See **TABLE 8.8**.

Vitamin A has two dietary forms: preformed vitamin A (retinol and its esterified form, retinyl ester) and provitamin A carotenoids.[119] Preformed vitamin A is found in foods from animal sources such as dairy products, fish, and meat. Provitamin A carotenoids are found in plants and must be converted into vitamin A in the body. Common provitamin A carotenoids include beta-carotene, alpha-carotene, and beta-cryptoxanthin. Both forms of vitamin A must be processed intracellularly into retinal and retinoic acid, the active forms of vitamin A.[120] **TABLE 8.9** shows the RDAs for vitamin A.

## Plasma Levels

Serum or plasma concentrations of carotenoids are considered among the best biological markers for fruit and vegetable intake. Performing a hepatic biopsy is the most accurate way to determine inadequate vitamin A intake. This invasive technique, however, is not an acceptable method for population studies. For that reason, serum or plasma retinol is measured via the use of high-performance liquid chromatography (HPLC) with ultraviolet (UV) detection after the split from its carrier, retinol binding protein (RBP). Because retinol is tightly linked with RBP, the measurement of this transport protein through *enzyme-linked immunosorbent assay* (ELISA) has also been used to determine vitamin A levels. In most populations, serum RBP has been shown to be a proper proxy for retinol. Serum or plasma concentrations of carotenoids are measured by use of HPLC and visible light (450 nm) absorbance. Clinical laboratories normally use conventional units for serum concentrations of these fat-soluble micronutrients [$\mu$g per deciliter (dL)]. Serum levels less than 20 $\mu$g/dL imply deficiency. Those with serum concentrations of less than 10 $\mu$g/dL are considered severely deficient.[43] With vitamin A deficiency, serum carotene levels are normally low. As a result, low serum carotene can be used as a surrogate indicator of malabsorption and nutritional status.

Serum vitamin A concentrations are not infallible when measuring vitamin A stores. Serum retinol levels may be artificially low in individuals with severe PEM. These individuals lack the proper levels of dietary protein, energy, and zinc that are needed for the production of RBP.[45]

| **TABLE 8.8** Vitamin A deficiency | | | | |
|---|---|---|---|---|
| **Vitamin** | **Function** | **Deficiency Disorder** | **Main Food Sources** | **Excessive Consumption** |
| Vitamin A (retinol, retinal, retinoic acid) | Vision, epithelial differentiation, antioxidant | Night blindness, xerophthalmia, keratomalacia, Bitot's spot, follicular hyperkeratosis | Cod-liver oil, milk products, carrots, sweet potatoes, spinach, pumpkin, dark leafy green vegetables, butter, egg yolk | Not associated with major adverse effects. Consuming massive amounts in a short period of time can result in increased intracranial pressure, dizziness, nausea, headaches, skin irritation, joint and bone pain, and coma and can result in death. |

Modified from National Institutes of Health Office of Dietary Supplements. Vitamin A-Fact Sheet for Health Professionals. 2016. https://ods.od.nih.gov/factsheets/VitaminA-HealthProfessional/#en2. Accessed May 26, 2017.

**TABLE 8.9**  Recommended dietary allowances for vitamin A

| Age | Male (mcg RAE)* | Female (mcg RAE)* | Pregnancy (mcg) | Lactation (mcg) |
| --- | --- | --- | --- | --- |
| 0–6 months* | 400 | 400 | | |
| 7–12 months* | 500 | 500 | | |
| 1–3 years | 300 | 300 | | |
| 4–8 years | 400 | 400 | | |
| 9–13 years | 600 | 600 | | |
| 14–18 years | 900 | 700 | 750 | 1,200 |
| 19–50 years | 900 | 700 | 770 | 1,300 |
| 51+ years | 900 | 700 | | |

*mcg RAE = micrograms retinol activity equivalent.
Modified from Institute of Medicine, Food and Nutrition Board. Dietary reference intakes: vitamin A, vitamin K, arsenic, boron, chromium, copper, iodine, iron, manganese, molybdenum, nickel, silicon, vanadium and zinc. Washington, D.C.: National Academy Press. 2001. https://www.nap.edu/catalog/11537/dietary-reference-intakes-the-essential-guide-to-nutrient-requirements. Accessed May 25, 2017.

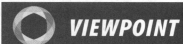 **VIEWPOINT**

## Nutrition and a Professional Chef

*Ari S. Rubinoff*

We are fascinated with food. We are constantly flooded with images of food through magazines, televised media, and social media. Some of us love to cook and feel a special connection to either Grandma's recipe for that soufflé that everybody loved at last week's dinner party or that special restaurant or aroma that wakes up fond memories of a special night out or celebratory family gathering.

It is safe to say that food plays an important part of our lifestyle both mentally and physically. Eating the right types and amounts of foods are part of a healthy lifestyle, which also involves maintaining a healthy weight, being physically active, and learning about what you are eating. With the constant barrage of nutritional trends such as organic, farm to table, more proteins, fewer carbs, vegetarian, low fat, raw, and paleo, it can be confusing as to what proper nutrition is about. How can we simply just eat healthful, wholesome foods? Add to that confusion people who have food allergies or medically required dietary restrictions, such as the patron with diabetes who needs an accurate carbohydrate count or

the customer who needs a low- or no-salt diet? It is the job of the chef, along with a trained registered dietitian nutritionist, to figure that out and create foods, recipes, and entire menus for customers that meet their cultural, health, and personal taste preferences.

The typical American purchases food—whether breakfast, lunch, dinner, or a snack—from a food-service operation three to five times a week.[1] As a trained chef working in the industry, I can tell you that the days of serving steamed carrots and house salads as a healthy alternative are long past. Not only are chefs responsible for the nutritional value of the food they serve but also the flavor of that food. More and more of my customers are as concerned about where their food came from as what is in it. We have to be creative and educated in what we are serving. As a food-service professional, I am accountable to my customers to practice contemporary cooking techniques that provide a balanced diet that is moderate in rich ingredients and well prepared without sacrificing taste or quality. The chefs that work alongside me are also responsible for preparing nutritious food that is well balanced so my guests can maintain their current nutritional lifestyles.

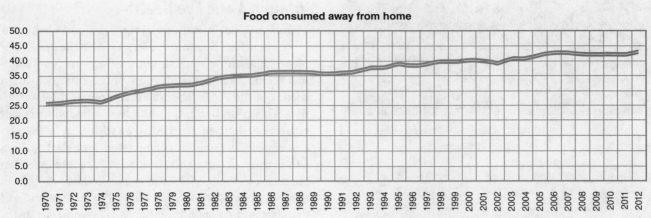

**Food consumed away from home**

Data from United States Department of Agriculture Economic Research Service. https://www.ers.usda.gov/topics/food-choices-health/food-consumption-demand/food-away-from-home.aspx Retrieved 12/14/17.

It is well accepted that healthful food choices are essential to living a balanced life. More than 40% of food in the American diet is prepared away from home.[2] In 2015, for the first time Americans spent more money eating out than they did buying groceries.[3]

With the increasing number of people eating out, the need for foods of high nutritional value is as essential as the taste of the food we serve. It is also essential to the survival of many food businesses. In today's food-service environment, special requests for what "not" to include in dishes are as common as what patrons do want in their foods. As a chef in today's industry, it is my goal to prepare food to meet each individual request and to present dishes with the highest level of quality and professionalism.

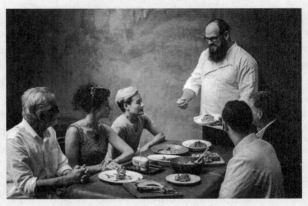

### References

1. Drummond KE, Before L. *Nutrition for Foodservice and Culinary Professionals*. 8th ed. New York, NY: Wiley; 2013.
2. USDA Economic Research Service Food-Away -From Home. https://www.ers.usda.gov/topics /food-choices-health/food-consumption-demand /food-away-from-home.aspx.
3. Jamrisko M. Americans' spending on dining out just overtook grocery sales for the first time ever. Bloomberg Markets. https://www.bloomberg.com/news /articles/2015-04-14/americans-spending-on-dining -out-just-overtook-grocery-sales-for-the-first-time-ever.

## Relative Dose Response

For segments of the world population with high levels of vitamin A deficiency, the WHO has outlined vitamin-replacement tactics. Periodic supplementation using the doses outlined in **TABLE 8.10** is advocated for segments of the population with widespread vitamin A deficiency.[122]

Pregnant women who reside in areas with health problems related to vitamin A deficits should receive small and frequent doses not exceeding 10,000 international units (IU) or 25,000 IU weekly for 12 weeks during pregnancy.[123]

Providing vitamin A supplementation to newborns, infants one to five months old, and new mothers living in areas at high risk for deficiency is no longer the standard.[122,123] In many studies and systematic reviews, the use of vitamin A supplementation did not yield reliable health benefits; in some instances, side effects were observed in infants.[124] Supplementation for newborns has been especially controversial

**TABLE 8.10** Vitamin A dose recommendation for a population with widespread deficiency

| Age Group (Months) | Dose Recommendation (IU Orally) | Number of Doses |
|---|---|---|
| Infants 6–12 | 100,000 (30 mg retinol equivalent) | One |
| Children 12–59 | 200,000 (60 mg retinol equivalent) | Provide every 4–6 months |

IU= International units.
Reprinted from World Health Organization, World Health Organization Guideline: Vitamin A supplementation for infants and children 6-59 months of age (2011), © 2011.

because of varied results from numerous large studies.[125] A study conducted in India advocated a modest benefit for survival in young infants receiving vitamin A supplementation: risk ratio 0.9, 95% confidence interval (CI) 0.81–1.00. A comparable study conducted in Ghana and Tanzania yielded no benefit and pointed toward higher risks of mortality in those receiving vitamin A supplementation.[126–128]

The WHO has outlined vitamin A supplementation guidelines for children assessed at high risk for deficiencies (such as those with measles, diarrhea, respiratory disease, or severe malnutrition) and who live in high-risk areas and have not received supplementation for the previous four months. See **TABLE 8.11**.

**TABLE 8.11** Vitamin A supplement recommendation for children

| Age Group (Months) | Dose Recommendation (IU, Oral Doses) |
|---|---|
| Infants <6 | 50,000 (30 mg retinol equivalent) |
| Infants 6–12 | 100,000 (60 mg retinol equivalent) |
| Children >12 | 200,000 (60 mg retinol equivalent) |

IU= International units.
Reprinted from World Health Organization, Vitamin A supplements: a guide to their use in the treatment and prevention of vitamin A deficiency and xerophthalmia, 2nd Edition (1997), © 1997.

## Vitamin A and Eye Health

Maintaining adequate body levels of vitamin A helps promote eye health. Vitamin A plays a role in the prevention of xerophthalmia and phototransduction. *Xerophthalmia* refers to abnormal dryness of the conjunctiva and cornea of the eye, with inflammation and ridge formation. This condition is typically seen in individuals with vitamin A deficiency. **Phototransduction** is the process by which the light is converted into electrical signals in the rod, cone, and photosensitive ganglion cells of the retina of the eye. The rod cells and the cone cells are retinal-specialized photoreceptors. The cone cells absorb the light and color in bright light. The rod cells distinguish motion and are sensitive for night vision.[129]

Treatment of xerophthalmia involves providing three doses of vitamin A at the age and dose described in Table 8.11. Adolescents and adults should receive 200,000 IU orally.[130] The first does is provided at the time the diagnosis is made. The second dose is given the next day, and the third is provided two weeks later.[130]

Age-related macular degeneration (AMD) is one of the main reasons older adults lose their sight. AMD's etiology is unknown, but it is believed that oxidative stress over time plays a role. The Age-Related Eye Disease Study (AREDS) randomized controlled trial (RCT) reports that individuals at high risk for developing AMD can decrease their disease risk by 25% by consuming a dietary supplement with beta-carotene. In this RCT, participants received a supplement that contained 15 mg beta-carotene with vitamin E (400 IU dl-alpha-tocopheryl acetate), vitamin C (500 mg), zinc (80 mg), and copper (2 mg).[131] A follow-up AREDS2 study validated the value of this supplement in decreasing the progression of AMD over a median follow-up phase of five years. This study also reported that adding lutein (10 mg) and zeaxanthin (2 mg) or omega-3 fatty acids to the original supplement did not provide additional benefits.[132]

## Liver-Store Measurements

The requirements for vitamin A are based on the assurance of adequate liver stores of vitamin A. The tolerable upper intake level (UL) is based on liver abnormalities as the critical endpoint.

Some 80% to 90% of the body's vitamin A is stored in the liver. From there it is released into circulation via a process dependent on RBP. The liver is responsible for vitamin A oxidation and catabolism, as well as for retinol distribution to target tissues.[133] Approximately 50%–90% of the retinol consumed is absorbed and transported to the liver by chylomicrons and stored as retinyl in Ito cells, together with lipids. There is a direct correlation between liver levels and serum levels of vitamin A. As the level of vitamin A decreases in the liver, so does the serum concentration.[134] Excess vitamin A is stored in the liver. Most of the vitamin A metabolites are eliminated in the urine; some vitamin A is also excreted in the bile. Amounts excreted through bile increase as the vitamin A in the liver surpasses a critical level. This functions as a defensive mechanism for decreasing the risk of nutrient overload.[45]

Individuals with increased alcohol intake, history of liver disease, hyperlipidemia, or severe PEM can be especially vulnerable to adverse effects of excessive preformed vitamin A ingestion. The UL for vitamin A defined for the population might not apply to this group. The UL is not intended for application to groups of malnourished people prophylactically receiving vitamin A either occasionally, or through fortification, or as a way to avert vitamin A deficit.[45]

## Retinol Isotope Dilution

Performing a liver biopsy—the gold standard for measuring vitamin A—is not a convenient method. This is why retinol isotope dilution equations are used to determine vitamin A status and the efficacy of vitamin A intervention programs. This is a much less invasive and feasible method.[135]

The process of isotope dilution requires providing a tracer dose of vitamin A branded with either radioactive (tritium and $^{14}C$) or stable (deuterium and $^{13}C$) isotopes, permitting the tracer to mix with the body pool of vitamin A, and then measuring the tracer-to-tracee ratio after mixing has taken place. The following are key assumptions in the isotope-dilution test:[135]

- The tracer dose mixes fully with the tracee body pool.
- The tracer performs indistinctly from the tracee in the system.
- The tracer is measurable by analytical methods in the framework of the tracee.
- The tracer does not disturb the system being studied.
- The tracee system is a single pool in steady state (tracee mass is constant).

Liver reserves analyzed with $[^{13}C]$ retinol isotope dilution were favorably correlated with liver reserves ($r = 0.98$) in rats provided with low and moderate doses of vitamin A and in nonhuman primates with hypervitaminosis A.[136,137]

## Vitamin D Levels

Vitamin D (calciferol) includes a group of fat-soluble secosterols found naturally in a small number of foods such as fish-liver oils, fatty fishes, mushrooms, egg yolks, and liver. The two main physiologically significant forms of vitamin D are $D_2$ (ergocalciferol) and $D_3$ (cholecalciferol). Vitamin $D_3$ is photosynthesized in the skin of humans via sun exposure by the action of solar UV B radiation on 7-dehydrocholesterol already present in the skin.[43,138]

Vitamin $D_2$ is manufactured by UV irradiation of ergosterol, which is present in molds, yeast, and higher-order plants. In geographic locations where regular sun exposure is not a problem, dietary vitamin D intake is of insignificant importance. Latitude, season, aging, sunscreen use, and skin color affect the manufacture of vitamin $D_3$ by the skin. In the United States, most of the dietary intake of vitamin D comes from fortified milk products and other fortified foods such as breakfast cereals and orange juice.[100]

Vitamin D synthesized through the skin or consumed via the diet is biologically inert and requires enzymatic conversion into an active metabolite. Vitamin D is transformed enzymatically in the liver to 25-hydroxyvitamin D (25[OH]D), the chief circulating form of vitamin D, and then in the kidney to 1,25-dihydroxyvitamin D, the active form of vitamin D.[100] The active form of vitamin D is believed to be responsible for most, if not all, of the biologic functions in the body.[43] See **FIGURE 8.3**. The production of 25(OH) vitamin D in the liver is driven by the amount of vitamin D available from dietary intake and sun exposure. Production of $1,25(OH)_2$ vitamin D in the kidney is closely regulated by mineral requirements. In the liver, vitamin D-25-hydroxylase is downregulated by vitamin D and its metabolites. This action controls for any surge in the circulating level of 25(OH) vitamin D after dietary intake or after vitamin D production because of sun exposure. In the kidney, in response to serum calcium and phosphorus levels, the manufacture of $1,25(OH)_2$ vitamin D is controlled by the action of PTH.[43,139,140]

The main role of vitamin D (1,25-dihydroxyvitamin D) is to preserve serum calcium and phosphorus levels within the normal range by promoting the effectiveness of the small intestine to absorb these minerals from the diet.[139,140] When dietary calcium intake is insufficient to meet the body's calcium needs, $1,25(OH)_2$ vitamin D and PTH activate calcium stores from the bone. In the kidney, $1,25(OH)_2$ vitamin D promotes calcium reabsorption by the distal renal tubules.[43]

Vitamin D is responsible for other functions in the body, such as modulation of cell growth, neuromuscular and immune activity, and decreasing inflammation. Many genes encoding proteins that control cell proliferation, differentiation, and apoptosis are regulated in part by vitamin D. Many cells have vitamin D receptors, and some convert 25(OH) vitamin D to $1,25(OH)_2$ vitamin D.[100,141,142]

## Serum Levels

The serum level of 25(OH) vitamin D is the best indicator of vitamin D status. It measures vitamin D

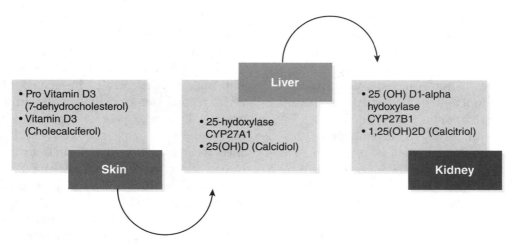

**FIGURE 8.3** Vitamin D transformation.

Data from Center for Disease Control and Prevention, National Center for Environmental Health Division of Laboratory Sciences. Second National Report on Biochemical Indicators of Diet and Nutrition in the U.S. Population 2012. 2013. https://www.cdc.gov/nutritionreport/pdf/nutrition_book_complete508_final.pdf. Accessed May 14, 2017. Courtesy of Nancy Munoz.

created cutaneously as well as the nutrient obtained from food and supplements with a long circulating half-life of five days.[143] 25(OH) vitamin D serves as a biomarker of exposure, but it is not clear to what extent it also serves as a biomarker of effect in terms of health status. Serum 25(OH) vitamin D levels do not indicate the amount of vitamin D stored in body tissues.[100]

Circulating 1,25(OH)$_2$vitamin D is normally not a good indicator of vitamin D status because of its short half-life of 15 hours. Serum levels of 1,25(OH)$_2$ vitamin D are tightly controlled by PTH, calcium, and phosphate.[143] Levels of 1,25(OH)$_2$vitamin D do not usually drop until vitamin D deficiency is severe.[43]

## Vitamin D Deficiency

Vitamin D deficiency is categorized by poor bone mineralization or by demineralization of the skeleton. Among children, vitamin D deficiency is seen as a bone deformity known as *rickets*. In adults, vitamin D deficiency is characterized by a mineralization defect in the skeleton, causing osteomalacia, contributing to secondary hyperparathyroidism and resulting in osteopenia and osteoporosis. See **TABLE 8.12**.

Other roles for vitamin D outside of bone health are currently being researched, including effects on muscle strength, the risk for cancer, and the risk for type 2 diabetes.[144] The Agency for Healthcare Research and Quality examined the effectiveness and safety of vitamin D on outcomes associated with bone health. The report advocates that vitamin D supplementation has positive effects on bone health in postmenopausal women and older men.[145] Evaluation of vitamin D levels and health outcomes discovered no significant relationships between vitamin D status and total cancer mortality, nor did it find any conclusive evidence for the association of vitamin D status with cancer risk or outcomes.[146] Research supports no clear

| **TABLE 8.12** Vitamin D deficiency | | | | |
|---|---|---|---|---|
| **Vitamin** | **Function** | **Deficiency Disorder** | **Main Food Sources** | **Excessive Consumption** |
| D (cholecalciferol, ergocalciferol) | Prohormone for calcium regulation | Rickets, osteomalacia, osteopenia, osteoporosis, craniotabes | Cod-liver oil, fatty fish, milk, egg yolk, liver, maitake mushrooms, fortified cereals | Contributes to anorexia, weight loss, polyuria, and heart arrhythmias. More serious adverse effects include increased blood levels of calcium, which leads to vascular and tissue calcification as well as heart, blood vessel, and kidney damage. |

Modified from National Institute of Health Office of Dietary Supplements. Vitamin D- The fact sheet for health professionals. 2016. https://ods.od.nih.gov/factsheets/VitaminD-HealthProfessional/#en1. Accessed May 26, 2017.

**TABLE 8.13** Recommended dietary allowances for Vitamin D

| Age | Male (IU/mcg) | Female (IU/mcg) | Pregnancy (IU/mcg) | Lactation (IU/mcg) |
|---|---|---|---|---|
| 0–12 months* | 400/10 | 400/10 | | |
| 1–13 years | 600/15 | 600/15 | | |
| 14–18 years | 600/15 | 600/15 | 600/15 | 600/15 |
| 19–50 years | 600/15 | 600/15 | 600/15 | 600/15 |
| 51–70 years | 600/15 | 600/15 | | |
| 70+ years | 800/20 | 800/20 | | |

*Adequate intake (AI).

Modified from National Institute of Health Office of Dietary Supplements. Vitamin D- The fact sheet for health professionals. 2016. https://ods.od.nih.gov/factsheets/VitaminD-HealthProfessional/#en1. Accessed May 26, 2017.

association between vitamin D status and cardiometabolic outcomes involving fasting glucose, blood pressure, myocardial infarction, or stroke. RCTs displayed no clinically significant reliable effects of vitamin D supplementation at the dosages given.[147]

The Food and Nutrition Board (FNB) of the National Academies of Sciences, Engineering, and Medicine established an RDA for vitamin D based on a daily intake that is adequate to support bone health and normal calcium metabolism in healthy people. RDAs for vitamin D are listed in both IUs and micrograms (mcg). Even though sunlight can be a main source of vitamin D for a segment of the population, the vitamin D RDAs are defined on the basis of insignificant sun contact. See **TABLE 8.13**.

## Vitamin C Levels

Ascorbic acid (vitamin C) is a water-soluble vitamin that functions as an antioxidant and a cofactor in enzymatic and hormonal processes. Vitamin C is involved in the biosynthesis of carnitine, neurotransmitters, collagen, and other components of connective tissue, and it regulates the absorption, transport, and storage of iron. The adult requirement for vitamin C is based on the amount of the nutrient needed to deliver antioxidant defense. The UL for adverse effects is based on the amount that triggers osmotic diarrhea and gastrointestinal disturbances.[2,148]

Current research is exploring the potential role of vitamin C in limiting the harmful effects of free radicals and preventing or delaying certain cancers and the development of cardiovascular disease and other illnesses in which oxidative stress appears to have a causal role. Aside from its biosynthetic and antioxidant role, vitamin C supports the immune system and increases the absorption of nonheme iron.[2,148]

Vitamin C deficiency is known to cause scurvy. Signs and symptoms of scurvy include fatigue, connective-tissue weakness, bleeding gums, and capillary fragility. Vitamin C deficiency is not a problem in the United States and Canada. The risk for developing adverse effects because of excessive consumption seems to be minimal even at the highest usual vitamin C intakes.[148–152]

**TABLE 8.14** lists the current RDAs for vitamin C.[2] The RDAs for vitamin C were developed based on its known physiological and antioxidant role in white blood cells, which are higher than the requirements to prevent signs and symptoms of deficiency.[2,152] For infants, the FNB established an adequate intake (AI) level for vitamin C.

## Assessing Vitamin C Levels

Practically 70%–90% of the vitamin C consumed is absorbed by the body at an average intake of 30–180 milligrams per day (mg/d). Vitamin C consumed after the plasma has reached a point of saturation (approximately 70 $\mu$mol/L) will probably be eliminated as unmetabolized ascorbic acid in the urine. When intake is greater than 1 g/day, absorption of vitamin C falls to <50% and unmetabolized ascorbic acid is excreted in the urine.[2,43] Vitamin C concentration can be evaluated by determining total ascorbic acid (oxidized and reduced) in serum or plasma, buffy coat, or leucocytes. Ascorbic acid in plasma is termed an *index* of the circulating vitamin accessible to tissues.

**TABLE 8.14** Recommended dietary allowances for vitamin C

| Age | Male (mg) | Female (mg) | Pregnancy (mg) | Lactation (mg) |
|---|---|---|---|---|
| 0–6 months* | 40 | 40 | | |
| 7–12 months* | 50 | 50 | | |
| 1–3 years | 15 | 15 | | |
| 4–8 years | 25 | 25 | | |
| 9–13 years | 45 | 45 | | |
| 14–18 years | 75 | 65 | 80 | 115 |
| 19+ years | 90 | 75 | 85 | 120 |

Smokers: Individuals who smoke require 35 mg/day more vitamin C than nonsmokers.

*Adequate intake.

Modified from National Institute of Health Office of Dietary Supplements. Vitamin C-Fact Sheet for Health Professionals. 2016. https://ods.od.nih.gov/factsheets/VitaminC-HealthProfessional/. Accessed May 28, 2017.

In leucocytes, particularly for polymorphonuclear leucocytes, ascorbic acid is assumed to be a good indicator of tissue stores.[43]

Because high-performance liquid chromatography methods with electrochemical detection offer needed sensitivity and specificity, they are commonly used to quantify serum vitamin C levels. Older spectrophotometric methods were prone to hindrances from several elements such as riboflavin and aspirin. SRM 970, a multilevel standard reference material, is available from the National Institute of Standards and Technology (NIST) for human serum, with certified values for ascorbic acid. The Micronutrients Measurement Quality Assurance Program, supported by the NIST, sponsors interlaboratory comparison studies intended to ensure high-quality measurements of serum vitamin C.[43]

## Vitamin C Deficiency

Vitamin C deficiency is typically expressed as plasma or serum levels <11.4 $\mu$mol/L (micromoles per liter), or the concentration at which evidence of scurvy is evident. Serum ascorbic acid levels 11.4 $\mu$mol/L to 23 $\mu$mol/L are considered low.[99]

The timeline for signs and symptoms of scurvy to appear are dependent on overall vitamin C body reserves. Generally, scurvy symptoms are evident within one month of minimal to no vitamin C intake (< 10 mg/day). Scurvy symptoms include weakness, fatigue, aches and pains, and gum inflammation.[148,152,153] As the vitamin C deficit advances, collagen synthesis becomes compromised and connective tissues become debilitated, contributing to petechiae, ecchymoses, purpura, joint pain, poor wound healing, hyperkeratosis, and corkscrew hairs.[148,150–152] Other symptoms of scurvy involve depression, swollen and bleeding gums, and loss of teeth as a result of tissue and capillary brittleness.[2,148] Iron-deficiency anemia may occur with vitamin C deficiency because of increased bleeding and decreased nonheme-iron absorption. Children can have signs and symptoms of bone disease. If untreated, scurvy can be fatal.[148,154] See **TABLE 8.15**.

In this day and age, the incidence of vitamin C deficiency and scurvy are rare in developed countries. Obvious deficit symptoms happen only if vitamin C consumption falls to <10 mg/day for many weeks.[148,154] Although vitamin C deficiencies are rare in developed countries, they can still happen in people with limited food variety. NHANES 2003–2004 data reported that children and older adults had the highest serum concentrations of this vitamin. When compared to nonsmokers, the mean level of vitamin C was one-third lower for adult smokers.[43,155]

## Vitamin B$_6$ Levels

Vitamin B$_6$ (pyridoxine and related compounds) is a coenzyme involved in the metabolism of amino acids, glycogen, and sphingoid bases. Vitamin B$_6$

**TABLE 8.15** Vitamin C deficiency

| Vitamin | Function | Deficiency Disorder | Main Food Sources | Excessive Consumption |
|---|---|---|---|---|
| Vitamin C (ascorbate) | Antioxidant, collagen synthesis | Scurvy—fatigue, petechiae, ecchymoses, bleeding gums, depression, dry skin, impaired wound healing | Citric fruits, peppers, papaya, broccoli, brussel sprouts, strawberries, paprika, kohlrabi | Signs associated with excessive consumption include nausea, vomiting, heartburn, stomach cramps, and headache. Amounts higher than 2000 mg daily are possibly unsafe and have been associated with kidney stones and severe diarrhea. |

Modified from National Institute of Health Office of Dietary Supplements. Vitamin C-Fact Sheet for Health Professionals. 2016. https://ods.od.nih.gov/factsheets/VitaminC-HealthProfessional/. Accessed May 28, 2017.

includes a group of six related compounds: pyridoxal (PL), pyridoxine 5'-phosphate (PN), pyridoxamine (PM), and their respective 5-phosphates [pyridoxal 5'-phosphate (PLP), pyridoxine 5'-phosphate (PNP), and pyridoxamine 5'-phosphate (PMP)]. PLP and PM are the forms found in animal tissue, whereas PN and PPN are seen in plant sources, sometimes in the form of glucoside. The main measure used to appraise the requirements for vitamin $B_6$ is a plasma pyridoxal 5-phosphate value of at least 20 nmol/L. The UL uses sensory neuropathy as the benchmark adverse effect.

The clinical signs and symptoms of vitamin $B_6$ deficit are only seen during depletion with minuscule levels of the vitamin. There have been no reports of deficiency at intakes of 0.5 mg/day or more. No adverse effects have been connected with high consumption of the vitamin from food sources. Extremely large oral doses of supplementary pyridoxine, defined as 2,000 mg/day or more on a prolonged basis, have been linked with the signs and symptoms of sensory neuropathy and dermatological lacerations.[43,155]

Dietary Reference Intakes for infants from birth to 12 months were defined as AI. See **TABLE 8.16**.[156,157]

**TABLE 8.16** Recommended dietary allowances for Vitamin $B_6$

| Age | Male (mg) | Female (mg) | Pregnancy (mg) | Lactation (mg) |
|---|---|---|---|---|
| Birth–6 months* | 0.1 | 0.1 | | |
| 7–12 months* | 0.3 | 0.3 | | |
| 1–3 years | 0.5 | - | | |
| 4–8 years | 0.6 | 0.6 | | |
| 9–13 years | 1.0 | 1.0 | | |
| 14–18 years | 1.3 | 1.2 | 1.9 | 2.0 |
| 19–50 years | 1.3 | 1.3 | 1.9 | 2.0 |
| 51+ years | 1.7 | 1.5 | | |

*Adequate intake.
Modified from National Institute of Health Office of Dietary Supplements. Vitamin B6- Dietary Supplement Fact Sheet. 2016. https://ods.od.nih.gov/factsheets/VitaminB6-HealthProfessional/. Accessed May 28, 2017.

## Assessing Vitamin B₆ Levels

Vitamin B₆ serum levels are analyzed by HPLC with fluorometric detection. Chemical derivatization is most often used to boost PLP fluorescence.[158] Enzymatic and microbiological methods have also been used.[159] Other methods being used include liquid chromatography–mass spectrometry (LC-MS/MS).[160]

## Vitamin B₆ Deficiency

As previously mentioned, vitamin B₆ deficiency is uncommon. Insufficient vitamin B₆ status is generally related with low levels of other B vitamins, including vitamin B₁₂ and folic acid. Vitamin B₆ deficiency produces organic changes that become more defined as the deficiency further develops.[157,161]

Vitamin B₆ deficit can be a precursor for microcytic anemia, electroencephalographic abnormalities, dermatitis with cheilosis and glossitis, depression and confusion, and immunocompromised system. Adults with marginal vitamin B₆ levels or slight deficiency might be asymptomatic for many months or even years. Signs and symptoms for infants with vitamin B₆ deficiency include irritability, uncharacteristically acute hearing, and convulsive seizures.[157,161]

End-stage renal disease (ESRD), chronic renal injury, and other kidney diseases can contribute to vitamin B₆ deficiency.[162] Malabsorption syndromes such as celiac disease, Crohn's disease, and ulcerative colitis; and genetic diseases such as homocystinuria, can cause vitamin B₆ deficiency.[157,161] See **TABLE 8.17**.

## Folate Levels

Folate is a B vitamin that works as a coenzyme in the breakdown of nucleic and amino acids. This nutrient is critically important through periods of rapid cell division and growth, such as throughout pregnancy and infancy. *Folate* is a term that describes both the natural form of the vitamin—food folate or pteroyl-polyglutamates—and the synthetic, monoglutamate form (folic acid). The monoglutamate form is used for fortified foods and nutritional supplements.[163,164]

The nutrition requirements for folate are determined based on the amount of dietary folate equivalents (DFEs), with standards corrected for variances in the absorption of food folate and folic acid necessary to maintain erythrocyte folate. DFEs adapt for the almost 50% decreased bioavailability of food folate (as opposed to folic acid). The UL critical point is founded on the exacerbation of neuropathy in vitamin B₁₂–deficient individuals. The UL is based on total intake from fortified food or dietary supplements and does not account for naturally occurring food folate.[163,164]

During childbearing years, women must consume 400 mg of folic acid/day to reduce the risk for neural tube defects (NTDs). It must be pointed out that the recommendation specifies folic acid (the supplemental form), which has a higher bioavailability than folate (the form occurring naturally in whole foods). In countries where foods are not fortified with folic acid, a multivitamin with 400 mg of folic acid, in addition to the folate consumed through a healthful diet, is recommended.[163,164]

Approximately 85% of folic acid, when taken with food, is absorbed by the body. Of the folate naturally occurring in food, only 50% is bioavailable. Folate intake is measured in micrograms (mcg) of dietary DFEs. See **TABLE 8.18** for a list of the current RDAs for folate. Based on the different absorption rate of folic acid and folate, 1 mcg DFE is the equivalent of 1 mcg food folate, 1 mcg DFE is calculated to provide 0.6 mcg folic acid from fortified foods and dietary supplement when taken with food, and 1 mcg DFE

| **TABLE 8.17** Vitamin B₆ deficiency | | | | |
|---|---|---|---|---|
| **Vitamin** | **Function** | **Deficiency Disorder** | **Main Food Sources** | **Excessive Consumption** |
| B₆ (proxidine, pyridoxal) | Transaminase cofactor | Anemia, weakness, insomnia, difficulty walking, nasolabial seborrheic dermatitis, cheilosis, stomatitis | Bananas, chickpeas, fortified cereals, yeast, potatoes, brown rice, salmon, chicken, tuna, liver | High consumption of vitamin B₆ from food sources has not been associated with adverse effects. Intake of 1–6 g oral pyridoxine/day for 12–40 months can contribute to severe and progressive sensory neuropathy and ataxia. |

Modified from National Institute of Health Office of Dietary Supplements. Vitamin B6- Dietary Supplement Fact Sheet. 2016. https://ods.od.nih.gov/factsheets/VitaminB6-HealthProfessional/. Accessed May 28, 2017.

**TABLE 8.18** Recommended dietary folate intake

| Age | Male (mcg DFE) | Female (mcg DFE) | Pregnant (mcg DFE) | Lactating (mcg DFE) |
|---|---|---|---|---|
| Birth–6 months* | 65* | 65* | | |
| 7–12 months* | 80* | 80* | | |
| 1–3 years | 150 | 150 | | |
| 4–8 years | 200 | 200 | | |
| 9–13 years | 300 | 300 | | |
| 14–18 years | 400 | 400 | 600 | 500 |
| 19+ years | 400 | 400 | 600 | 500 |

*For infants, up to 12 months of age AI for folate is the reference point for intake.

Modified from Otten JJ, Hellwig JP, Meyers LD. Folate. In Otten JJ, Hellwig JP, Meyers LD, eds. *Dietary Reference Intakes: The Essential Guide to Nutrient Requirements*. Washington, DC: National Academies Press. 2006:244-253.

provides 0.5 mcg folic acid from a dietary supplement taken on an empty stomach.[163] For infants up to 12 months of age, the AI for folate is the reference point for intake. The AI for infants encompasses the average intake of folate in healthy breast-fed infants in the United States.[163]

## Assessing Folate Levels

The body's content of folate is estimated to be 10–30 mg, of which approximately 50% is stored in the liver and the remainder in blood and body tissues. Folate levels are measured via assessing serum or plasma folate. Clinical laboratories normally use ng/mL for calculating concentrations of folate. A level >3 ng/mL is an indication of adequate intake.[163] Because this indicator is sensitive to recent dietary intake, it might not truly reflect the body's long-term folate status. The use of erythrocyte folate concentration measures long-term folate intake. An erythrocyte folate level >140 ng/mL implies adequate folate status.[43,163]

A composite of serum or erythrocyte concentration and markers of metabolic function are also used to evaluate folate status. Plasma homocysteine level is a regularly used functional indicator of folate status. Note that homocysteine levels are not especially specific markers of folate status, because the results can be affected by conditions such as kidney disease, vitamin 12, and other micronutrient deficits.[43,163]

In a research environment, chromatography-based methods, combined with LC-MS/MS, are used to quantify individual forms of folate in serum or whole blood.[43,165] International reference materials for serum folate from NIST and the National Institute for Biological Standards and Control (NIBSC), with LC-MS/MS, are available. A reference material (standard) for whole-blood folate is available from the NIBSC (95/528). Consensus of numerous protein-binding and microbiological tests were used to determine the standards for whole-blood folate.[43,165]

## Folate Deficiency

Isolated folate deficiency is rare. Folate deficiency is usually seen with other nutrient deficiencies such as vitamin $B_6$ and $B_{12}$ deficiencies. Contributors to folate deficiency include poor-quality diets, excessive alcohol consumption, and sometimes malabsorption disorders. Megaloblastic anemia is the main clinical indication of folate and vitamin $B_{12}$ deficiency.[166] Individuals suffering from megaloblastic anemia normally present with weakness, fatigue, difficulty concentrating, irritability, headache, heart palpitations, and shortness of breath.[163] See **TABLE 8.19**.

Folate deficiency can also present as superficial ulcerations in the tongue and oral mucosa as well as changes in skin, hair, and fingernail coloration and raised blood homocysteine levels.[163,166]

Women who consume less than adequate folate are at higher risk for delivering infants with NTDs. These are birth defects of the brain, spine, or spinal cord. These develop in the first month of pregnancy.

**TABLE 8.19** Folate deficiency

| Vitamin | Function | Deficiency Disorder | Main Food Sources | Excessive Consumption |
|---------|----------|--------------------|--------------------|-----------------------|
| Folate | One-carbon transfer | Megaloblastic anemia, neural tube defects | Liver, spinach, avocado, lentils, fortified cereals, enriched rice | High consumption of folic acid increases the risk for or exacerbates the anemia and cognitive symptoms associated with vitamin $B_{12}$ deficiency. |

Data from National Institute of Health Office of Dietary Supplements. Vitamin $B_6$—Dietary supplement fact sheet; 2016. https://ods.od.nih.gov/factsheets/VitaminB$_6$-HealthProfessional/.

The two most common neural tube defects are spina bifida and anencephaly.[163] Inadequate folate intake has also been related to low infant birthweight, preterm delivery, and fetal growth retardation.[167]

Malabsorption disorders can increase the risk for folate deficiency. These include tropical sprue, celiac disease, and inflammatory bowel disease. Decreased gastric acid secretion resulting from atrophic gastritis, gastric surgery, and other conditions can also diminish folate absorption.[166]

## Folate and Population Health

Surveillance of the effect of the American folic-acid fortification program of enriched grains and cereal products on serum and RBC folate levels is important to public health. Serum folate levels have increased by more than 50%, and RBC folate concentrations have increased by about 50% after the introduction of fortification in 1998. From 1999 to 2006, the prevalence of low serum (<2 ng/mL) and RBC folate (<95 ng/mL) concentrations was less than 1% of the American population. This included women of childbearing age, regardless of race or ethnicity. Folate deficiency is virtually nonexistent in the general population. Incidence of folate deficiency might be limited to individuals with malabsorption, alcoholism, or use of certain drugs.[43]

## Vitamin B$_{12}$ Levels

Vitamin $B_{12}$ is a water-soluble vitamin that occurs in several forms and contains the mineral cobalt. Compounds with vitamin $B_{12}$ are referred to as *cobalamin*. Methylcobalamin and 5-deoxyadenosylcobalamin are the forms of vitamin $B_{12}$ that are active in human metabolism.[168] It functions as a coenzyme for an important methyl transfer reaction that changes homocysteine to methionine and for a distinct process that transforms L-methylmalonyl-coenzyme A to succinylcoenzyme A.[43]

Vitamin $B_{12}$ occurs naturally in animal foods such as fish, meat, poultry, eggs, milk, and milk products. The *Dietary Guidelines for Americans* identify vitamin $B_{12}$ as a nutrient of concern for certain segments of the population. The dietary guidelines advise individuals 50 years of age and older to eat foods fortified with vitamin $B_{12}$ or take a dietary supplement.[46]

Bound to protein in food, vitamin $B_{12}$ is made available to the body by the reaction of hydrochloric protease in the stomach. The vitamin $B_{12}$ that is added to fortified foods and nutritional supplement is in bioavailable (free) form. The bioavailable form of vitamin $B_{12}$ combines with intrinsic factor for the nutrient to be absorbed by the body. Around 56% of every 1 mcg oral intake is absorbed. Absorption does decrease considerably when the capacity of intrinsic-factor molecules (the carriers for vitamin $B_{12}$) is exceeded.[168]

See **TABLE 8.20** for a list of the current RDAs for vitamin $B_{12}$. For infants up to 12 months of age, AI for folate is the reference point for intake. The AI for infants encompasses the average intake of folate in healthy breast-fed infants in the United States.[168]

## Assessing Vitamin B$_{12}$ Levels

Vitamin $B_{12}$ status is assessed by serum vitamin $B_{12}$ levels. Results of <170–250 pg/mL (120–180 picomol/L) for adults indicates a vitamin $B_{12}$ deficiency.[168] Evidence shows that serum vitamin $B_{12}$ levels may not be a true reflection of intracellular concentrations.[169] A high serum homocysteine level, defined as >13 micromol/L, might also imply a vitamin $B_{12}$ deficit.[170] The use of homocysteine as an indicator of vitamin $B_{12}$ has poor specificity because this parameter is influenced by factors such as low vitamin $B_6$ and folate levels.[168] High levels of methylmalonic acid, >0.4 micromol/L, possibly indicate more reliably vitamin $B_{12}$ levels because this is indicative of a metabolic change that is highly specific to vitamin $B_{12}$ deficiency.[168–170]

**TABLE 8.20** Recommended dietary allowances for vitamin $B_{12}$

| Age | Male (mcg) | Female (mcg) | Pregnancy (mcg) | Lactation (mcg) |
|---|---|---|---|---|
| 0–6 months* | 0.4 | 0.4 | | |
| 7–12 months* | 0.5 | 0.5 | | |
| 1–3 years | 0.9 | 0.9 | | |
| 4–8 years | 1.2 | 1.2 | | |
| 9–13 years | 1.8 | 1.8 | | |
| 14+ years | 2.4 | 2.4 | 2.6 | 2.8 |

*Adequate intake.

Data from National Academies of Science Engeneering and Medicne. Dietary Reference Intakes: The Essential Guide to Nutrient Requirements- Vitamin B12. The National Academies Press. file://Users/nancymunoz/Downloads/182-187.pdf. Accessed May 29, 2017. 2006.

Serum vitamin $B_{12}$ is generally assessed by competitive protein-binding test.[171] Research methods for homocysteine assessment are HPLC with fluorescence detection or in tandem mass spectrometry. Clinical assessment methods are based on immunoassay or enzymatic standards.[172] International reference materials include NIBSC 03/178 for serum vitamin $B_{12}$ (consensus value) and NIST SRM 1955 and 1950 for plasma homocysteine via certified concentration by LC-MS/MS or gas chromatography–mass spectroscopy (GC-MS).[43]

## Vitamin $B_{12}$ Deficiency

The main causes for the development of vitamin $B_{12}$ deficiency include malabsorption of vitamin $B_{12}$ from food, pernicious anemia, postsurgical malabsorption, and dietary deficiencies. Vitamin $B_{12}$ deficiency is depicted by megaloblastic anemia, fatigue, weakness, constipation, loss of appetite, and weight loss.[168] Other symptoms of vitamin $B_{12}$ deficiency include numbness and tingling in the hands and feet, difficulty maintaining balance, depression, confusion, dementia, poor memory, and soreness of the mouth or tongue.[173] In infants, signs of vitamin $B_{12}$ include failure to thrive, movement disorders, developmental delays, and megaloblastic anemia.[174] These symptoms are not unique to vitamin $B_{12}$ deficiency. See **TABLE 8.21**.

In older adults, atrophic gastritis reduces the secretion of hydrochloric acid in the stomach. This

**TABLE 8.21** Vitamin $B_{12}$ deficiency

| Vitamin | Function | Deficiency Disorder | Main Food Sources | Excessive Consumption |
|---|---|---|---|---|
| $B_{12}$ (cobalamin) | One-carbon transfer | Megaloblastic anemia (pernicious anemia), neurologic symptoms (subacute combined degeneration) | Clams, salmon, liver, egg yolk, meat, lentils, spinach, fortified cereals | Increase in rates of restenosis after stent placement and vitamin $B_{12}$ supplementation. Other adverse effects include nausea, difficulty swallowing, and diarrhea. Treatment of vitamin $B_{12}$ deficiency may lead to an increase in blood volume and the number of red blood cells. In people with low serum levels of potassium, the correction of megaloblastic anemia with vitamin $B_{12}$ may result in fatally low potassium levels. |

Data from National Academies of Science Engineering and Medicine. Dietary Reference Intakes: The Essential Guide to Nutrient Requirements- Vitamin B12. The National Academies Press
https://www.nap.edu/catalog/11537/dietary-reference-intakes-the-essential-guide-to-nutrient-requirements Accessed May 29, 2017. 2006.

contributes to decreased vitamin B$_{12}$ absorption.[168] Diminished hydrochloric acid levels can also promote the increased growth of normal intestinal bacteria that use vitamin B$_{12}$. This reaction further reduces the amount of vitamin B$_{12}$ available to the body.[168]

Although individuals who suffer from atrophic gastritis are unable to absorb the vitamin B$_{12}$ provided in food, they can absorb the synthetic vitamin B$_{12}$ added to fortified foods and dietary supplements. As a result, the HMD recommends that adults 50 years of age and older acquire most of their vitamin B$_{12}$ from vitamin supplements or fortified foods.[168]

The most common treatment for vitamin B$_{12}$ deficiency is the use of vitamin B$_{12}$ injections. This method sidesteps possible barriers for absorption. Note that high doses of oral vitamin B$_{12}$ can also be effective. Review of the literature supports the belief that oral vitamin B$_{12}$ can be as effective as injections.[174] The determinant of whether to take vitamin B$_{12}$ treatment via injection or oral dose is the individual's ability to absorb vitamin B$_{12}$, the practice of using injections has not changed in most countries.[175]

> **Recap** Data on actual vitamin consumption are necessary as a component of an individual's nutrition assessment and for national food and health policy planning. Biochemical assessment that measures individual and population nutritional status is an important assessment component.

# ▸ Blood Chemistry Studies

> **Preview** Biochemical tests are used to diagnose diseases and conditions.

A blood chemistry study is performed on a blood sample to determine the amount of a target substance in the body. Target substances include electrolytes such as sodium, potassium, and chloride; proteins such as albumin; and other substances such as blood glucose levels and enzymes. Blood chemistry levels provide information about how well the body's organs work, its nutritional status, and other assessment parameters. Abnormal results of a blood component can be an indication of illness or of particular interest, a nutrient deficit. Blood chemistry studies are also used to monitor the results of interventions. These can be used before, during, and after an intervention to help

collect data. Blood chemistry study is synonymous with blood chemistry test.

## Alanine Aminotransferase

The alanine aminotransferase (ALT) test is generally used to identify liver injury. It is frequently prescribed in combination with aspartate aminotransferase as part of a liver panel or comprehensive metabolic panel (CMP).[176]

ALT is an enzyme located mainly in liver and kidney cells. When the liver is injured, ALT is discharged into the blood. ALT results are regularly compared to the values of other tests such as alkaline phosphatase, total protein, and bilirubin to help establish which type of liver disease is present. This test is also used to monitor the treatment provided to individuals with liver disease as a way to measure whether the treatment is working.[176]

Normal ALT results range from 29 IU/L to 33 IU/L for males and 19 IU/L to 25 IU/L for females. A low level of ALT in the blood is considered to be normal. Extremely high levels of ALT, defined as more than 10 times the normal level, are associated with acute hepatitis, often linked to a viral infection. In acute hepatitis, ALT results can be high for approximately 1–2 months. Levels of ALT may also be significantly elevated, as high as more than 100 times normal, because of exposure to drugs or other elements that are toxic to the liver or in conditions that cause diminished blood circulation to the liver.[176]

ALT levels are moderately high in chronic hepatitis. Other contributors to moderately high levels of ALT involve obstruction of bile ducts, cirrhosis, heart damage, alcohol abuse, and liver tumors.[176]

## Total Protein and Albumin

Total protein and albumin assays are regularly included in the panels of tests performed as part of a health examination, such as a CMP. Total protein and albumin tests can be ordered to help diagnose disease, monitor changes in health status, and act as a screen that may indicate the need for other follow-up tests.[177]

Proteins are the building blocks of all cells and tissues. They are essential for body growth, development, and health promotion. They form the structural part of most organs and make up enzymes and hormones that regulate body functions. Total protein and albumin determines the total amount of the different forms of proteins in the blood serum.[177]

As previously mentioned, albumin and globulin are the two types of proteins found in the blood.

Albumin accounts for nearly 60% of the total blood protein. Produced by the liver, albumin is needed for several functions that act as a carrier for several small molecules and ions, as well as a source of amino acids for tissue metabolism, and as the principle constituent needed to maintain osmotic pressure. The remaining 40% of proteins in the plasma are denoted as globulins. Globulin proteins include enzymes, antibodies, hormones, carrier proteins, and numerous other types of proteins. The level of total protein in the blood is normally a relatively stable value, reflecting a balance in loss of old protein molecules and production of new protein molecules.[177]

Total protein may decrease in conditions in which the creation of albumin and globulin is weakened, such as with severe disease. Levels are also decreased in the presence of conditions that promote protein catabolism or protein loss as in the case of kidney injury. Conditions that increase plasma volume, such as heart failure, also decrease total protein levels. Total protein levels are increased during inflammation, multiple myeloma, and dehydration.[177]

## Bilirubin

Bilirubin is an orange-yellow waste product chiefly produced by the normal breakdown of heme, a component of hemoglobin found in RBCs. Bilirubin is processed by the liver to be eliminated by the body. The bilirubin test measures the quantity of bilirubin in the blood and is used to evaluate an individual's liver function and assist in the diagnosis of hemolytic anemias.[178,179]

Nearly 250 mg to 350 mg of bilirubin is manufactured in a healthy adult every day. The majority of bilirubin in the blood, approximately 85%, occurs as a result of damaged RBCs. The remaining 15% is derived from the bone marrow or liver. The body produces conjugated and unconjugated bilirubin. Conjugated bilirubin occurs when the heme molecule is released from hemoglobin because of RBC degradation. Conjugated bilirubin develops when the unconjugated bilirubin is carried by proteins to the liver and glucose molecules attach to bilirubin.[178,179]

If the bilirubin level rises in the blood, an individual becomes jaundiced. The yellow pigment is normally seen in the skin and the whites of the eyes. This test is used to define different conditions. Unconjugated bilirubin is increased in individuals with hemolysis, pernicious anemia, and cirrhosis of the liver. High levels of conjugated bilirubin is seen in episodes of acute hepatitis. In newborns, a high bilirubin level can be a temporary condition that resolves in a couple of days.

If bilirubin levels are critically high, further testing should occur because increased concentrations can be indicative of blood type incompatibility, congenital infection, hypoxia, or liver disease in the newborn. Overall, higher bilirubin levels are found in males and African Americans.[179]

Normal range is 0 to 0.3mg/dL of conjugated bilirubin. Total bilirubin range is defined as 0.3 to 1.9 mg/dL. Overall, normal ranges vary among different laboratories.[178]

## Blood Urea Nitrogen

Blood urea nitrogen (BUN) is used to assess kidney function. This laboratory test is used to help diagnose kidney injury and to monitor the effectiveness of dialysis and other interventions used in the presence of kidney injury. BUN is mainly used with a creatinine test as part of a renal panel, BMP, or CMP.[180]

Urea is a waste product of protein synthesis into amino acids. This reaction produces ammonia, which is metabolized into a less noxious form of urea. The BUN test quantifies the amount of urea nitrogen present in the blood. Liver and kidney diseases can affect the amount of urea in the blood. High levels of urea in the blood occur when the liver overproduces urea or when the kidneys are unable to filter the amount being created. When damage in the liver hinders urea production, BUN levels decrease.[180]

High BUN levels imply compromised kidney function. This can be related to acute or chronic kidney disease, damage, or failure. It can also occur in the presence of conditions that reduce the blood flow to the kidneys, including heart failure, shock, stress, severe burns, conditions that create a decreased urine flow, and dehydration. Increased BUN can also occur as a result of catabolism, extremely high dietary protein intake, or gastrointestinal bleeding. Decreased BUN levels are not especially common and are normally not a cause for worry. Although BUN levels might be low in the presence of liver disease, malnutrition, and overhydration, this laboratory value is not used to assess these conditions. The normal range for BUN is 6 to 20 mg/dL. Normal values vary among different laboratories.[180]

## Creatinine

Creatinine is a blood waste product. It is produced as a result of protein synthesis and muscle breakdown in the body, which occurs at a fairly constant rate. The amount manufactured varies based on the individual's size and muscle mass. As a result, creatinine levels are higher in men (as compared to women and children).[181]

Creatinine is filtered from the blood via the kidneys and excreted via urine. Individuals with kidney disease present increased creatinine blood levels. Blood serum and urine creatinine tests are used to assess kidney function.[181]

Blood creatinine levels are often used with other laboratory tests such as the 24-hour urine test to develop calculations that are used in evaluating kidney function. It is also commonly prescribed with a BUN or as part of a CMP or BMP. Creatinine and BUN levels are useful not only in diagnosing kidney injury but also in monitoring the progression of kidney dysfunction and the effectiveness of the interventions in place.[181]

Calculations performed using creatinine levels in the diagnosis of kidney function include estimated glomerular filtration rate and creatinine clearance. To calculate eGFR, the individual's age, weight, gender, and creatinine concentrations are used. In adults, suggested calculations for estimating glomerular filtration rate (GFR) from serum creatinine involve the modification of diet in renal disease (MDRD) study equation (isotope dilution mass spectrometry, traceable version) and the chronic kidney disease epidemiology collaboration (CKD-EPI) equation.[181,182] See **TABLE 8.22**.

The eGFR is also used to classify kidney injury stages. See **TABLE 8.23**. The creatinine clearance measures the kidneys' effectiveness in sifting smaller molecules (such as creatinine) out of the blood.[181,182]

## Calcium

Blood calcium levels are used to screen, diagnose, or monitor various illnesses involving an individual's teeth, heart, nerves, kidneys, and bones. It is commonly used

**TABLE 8.22** GFR calculators for adults (used in the united states)

| Name | Formula for Calculation |
|------|------------------------|
| MDRD for adults (conventional units) | GFR (mL/min/1.73 m²) = 175 $\times (S_{cr})^{-1.154}$ $\times (Age)^{-0.203}$ $\times$ (0.742 if female) $\times$ (1.212 if African American) (conventional units) |
| CKD-EPI Adults (conventional units) | GFR = 141 $\times$ min $(S_{cr}/\kappa, 1)^{\alpha}$ $\times$ max $(S_{cr}/\kappa, 1)^{-1.209}$ $\times 0.993^{Age}$ $\times$ 1.018 (if female) $\times$ 1.159 (if black) |

MDRD = modification of diet in renal disease.

CKD-EPI = chronic kidney disease epidemiology collaboration.

Data from National Institute of Health National Institute of Diabetes and Digestive and Kidney Diseases. Glomelular Filtration Rate Calculators. National Institute of Health National Institute of Diabetes and Digestivr and Kidney Diseases. 2017. https://www.niddk.nih.gov/health-information/health-communication-programs/nkdep/lab-evaluation/gfr-calculators/Pages/gfr-calculators.aspx. Accessed June 1, 2017.

**TABLE 8.23** Stages of kidney injury

| (GFR)* | Description | Stage |
|--------|-------------|-------|
| > 90 | Risk factors for kidney disease (e.g., diabetes, high blood pressure, family history, older age, ethnic group) | At increased risk |
| 90+ | Kidney damage with normal kidney function | 1 |
| 89–60 | Kidney damage with mild loss of kidney function | 2 |
| 59–44 | Mild to moderate loss of kidney function | 3a |
| 44–30 | Moderate to severe loss of kidney function | 3b |
| 29–15 | Severe loss of kidney function | 4 |
| < 15 | Kidney failure | 5 |

*Glomerular filtration rate.

Data from National Kidney Foundation. https://www.kidney.org/atoz/content/about-chronic-kidney-disease Access 6/3/2017.

in persons suffering from hyperactive or hypoactive thyroid disorders and malabsorption. A total calcium level is usually included in a CMP and BMP.[183]

Normal calcium level values range from 8.5 to 10.2 mg/dL (2.13 to 2.55 millimol/L). This range might be different among laboratories. Abnormal calcium result is an indication of some sort of disorder in the body. To assist in the diagnosis of underlying disease, different tests can be prescribed to measure ionized calcium, urine calcium, phosphorus, magnesium, vitamin D, parathyroid hormone, and PTH-related peptide. PTH and vitamin D control calcium concentrations in the blood within a tight range of values.[184]

High levels of calcium in the blood can occur as a result of different conditions altering an individual's health status. A higher-than-normal level of calcium can occur as a result of many health conditions. Some of the conditions that contribute to high levels of calcium include being bedbound for long periods of time, overconsumption of dietary calcium and vitamin D, and the presence of hyperparathyroidism. Infections that produce granulomas such as tuberculosis and fungal and myocardial infections can also contribute to increased calcium levels. Abnormally high calcium levels are frequently seen in conjunction with multiple myeloma, T-cell lymphoma, metastatic bone tumor, and other types of cancer. Paget syndrome, sarcoidosis, tumors that produce parathyroid gland–like reactions, and the use of medications such as lithium, tamoxifen, and thiazides are also contributors to high calcium levels.[183]

Low calcium levels are often the result of disarrays that interfere with the absorption of nutrients in the intestines, hyperparathyroidism, and kidney injury. Other contributors to decreased calcium levels include hypoalbuminemia, liver disease, hypomagnesemia, pancreatitis, and vitamin D deficit.[184]

The total calcium level is the most commonly used test to appraise calcium status. This is a good indicator of the quantity of free calcium present in the blood. Ionized calcium measure is used for individuals in which total calcium is not a good indicator of calcium status. In patients who are critically ill, those receiving transfusions and intravenous fluids, undergoing major surgery, and with hypoalbuminemia-ionized calcium, this is the preferred test. Large fluctuations in ionized calcium must be monitored because they can result in tachycardia, bradycardia, muscle spasms, altered cognition, and coma.[183]

## Carbon Dioxide

A carbon dioxide ($CO_2$) test is also referred as total $CO_2$ test ($TCO_2$ test), bicarbonate test, $HCO_3$ test, and $CO_2$ test serum. It measures the amount of carbon dioxide in the blood serum. This test is mostly prescribed as a component of an electrolyte panel, BMP, or CMP. Changes in $CO_2$ level is an indication of fluid shift (losing fluids or retaining fluids). This creates an electrolyte imbalance. $CO_2$ blood concentrations are influenced by kidney and lung function. The kidneys assist in maintaining bicarbonate-level homeostasis.[185,186]

The normal range for $CO_2$ is 23–29 milliequivalents per liter (mEq/L). Normal values can vary by testing location. This test may be prescribed in the presence of signs and symptoms of acidosis or alkalosis or with acute conditions and symptoms such as prolonged vomiting or diarrhea, weakness, fatigue, or respiratory distress. As part of an electrolyte panel or BMP, $CO_2$ levels can be used to monitor individuals taking medications that can cause electrolyte imbalance. These are also used to monitor conditions such as hypertension, heart failure, liver disease, and kidney injury.[185,186]

An abnormal $CO_2$ result is indicative of the body's inability to maintain acid–base balance. This can occur as a result of the body not being able to eliminate carbon dioxide through the lungs or the kidneys or the presence of an electrolyte imbalance (especially potassium deficiency).[185,186] **TABLE 8.24** lists conditions in which abnormal $CO_2$ levels are seen.

| **TABLE 8.24** Conditions contributing to abnormal $CO_2$ concentrations | |
|---|---|
| **Above-Normal Concentrations** | **Below-Normal Concentrations** |
| Addison's disease | Conn's syndrome |
| Diarrhea | Cushing's syndrome |
| Diabetic ketoacidosis | Hyperaldosteronism |
| Ethylene glycol or methanol poisoning | Lung diseases, including COPD* |
| Ethylene glycol poisoning | Metabolic alkalosis |
| Kidney disease | Severe prolonged vomiting or diarrhea (or both) |
| Lactic acidosis | |
| Metabolic acidosis | |
| Salicylate toxicity (such as aspirin overdose) | |
| Shock | |

*Chronic obstructive pulmonary disease.
Data from National Library of Medicine. CO2 blood test. medline Plus. 2017. https://medlineplus.gov/ency/article/003469.htm. Accessed June 3, 2017.

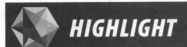
## HIGHLIGHT

## What Is a Basic Metabolic Panel?

A basic metabolic panel is a slate of eight tests utilized to evaluate an individual's metabolism. It includes kidney function, blood glucose level, electrolytes and acid base balance.

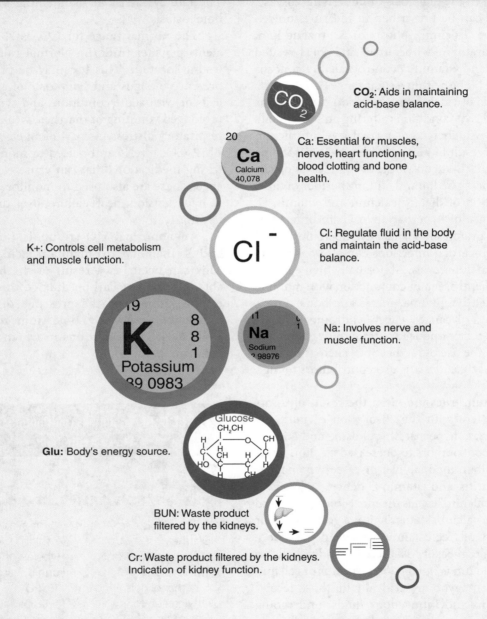

$CO_2$: Aids in maintaining acid-base balance.

Ca: Essential for muscles, nerves, heart functioning, blood clotting and bone health.

Cl: Regulate fluid in the body and maintain the acid-base balance.

K+: Controls cell metabolism and muscle function.

Na: Involves nerve and muscle function.

Glu: Body's energy source.

BUN: Waste product filtered by the kidneys.

Cr: Waste product filtered by the kidneys. Indication of kidney function.

Abbreviations: Sodium (Na), Potassium (K), Chloride (Cl), Carbon Dioxide Content ($CO_2$). Blood Urea Nitrogen (BUN). Serum Creatinine (Cr), Serum Glucose (Glu). Calcium (Ca).

Data from American Association of Clinical Chemistry. Basic Metabolic Panel. American Association of Clinical Chemistry. 2017 https://labtestsonline.org/understanding/analytes/bmp/tab/glance/ Accessed June 10, 2017.

## Chloride

Chloride is a negatively charged electrolyte that helps maintain proper hydration and acid balance in the body, along with potassium, sodium, and $CO_2$. A chloride blood test helps identify abnormal levels of chloride in the body.[187]

A chloride blood test is normally not ordered as a standalone test. It is usually requested with other electrolyte tests to help determine the cause of signs and symptoms such as vomiting, diarrhea, weakness, and respiratory distress.[187]

Normal chloride ranges from 96 to 106 milliequivalents per liter (mEq/L) or 96 to 106 millimoles per liter (millimol/L). As with other laboratory results, the normal range can vary by testing facility.[187] See **TABLE 8.25** for a list conditions contributing to abnormal chloride levels.

## Cholesterol

A cholesterol test is conducted as a standalone test or as a component of a lipid profile. This test is used as a predictive tool to assess the risk of developing heart disease and to determine interventions based on risk level. When ordered as a component of a lipid profile, this test is useful in monitoring the effectiveness of the treatment in place. A lipid panel includes the testing of high-density lipoprotein cholesterol (HDL-C), low-density lipoprotein cholesterol (LDL-C), and serum triglycerides.

As a preventive health measure, adults with no identified risk for heart disease should test their blood cholesterol every four years. For individuals at risk of developing heart disease, this test should be done more often. Risks for heart disease are listed in **TABLE 8.26**. Children should be tested for cholesterol levels once between ages 9 and 11 years, and once again between ages 17 and 21 years. Those screened at increased level for developing heart disease should be tested more often.

Cholesterol concentrations are also used as part of the lipid profile panel to monitor the effectiveness of lipid-lowering lifestyle changes and medications. The American College of Cardiology and the American Heart Association guidelines for 2013 support the use of lipid profile testing every four to 12 weeks past the start of statin therapy and every three to 12 weeks thereafter to monitor the treatment's effectiveness.[188]

Overall, cholesterol levels are classified in three categories of risk: desirable, borderline high, and high. A cholesterol level below 200 mg/dL is considered desirable and is associated with a low risk for heart disease. A range between 200 mg/dL and 239 mg/dL is defined as borderline high and considered a moderate risk. For this risk level, evaluating LDL-C and HDL-C is a part of the assessment to determine if treatment is needed. A high risk of disease development involves a cholesterol level >240 mg/dL. This level requires in-depth assessment to define the causative factor.[188]

## Triglycerides

Triglyceride tests are also used to determine risk for developing heart disease and to monitor the effectiveness of interventions. Triglycerides are a component of the lipid profile test. The guidelines discussed

| **TABLE 8.25** Conditions contributing to abnormal chloride concentrations | |
|---|---|
| **Above-Normal Concentrations** | **Below-Normal Concentrations** |
| Use of carbonic anhydrase inhibitors<br>Diarrhea<br>Metabolic acidosis<br>Respiratory alkalosis<br>Renal tubular acidosis | Addison's disease<br>Bartter syndrome<br>Burns<br>Heart failure<br>Dehydration<br>Profuse sweating<br>Hyperaldosteronism<br>Metabolic alkalosis<br>Respiratory acidosis<br>Syndrome of inappropriate diuretic hormone secretion (SIADH)<br>Vomiting |

Data from US National Library of Medicine. Chloride test - blood. Medline Plus. 2017. https://medlineplus.gov/ency/article/003485.htm. Accessed June 3, 2017.

| **TABLE 8.26** Risks for developing heart disease | |
|---|---|
| **Major Risks for Developing Heart Disease** | |
| Cigarette smoking<br>Overweight<br>Obese<br>Unhealthy diet<br>Sedentary lifestyle<br>Age<br>■ Men 45 years or older<br>■ Women 55 years or older | Hypertension<br>Taking hypertensive medications<br>Family history of premature heart disease<br>Having preexisting heart disease<br>History of heart attack<br>Diabetes or Prediabetes |

Data from US National Library of Medicine. Cholesterol. Medline Plus. 2016. https://medlineplus.gov/cholesterol.html Accessed June 3, 2017.

for cholesterol screening and testing also apply to triglycerides testing.[188]

For adults, serum triglyceride concentration < 150 mg/dL is considered desirable. Levels between 150 mg/dL and 199 mg/dL is considered borderline high, 200–499 mg/dL is high, and > 500 mg/dL is considered very high. Individuals with triglyceride levels > 1,000 mg/dL are at risk of developing pancreatitis. These individuals need immediate treatment. Individuals with uncontrolled blood sugars can also have very high triglycerides.[188]

## Glucose

A blood glucose test is used to screen individuals who are at risk of developing diabetes before signs and symptoms are evident, diagnosing prediabetes and gestational diabetes, and identifying hyperglycemia and hypoglycemia. Blood glucose levels are also used as a monitoring tool for those already diagnosed with diabetes mellitus (DM).[189]

Depending on the purpose, there are several testing protocols to choose from. To diagnose type 1 and type 2 diabetes (T1D and T2D), one of three tests can be used: fasting blood glucose (FBG), two-hour tolerance test (GTT), and hemoglobin A1C (A1C). The FBG test measures the amount of serum glucose after a person has fasted for at least eight hours. A GTT involves an FBG and the consumption of a 75-g glucose beverage. Two hours later, another blood sample is drawn. The expectation is that the body will release insulin to process the glucose generated by consuming the carbohydrate-loaded beverage. The A1C is another blood test that can be used instead of the FBG test for screening and diagnosing DM. Once the initial test is abnormal, the test is repeated on a different day. If both tests are abnormal, then a diagnosis is confirmed.[189]

To screen for gestational diabetes (GDM), pregnant women are tested somewhere between the 24th and 28th weeks of pregnancy. Either the one- or two-step approach is used. The one-step two-hour glucose tolerance test (OGTT) involves an FBG level followed by consuming a 75-g dose of glucose beverage. The blood sugar level is tested one hour and two hours after the glucose beverage is consumed. If one of the tests results in increased levels, a diagnosis of GDM is assigned. For a two-step blood glucose test, the woman is given 50-g glucose drink and blood sugars are tested after one hour. If this test is abnormal, a three-hour oral blood glucose tolerance is performed. To complete this test, after an FBG, the woman is given a 100-g glucose dose and blood sugars

are measured after one, two, and three hours. If two of the blood sugars are high, then a GDM diagnosis is assigned. Once diagnosed, those with DM often test their blood sugars daily and sometimes more often. This is normally done with the use of glucose meters and testing strips.[189]

Many organizations, including the American Diabetes Association and the USPSTF, endorse diabetes screening for those 45 years of age and older or when a person of any age has risk factors (see **TABLE 8.27**).

High blood glucose levels are normally associated with DM. Other diseases such as infection, kidney disease, and acute stress can also contribute to increased blood glucose levels. In individuals with signs and symptoms of DM, a random blood (nonfasting) sample of 200 mg/dL or greater suggests DM.[189]

In a person with signs and symptoms of DM or hyperglycemia, a nonfasting glucose level (random blood sample) that is equal to or greater than 200 mg/dL indicates DM. See **TABLE 8.28**.[189]

A decreased glucose level might indicate hypoglycemia,[190] a condition that presents with unusually low blood glucose levels that can result in unconsciousness and death. This is an important consideration for individuals with DM and investigators researching diabetes treatment.[191] The ADA defines

---

**TABLE 8.27** Major risk factors for developing diabetes mellitus (DM)

- Overweight, obese, or sedentary lifestyle
- Family history of DM
- A woman with history of gestational diabetes and delivering an infant 9 pounds or larger
- History of polycystic ovarian syndrome
- Ethnic backgrounds or races considered at high risk: African American, Latino, Native American, Asian American, Pacific Islander
- Hypertension

- Taking medication for hypertension
- Low HDL cholesterol level (less than 35 mg/dL) or a high triglyceride level (more than 250 mg/dL) or both
- A1C equal to or above 5.7%
- History of prediabetes
- History of cardiovascular disease

Data from American Diabetes Association. American Diabetes Association Standards of Medical Care in Diabetesd2017. Diabetes Care. 2017;40(Supplement 1):146. https://professional.diabetes.org/sites/professional.diabetes.org/files/media/dc_40_s1_final.pdf. Accessed June 3, 2017.

**TABLE 8.28** Fasting blood glucose

| Glucose Level (mg/dL) | Indication |
|---|---|
| 70–99 | Normal fasting glucose |
| 100–125 | Prediabetes (impaired fasting glucose) |
| ≥126 on more than one testing occasion | Diabetes |

Data from Blood Sugar Test Blood. Medline Plus. https://medlineplus.gov/ency/article/003482.htm Accessed 6/2/2017

that a level of < 3.0 mmol/l (54 mg/dl) is a serious, clinically important hypoglycemia, whether or not that level is associated with symptoms.[191] Individuals with this condition show signs and symptoms such as sweating, palpitation, hunger, and anxiety. Eventually the low blood glucose levels affect the brain and provoke symptoms such as confusion, hallucinations, blurred vision, and possibly coma and death.[189] Conditions such as adrenal insufficiency, severe liver disease, insulin overdose, and starvation contribute to hypoglycemia.[189]

## Phosphorus

Phosphorus tests are commonly prescribed with other tests such PTH and vitamin D. Phosphorus levels—also known as PO4, P, and phosphate—are used to diagnose and monitor treatments for conditions that contribute to calcium and PO4 imbalances. PO4 is normally tested via serum level, although urine samples are used to assess the amount of PO4 excreted by the kidneys.

Mildly abnormal PO4 levels produce no symptoms. PO4 levels are usually tested as a result of abnormal calcium effects such as fatigue, muscle weakness, cramping, or bone health symptoms. Phosphorus levels can also be prescribed as a result of kidney injury and gastrointestinal disturbances.[192]

Normal PO4 standards range from 2.4 to 4.1 mg/dL. Values can vary by testing site. Low levels are associated with alcoholism, hypercalcemia, hyperparathyroidism, malnutrition, and vitamin D deficiency. High levels are present in diabetic ketoacidosis, kidney failure, liver disease, overconsumption of vitamin D, high PO4 consumption, and use of medications containing phosphate.[192]

## Potassium

A potassium (K) test is used to identify hyperkalemia and hypokalemia. It is a component of the electrolyte panel, BMP, and CMP. This electrolyte is essential for cell metabolism. It plays a vital role in transporting nutrients, communicates messages between nerves and muscles, and controls the heart's electrical activity.

Potassium level tests are essential in diagnosing and managing kidney injury. Other conditions that contribute to abnormal potassium levels include vomiting and profuse sweating. Potassium as a standalone laboratory value is used in diagnosing and managing heart conditions and monitoring the effects of mediations that cause potassium loss (such as diuretics) or retention.[193]

The normal potassium concentrations range from 3.7 mEq/L to 5.2 mEq/L. Normal values can be different, depending on the testing facility. See **TABLE 8.29**.

**TABLE 8.29** Conditions contributing to abnormal potassium concentrations

| Hyperkalemia | Hypokalemia |
|---|---|
| ■ Kidney disease<br>■ Addison's disease<br>■ Injury to tissue<br>■ Infection<br>■ Diabetes<br>■ Dehydration<br>■ High potassium intake via diet<br>■ Excessive IV potassium<br>■ Certain drugs can also cause high potassium in a small percentage of people<br>■ Nonsteroidal anti-inflammatory drugs (NSAIDs), ACE inhibitors, beta blockers, angiotensin-converting enzyme inhibitors, and potassium-sparing diuretics | ■ Diarrhea<br>■ Vomiting<br>■ Conn syndrome (hyperaldosteronism)<br>■ Complication of acetaminophen overdose<br>■ Insulin therapy<br>■ Use of potassium-wasting diuretics<br>■ In addition, certain drugs such as corticosteroids, beta-adrenergic agonists, alpha-adrenergic antagonists, antibiotics, and the antifungal agent amphotericin B |

Data from US National Library of Medicine. Potassium. Medline Plus. 2016. https://medlineplus.gov/ency/article/003484.htm. Accessed June 3, 2017.

## Sodium

Sodium (Na) is the major component of extracellular fluid. It is an electrolyte essential for all body functions, including regulation of acid–base balance, tissue osmolality, and enzyme activity. It is present in all body fluids. As such, it plays an essential role for the retention of body water by maintaining osmotic pressure.[194]

A serum sodium test can be used to identify and to monitor treatment for dehydration, edema, hypernatremia, and hyponatremia. This test can also be ordered to pinpoint electrolyte imbalances as well as illnesses related to hypertension, heart failure, liver, kidney injury, and other conditions.[194]

Normal Na values are 137–147 mmol/L. Hyponatremia can occur as a result of Na losses related to diarrhea, vomiting, profuse sweating, use of diuretics, kidney injury, and Addison's disease. Excessive fluid consumption and the presence of edema also contribute to low Na levels. Edema can occur as a result of heart failure, cirrhosis, and kidney conditions that contribute to protein loss. Fluid retention also occurs as a result of high levels of antidiuretic hormone in the body. Hypernatremia is most often caused by dehydration, Cushing's syndrome, or diabetes insipidus.[194]

Sodium urine levels should be assessed in association with serum blood results. The body typically removes excess sodium throughout the day. High urine Na levels can be a result of increased serum Na levels. If the increased urine Na level is elevated to true Na losses, the blood serum Na levels will be normal to low. When abnormal Na levels are related to decreased intake, both Na and urine Na levels will be low.[194]

**Recap** Biochemical studies are an important component of conducting population studies and completing assessments on individuals. Blood and urine levels echo the amount of nutrients and dietary compounds found in the body or passing through the body from food and supplement intake.

## ▶ Chapter Summary

The use of biomarkers is common in both clinical research and clinical practice. Some biomarkers have accurately forecast pertinent clinical outcomes across a range of treatments and populations. For others, the validity is assumed.[10]

In the clinical setting, the laboratory tests most commonly used in the assessment of individuals are measurements of serum protein concentrations—specifically, albumin, prealbumin, and transferrin. Of the three proteins, albumin has been the most extensively researched. Serum albumin and prealbumin are no longer considered reliable indicators of nutritional status. Many clinical variables including hydration status, organ function, infection, and metabolic stress affect albumin results, so this protein has been deemed a better marker of the severity of disease and inflammation than of nutritional status.[13] We now know that these assessment parameters are indicators of severity of disease and not sensitive indicators of nutritional status.

Biochemical assessment parameters are influenced by non-nutrition aspects related to disease process, physiology, and environmental factors, to name a few. Data obtained from other assessment sources such as diet history and anthropometric references help frame the results obtained from biochemical assessments.

Blood or urine levels of biochemical markers (or both) can be useful in evaluating the adequacy of intake for individuals and the American population as a whole. These indicators can suggest cumulative intakes from foods, some fortified with micronutrients (such as iron, thiamin, riboflavin, niacin, and folate), and from dietary supplements that contain vitamins, minerals, or both. Blood and urine concentrations of biochemical indicators can be influenced by factors other than diet, such as diseases.[43]

Nutritional deficiencies are well documented and have specific signs and symptoms. The CDC reports that biochemical concentrations below optimum levels have been linked to adverse health effects. Diseases associated with less-than-desirable biochemical levels include cardiovascular disease, stroke, impaired cognitive function, cancer, eye diseases, and poor bone health. Consuming excessive amounts of nutrients can show signs and symptoms of toxicity.[43]

Vitamins are organic chemical compounds that are essential in small amounts for normal body functioning, disease prevention, and well-being. Vitamins and minerals must be ingested (with the exception of vitamin D) because they cannot be synthesized by the body. There are many contributors to vitamin deficiencies. In its basic form, a vitamin deficiency is linked to diet. In many countries around the world, individuals with scarce resources do not eat adequate amounts of nutrient-rich foods such as meat, eggs, fish, milk, legumes, fruits, and vegetables.

HMD has documented the absence of nutrition biochemical markers as a knowledge gap that requires further research. The current knowledge gap includes the need for predictive biomarkers that can forecast functional outcomes and chronic diseases, as well as the need to improve dietary assessment and planning methods.[2] Nutrition biomarkers have their own set of limitations. This includes cost and the degree of invasiveness.[6]

---

 **CASE STUDY**

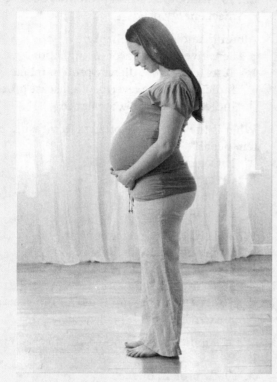

© Amble Design/Shutterstock.

Maria is a 28-year-old woman visiting your outpatient clinic for the first time. She complains of feeling extremely tired for most of the past 4–6 months. She is 6 months pregnant with her second child. Maria is not being examined by a physician on a regular basis and is not taking prenatal vitamins. A nutrition-focused physical exam yields pale conjunctiva and spooning nails. Her laboratory history includes the following results:

- Hg: 7.1 g/dL
- HCT: 23%
- Mean corpuscular volume: 110 fl (normal = 85–95 fl)
- Serum ferritin: < 15 ng/mL
- Transferrin: < 10%

### Questions:

1. How reliable is a physical examination in diagnosing anemia?
2. What are the lab values describing?
3. How does the MCV help you in a diagnostic workup of anemia?
4. Do the other laboratory results such as Hg, HCT, and ferritin add to the diagnosis? Explain.
5. What other tests would help confirm iron deficiency?
6. What is ferritin? How do you interpret low and high ferritin values?
7. The attending physician in the clinic wishes to order vitamin B12 and folate tests to ensure a complete laboratory profile. Is this indicated? Explain your answer.

# Learning Portfolio

## Key Terms

Biomarker assessment
Conditionally indispensable amino acids
Creatinine clearance
Creatinine height index (CHI)
Dispensable amino acids
Erythropoiesis
Estimated glomerular filtration rate (eGFR)
Hemochromatosis

Hemolysis
Hypervitaminosis
Hypoparathyroidism
Indispensable amino acids
Nitrogen balance
Nonprotein calories
Nutritional biomarker
Phototransduction

## Study Questions

1. The use of biomarker indicators is:
   a. A subjective way to evaluate nutritional status.
   b. An objective approach to measure nutritional status.
   c. An assessment method to quantify all dietary intake.
   d. A precise way to account for self-reported data.

2. One limitation of using nutrition biomarker includes:
   a. Nutrition biomarkers are not especially reliable.
   b. Nutrition biomarkers only measure vitamin intake.
   c. Nutrition biomarkers are expensive to use.
   d. Nutrition biomarkers are noninvasive.

3. In nutrition-related research a biomarker is defined as:
   a. A distinct molecule found in blood or other body fluids that is a sign of disease, process, or condition.
   b. A chemical used to measure an individual's level of health.
   c. A substrate to measure organ performance.
   d. A body chemical used to measure how well the body metabolizes food.

4. In the clinical setting, which are the most commonly used laboratory test to measure protein concentrations?
   a. Albumin, transferrin, creatinine
   b. Creatinine, prealbumin, creatinine height index
   c. Transferrin, creatinine, albumin
   d. Prealbumin, transferrin, albumin

5. A creatinine test is used to measure:
   a. Protein levels.
   b. Kidney function.
   c. Liver function.
   d. Urine clearance.

6. The RDA for dietary protein was established based on:
   a. Research on nitrogen balance at the time the RDA was published.
   b. Research on prealbumin levels at the time the RDA was published.
   c. Research on albumin levels at the time the RDA was published.
   d. Research on creatinine balance at the time the RDA was published.

7. Why must individuals meet their nonprotein needs?
   a. To ensure that the individual's carbohydrate needs are met
   b. To promote sufficient nitrogen intake
   c. To support sufficient vitamin and mineral intake to support needs
   d. To ensure the carbon protein is not used to meet energy needs

8. Albumin and prealbumin are:
   a. Sensitive indicators of malnutrition.
   b. Tests to measure dietary protein intake.
   c. Indicators of the severity of a disease process.
   d. Indicators of nitrogen balance.

9. What is the acceptable process to measure protein needs?
   a. Nitrogen balance
   b. Creatinine height index
   c. Creatinine clearance
   d. Urea nitrogen

10. What is the function of albumin?
    a. To maintain blood pressure
    b. To transport tyroxine
    c. To transport iron
    d. To act as a carrier molecule for minerals and hormones

11. What conditions are known to affect albumin levels?
    a. Daily protein intake
    b. Inflammatory conditions
    c. The body's hormone level
    d. Daily caloric intake

12. Prealbumin has a half-life of:
    a. Two to three days.
    b. 12 hours.
    c. 14 to 20 days.
    d. Three to five days.

13. Prealbumin levels appear to be high with episodes of:
    a. Postsurgical complications.
    b. The presence of hepatic disease.
    c. Acute catabolic states.
    d. Renal failure.

14. Transferrin levels are decreased in the presence of:
    a. Iron deficiency anemia.
    b. Heart failure.
    c. Low albumin levels.
    d. Hodgkin's disease.

15. Retinol binding capacity circulates in the blood bound to:
    a. Creatinine.
    b. Vitamin A.
    c. Vitamin C.
    d. Prealbumin.

16. Most of the body's iron is stored in:
    a. The bones.
    b. The blood.
    c. Hemoglobin molecules.
    d. The enamel of the teeth.

17. According to the World Health Organization, how many cases of anemia worldwide are the result of iron deficiencies?
    a. 0.5 billion to 1.6 billion
    b. 3.3 billion to 5.2 billion
    c. 1.5 million to 2.0 million
    d. 1.2 million to 2.3 million

18. What happens during stage one iron deficiency?
    a. We see impaired erythropoiesis.
    b. Bone marrow iron stores are low, but hemoglobin and serum iron are within normal levels.
    c. The transferrin level is increased (>8.5 mg/L), and serum iron and transferrin saturation are reduced to < 50 $\mu$g/dL.
    d. Anemia is present even though RBCs appear to be normal.

19. What is one of the first changes seen in individuals with iron-deficiency anemia?
    a. High hematocrit level
    b. High MCV
    c. Low hemoglobin
    d. Low ferritin

20. TIBC is used to measure:
    a. The amount of oxygen in the blood.
    b. Either iron deficiency or iron overload.
    c. Iron reserves.
    d. Transferrin ratios to iron.

21. What is mean corpuscular hemoglobin?
    a. The average amount of hemoglobin by weight in the RBCs of a blood sample
    b. The packed spun volume of blood that contains intact RBCs calculated as a percentage
    c. Determines the oxygen carrying capacity of the blood
    d. Measures the average size of RBCs, which helps define the type of anemia present

22. Which mineral is essential for normal growth and development during pregnancy, childhood, and adolescence and is needed to maintain adequate sense of taste and smell?
    a. Calcium
    b. Iodine
    c. Zinc
    d. Phosphorus

23. The calcium RDA was determined based on:
    a. The amount of calcium needed for the average healthy male.
    b. The amounts of calcium needed for bone health.
    c. The amount of calcium needed for teeth enamel.
    d. The amount of calcium needed during pregnancy.

24. Worldwide, what are the mains sources of iodine?
    a. Table salt and scallops
    b. Seafood and table salt
    c. Iodized salt and seafood
    d. Iodized salt and fish

25. Vitamin A is:
    a. A chemical organic compound essential, in small amounts, for normal body functioning.
    b. A trace element that is a vital component of thyroid hormones.
    c. One of the most abundant vitamins in the body and involved in vascular contraction and vasodilation.
    d. A group of fat-soluble retinoids, including retinol, retinal, and retinyl esters.

26. The two main forms of vitamin D are:
    a. Vitamin D and $D_2$ (ergocalciferol).
    b. 25-hydroxyvitamin D and vitamin $D_3$ (cholecalciferol).
    c. $D_2$ (ergocalciferol) and $D_3$ (cholecalciferol).
    d. 25(OH)D and $D_2$ (ergocalciferol).

27. Vitamin C is an important vitamin due to its involvement in?
    a. The biosynthesis of carnitine, neurotransmitters, collagen, and other components of connective tissue.
    b. The metabolism of amino acids, glycogen, and sphingoid bases.
    c. Promoting acid–base balance.
    d. Transforming pyridoxal, pyridoxine, pyridoxamine, and their respective 5-phosphates into water-soluble substances.

28. A vitamin $B_6$ deficiency is a precursor of:
    a. Microcytic anemia.
    b. Iron-deficiency anemia.

  c. Macrocytic anemia.
  d. Thalassemia anemia.

29. What percentage of folic acid is absorbed by the body when the folic acid is taken with food?
  a. 95
  b. 90
  c. 85
  d. 100

30. The main causes of vitamin $B_{12}$ deficiency include:
  a. Megaloblastic anemia and decreased transferrin.
  b. Iron-deficiency anemia and $B_6$ malabsorption from food.
  c. Vitamin C and vitamin $B_{12}$ malabsorption from food.
  d. Vitamin $B_{12}$ malabsorption from food and pernicious anemia.

## Discussion Questions

1. What is the definition of biochemical marker?
2. Describe the laboratory tests most commonly used in a clinical setting to assess an individual's protein stores?
3. What is the value of using biochemical markers for mineral levels? Give two examples and discuss how the use of mineral biomarkers is used to identify deficiencies and monitor public health.
4. Identify and discuss two vitamins whose deficiency affect worldwide health. Discuss how prevalent the problem is and review the data used to assess the problem.
5. Describe hyponatremia, hyponatremia, hyperkalemia, and hypokalemia. What test can be used to identify each of these conditions?

## Activities

1. Visit the American Association for Clinical Chemistry section for health professionals (https://labtestsonline.org/for-health-professionals/). Select an article from "The Latest News" and provide an executive summary for the instructor and a three-minute verbal synopsis to the class. Why is this an important topic?
2. Vitamins have been linked to the prevention and treatment of many conditions, including breast cancer, cardiovascular disease, and even obesity. Locate a research study from a peer-reviewed source that addresses vitamin health claims. What is the claim being researched? What was the conclusion? How does this research affect the health of individuals and populations? Does this research study affect practice? Why? Why not?

## Online Resources

### CDC's Second Nutrition Report: Infographic

The second national report on biochemical indicators of diet and nutrition in the U.S. population (2012) from the Centers for Disease Control and Prevention: https://www.cdc.gov/nutritionreport/infographic .html.

### CDC: Anemia or Iron Deficiency

https://www.cdc.gov/nchs/fastats/anemia.htm

### NIH: Dietary Supplements

https://ods.od.nih.gov/

### National Institutes of Health: Nutrient Recommendations

https://ods.od.nih.gov/Health_Information/Dietary _Reference_Intakes.aspx

### National Academies of Sciences, Engineering, and Medicine: Food and Nutrition Board

http://nationalacademies.org/hmd/about-hmd /leadership-staff/hmd-staff-leadership-boards/food -and-nutrition-board.aspx

### National Academies of Science, Engineering, and Medicine: Dietary Reference Intakes

https://www.nap.edu/catalog/9956/dietary-reference -intakes-applications-in-dietary-assessment#toc

### CDC: National Health and Nutrition Examination Survey

https://www.cdc.gov/nchs/nhanes/index.htm

### U.S. Department of Agriculture: ChooseMyPlate

https://www.choosemyplate.gov/

**USDA ChooseMyPlate: Dietary Guidelines 2015–2020**

https://www.choosemyplate.gov/dietary-guidelines

**American Association for Clinical Chemistry: Lab Tests Online**

https://labtestsonline.org/

# References

1. Pfeiffer CM, Schleicher RL, Johnson CL, Coates PM. Assessing vitamin status in large population surveys by measuring biomarkers and dietary intake—two case studies: folate and vitamin D. *Food Nutr Res.* 2012; 56:5944.
2. National Academy of Sciences Engineering and Medicine. Dietary reference intakes: research synthesis workshop summary: Vitamin C. 2007. file:///Users/nancymunoz/Downloads/202-210.pdf. Accessed May 28, 2017.
3. Hardin DS. Validating dietary intake with biochemical markers. *J Am Diet Assoc.* 2009; 109(10):1698-1699.
4. McCabe-Sellers B. Advancing the art and science of dietary assessment through technology. *J Am Diet Assoc.* 2010; 110(1):52-54.
5. Monsen ER. *Research Successful Approaches.* 2nd ed. Chicago, IL: American Dietetic Association; 2003:1-482.
6. Thompson FE, Subar AF, Loria CM, Reedy JL, Baranowski T. Need for technological innovation in dietary assessment. *J Am Diet Assoc.* 2010; 110(1):48-51.
7. Combs GF, Trumbo PR, McKinley MC, et al. Biomarkers in nutrition: New frontiers in research and application. *Ann NY Acad Sci.* 2013; 1278(1):1-10.
8. Potischman N. Biologic and methodologic issues for nutritional biomarkers. *J Nutr.* 2003; 133(Suppl 3):875S–880S.
9. Biomarkers Definition Working Group. Biomarkers and surrogate endpoints: preferred definitions and conceptual framework. *Clin Pharmacol Ther.* 2001; 69:89.
10. Strimbu K, Tavel JA. What are biomarkers? *Curr Opin HIV AIDS.* 2010; 5(6):463-466.
11. Raiten DJ, Namasté S, Brabin B, et al. Executive summary: Biomarkers of nutrition for development: building a consensus. *Am J Clin Nutr.* 2011; 94(2):633S–650S.
12. Jellinge ME, Henriksen DP, Hallas P, Brabrand M. Hypoalbuminemia is a strong predictor of 30-day all-cause mortality in acutely admitted medical patients: A prospective, observational, cohort study. *PLoS One.* 2014; 9(8):e105983.
13. Jeejeebhoy KN. Nutritional assessment. *Nutrition.* 2000; 16(7-8):585-590.
14. Cross AJ, Major JM, Sinha R. Urinary biomarkers of meat consumption. *Cancer Epidemiol Biomarkers Prev.* 2011; 20(6):1107-1111.
15. American Association of Clinical Chemistry. *Creatinine.* 2017. https://labtestsonline.org/understanding/analytes/creatinine/tab/test/-what.
16. Creatinine height index. *Mosby's Medical Dictionary.* 8th ed. New York, NY: Elsevier; 2009. http://medical-dictionary.thefreedictionary.com/creatinine+height+index.
17. Alpers DH, Stenson WF, Taylor BE, Bier DM. *Manual of Nutritional Therapeutics.* 5th ed. Philadelphia, PA: Wolters Kluwer/Lippincott Williams and Wilkins; 2008. https://books.google.com/books?id=b0iiYNob_WwC&pg=PA104&lpg=PA104&dq=what+is+creatinine+height+index&source=bl&ots=wk9bymegzE&sig=n9R5UdmILm1eCrjAFhvNSc1So38&hl=en&sa=X&ved=0ahUKEwiQ6aKeqOXTAhVY2GMKHf26DCw4ChDoAQg-MAU-v=onepage&q=what%20is%20creatinine%20height%20index&f=false.
18. National Academy of Sciences Engineering and Medicine. *Dietary Reference Intake- Protein and Amino Acids.* 2005. https://www.nap.edu/read/10490/chapter/12.
19. Courtney-Martin G, Ball RO, Pencharz PB, Elango R. Protein requirements during aging. *Nutrients.* 2016; 8(8):492.
20. Duffy B, Gunn T, Collinge J, Pencharz PB. The effect of varying protein quality and energy intake on the nitrogen metabolism of parenterally fed very low birthweight (less than 1600 g) infants. *Pediatr Res.* 1981; 15(7):1040-1044.
21. World Health Organization (WHO). Maternal, newborn, child and adolescent health: Malnutrition. 2017. http://www.who.int/maternal_child_adolescent/topics/child/malnutrition/en/.
22. Tierney EP, Sage RJ, Shwayder T. Kwashiorkor from a severe dietary restriction in an 8-month infant in suburban Detroit, Michigan: Case report and review of the literature. *Int J Dermatol.* 2010; 49(5):500-506.
23. Corish CA, Kennedy NP. Protein-energy undernutrition in hospital in-patients. *Br J Nutr.* 2000; 83(6):575-591.
24. *Merriam Webster Dictionary.* Nitrogen balance. 2017. https://www.merriam-webster.com/dictionary/nitrogen balance.
25. Meakins TS, Jackson AA. Salvage of exogenous urea nitrogen enhances nitrogen balance in normal men consuming marginally inadequate protein diets. *Clin Sci (Lond).* 1996; 90:215–255.
26. Zello GA, Pencharz PB, Ball RO. Phenylalanine flux, oxidation, and conversion to tyrosine in humans studied with L-[1-13C] phenylalanine. *Am J Physiol.* 1990; 259:E835-E843.
27. Rand WM, Young VR. Statistical analysis of nitrogen balance data with reference to the lysine requirement in adults. *J Nutr.* 1999; 129(10):1920–1926.
28. Doweiko JP, Nompleggi DJ. The role of albumin in human physiology and pathophysiology, part III: Albumin and disease states. *J Parenter Enteral Nutr.* 1991; 15:476–483.
29. Raguso CA, Dupertuis YM, Pichard C. The role of visceral proteins in the nutritional assessment of intensive care unit patients. *Curr Opin Clin Nutr Metab Care.* 2003; 6(2):211–216.
30. Bharadwaj S, Ginoya S, Tandon P, et al. Malnutrition: Laboratory markers vs nutritional assessment. *Gastroenterol Rep.* 2016; 4(4):272–280. https://www.ncbi.nlm.nih.gov/pubmed/27174435.
31. Pronsky Z, Crowe JP. *Food and Medication Interactions.* 17th ed. Birchrunville, PA: Food Medication Interactions; 2012.
32. Fuhrman MP, Charney P, Mueller CM. Hepatic proteins and nutrition assessment. *J Am Diet Assoc.* 2004; 104:1258–1264.
33. Finucane P, Rudra T, Hsu R, et al. Markers of the nutritional status in acutely ill elderly patients. *Gerontology.* 1988; 34:304–310.
34. Gibson RS. Assessment of protein status. In: Gibson RS, ed. *Principles of Nutritional Assessment.* New York, NY: Oxford University Press; 1990.
35. Ronne H, Ocklind C. Ligand-dependent regulation of intracellular protein transport: Effect of vitamin A on the secretion of retinol-binding protein. *J Cell Biol.* 1983; 96(3):907–910.
36. Davis JT, DE O. Retinol processing by the peritubular cell from rat testis. *Biol Reprod.* 1995; 52(2):356–364.

37. Davis JT, Ong DE. Synthesis and secretion of retinol-binding protein by cultured rat Sertoli cells. *Biol Reprod.* 1992; 47(4):528–533.

38. Jaworowski A, Fang Z, Khong TF, et al. Protein synthesis and secretion by cultured retinal pigment epithelia. *Biochim Biophys Acta.* 1995; 1245(1):121–129.

39. MacDonald PN, Bok D, Ong DE. Localization of cellular retinol-binding protein and retinol-binding protein in cells comprising the blood-brain barrier of rat and human. *Proc Natl Acad Sci USA.* 1990; 87(11):4265–4269.

40. Newcomer ME, Ong DE. Retinol binding protein and its interaction with transthyretin. In: *Madame Curie Bioscience Database [Internet].* Austin, TX: Landes Bioscience. https://www.ncbi.nlm.nih.gov/books/NBK6223/.

41. Yang Q, Graham TE, Mody N, et al. Serum retinol binding protein 4 contributes to insulin resistance in obesity and type 2 diabetes. *Nature.* 2005; 436:356–362.

42. Zabetian-Targhi F, Mahmoudi MJ, Rezaei N, Mahmoudi M. Retinol binding protein 4 in relation to diet, inflammation, immunity, and cardiovascular diseases. *Adv Nutr.* 2015; 6: 748–762.

43. Centers for Disease Control and Prevention (CDC). *Second National Report on Biochemical Indicators of Diet and Nutrition in the U.S. Population 2012.* https://www.cdc.gov/nutritionreport/pdf/nutrition_book_complete508_final.pdf.

44. Miret S, Simpson RJ, McKie AT. Physiology and molecular biology of dietary iron absorption. *Annu Rev Nutr.* 2003; 23:283–301.

45. Institute of Medicine, Food, and Nutrition Board. *Dietary Reference Intakes: Vitamin A, Vitamin K, Arsenic, Boron, Chromium, Copper, Iodine, Iron, Manganese, Molybdenum, Nickel, Silicon, Vanadium, and Zinc.* Washington, DC: National Academy Press; 2001. https://www.nap.edu/catalog/11537/dietary-reference-intakes-the-essential-guide-to-nutrient-requirements.

46. US Department of Agriculture. Scientific Report of the 2015 Dietary Guidelines Advisory Committee. 2015. https://health.gov/dietaryguidelines/2015-scientific-report/pdfs/scientific-report-of-the-2015-dietary-guidelines-advisory-committee.pdf.

47. Stoltzfus RJ. Iron deficiency: Global prevalence and consequences. *Food Nutr Bull.* 2003; (4 Suppl):S99-S103. https://www.uptodate.com/contents/iron-deficiency-in-infants-and-young-children-screening-prevention-clinical-manifestations-and-diagnosis/abstract/1,2.

48. WHO. Worldwide Prevalence of Anaemia 1993–2005: WHO Global Database on Anemia. 2008. http://apps.who.int/iris/bitstream/10665/43894/1/9789241596657_eng.pdf.

49. Braunstein EM. Merck Manual—iron Deficiency Anemia. 2017. http://www.merckmanuals.com/professional/hematology-and-oncology/anemias-caused-by-deficient-erythropoiesis/iron-deficiency-anemia.

50. Haas JD, Brownlie T IV. Iron deficiency and reduced work capacity: A critical review of the research to determine a causal relationship. *J Nutr.* 2001; 131(2S-2):676S-688S.

51. Schorr TO, Hediger ML. Anemia and iron-deficiency anemia: Compilation of data on pregnancy outcome. *Am J Clin Nutr.* 1994; 59:(2 suppl):492S-500S.

52. Grantham-McGregor S, Ani C. A review of studies on the effect of iron deficiency on cognitive development in children. *J Nutr.* 2001; 131:(2S-2):649S–666S.

53. Beard J. Indicators of the iron status of the population: Free erythrocyte protoporphyrin and zinc protoporphyrin; serum and plasma iron, total iron binding capacity and transferrin saturation; and serum transferrin receptor. In: WHO/CDC. *Assessing the Iron Status of Populations: Report of a Joint World Health Organization/Centers for Disease Control and Prevention Technical Consultation on the Assessment of Iron Status at the Population Level.* Geneva: World Health Organization; 2007. http://www.who.int/nutrition/publications/micronutrients/anaemia_iron_deficiency/9789241596107/en/.

54. Pietrangelo A. Hereditary hemochromatosis—a new look at an old disease. *N Engl J Med.* 2004; 350(23):2383–2397.

55. Meyron-Holtz EG, Moshe-Belizowski S, Cohen LA. A possible role for secreted ferritin in tissue iron distribution. *J Neural Transm (Vienna).* 2011; 118(3):337–347.

56. WHO/UNICEF/UNU. *Iron Deficiency Anaemia: Assessment, Prevention, and Control. A Guide For Programme Managers.* Geneva: World Health Organization; 2011. http://www.who.int/nutrition/publications/micronutrients/anaemia_iron_deficiency/WHO_NHD_01.3/en/.

57. Moore C, Ormseth M, Fuchs H. Causes and significance of markedly elevated serum ferritin levels in an academic medical center. *J Clin Rheumatol.* 2013; 19(6):324–328.

58. Wians FH, Urban JE, Keffer JH, Kroft SH. Discriminating between iron deficiency anemia and anemia of chronic disease using traditional indices of iron status vs transferrin receptor concentration. *Am J Clin Pathol.* 2001; 115(1):112–118.

59. Weiss G, Goodnough LT. Anemia of chronic disease. *N Engl J Med.* 2005; 352(10):1011–1023.

60. Finch CA, Huebers H. Perspectives in iron metabolism. *N Engl J Med.* 1982; 306(25):1520-1528.

61. Braunstein EM. Merck Manual—Iron Deficiency Anemia. 2017. http://www.merckmanuals.com/professional/hematology-and-oncology/anemias-caused-by-deficient-erythropoiesis/iron-deficiency-anemia.

62. Anderson KE, Sassa S, Peterson CM, Kappas A. Increased erythrocyte uroporphyrinogen-l-synthetase, delta-aminolevulinic acid dehydratase and protoporphyrin in hemolytic anemias. *Am J Med.* 1977; 63(3):359–364.

63. Benz EJ. Disorders of hemoglobin. In: Kasper D, Fauci A, Hauser S, Longo D, Jameson J, Loscalzo J. eds. *Harrison's Principles of Internal Medicine.* 19th ed. New York, NY: McGraw-Hill; 2017. http://accessmedicine.mhmedical.com/content.aspx?bookid=1130&sectionid=79731188.

64. Gallagher PG. The red blood cell membrane and its disorders: Hereditary spherocytosis, elliptocytosis, and related diseases. In: Kaushansky K, Lichtman MA, Beutler E, Kipps TJ, Seligsohn U, Prchal JT, eds. *Williams Hematology.* 8th ed. New York, NY: McGraw Hill; 2010; 617–646.

65. Gehrs BC, Friedberg RC. Autoimmune hemolytic anemia. *Am J Hematol.* 2002; 69(4):258–271.

66. Schick P. Hemolytic anemia. 2016. http://emedicine.medscape.com/article/201066-overview?pa=UrKztP%2FwAgnnZuXAA40p1sRU1AG3dtUDcrfPQ8EpedOOH8CAi2jrbjp1im2DedctW7ArB8PRZz0YZIdSDBS0bichrzF%2F7vlnSF6AEX%2F09M8%3D - a5.

67. Mais DD. Diseases of red blood cells. In: Laposata M, ed. *Laboratory Medicine: The Diagnosis of Disease in the Clinical Laboratory.* New York, NY: McGraw-Hill; 2014. http://accessmedicine.mhmedical.com/content.aspx?bookid=1069&sectionid=60776350.

68. Cario H. Childhood polycythemias/erythrocytoses: Classification, diagnosis, clinical presentation, and treatment. *Ann Hematol.* 2005; 84(3):137–145.

69. Kemp WL, Burns DK, Brown TG. Hematopathology. In: *Pathology: The Big Picture.* New York, NY: McGraw-Hill; 2008.

70. Ryan DH. Examination of blood cells. In: Kaushansky K, Lichtman MA, Prchal JT, Levi MM, Press OW, Burns LJ, Caligiuri M. eds. *Williams Hematology*. 9th ed. New York, NY: McGraw-Hill; 2017. http://accessmedicine.mhmedical.com/content.aspx?bookid=1581&sectionid=108034325.

71. England JM, Walford DM, Waters DA. Re-assessment of the reliability of the haematocrit. *Br J Haematol*. 1972; 23:247–256.

72. Fairbanks VF. Nonequivalence of automated and manual hematocrit and erythrocyte indices. *Am J Clin Pathol*. 1980; 73:55–62.

73. Schwartz CR, Garrison MW. Interpretation of clinical laboratory tests. In: Alldredge BK, Corelli RL, Ernst ME, eds. *Koda-Kimble & Young's Applied Therapeutics: The Clinical Use of Drugs*. 10th ed. Baltimore, MD: Lippincott Williams & Wilkins; 2013;16–41.

74. Whalen KL, Borja-Hart N. Interpretation of clinical laboratory data. In: Nemire RE, Kier KL, Assa-Eley M, eds. *Pharmacy Student Survival Guide*, 3rd ed. New York, NY: McGraw-Hill; 2014. http://accesspharmacy.mhmedical.com/content.aspx?bookid=1593&sectionid=99824844.

75. US Department of Health and Human Services, National Institutes of Health, National Heart Lung and Blood Institute. *Your Guide to Anemia: Healthy Lifestyle Changes*; 2011. https://www.nhlbi.nih.gov/files/docs/public/blood/anemia-yg.pdf.

76. Weiss GB, Bessman JD. Spurious automated red cell values in warm autoimmune hemolytic anemia. *Am J Hematol*. 1984; 17(4):433–435.

77. Schrier SL. Approach to the adult patient with anemia. UpToDate. 2016. https://www.uptodate.com/contents/approach-to-the-adult-patient-with-anemia?source=machineLearning&search=Mean%20Corpuscular%20Volume&selectedTitle=2~80&sectionRank=1&anchor=H35 - H35.

78. Schrier SL. Causes and diagnosis of iron deficiency and iron deficiency anemia in adults. UpToDate. 2017. https://www.uptodate.com/contents/causes-and-diagnosis-of-iron-deficiency-and-iron-deficiency-anemia-in-adults?source=search_result&search=The%20Centers%20for%20Disease%20Control%20and%20Prevention%20(CDC)%20in%20the%20United%20States%20has%20developed%20guidelines%20for%20screening%20various%20patient%20groups%20for%20iron%20deficiency&selectedTitle=1~150 - H37.

79. CDC. Recommendations to prevent and control iron deficiency in the United States. *MMWR Recomm Rep*. 1998; 47(RR-3):1–29.

80. US Preventive Services Task Force. Final Update Summary: Iron Deficiency Anemia in Pregnant Women: Screening and Supplementation. 2015. https://www.uspreventiveservicestaskforce.org/Page/Document/UpdateSummaryFinal/iron-deficiency-anemia-in-pregnant-women-screening-and-supplementation.

81. Prasad AS. Clinical manifestations of zinc deficiency. *Annu Rev Nutr*. 1985; 5:341–363.

82. Institute of Medicine, Food, and Nutrition Board. *Dietary Reference Intakes: Vitamin A, Vitamin K, Arsenic, Boron, Chromium, Copper, Iodine, Iron, Manganese, Molybdenum, Nickel, Silicon, Vanadium, and Zinc*. Washington, DC: National Academy Press; 2001. https://www.nap.edu/catalog/11537/dietary-reference-intakes-the-essential-guide-to-nutrient-requirements.

83. Prasad AS. Zinc: An overview. *Nutrition*. 1995; 11:93–99.

84. Heyneman CA. Zinc deficiency and taste disorders. *Ann Pharmacother*. 1996; 30(2):186–187.

85. Simmer K, Thompson RP. Zinc in the fetus and newborn. *Acta Paediatr Scand Suppl*. 1985; 319:158–163.

86. Fabris N, Mocchegiani E. Zinc, human diseases, and aging. *Aging (Milano)*. 1995; 7(2):77–93.

87. Maret W, Sandstead HH. Zinc requirements and the risks and benefits of zinc supplementation. *J Trace Elem Med Biol*. 2006; 20(1):3–18.

88. Rink L, Gabriel P. Zinc and the immune system. *Proc Nutr Soc*. 2000; 59(4):541–552.

89. National Institutes of Health Office of Dietary Supplements. Zinc fact sheet. 2016. https://ods.od.nih.gov/factsheets/Zinc-HealthProfessional/.

90. Alaimo K, McDowell MA, Briefel RR, et al. Dietary intake of vitamins, minerals, and fiber of persons ages 2 months and over in the United States: Third National Health and Nutrition Examination Survey, Phase 1, 1988-91. *Adv Data*. 1994; 14(258):1–28.

91. Interagency Board for Nutrition Monitoring and Related Research. *Third Report on Nutrition Monitoring in the United States*. Washington, DC: US Government Printing Office; 1995.

92. Ervin RB, Kennedy-Stephenson J. Mineral intakes of elderly adult supplement and non-supplement users in the third national health and nutrition examination survey. *J Nutr*. 2002; 132(11):3422–3427.

93. Oakes EJ, Lyon TD, Duncan A, Gray A, Talwar D, O'Reilly DS. Acute inflammatory response does not affect erythrocyte concentrations of copper, zinc and selenium. *Clin Nutr*. 2008; 27(1):115–120.

94. Pazirandeh S. Overview of dietary trace minerals. UpToDate. 2016. https://www.uptodate.com/contents/overview-of-dietary-trace-minerals?source=search_result&search=zinc%20plasma%20concentration&selectedTitle=1~150 - H58.

95. Sachdev HP, Mittal NK, Yadav HS. Oral zinc supplementation in persistent diarrhoea in infants. *Ann Trop Paediatr*. 1990; 10(1):63–69.

96. King JC, Shames DM, Lowe NM, et al. Effect of acute zinc depletion on zinc homeostasis and plasma zinc kinetics in men. *Am J Clin Nutr*. 2001; 74(1):116–124.

97. Pinna K, Woodhouse LR, Sutherland B, Shames DM, King JC. Exchangeable zinc pool masses and turnover are maintained in healthy men with low zinc intakes. *J Nutr*. 2001; 131(9):2288–2294.

98. Hambidge KM. Hair analyses: Worthless for vitamins, limited for minerals. *Am J Clin Nutr*. 1982; 36(5):943–949.

99. Gibson RS. *Principles of Nutritional Assessment*. 2nd ed. New York, NY: Oxford University Press; 2005.

100. Ross AC, Abrams SA, Aloia JF, et al. *Committee to Review Dietary Reference Intakes for Vitamin D and Calcium. Dietary Reference Intakes for Calcium and Vitamin D*. Washington, DC: National Academy Press; 2011.

101. National Institute of Health Office of Dietary Supplements. Calcium. https://ods.od.nih.gov/factsheets/Calcium-Health Professional/.

102. US Department of Agriculture/Economic Research Service. Dairy products: Per capita consumption, United States (Annual). 2016. https://www.ers.usda.gov/data-products/dairy-data/.

103. National Academies of Science, Engeneering, and Medicine. *DRI Dietary reference Intakes for Calcium and Vitamin D*. Washington, DC: The National Academies Press; 2011. https://www.nap.edu/download/13050.

104. Andon MB, Peacock M, Kanerva RL, De Castro JAS. Calcium absorption from apple and orange juice fortified with calcium citrate malate (CCM). *J Am Coll Nutr.* 1996; 15(3):313–316.

105. Weaver CM, Heaney RP. Calcium. In: Shils ME, Shike M, Ross AC, Caballero B, Cousins RJ, eds. *Modern Nutrition in Health and Disease.* 10th ed. Baltimore, MD: Lippincott Williams & Wilkins; 2006; 194–210.

106. Cooper MS, Gittoes NJ. Diagnosis and management of hypocalcaemia. *BMJ.* 2008; 336(7656):1298–1302.

107. Shoback D. Hypocalcemia: definition, etiology, pathogenesis, diagnosis, and management. In: Rosen CJ, ed. *Primer on the metabolic bone diseases and disorders of mineral metabolism.* 7th ed. Hoboken, NJ: American Society for Bone and Mineral Research; 2008.

108. Kelly A, Levine MA. Hypocalcemia in the critically ill patient. *J Intensive Care Med.* 2013; 28(3):166–177.

109. Goltzman D. Diagnostic approach to hypocalcemia. UpTo Date. 2016. https://www.uptodate.com/contents/diagnostic-approach-to-hypocalcemia.

110. Weaver CM, Proulx WR, Heaney RP. Choices for achieving adequate dietary calcium with a vegetarian diet. *Am J Clin Nutr.* 1999; 70(3 suppl):543S-548S.

111. Heaney RP. Bone mass, nutrition, and other lifestyle factors. *Nutr Rev.* 1996; 54(4 pt 2):S3-S10.

112. Kerstetter JE, O'Brien KO, Caseria DM, Wall DE, Insogna KL. The impact of dietary protein on calcium absorption and kinetic measures of bone turnover in women. *J Clin Endocrinol Metab.* 2005; 90(1):26–31.

113. Barrett-Connor E, Chang JC, Edelstein SL. Coffee-associated osteoporosis offset by daily milk consumption. *JAMA.* 1994; 271(4):280-283.

114. Murray CW, Egan SK, Kim H, Beru N, Bolger PM. US Food and Drug Administration's Total Diet Study: Dietary intake of perchlorate and iodine. *J Expo Sci Environ Epidemiol.* 2008; 18(6):571–580.

115. Beers MH. Vitamin deficiency, dependency, and toxicity. In: *Merck Manual of Diagnosis and Therapy.* 18th ed. Whitehouse Station (NJ): Merck & Co.; 2006. http://www.merckmanuals.com/professional/nutritional-disorders/vitamin-deficiency-dependency,-and-toxicity.

116. WHO. *Assessment of Iodine Deficiency Disorders and Monitoring Their Elimination: A Guide for Programme Managers.* 3rd ed. Geneva: WHO; 2007. http://apps.who.int/iris/handle/10665/43781.

117. Andersen S, Karmisholt J, Pedersen KM, Laurberg PR. Reliability of studies of iodine intake and recommendations for number of samples in groups and in individuals. *Br J Nutr.* 2008; 99(4):813–818.

118. United Call to Action. *Investing in the Future: Vitamin and Mineral Deficiencies. Global Report Summary 2009;* 2010. http://www.unitedcalltoaction.org/documents/Investing_in_the_future.pdf.

119. Johnson EJ, Russell RM. Beta-carotene. In: Coates PM, Betz JM, Blackman MR, et al., eds. *Encyclopedia of Dietary Supplements.* 2nd ed. New York, NY: Informa Healthcare; 2010; 115–120.

120. Ross CA. Vitamin A. In: Coates PM, Betz JM, Blackman MR, et al., eds. *Encyclopedia of Dietary Supplements.* 2nd ed. New York, NY: Informa Healthcare; 2010; 778–791.

121. Roodhooft JM. Leading causes of blindness worldwide. *Bull Soc Belge Ophthalmol.* 2002; 283:19–25.

122. WHO. World Health Organization Guideline: Vitamin A supplementation for infants and children 6-59 months of age (2011). 2011. http://www.who.int/nutrition/publications/micronutrients/guidelines/vas_6to59_months/en/.

123. WHO. *Guideline: Vitamin A Supplementation in Pregnant Women.* Geneva: WHO; 2011. http://www.who.int/nutrition/publications/micronutrients/guidelines/vas_pregnant/en/.

124. Imdad A, Ahmed Z, Bhutta ZA. Vitamin A supplementation for the prevention of morbidity and mortality in infants one to six months of age. *Cochrane Database Syst Rev.* 2016:9:CD007480. [ePub ahead of print]

125. Haider BA, Bhutta ZA. Neonatal vitamin A supplementation for the prevention of mortality and morbidity in term neonates in developing countries. *Cochrane Database Syst Rev.* 2011;(10):CD006980.

126. Mazumder S, Taneja S, Bhatia K, et al. Efficacy of early neonatal supplementation with vitamin A to reduce mortality in infancy in Haryana, India (Neovita): A randomised, double-blind, placebo-controlled trial. *Lancet.* 2015; 385(9975):1333–1342.

127. Masanja H, Smith ER, Muhihi A, et al. Effect of neonatal vitamin A supplementation on mortality in infants in Tanzania (Neovita): A randomised, double-blind, placebo-controlled trial. *Lancet*; 2015; 385(9975):1324–1332.

128. Edmond KM, Newton S, Shannon C, et al. Effect of early neonatal vitamin A supplementation on mortality during infancy in Ghana (Neovita): A randomised, double-blind, placebo-controlled trial. *Lancet.* 2015; 385(9975):1315–1323.

129. Saari JC. Retinoids in photosensitive systems. In: Sporn MB, Roberts AB, Goodman DS, eds. *The Retinoids: Biology, Chemistry, and Medicine.* New York, NY: Raven Press; 1994: 351.

130. WHO. *Vitamin A Supplements: A Guide to Their Use in the Treatment and Prevention of Vitamin A Deficiency and Xerophthalmia.* 2nd ed. Geneva: WHO; 1997. http://apps.who.int/iris/handle/10665/41947.

131. Age-Related Eye Disease Study Research Group. A randomized, placebo-controlled, clinical trial of high-dose supplementation with vitamins C and E, beta carotene, and zinc for age-related macular degeneration and vision loss: AREDS report no. 8. *Arch Ophthalmol.* 2001; 119(1):1417–1436.

132. The Age-Related Eye Disease Study 2 Research Group. Lutein + zeaxanthin and omega-3 fatty acids for age-related macular degeneration: the Age-Related Eye Disease Study 2 (AREDS2) randomized clinical trial. *JAMA.* 2013; 309(19):2005–2015.

133. Dawson HD, Yamamoto Y, Zolfaghari R, et al. Regulation of hepatic vitamin A storage in a rat model of controlled vitamin A status during aging. *J Nutr.* 2000; 130(5):1280-1286.

134. Leo MA, Lieber CS. Alcohol, vitamin A, and beta-carotene: Adverse interactions, including hepatotoxicity and carcinogenicity. *Am J Clin Nutr.* 1999; 69(6): 1071–1085.

135. Haskell MJ, Ribaya-Mercado JD. Vitamin A Tracer Task Force. *Handbook on Vitamin A Tracer Dilution Methods to Assess Status and Evaluate Intervention Programs.* Washington, DC: HarvestPlus. 2005. https://assets.publishing.service.gov.uk/media/57a08c83e5274a31e000127a/tech05.pdf.

136. Tanumihardjo SA. Vitamin A status assessment in rats with (13)C(4)-retinyl acetate and gas chromatography/combustion/isotope ratio mass spectrometry. *J Nutr.* 2000; 130(11):2844–2849.

137. Escaron AL, Green MH, Howe JA, Tanumihardjo SA. Mathematical modeling of serum 13C-retinol in captive rhesus monkeys provides new insights on hypervitaminosis A. *J Nutr.* 2009; 139(10):2000–2006.

138. Fieser LF, Fieser M. Vitamin D. In: *Steroids.* New York, NY: Reinhold Publishing; 1959; 90–168.

139. DeLuca HF. The vitamin D story: a collaborative effort of basic science and clinical medicine. *FASEB J.* 1988; 2(3): 224–236.

140. Reichel H, Koeffler HP, Norman AW. The role of the vitamin D endocrine system in health and disease. *N Engl J Med.* 1989; 320(15):980–991. 1989.

141. Holick MF. Vitamin D. In: Shils ME, Shike M, Ross AC, Caballero B, Cousins RJ, eds. *Modern Nutrition in Health and Disease.* 10th ed. Philadelphia, PA: Lippincott Williams & Wilkins; 2006.

142. Norman AW, Henry HH. Vitamin D. In: Bowman BA, Russell RM, eds. *Present Knowledge in Nutrition.* 9th ed. Washington, DC: ILSI Press; 2006.

143. Jones G. Pharmacokinetics of vitamin D toxicity. *Am J Clin Nutr.* 2008; 88(2):582S-586S.

144. National Institute of Health Office of Dietary Supplements. Vitamin D: The Fact Sheet for Health Professionals; 2016. https://ods.od.nih.gov/factsheets/VitaminD-Health Professional/.

145. Cranney A, Horsley T, O'Donnell S, et al. Effectiveness and safety of vitamin D in relation to bone health. *Evid Rep Technol Assess.* No. 158 AHRQ Publication No. 07-E013. Rockville, MD: Agency for Healthcare Research and Quality; 2007.

146. Chung M, Balk EM, Brendel M, et al. Vitamin D and calcium: A systematic review of health outcomes. *Evid Rep Technol Assess.* No. 183. AHRQ Publication No. 09-E015. Rockville, MD: Agency for Healthcare Research and Quality; 2009.

147. Pittas AG, Chung M, Trikalinos T, et al. Systematic review: Vitamin D and cardiometabolic outcomes. *Ann Intern Med.* 2010; 152(5):307–314.

148. National Institutes of Health Office of Dietary Supplements. Vitamin C: Fact Sheet for Health Professionals; 2016. https://ods.od.nih.gov/factsheets/VitaminC-HealthProfessional/.

149. National Academies of Science, Engineering, and Medicine. *Dietary Reference Intakes: The Essential Guide to Nutrient Requirements.* Washington, DC: The National Academies Press; 2006. https://www.nap.edu/catalog/11537/dietary-reference-intakes-the-essential-guide-to-nutrient-requirements.

150. Li Y, Schellhorn HE. New developments and novel therapeutic perspectives for vitamin C. *J Nutr.* 2007; 137(10):2171–2184.

151. Carr AC, Frei B. Toward a new recommended dietary allowance for vitamin C based on antioxidant and health effects in humans. *Am J Clin Nutr.* 1999; 69:1086–1107.

152. Jacob RA, Sotoudeh G. Vitamin C function and status in chronic disease. *Nutr Clin Care.* 2002; 5(2):66–74.

153. Wang AH, Still C. Old world meets modern: a case report of scurvy. *Nutr Clin Pract.* 2007; 22(4):445–448.

154. Weinstein M, Babyn P, Zlotkin S. An orange a day keeps the doctor away: Scurvy in the year 2000. *Pediatrics.* 2001; 108(3):E55.

155. Schleicher RL, Carroll MD, Ford ES, Lacher DA. Serum vitamin C and the prevalence of vitamin C deficiency in the United States: 2003-2004 National Health and Nutrition Examination Survey (NHANES). *Am J Clin Nutr.* 2009; 90(5):1252–1263.

156. National Academies of Science, Engineering, and Medicine. Vitamin B$_6$. In: *Dietary Reference Intakes: The Essential Guide to Nutrient Requirements.* Washington, DC: The National Academies Press; 2006. https://www.nap.edu/catalog/11537/dietary-reference-intakes-the-essential-guide-to-nutrient-requirements.

157. National Institute of Health Office of Dietary Supplements. Vitamin B$_6$: Dietary Supplement Fact Sheet; 2016. https://ods.od.nih.gov/factsheets/VitaminB6-HealthProfessional/.

158. Rybak ME, Pfeiffer CM. Clinical analysis of vitamin B(6): determination of pyridoxal 5'-phosphate and 4-pyridoxic acid in human serum by reversed-phase high-performance liquid chromatography with chlorite postcolumn derivatization. *Anal Biochem.* 2004; 333(2):336–344.

159. Coburn SP. Vitamin B$_6$. In: Song WO, Beecher GR, Eitenmiller RR, eds. *Modern Analytical Methodologies in Fat- and Water-Soluble Vitamins.* New York, NY: John Wiley & Sons; 2000: 291–311.

160. Rybak ME, Jain RB, Pfeiffer CM. Clinical vitamin B$_6$ analysis: An interlaboratory comparison of pyridoxal 5'-phosphate measurements in serum. *Clin Chem.* 2005; 51(7):1223–1231.

161. McCormick D. Vitamin B$_6$. In: Bowman B, Russell R, eds. *Present Knowledge in Nutrition.* 9th ed. Washington, DC: International Life Sciences Institute; 2006.

162. Mackey A, Davis S, Gregory JV. Vitamin B$_6$. In: Shils M, Shike M, Ross A, Caballero B, Cousins R, eds. *Modern Nutrition in Health and Disease.* 10th ed. Baltimore, MD: Lippincott Williams & Wilkins; 2005.

163. National Academies of Science, Engeneering, and Medicne. Folate. In: *Dietary Reference Intakes: The Essential Guide to Nutrient Requirements*; 2006. Washington, DC: The National Academies Press. https://www.nap.edu/catalog/11537/dietary-reference-intakes-the-essential-guide-to-nutrient-requirements.

164. National Institute of Health Office of Dietary Supplements. Folate: Fact sheet for health professionals; 2016. https://ods.od.nih.gov/factsheets/VitaminC-HealthProfessional/.

165. Pfeiffer CM, Fazili Z, Zhang M. Folate analytical methodology. In: Bailey LB, ed. *Folate in Health and Disease.* 2nd ed. Boca Raton, FL: CRC Press, Taylor & Francis Group; 2010: 517–574.

166. Carmel R. Folic acid. In: Shils M, Shike M, Ross A, Caballero B, Cousins R, eds. *Modern Nutrition in Health and Disease.* Baltimore, MD: Lippincott Williams & Wilkins; 2005: 470–481.

167. Scholl TO, Johnson WG. Folic acid: influence on the outcome of pregnancy. *Am J Clin Nutr.* 2000; 71(5 suppl):1295S-1303S.

168. National Academies of Science, Engeneering, and Medicne. Vitamin B$_{12}$. In: *Dietary Reference Intakes: The Essential Guide to Nutrient Requirements.* Washington, DC: The National Academies Press; 2006. https://www.nap.edu/catalog/11537/dietary-reference-intakes-the-essential-guide-to-nutrient-requirements.

169. Clarke R. B-vitamins and prevention of dementia. *Proc Nutr Soc.* 2008; 67(1):75–81.

170. Andrès E, Federici L, Affenberger S, et al. B$_{12}$ deficiency: A look beyond pernicious anemia. *J Fam Pract.* 2007; 56(7):537–542.

171. Carmel R. Biomarkers of cobalamin (vitamin B-12) status in the epidemiologic setting: a critical overview of context, applications, and performance characteristics of cobalamin, methylmalonic acid, and holotranscobalamin II. *Am J Clin Nutr.* 2011; 94(1):348S–358S.

172. Refsum H, Smith AD, Ueland PM, et al. Facts and recommendations about total homocysteine determinations: an expert opinion. *Clin Chem*. 2004; 50(1):3–32.

173. Bottiglieri T. Folate, vitamin B$_{12}$, and neuropsychiatric disorders. *Nutr Rev*. 1996; 54(12):382–390.

174. National Institute of Health Office of Dietary Supplements. Vitamin B$_{12}$: Dietary supplement fact sheet; 2016. https://ods.od.nih.gov/factsheets/VitaminB12-HealthProfessional/.

175. Vidal-Aladall J, Butler CC, Cannings-John R, et al. Oral vitamin B$_{12}$ versus intramuscular vitamin B$_{12}$ for vitamin B$_{12}$ deficiency. *Cochrane Database Syst Rev*. 2005; 20(3):CD004655.

176. Friedman LS. Approach to the patient with abnormal liver biochemical and function tests. UpToDate; 2017. https://www.uptodate.com/contents/approach-to-the-patient-with-abnormal-liver-biochemical-and-function-tests?source=search_result&search=alanine%20aminotransferase&selectedTitle=1~150.

177. American Association of Clinical Chemistry. Total Protein and albumin/globulin (A/G) ratio. Washington, DC: American Association of Clinical Chemistry; 2016. https://labtestsonline.org/understanding/analytes/tp/tab/test.

178. US National Library of Medicine. Bilirubin blood test. Medline Plus; 2015. https://medlineplus.gov/ency/article/003479.htm.

179. American Association of Clinical Chemistry. Bilirubin; 2015. https://labtestsonline.org/understanding/analytes/bilirubin/tab/glance/.

180. American Association of Clinical Chemistry. Blood urea nitrogen; 2016. https://labtestsonline.org/understanding/analytes/bun/tab/glance.

181. American Association of Clinical Chemistry. Creatinine; 2015. https://labtestsonline.org/understanding/analytes/creatinine/tab/test.

182. National Institute of Health National Institute of Diabetes and Digestive and Kidney Diseases. Glomelular filtration rate (GFR) calculators; 2017. https://www.niddk.nih.gov/health-information/health-communication-programs/nkdep/lab-evaluation/gfr-calculators/Pages/gfr-calculators.aspx.

183. American Association of Clinical Chemistry. Calcium; 2017. https://labtestsonline.org/understanding/analytes/calcium/tab/test/.

184. National Library of Medicine. Calcium blood test. Medline Plus; 2015. https://medlineplus.gov/ency/article/003477.htm.

185. National Library of Medicine. CO$_2$ blood test. MedlinePlus; 2017. https://medlineplus.gov/ency/article/003469.htm.

186. American Association of Clinical Chemistry. Bicarbonate; 2016. https://labtestsonline.org/understanding/analytes/co2/tab/glance/.

187. US National Library of Medicine. Chloride test—blood. Medline Plus; 2017. https://medlineplus.gov/ency/article/003485.htm.

188. Stone NJ, Robinson J, Lichtenstein AH, et al. 2013 ACC/AHA guideline on the treatment of blood cholesterol to reduce atherosclerotic cardiovascular risk in adults: A report of the American College of Cardiology/American Heart Association Task Force on Practice Guidelines. *Circulation*. 2013. http://circ.ahajournals.org/content/circulationaha/early/2013/11/11/01.cir.0000437738.63853.7a.full.pdf.

189. American Diabetes Association. Standards of medical care in diabetes 2017. *Diabetes Care*. 2017; 40(suppl 1):S1-S132. https://professional.diabetes.org/sites/professional.diabetes.org/files/media/dc_40_s1_final.pdf..

190. Seaquist ER, Anderson J, Childs B, et al. Hypoglycemia and diabetes: A report of a workgroup of the American Diabetes Association and The Endocrine Society. *Diabetes Care*. 2013; 36(5):1384-1395. https://www.ncbi.nlm.nih.gov/pmc/articles/PMC3631867/.

191. Gubitosi-Klug RA, Braffett BH, White NH, et al. The Diabetes Control and Complications Trial (DCCT)/Epidemiology of Diabetes Interventions and Complications (EDIC) research group. *Diabetes Care*. 2017; 40(8):1010–1016. http://care.diabetesjournals.org/content/40/8/1010.

192. US National Library of Medicine. Phosphorus blood test. MedlinePlus; 2017. https://medlineplus.gov/ency/article/003478.htm.

193. US National Library of Medicine. Potassium. MedlinePlus; 2016. https://medlineplus.gov/ency/article/003484.htm.

194. US National Library of Medicine. Sodium. MedlinePlus; 2017. https://medlineplus.gov/sodium.html-summary.

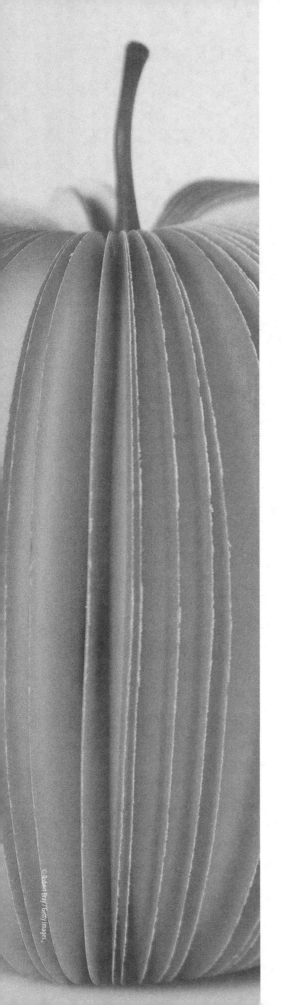

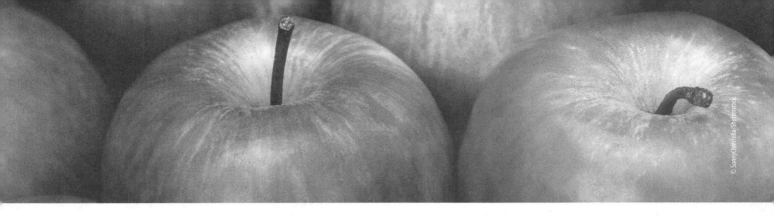

# CHAPTER 9

# Clinical Assessment of Nutritional Status

**Phyllis Famularo**, DCN, RD, CSG, LDN, FAND

## LEARNING OBJECTIVES

After reading this chapter, the learner will be able to:

1. Understand the components of a complete nutritional assessment.
2. Explain how the nutritional status assessment will vary based on the care setting, including acute care, long-term care, rehabilitation setting or community-dwelling patient or client.
3. Express the rationale for obtaining a client history when completing a nutritional assessment.
4. Identify and discuss the information collected in a client history.
5. Define the limitations of completing a food- and nutrition-related history.
6. Indicate how the findings from the nutrition-focused physical exam are used to define the nutritional status of the client.
7. Explain the differences between starvation-related malnutrition, chronic disease-related malnutrition, and acute disease- or injury-related malnutrition.
8. Determine energy requirements for healthy and unhealthy clients.
9. Describe the methods used for estimating protein requirements.
10. Calculate fluid needs for individuals as part of the nutrition-assessment process.
11. Create an awareness of the psychological and behavioral characteristics of an individual with eating disorders.
12. Discuss the impact of HIV on nutrition status.
13. Understand the process for completing the MNA, the MUST, and the SGA.

## ▶ Introduction

A complete and thorough nutritional assessment is critical in determining the most appropriate nutritional plan of care for a patient, resident, or client. A nutritional assessment should have multiple components, including a **client history**, a food- and nutrition-related history, medication regimen, anthropometrics, laboratory and related medical tests, and nutrition-focused physical findings. The last component should include oral status and psychosocial aspects that can affect nutritional status. By using all of the available data, the clinician will be able to recommend and implement nutritional interventions that will lead to improved nutritional status or disease management. In addition to reviewing the components of a nutritional assessment, this chapter gives special consideration to the process for conducting a nutrition-focused physical examination and evaluating individuals for **malnutrition**. The chapter also presents information on the nutritional aspects and management of diseases such as human immunodeficiency virus and eating disorders, as well as the use of validated nutrition-screening and assessment tools.

## ▶ Nutritional Assessment

**Preview**   Adequate nutritional intake is essential to maintaining health, functional status, and overall quality of life. The burden of chronic disease can be ameliorated by consuming an appropriate combination of essential nutrients that incorporate a combination of carbohydrates, protein, fat, fluids, and micronutrients, including vitamins and minerals.

**Nutritional status** can be defined as "the health status of individuals or population groups as influenced by their intake and utilization of nutrients."[1] An individual's nutritional status can be determined by evaluating diet patterns and quality, the process of food and fluid intake, digestion, nutrient absorption, metabolism, and the excretion of waste products. Any factors that affect the intake and use of nutrients can affect nutritional status and health.

To determine if nutritional intake is meeting the individual's needs, a nutritional assessment should be completed. Differences in healthcare settings and target populations guides the process used to complete such an assessment. Its findings, however, will help define a nutrition prescription that will address the individual's nutritional needs and help promote maintenance or improvement of his or her nutritional status.

### Nutrition Screening

Although a full nutritional assessment is the approach of choice in determining nutritional status, **nutrition screening** is the first-line process of identifying patients, clients, or groups that are at nutritional risk and will benefit from nutrition assessment and intervention by a nutrition professional.[2] Because of the limited nutrition resources in the community setting, a nutrition screen may be an acceptable approach for recognizing individuals at nutritional risk. In addition, the large number of admissions to acute-care facilities makes a nutritional screen highly recommended within the first 24 hours of admission so that nutritional risk can be identified and treatment implemented.[3] In the long-term care setting as well as rehabilitation centers that accept Medicare and Medicaid funds, a full nutrition assessment is required for all admissions as described in the regulations set forth by the Centers for Medicare and Medicaid (CMS).[4]

Many validated nutrition-screening tools have been developed and are available for members of the inter-professional team to use. The Academy of Nutrition and Dietetics (the Academy) has completed an evidence analysis to help define the sensitivity, specificity, and reliability of some of the available screens in identifying nutrition risks for different patient populations.[5] Sensitivity, specificity, and reliability can be defined as follows[6]:

- *Sensitivity.* How effective is the screening tool in detecting a disease or condition? The higher the sensitivity of a nutrition-screening tool, the fewer cases of nutrition risk that will go undetected.
- *Specificity.* How often does the screening tool give negative results in those who are free of the disease or condition? The higher the specificity of a nutrition-screening tool, the fewer well-nourished persons who are incorrectly labeled as at nutritional risk, and the fewer resources that are wasted on those who need no intervention.
- *Reliability.* Are results obtained by different investigators consistent when repeated with the same subjects?

A screening tool should be easy to administer and score, transferable from one care setting to another, effective in identifying the need for nutrition-assessment completion, and cost-effective. The use of screening tools facilitates early intervention for those at nutritional risk and includes relevant data on risk factors and the interpretation of data for intervention or treatment.[7] The **Mini Nutritional Assessment (MNA)** and the **Malnutrition Universal Screening Tool (MUST)** are two examples of validated instruments used to determine nutritional risk. These tools are discussed in detail later in this chapter.

## Nutritional Assessment Purpose

The purpose of a nutritional assessment is to acquire, validate, and interpret data needed to identify nutrition-related problems, their root causes, and their relevance to overall health status. A **nutritional assessment** has been defined by the American Society of Enteral and Parenteral Nutrition (ASPEN) as "a comprehensive approach to diagnosing nutrition problems that uses a combination of the following: medical, nutrition, and medication histories; physical examination; anthropometric measurements; and laboratory data."[8] After completing the assessment, the nutrition professional identifies nutritional problems and develops a plan of care with specific interventions to maintain or improve nutritional outcomes. To facilitate nutrition care across health care settings, the Academy has developed the International Dietetics and Nutrition Terminology (IDNT), a standardized language for nutrition professionals. Using this language and evidence-based practice, registered dietitian nutritionists (RDNs) provide medical nutrition therapy (MNT) using nutrition assessment, nutrition diagnoses, interventions, and monitoring and evaluation standards across the continuum of health care.[9]

## Components of Nutritional Assessment

Data collection for a nutritional assessment includes securing anthropometric and biochemical data; clinical assessment information, including client history, medical history, signs and symptoms, and medication use; and food and diet history. The mnemonic ABCD can be used to remember the four main components of the nutritional assessment:

> A—Anthropometric
> B—Biochemical
> C—Clinical assessment
> D—Dietary or food- and nutrition-related history

## Anthropometry

**Anthropometry** is the study of the measurement of the human body in terms of the dimensions of bone, muscle, and adipose (fat) tissue. This includes the measurement of weight, height, weight changes, and body composition, including **body mass index (BMI)**, which is used to determine how the patient compares to reference standards. Results can indicate normal, undernutrition or malnutrition, or overnutrition (overweight and obese). Anthropometric measurements can be used to compare an individual to assess and monitor his or her nutritional status against standards for a population and relevant health studies. The anthropometric measurements most commonly used are height and weight, various circumference measurements, and skinfold thickness. More complex methods include bioelectrical impedance, dual-energy x-ray absorptiometry (DXA), body density, and total body water estimates that are not readily available in clinical settings.[10]

## Weight Measurement

Body weight is one of the easiest and most routinely collected anthropometric measures. Weight is used to monitor the patient's or individual's nutritional status and is and is a rough estimate of energy stores.[11] Weight does not, however, provide information on actual body composition.[12] Because weight can be easily and noninvasively measured, it remains an important measurement in assessing nutritional status and determining energy requirements. Accurate weight measures are critical for the initial nutritional evaluation and subsequent assessments of the patient or individual. In addition, accurate weights are necessary to accurately dose chemotherapeutic agents, anesthetics, and other medications. A variety of conditions may make many patients unable to stand on a regular bathroom or upright beam scale. Also available are a variety of scales that allow an individual to stay seated or facilitates the weight to be obtained while the individual is in bed. Proper technique must be used because dangling limbs and improper zeroing can lead to wide fluctuations in weight measurements. It is important to weigh the patient in the same type of clothing, at the same time of the day, before eating and after voiding.[11] It is recommended that a patient who receives diuretic therapy or has varying edema be weighed in the morning shortly after rising; however, this may be not be possible for some patients or individuals, depending on the care setting. A scale-calibration schedule is critical, as is a battery-charging schedule for digital scales. Frequent training of staff that completes weight measurements is also essential.[13] Research conducted in acute-and long-term care settings has found that recorded weights can be inaccurate, and sometimes weights are not obtained at all.

Body weight measurements can be compared to reference standards published by the National

Center for Health Statistics, which provides data for infants, children, and adults using information from the National Health and Nutrition Examination Survey (NHANES).[14] Weight measurement data are divided into three-month increments for infants, one-year increments for children up to age 19 years, and 10-year increments for adults 20 years of age and older. It provides fifth percentile through 95th percentile data for weights of any given height. The final age grouping for adults is 80 years and older. Although these weight reference tables do not provide "ideal" weights for health, they represent the weight statuses of children and adults living in the United States today.

## Weight Changes

Evaluation of weight changes is an important component when completing a nutrition assessment. Changes in weight, both losses and gains, have been shown to be predictive of negative health outcomes in adults. In a study of older adults, weight loss and weight cycling (alternating weight gain and weight loss) were noted to significantly affect mobility and mortality when compared to those with stable weights or weight gains.[15] Weight gain has also been identified as an indicator of mortality in the intensive care unit (ICU) or in patients with heart failure.[16,17] When assessing individuals with weight loss, the weight loss must be evaluated within the framework in which it occurred, such as in the context of acute illness or injury, chronic illness, and social or environmental circumstances. In acute illness or injury, a weight loss of more than 2% in one week, 5% in one month, and 7.5% in three months is considered severe. Weight loss is severe in chronic disease (organ failure, cancer, rheumatoid arthritis, etc.) and in the context of social or environmental circumstances (anorexia or starvation) if weight loss is more than 5% in one month, 7.5% in three months, 10% in 6 months, and 20% in one year. In long-term care communities (nursing homes) regulated by the CMS, significant weight loss is defined at 5% or more in one month and 10% or more in six months.

Because of the potential for poor outcomes in patients who have significant weight changes, weights should be taken at admission and monitored at routine intervals based on the clinical setting so that timely nutritional interventions can be put into place. When weight does change, it is important to investigate its root cause and determine the appropriate interventions.[18] For example, if a nursing home resident seems to have difficulty chewing and has experienced weight

loss, then the appropriate intervention would be to provide softer foods and refer for a dental consult rather than provide a nutritional supplement between meals. The supplement may improve the caloric intake, but it will not address the chewing problem. For a patient with weight loss and difficulty chewing in an acute-care setting, a softer diet consistency and an oral nutritional supplement may be the appropriate intervention because of the significantly shorter length of stay. Quickly improving the patient's intake and weight status may help prevent readmission to the hospital.

## Height Measurement

An accurate measurement of height is needed because many of the indicators of appropriate body weight require an individual's height.[11] Although the easiest method of obtaining height is a standing-height measurement using a stadiometer (standing scale), this may not always be feasible or accurate because of illness, kyphosis, and limited mobility. Several predictive methods can be used when an individual is unable to stand for a height measurement, and four methods have been reported for measuring height when an individual cannot be measured on a stadiometer: arm span (or a variation called *demispan*), knee height, forearm length (or ulnar length), and segmental measurement.

■ *Arm span.* Arm span is correlated with height in both men and women (±10%).[19] This can be accomplished by having the patient extend both arms at the level of the shoulder with the back pressed against a flat surface for maximum accuracy. The measurement is taken from the longest fingertip on one hand to the longest fingertip on the other hand.[20] In the demispan, the distance is measured from the sternal notch to the tip of the longest fingertip and doubled to estimate stature. The demispan can be used for patients who cannot easily extend both arms, such as those who are contracted or have hemiplegia on one side of the body.[21]

■ *Knee height.* While the patient is supine, both the knee and the ankle are held at 90-degree angles. One blade of a sliding broad-blade caliper is placed under the heel of the foot, and the other blade is placed on the anterior surface of the thigh. The shaft of the caliper is held parallel to the long axis of the lower leg, and pressure is applied to compress the tissue. Height (in cm) is then calculated as follows[21]:

Females: Height in cm = $84.88 - (0.24 \times \text{age})$
$+ (1.83 \times \text{knee height})$

| HEIGHT (m) | | | | | | | | | | | | | | |
|---|---|---|---|---|---|---|---|---|---|---|---|---|---|---|
| Men (<65 years) | 1.94 | 1.93 | 1.91 | 1.89 | 1.87 | 1.85 | 1.84 | 1.82 | 1.80 | 1.78 | 1.76 | 1.75 | 1.73 | 1.71 |
| Men (>65 years) | 1.87 | 1.86 | 1.84 | 1.82 | 1.81 | 1.79 | 1.78 | 1.76 | 1.75 | 1.73 | 1.71 | 1.70 | 1.68 | 1.67 |
| Ulna length (cm) | 32.0 | 31.5 | 31.0 | 30.5 | 30.0 | 29.5 | 29.0 | 28.5 | 28.0 | 27.5 | 27.0 | 26.5 | 26.0 | 25.5 |
| Women (<65 years) | 1.84 | 1.83 | 1.81 | 1.80 | 1.79 | 1.77 | 1.76 | 1.75 | 1.73 | 1.72 | 1.70 | 1.69 | 1.68 | 1.66 |
| Women (>65 years) | 1.84 | 1.83 | 1.81 | 1.79 | 1.78 | 1.76 | 1.75 | 1.73 | 1.71 | 1.70 | 1.68 | 1.66 | 1.65 | 1.63 |
| Men (<65 years) | 1.69 | 1.67 | 1.66 | 1.64 | 1.62 | 1.60 | 1.58 | 1.57 | 1.55 | 1.53 | 1.51 | 1.49 | 1.48 | 1.46 |
| Men (>65 years) | 1.65 | 1.63 | 1.62 | 1.60 | 1.59 | 1.57 | 1.56 | 1.54 | 1.52 | 1.51 | 1.49 | 1.48 | 1.46 | 1.45 |
| Ulna length (cm) | 25.5 | 24.5 | 24.0 | 23.5 | 23.0 | 22.5 | 22.0 | 21.5 | 21.0 | 20.5 | 20.0 | 19.5 | 19.0 | 18.5 |
| Women (<65 years) | 1.65 | 1.63 | 1.62 | 1.61 | 1.59 | 1.58 | 1.56 | 1.55 | 1.54 | 1.52 | 1.51 | 1.50 | 1.48 | 1.47 |
| Women (>65 years) | 1.61 | 1.60 | 1.58 | 1.56 | 1.55 | 1.53 | 1.52 | 1.50 | 1.48 | 1.47 | 1.45 | 1.44 | 1.42 | 1.40 |

**FIGURE 9.1** Estimating height from ulna length.

Reproduced from Estimating height in bedridden patients. RxKinetics. http://www.rxkinetics.com/height_estimate.html. Date unknown. Accessed January 7, 2017.

Males: Height in cm = 64.19 – (0.04 × age) + (2.02 × knee height)

- *Forearm or ulnar length.* This method can also be used in patients who have osteoporosis, kyphosis, or arthritis. Forearm length can be measured by calculating the distance between the olecranon and the styloid process of the ulna. Ulnar length must be converted to height (**FIGURE 9.1**).[22] A study using this method reported that although height decreases with age, arm measurements do not change to the same degree.[23]
- *Segmental measurement.* This method can be used for individuals who have severe neuromuscular deformities, as in cerebral palsy. Segment lengths should be measured between specific bony landmarks and as vertical distances between a flat surface and a bony landmark (heel to knee, knee to hip, hip to shoulder, and shoulder to top of head). The sectional measurements are then totaled to determine stature. Segments should not be measured from joint creases. This method has potential for error and there is only fair to poor agreement with actual height.[24]

## Body Composition
### Body Mass Index

Once accurate weight and height measurements have been obtained, BMI, a weight-to-height ratio, is calculated by dividing weight in kilograms by the square of a patient's height in meters. The result indicates whether the patient is overweight, normoweight, or underweight. A limitation of this measurement is that BMI does not measure body fat directly.

However, research has shown that BMI is moderately correlated with more-direct measures of body fat, including skinfold thickness and bioelectrical impedance.[25,26] See **TABLE 9.1** for BMI calculations. The Centers for Disease Control and Prevention (CDC) has issued the BMI recommendations for adult 20 years of age and older for both men and women. Individuals with BMIs of less than 18.5 are classified as underweight. Those with BMIs between 18.5 and 24.9 are considered normal or at normal or healthy weights. A BMI of 30 or above is considered obese. Individuals who have BMIs of 30 or higher are at increased risk for developing diseases and health conditions such as:[27,28]

- All causes of death (increased mortality)
- Hypertension
- Dyslipidemia
- Type 2 diabetes
- Coronary heart disease
- Cardiovascular accident
- Gallbladder disease
- Osteoarthritis
- Sleep apnea and breathing problems
- Chronic inflammation and increased oxidative stress
- Some cancers (endometrial, breast, colon, kidney, gallbladder, and liver)
- Low quality of life
- Mental illness such as clinical depression, anxiety, and other mental disorders; and
- Body pain and difficulty with physical functioning

The prevalence of obesity in the United States was identified as 36.5% in 2011–2014. More than one-third of all adults in the United States have a BMI of 30 or greater. Although the rate of obesity has been increasing since the 1970s, this trend has leveled off

| **TABLE 9.1** Calculation of body mass index (BMI) | |
|---|---|
| **Measurement Units** | **Formula and Calculation** |
| Kilograms and meters (or centimeters) | Formula: weight (kg) ÷ [height (m)]$^2$<br>With the metric system, the formula for BMI is weight in kilograms divided by height in meters squared. Because height is commonly measured in centimeters, divide height in centimeters by 100 to obtain height in meters.<br>Example: Weight = 68 kg; height = 165 cm (1.65 m)<br>Calculation: $68 \div (1.65)^2 = 24.98$ |
| Pounds and inches | Formula: weight (lb) ÷ [height (in)]$^2$ × 703<br>Calculate BMI by dividing weight in pounds (lbs) by height in inches (in) squared and multiplying by a conversion factor of 703.<br>Example: Weight = 150 lbs; height = 5′5″ (65″)<br>Calculation: $[150 \div (65)^2] \times 703 = 24.96$ |

Modified from Centers for Disease Control and Prevention (CDC). Available at: https://www.cdc.gov/healthyweight/assessing/bmi/adult_bmi/index.html. Accessed January 19, 2017.

for all groups except women greater than 60 years of age.[29]

In recent years, BMI has been questioned as a significant factor in determining the nutrition status and mortality risk for older adults. The Nutrition Screening Initiative included the use of BMI and states that elderly persons with a BMI of more than 27 or less than 24 may be at increased risk for poor nutritional status. A meta-analysis of eight studies that included 370,416 subjects indicated that a BMI less than 22 was associated with a higher mortality risk in those ages 65 years and older. At higher ranges of BMI, mortality increased for younger adults at a BMI of 28.0 to 28.9, but did not tend to significantly increase in older adults.[30]

## Skinfold and Circumference Measurements

BMI does not provide specific information about body composition, but skinfold and circumference measurements can be used to evaluate the actual composition of lean muscle tissue and adipose tissue. A nutritional assessment should include skinfold and circumference measurements, especially if malnutrition is suspected.

### Skinfold Measures

These measurements are relatively easy to measure and noninvasive. Unlike body weight, they are also less affected by hydration status. Skinfold measurements generally correlate with more-complex body-composition measurements, including air-displacement plethysmography (ADP) and bioelectrical impedance (BIA).[31] Measurements are made using a skinfold caliper at the following body sites: triceps, biceps, subscapular, and suprailiac. Using the same side of the body for both skinfold and circumference measurements for an individual is recommended. Standardized methods have been developed to measure skinfold at each body site with trained clinicians conducting the measurements. For example, the triceps skinfold (TSF) is measured at a point midway between the lateral projection of the acromial process of the scapula and the inferior margin of the olecranon. With the individual's elbow flexed to 90 degrees, the midway point is determined using a tape measure on the posterior of the arm and then marked. If possible, the person should be standing; otherwise, he or she should be sitting upright in a chair. For the measurement, the skinfold is measured with the arm hanging loosely at the side. The triceps skinfold is picked up with the left thumb and index finger, approximately 1 cm from the marked location on the triceps. The skinfold is held for the duration of the measurement.[32] Standardized equations have been developed to predict body fat and calculate fat-free mass (FFM) using one or more skinfold measurements.[33] Skinfold measurements are thought to be comparable to more sophisticated techniques to assess for body fat, but recommendations also suggest that equations may need to be modified to address body-composition differences in obese subjects and various ethnic groups.[34]

### Arm Circumference

Circumference measurements can be used alone or in combination with skinfold measurements or other circumferences to help evaluate nutritional status. The only tool required to measure arm circumference is a flexible tape measure in either metric or imperial measure. (If imperial measure is used, it will need to be converted to metric.) The mid–upper arm-circumference (MUAC) is measured at the same location used for the triceps skinfold. The measurement is taken with the elbow extended and the arm relaxed to the side of the body, with the palm facing the thigh.[11] MUAC data are available from the NHANES 2003–2006 for both adults and children by both age and gender in the United States and is expressed as means and percentiles. These data are collected to add to the knowledge about trends in child growth and development and trends in the distribution of body measurements in the American population.[35] The MUAC and the triceps skinfold measurements can be used to calculate the arm-muscle circumference (AMC) and the arm-muscle area (AMA), both of which estimate the amount of muscle or lean body mass (LBM) in the body. The following equation is used to calculate AMC and AMA and have been used to develop reference standards:

$$\text{AMC (cm)} = \text{MUAC (cm)} - [3.14 \times \text{TSF (mm)}]$$
$$\text{AMA (cm}^2) = \text{AMC}^2 \div 12.56$$

### Calf Circumference

This circumference measurement is also monitored by the NHANES studies. The World Health Organization has recommended that calf circumference (CC) be used as a measure of nutritional status in older adults and is included as one of the anthropometric measurements used in the Mini Nutritional Status Assessment.[36,37] A study of 170 hospitalized older adult patients found a positive correlation between CC and BMI, AMC, TSF, MUAC, and AMA.[38] To measure CC, the subject should be sitting with the left leg hanging loosely or standing with his or her weight evenly distributed on both feet. Next, wrap the measuring tape around the calf at the widest part and note the measurement nearest to 0.1 cm. Take additional measurements above and below the point to ensure that the first measurement was the largest. For bed-bound patients, an alternate procedure is specified.[39] The person lies in a supine position with the left knee bent at a 90-degree angle. A CC of less than 31 cm is considered a risk factor for malnutrition. As with other circumference measurements, CC can be used alone or in combination with skinfold measurements to aid in evaluating nutritional status.

### Waist Circumference and Waist-to-Hip Ratio

Although waist circumference and BMI are interrelated, waist circumference provides an independent risk predictor beyond BMI measurements. Waist circumference is particularly meaningful in individuals who are categorized as normal or overweight by BMI standards. At BMIs equal to or more than 35, waist circumference has little additional predictive power of disease risk beyond that of BMI, so it is not necessary to measure waist circumference in individuals with BMIs 35 and above. The waist circumference at which there is high risk of disease, including cardiovascular disease, type 2 diabetes, dyslipidemia, and hypertension, are as follows: men > 102 cm (> 40 inches) and women > 88 cm (> 35 inches).[40] Monitoring waist circumference over time, along with BMI, can provide an estimate of increased abdominal fat even without a change in BMI. In some ethnic groups, including Asian Americans, waist circumference is a better predictor of disease risk than BMI.[41] Waist circumference can be measured as follows with a flexible tape measure. Start at the top of the hip bone and bring the tape measure all the way around, level with the belly button. Ensure that the tape is straight around the waist and not tight. The breath should not be held while being measured. Waist-to-hip ratio (WTH) is also predictive of disease risk and is determined by measuring the waist and hip circumferences and then dividing the waist circumference by the hip circumference. For men, normal risk is a ratio of 0.90 or less; for women, 0.8 or less. For both men and women, a WTH ratio above 1.0 is considered at risk for cardiovascular and other chronic diseases. Studies show that waist circumference is more predictive of cardiovascular disease risk while others have reported that WTH ratio is a more sensitive indicator of disease risk.[42,43] Both measurements have been found to be predictive of cardiovascular events.[44] **TABLE 9.2** shows how disease risk is associated with overweight and underweight statuses.

## Other Methods of Assessing Body Composition

More advanced techniques for measuring body composition are available. However, the equipment to complete the measurement, the time involved, and the requisite clinician training are factors that may limit the use of these techniques. These additional body-composition methods are used mainly in research studies and for specific conditions that require information regarding body composition.

### Bioelectrical Impedance Analysis

BIA is a relatively quick, simple, and noninvasive method to measure body composition (lean body

**TABLE 9.2** Overweight and obesity by BMI, waist circumference, and associated disease risk

| | BMI (kg/m$^2$) | Obesity Class | Disease Risk* Relative to Normal Weight and Waist Circumference | |
|---|---|---|---|---|
| | | | Men ≤102 cm (≤40 in) Women ≤88 cm (≤35 in) | Men >102 cm (>40 in); Women >88 cm (>35 in) |
| Underweight | 18.5 | NA | Average | Average |
| Normal+ | 18.5–24.9 | NA | Average | Average |
| Overweight | 25.0–29.9 | NA | Increased | High |
| Obesity | 30.0–34.9 35.0–39.9 | I II | High Very high | Very high Very high |
| Extreme Obesity | ≥ 40 | III | Extremely high | Extremely high |

*Disease risk for type 2 diabetes, hypertension, and CVD.
+Increased waist circumference can also be a marker for increased risk even in persons of normal weight.

Adapted from Clinical guidelines on the identification, evaluation, and treatment of overweight and obesity in adults: the evidence report. National Heart Lung and Blood Institute in cooperation with The National Institute of Diabetes and Digestive and Kidney Diseases. NIH Publication No. 98-4083. September, 1998.

mass and fat mass). The technique determines body composition by measuring electrical conductivity under the premise that electric current flows at different rates through the body, depending on its composition. The body is composed mostly of water and ions by which electrical current can flow. Alternately, the body contains nonconducting materials (body fat) that provides resistance to the flow of electrical current. The principal of BIA is that electric current passes through the body at a differential rate, depending on body composition. Impedance is a drop in voltage when a small constant current with a fixed frequency passes between electrodes spanning the body. The procedure is as follows: Electrodes are placed on the hands and feet while an electrical current is passed through the body. Adequate hydration is necessary to ensure proper estimation of fat-free mass. Based on the measurements, predictive equations are used to measure total body water, FFM, and body cell mass (BCM) using gender, age, weight, height, and race. It has been suggested that alternative BIA equations be developed for diverse populations.[45]

### Dual-Energy X-Ray Absorptiometry

DXA is used to measure body composition as well as bone-mineral density to assess the risk of osteoporosis. In 2008, the Center for Health Statistics released DXA data from an NHANES population-based sample using modern fan beam scanners. Reference values were provided for individuals from eight to 85 years old and separated for gender and ethnicity. The following data were provided: percent fat, fat mass/height$^2$, lean mass/height$^2$, appendicular lean mass/height$^2$, bone-mineral content, and bone-mineral density.[46] DXA tests are performed by a licensed radiologic technologist and involve passing two low-dose x-ray beams through the body that differentiate among fat-free tissue, fat tissue, and bone. The results provide a precise measurement of total body fat and its distribution. DXA is used to determine long-term alterations in body composition with aging and short-term changes as a result of interventions to modify body fat or LBM.[47,48]

### Air-Displacement Plethysmography

Underwater weighing (or hydrostatic weighing) is considered the gold standard for obtaining body composition. A BOD POD is an ADP that uses whole-body densitometry to determine body composition (fat vs. lean body mass). Similar in principle to underwater weighing (air is used rather than water), the BOD POD measures body mass (weight) using a precise scale; volume is determined when a patient sits inside the BOD POD. Body density can then be calculated as mass/volume. Once the overall density of the body is determined, the relative proportions of body fat and lean body mass are calculated.[49] Results obtained using ADP (BOD POD) are similar to the underwater

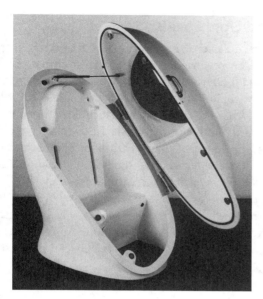

**FIGURE 9.2** BOD POD (air-displacement plethysmography).
Courtesy of COSMED USA, Inc.

weighing technique.[50] The benefit of ADP is that it can be used throughout the life cycle from infants to adults, with excellent accuracy.[51] See **FIGURE 9.2**.

## Biochemical Measures/Laboratory Data

In additional to anthropometric data, biochemical measures or laboratory data are necessary to complete a thorough nutritional assessment. Changes in biochemical data can be used to determine if nutrition interventions are effective, including adequacy of hydration, control of diabetes, and measures of nutritional adequacy or deficiency of specific micronutrients. Biochemical changes may be seen well before clinical signs of a nutrient deficiency occur. The nutrition professional should review the following laboratory tests: complete blood count (CBC); chemistry panel that includes electrolytes—sodium and potassium; glucose; blood urea nitrogen (BUN); creatinine; total protein; albumin; and blood lipids, including total cholesterol [high-density lipoproteins (HDLs) and low-density lipoproteins (LDLs) and triglycerides. Additional tests that may be useful to review are glycosylated hemoglobin (HbA1C); urinalysis; specific nutrient levels, including vitamin $B_{12}$; and iron, ferritin (storage iron), and folate.

## Protein Status

Albumin and prealbumin (transthyretin) have been determined to be poor indicators of protein status, and low serum levels reflect inflammation in the body rather than inadequate protein status.[52,53] Although the clinician will take note that albumin or prealbumin levels are low as a sign of potential inflammation,

conducting a **nutrition-focused physical examination (NFPE)** can provide a better indication of protein status.

## Nutritional Anemias

The results obtained by a CBC exam are evaluated to determine the presence of anemia. There are many different forms of anemia. The manifestation of low hemoglobin (Hgb) and hematocrit and a high or low mean corpuscular volume (MCV) may indicate the presence of a nutritional anemia. The healthcare provider may determine that additional laboratory tests are required to determine if the anemia could be nutritional in nature. Laboratory results such as serum iron (Fe), total iron-binding capacity, and serum ferritin may be indicated to rule out iron-deficiency anemia in the presence of low MCV (small or microcytic red blood cells). Serum vitamin $B_{12}$ and folate levels may be necessary if the MCV level is high (indicative of large or macrocytic red blood cells). The CBC can also indicate the presence of infection if the white blood cell count is elevated, which can correlate with a low albumin level and the presence of infection or inflammation.[54] Globally, iron deficiency is the most common nutrient deficiency. The CBC may also indicate a low total lymphocyte count (TLC), but many other factors can cause TLC to be low; therefore, its usefulness as an assessment of immune function and nutritional status is not reliable.[55]

## Electrolytes, Blood Urea Nitrogen, and Creatinine

The nutrition professional will need to review laboratory results for electrolytes, BUN, and creatinine to evaluate hydration status and kidney function. Elevated serum sodium (hypernatremia) may indicate dehydration, and a low sodium level (hyponatremia) can indicate overhydration or impairment in adrenal function. Abnormal sodium levels can also be the result of medication effects such as diuretics and some types of antidepressants. In some instances, fluid intake may need to be limited to increase serum sodium levels to normal.[56] Elevated BUN can be a sign of impaired kidney function as well as dehydration or excessive protein intake. An elevated creatinine is a sign of kidney dysfunction. The best marker of kidney function, however, is glomerular filtration rate (GFR), which uses serum creatinine, age, gender, and race to determine the presence and stage of kidney disease.[57] The GFR equation is as follows:

$$eGFR = 186 \times \text{serum creatinine}^{-1.154} \times \text{age}^{-0.203}$$
$$\times [1.210 \text{ if black}] \times [0.742 \text{ if female}]$$

## Laboratory Values for Diabetes Mellitus

The clinician should also review fasting blood glucose (FBG). Although FBG has limited value regarding diabetes management, elevated blood glucose may indicate the need to check the glycosylated (or glycated) hemoglobin level. HbA1C is a test that measures the long-term control of blood glucose. Excess glucose in the blood is bound to hemoglobin (Hgb), and because a red blood cell has a life of approximately 120 days, the HbA1C test can indicate the average blood glucose over the past three to four months.[58] The amount of glucose bound to Hgb is expressed as a percentage with levels as follows:

- 4.9–5.2%—Normal
- 5.3–5.4%—Intermediate
- 5.5–6.5%—Prediabetic
- ≥ 6.6%—Diabetes Mellitus

The estimated average glucose (eAG) is another way to interpret glycosylated hemoglobin results. **TABLE 9.3** provides a list of estimated average glucose results based on the data reported by the A1C. For instance, a patient with an A1C of 8% has an eAG of 183 mg/dL. This information can be useful for the patient because it helps translate A1C tests into numbers that would more closely represent daily glucometer readings.

**TABLE 9.3** Estimated average glucose

| HbA1C (%) | eAG (mg/dL) |
| --- | --- |
| 5 | 97 |
| 6 | 126 |
| 7 | 154 |
| 8 | 183 |
| 9 | 212 |
| 10 | 240 |
| 11 | 269 |
| 12 | 198 |

The relationship between A1C and eAG is described by the formula $28.7 \times A1C - 46.7 = eAG$.

Data from Nathan DM, Kuenen J, Borg R, Zheng H, Schoenfeld D, Heine RJ. Translating the A1C Assay Into Estimated Average Glucose Values. *Diabetes Care.* 2008;31(8):1-6.

## Blood Lipid Levels

Serum cholesterol, lipoprotein levels, and triglycerides should be reviewed. Elevated serum cholesterol and elevated LDL cholesterol levels are risk factors for cardiovascular disease. A total cholesterol above 240 mg/dL and an LDL cholesterol level greater than 160 mg/dL indicate high risk.[59] Low cholesterol levels can be a sign of malnutrition and be predictive of mortality in older adults—unless the patient is taking cholesterol-lowering medications.[60,61] Elevated serum triglycerides (TGs) can be caused by obesity, poorly controlled diabetes, hypothyroidism, kidney disease, or excessive alcohol consumption. As with elevated total and LDL cholesterol, high TGs can increase the risk of heart disease.

> **Recap** After anthropometric and laboratory data have been collected and reviewed, the nutrition professional will need to obtain additional information on the individual's food- and nutrition-related history to complete the data-collection process.

## ▶ Client History

> **Preview** The client history is an important component of a complete nutritional assessment as it provides information regarding acute and chronic medical conditions that can have an impact on nutrition status. Based on the IDNT reference manual, client history includes the following: personal history; medical, health, and family history; treatments and complementary or alternative medicine use; and social history.[9]

## Personal History

Personal history information pertinent to nutrition assessment includes age; gender; race or ethnicity; language spoken and written; literacy factors such as a language barrier or low literacy; educational level; physical disability, including impaired vision, hearing, or other; and mobility. These data are important to the nutritional assessment as the delivery of nutrition care and nutrition education and counseling may be affected by these factors. To express personal data or history, nutrition-assessment documentation may begin with, "Patient/client is a 65-year-old Spanish female with new-onset type 2 diabetes. Client speaks and reads English, 8th grade education level."

## Medical, Health, and Family History

Medical, health, and family history includes current and past medical diagnoses, conditions, and illnesses that can have an effect on nutritional status. The new or current diagnoses should be listed first, including the patient's or client's chief nutritional complaint, which includes indicators such as poor appetite, weight gain, difficulty swallowing, and unstable blood glucose. In addition to primary nutrition complaints, medical history should include body system diagnoses including cardiovascular, endocrine or metabolism, excretory, gastrointestinal, gynecological, hematological or oncological, immune system issues such as food allergies, integumentary (skin), musculoskeletal, neurological, psychological, and respiratory. Family medical history should also be assessed if pertinent to the primary nutrition complaint. For example, if the patient has new-onset type-2 diabetes, it would be important to know which family members have diabetes; this would also be relevant for patients with new diagnoses of hyperlipidemia and other conditions. An example of documentation related to medical and health history is: "Patient with a history of hypertension and elevated blood lipids. Patient reports that both parents were prescribed medication for hypertension and high cholesterol."

## Treatments

Treatments include both medical and surgical. Among the medical treatments are chemotherapy, dialysis, mechanical ventilation or oxygen therapy, ostomies, or current therapies such as occupational therapy, physical therapy, and speech therapy. Surgical treatments include coronary artery bypass, gastric bypass (type), intestinal resection, joint or orthopedic surgery or replacement, limb amputation, organ transplant, and total gastrectomy. In addition, palliative or end-of-life care is also considered under a treatment. A nutrition-assessment documentation might read, "Patient receiving dialysis three times weekly for end-stage kidney disease and experiencing decreased appetite due to fatigue and uremia."[9]

## Social History

Social history is important to gather because nonmedical factors can affect nutrition intake and the retention of nutrition education as well. Social indicators include socioeconomic factors, living or housing situations, domestic issues, social and medical support systems, geographic location of the home, occupation, religion, history of recent crisis, and daily stress level. For a patient receiving home care services, documentation of social history in the nutritional assessment may note, "Patient lives in own home alone and receives one meal per day from Meals on Wheels. Patient's family lives over 100 miles away and is only able to visit and purchase groceries every other week."

The client history can be obtained through the patient or client and by family interview, from the medical record, or by reference from the healthcare provider or other involved agency. The nutrition clinician will need to review the subjective data, the information the patient or family member shares, and objective data, or what the clinician detects based on the client medical history to form an assessment of the patient's overall nutritional status.[62]

The detail of the client history needed to form a complete nutrition assessment varies on the primary nutrition-related complaint. For example, if a patient reports constipation, then the nutrition clinician will need to be aware of the patient's usual bowel pattern or frequency because this varies significantly within the patient population.[63,64] Other important client history information necessary to evaluate the root cause and treatment of constipation would include concurrent disease state(s), the current medication regimen, supplement use, activity level, and previous medical conditions or surgeries.[65] Once the client history is obtained, food and fluid intake will be reviewed with the patient. This is covered in the next section.

> **Recap** The collection of the individuals' food- and nutrition-related history is an important component for the completion of a nutrition assessment. The patient's unique history can assist the nutrition professional in implementing nutrition interventions that will help the patient achieve nutritional goals.

## ▶ Food- and Nutrition-Related History

> **Preview** The **food- and nutrition-related history** is an important aspect of the nutrition assessment because it identifies current eating patterns and types and amounts of foods and beverages consumed. Previously called a diet history, the tool was developed in 1947 for use in food and nutrition research studies.[66]

## Components of Food- and Nutrition-Related History

Components of the food- and nutrition-related history include information on a typical day's eating pattern, including meals, beverages, and snacks; occasional alternative foods consumed; usual portion sizes; past changes in eating patterns; food preferences and dislikes; food allergies, intolerances, or aversions; and ethnic, cultural, and religious practices and preferences. In addition, food security should be assessed as well as transportation availability, cooking facilities, and health-related dietary restrictions. Medication regimen, alcohol consumption, and nutritional and non-nutritional supplement use should be gathered to provide a complete picture of the client's intake patterns. The diet history can be taken for a three-day period with one weekend day or for one day if time is a limiting factor.

Common questions used when gathering a food history include the following.

- How many times do you eat each day?
- When you arise, do you consume any food or beverages?
- When do you eat next? Avoid using names for meal or snack periods.
- How many servings of fruits and vegetables do you eat in a day?
- Do you eat meat, poultry, and fish?
- Do you have an intolerance to milk, dairy products, or other foods?
- Are there any foods that you avoid?
- Do you follow a meal plan prescribed by a health practitioner such as a fat-restricted or salt-restricted diet?
- What medications do you take (prescription and over-the-counter)?
- How much alcohol do you drink in a day?
- In the past month, have you skipped meals for any of the following reasons:[65]
  - Not enough food or money to buy food
  - No transportation to grocery stores
  - No working appliances (stove or kitchen utensils) to prepare food
  - No place to store perishable foods (refrigerator or freezer)
  - No access to congregate meal programs
  - Inability to prepare meals because of physical or cognitive impairments
- How many meals did you skip in the past week?

Questions should be specific and not judgmental about food-intake behaviors to promote open and honest answers to the interviewer's questions. For example, do not ask, "What do you eat for breakfast?" but rather, "Do you eat any food or beverages when you wake in the morning?" To view videos of nutrition professionals conducting food histories, refer to the Internet links at the end of the chapter.

Food histories can be modified based on the presenting medical condition(s) of the client or patient in order to obtain additional information that aids in planning for nutritional care. For example, for a client with diabetes, asking about specific meal and snack times, readiness to change nutrition-related behaviors, travel frequency, typical macronutrient intake, usual physical activity, appetite and gastrointestinal issues, and so on will add important information to the diet history.[65] A standardized diet history tool has been developed to support the diagnosis of food allergies.[67] A version is available for both pediatrics and adults. See **TABLE 9.4** for the pediatric version.

## Additional Methods to Determine Intake

Several other methods can be used to collect food-intake information if a food history is not completed because of time constraints, the individual is unable to provide the information, or data collection is required from multiple clients, as in epidemiological research. Direct observation of food and fluid intake, a 24-hour diet recall, a food-frequency questionnaire (FFQ), and diet checklists are additional options, depending on the setting and ability of individuals to participate. Observing meal intake can be useful in individuals who are not able to recall food intakes or provide a diet history. The nutrition professional or observer can witness for type and amount of foods consumed, intake of fluids, feeding ability, rate of eating, food preferences and dislikes, and ease of intake related to chewing and swallowing status.

## The 24-Hour Recall

The 24-hour food recall is a structured interview that attempts to capture all foods and beverages consumed over the previous 24-hour period. The trained interviewer uses open-ended questions to capture the time of day and portion sizes of food and beverages consumed. Food models, pictures, and other visual aids may be used to improve the accuracy of the recall. Supplement intake may also be included, although the interviewer asks questions about food and beverage intake first. A 24-hour recall generally takes about 20 to 60 minutes to complete.[68] Automated 24-hour recall systems are available for collecting interviewer-administered 24-hour dietary recalls in person or by telephone. The US Department of Agriculture's (USDA)

**TABLE 9.4** Pediatric diet history for food allergies

| | |
|---|---|
| 1 | Feeding history:   Breastfed;   formula fed;   N/A |
| 2 | If breastfed, review maternal diet; are there any foods being avoided or being consumed in excessive amounts? |
| 3 | a.  What type of infant formula or milk substitute is the child taking?<br>   ☐ Standard infant cow's milk formula with or without prebiotics/probiotics (circle)<br>   ☐ Partially/extensively hydrolyzed casein/whey formula: Type _____<br>   ☐ Partially/extensively hydrolyzed rice formula: Type _____<br>   ☐ Amino acid formula: Type _____<br>   ☐ Infant soy formula: Type _____<br>   ☐ Nonfortified soy formula: Type _____<br>   ☐ Fortified soya milk: Type _____<br>   ☐ Other milk: Fortified? Yes/No (circle): Type _____<br>b.  How much formula is taken per 24 hours? _____ |
| 4 | Have complementary foods been introduced into the diet of the child?   Yes   No (circle) |

| 5 | Food | Age | Format—in what form was food given? | Any problems with weaning or with particular foods, e.g., colic or reflux? |
|---|---|---|---|---|
| | Fruits | | | |
| | Vegetables | | | |
| | Rice/corn | | | |
| | Meat/chicken | | | |
| | Fats/oils | | | |
| | Cow's milk | | | |
| | Egg | | | |
| | Wheat | | | |
| | Cod or other white fish | | | |
| | Salmon or other oily fish | | | |
| | Shellfish | | | |
| | Soy | | | |
| | Tree nuts (specify type) | | | |
| | Seeds | | | |

*(continues)*

**TABLE 9.4** *(continued)*

| | | | |
|---|---|---|---|
| 6 | Is the child refusing food/to feed? | Yes | No |
| | If YES, is the refusal associated with back arching or distress crying? | Yes | No |
| 7 | Is the child experiencing early satiety or consuming only small portions? | Yes | No |
| 8 | Have foods been eliminated previously? | Yes | No |
| | If YES, was this helpful? | Yes | No |
| 9 | Are symptoms related to a specific food?<br>If no, complete Question 10 | Yes | No Possibly |
| 10 | If no specific food identified, list the meals preceding the most recent reaction and two other reactions including the most severe (think of age-related foods and possible cross-reacting foods to inhalant allergens) | | |

| Meal | Time of Onset of Symptoms (Minutes) | Symptom Type |
|---|---|---|
| | | |
| | | |

Adapted from: Skypala, IJ. The development of a standardized diet history tool to support the diagnosis of food allergy. Clin Translational Allergy. 2015;5:7.

Automated Multiple-Pass Method is a research-based, multiple-pass approach that uses five steps designed to enhance complete and accurate food recall and reduce respondent burden.[69] Automated self-administered tools are available as well, including the National Cancer Institute's Automated Self-Administered 24-hour (ASA24) dietary assessment tool.[68]

## Daily Food Checklist

A daily food checklist is another tool that can be used to gather and assess food and beverage intake. The tool provides a list of foods; over a one-day period, the respondent makes a check beside the food each time he or she eats it. The benefits of using a checklist are that the individual does not need to recall foods eaten the previous day and little effort is required to complete the list. The checklist can be used alone or in conjunction with another instrument such as the food-frequency questionnaire (FFQ) as the FFQ. The Observing Protein & Energy Nutrition (OPEN) study found that protein and energy intake estimates were closer to true intake when used in combination with an FFQ.[70] The National Institutes of Health have developed a seven-day automated checklist tool that can be completed online to facilitate data collection.[71]

## Food-Frequency Questionnaire

The FFQ is a defined list of foods and beverages with response categories to indicate usual intake of food over a certain time period. To assess total intake, an individual is asked about approximately 80–120 foods and beverages and usual portion size consumed is typically requested for each item. The FFQ can also include questions regarding supplement intake to determine whether the individual is completing 100% of the recommended daily intake for micronutrients. Generally, the FFQ is self-administered and can be completed in 30–60 minutes. It should be able to capture total dietary intake if the individual is able to complete it accurately.[71] The FFQ is generally used for large population studies, and many types have been developed based on varied ethnic groups. It is age appropriate for children and older adults and those that query specific types of food intakes, including dietary fiber, vitamin D, flavonoid intake, and others.

The NHANES has developed an FFQ that does not ask information regarding portion size to reduce respondent burden.[72]

> **Recap** From the information obtained from the client, the nutrition professional can determine both the qualitative and quantitative aspects of the individual's intake. Generally, the information collected from the diet history correlates with the client's nutritional status if the individual provides candid information. Diet histories do have some limitations; they can be time intensive and require a highly trained professional, preferably an RDN. In addition, the participant must be highly motivated to participate and be open and honest with the professional gathering the food-intake data. The client must also be able to remember the foods consumed in the past to provide an accurate assessment; individuals with acute illnesses or dementia may not be able to participate because of short-term memory loss.[73]

## ▶ Nutrition-Focused Physical Examination

> **Preview** The use of a nutrition-focused physical exam will help the nutrition professional validate and expand on the anthropometric and biochemical components, client history, and food- and nutrition-related histories.

### Why Conduct a Nutrition-Focused Physical Examination?

An NFPE is a critical component of a complete nutritional assessment because it provides information that cannot be gleaned from the food- and nutrition-related history, client history, anthropometric measurements, biochemical data, and medical tests and procedures. An NFPE includes evaluation of physical appearance, muscle and fat wasting, swallowing function, appetite, and affect, which can help determine nutritional status, signs of malnutrition, and nutrient deficiencies.[9] First, the NFPE can provide objective data in which the examiner may find physical aspects that were not included in the food history but can also be used to relate to findings from other healthcare professionals. Second, the NFPE can be used to organize information and determine whether findings are associated with a nutrition problem. The NPFE helps identify two general categories for potential nutrient deficiencies: macronutrients (energy, protein, fluids) and micronutrients (vitamins and minerals).[74]

Historically, a physical examination conducted by a physician, advanced-practice nurse, or physician's assistant has been conducted on patients seeking medical care. The physical findings from the exam would be used to identify medical problems that could be appropriately treated through patient education, physical therapy, medications, surgery, or other medical procedures. Unlike the medical examination, the NFPE is specifically a tool that can be used by nutrition professionals to complement the other aspects of the nutritional assessment and be used to develop a nutrition diagnosis versus a medical diagnosis. It is common knowledge that serum albumin and prealbumin are not sensitive indicators of protein status. Serum albumin and prealbumin levels are affected by several factors, including the patient's total body water, liver function, and renal losses. Albumin also tends to be depressed in inflammatory states in the body, caused by acute injury or trauma, infections, and chronic disease states such as arthritis, heart disease, wounds, and cancers, to name a few.[52,75] An NFPE is a way to determine if protein intake is adequate based on physical manifestations such as muscle wasting and fluid retention, as well as other physical findings.

### How to Conduct an NFPE

Physical characteristics that are pertinent when evaluating an individual's nutritional status include height and weight measurement and BMI, identification of edema and hydration status, identification of skin and mucosal changes, identification of fat loss, muscle wasting and loss of strength, identification of functional deficits, gastrointestinal factors that can affect the initiation of feedings, identification of nutritional neuropathies, and identification of psychological factors that can influence nutritional intake.[74]

The NFPE is a minimally invasive process. Techniques used in the NFPE include inspection, palpation and percussion. Inspection is the most commonly used technique. It involves observing various areas of the body with the unassisted eye and can include the use of a pen light to examine lesions or the oral cavity. Palpation is the process of using the hands to inspect the body. It can be used when examining subcutaneous fat loss in the triceps, muscle loss in the interosseous muscles in the hand, and skin turgor, and it can also be used to evaluate for pitting edema. Percussion is a method of tapping body parts with the fingers, hands, or a small instrument to assess for size, consistency, and borders of organs. Percussion can also assess the presence or absence of fluid in body areas.[76] This technique is when examining the abdomen, heart, and lungs.

Both the patient's external appearance and an evaluation of his or her skin, eyes, hair, oral cavity, abdomen, extremities, and nails can provide clues as to nutritional status and point toward nutritional deficiencies or factors that can affect nutritional intake.

An NFPE generally begins with a general observation of the body and skin, starting at the head and moving downward. Findings from overall appearance would include an observation of wasting or fat accumulation, as well as dermatitis, pigmentation changes, distended abdomen, liver enlargement, muscle wasting, presence of edema, and weakness of the extremities.[77] The initial inspection and observation will help the clinician determine areas that require additional examination.

## Skin

The skin is the largest organ of the body, and nutrition-focused findings may be noted in a variety of areas and conditions. Examination of the skin is conducted using inspection and palpation. Skin should be inspected for color and uniform appearance, symmetry, hygiene, lesions, tears, bruising, edema, rashes, and flakiness. Light palpation can be used to assess for moisture, temperature, texture, turgor, and mobility. To assess for skin turgor, a small area on the forearm or sternal area is pinched between the thumb and forefinger. If the skin readily returns to place when released, hydration is estimated to be adequate. If the skin does not quickly return to place, then the patient may have inadequate fluid intake or have edema (fluid retention) in the area assessed. A variety of skin lesions can indicate nutritional deficiencies, and the clinician should document a lesion's color(s), shape, texture, elevation, or depression, as well as the presence and quality of any exudate, including color, volume, odor, consistency, and location on the body.[78] **TABLE 9.5** indicates the physical-exam findings with the potential association of nutrient deficiencies or insufficiencies.

## Hair and Eyes

After completing the general observation of the patient and assessing skin status, the clinician should start looking at the patient from head to toe. Hair should be smooth and evenly distributed. Several signs of nutritional deficiencies and disease states can be determined from the hair. Coarse, dry, or brittle hair can be a sign of

| **TABLE 9.5** Nutrition-focused physical exam findings and associated nutritional deficiencies | | |
|---|---|---|
| | **Physical Exam Finding** | **Potential Association with Nutrient Deficiency** |
| Hair | Easily plucked without pain; dull; dry; lack of natural shine | Protein deficiency; malnutrition, essential fatty acid deficiency |
| | Corkscrew hair; unemerged coiled hairs | Vitamin C deficiency |
| | Lanugo (very fine soft hair all over body) | Calorie deficiency |
| | Color changes; depigmentation | Protein-calorie malnutrition; manganese, selenium, copper deficiency |
| Eyes | Xanthelasma (small yellowish lumps around eyes) | Hyperlipidemia |
| | Angular blepharitis (inflammation of eyelids, "grittiness" under eyelids) | Riboflavin, biotin, vitamin $B_6$, zinc deficiency |
| | Pale conjunctiva | Vitamin $B_6$, vitamin $B_{12}$, folate, iron, coper deficiency; anemias |
| | Night blindness, dry membranes, dull or soft cornea, infected/ulcerated eye | Vitamin A deficiency |
| | Keratomalacia; Bitot's spots (white or gray spots on conjunctiva) | Niacin, riboflavin, iron, vitamin $B_6$ deficiency |
| | Angular palpebritis (redness and fissures of eyelid corners) | |
| | Red and inflamed conjunctiva, swollen and sticky eyelids | |

**TABLE 9.5** *(continued)*

| | Physical Exam Finding | Potential Association with Nutrient Deficiency |
|---|---|---|
| Mouth, Gums, and Tongue | Soreness, burning | Riboflavin deficiency |
| | Angular stomatitis or cheilitis (redness, scars, swelling or fissures at the corner of the mouth | Riboflavin, niacin, iron, vitamin $B_6$, vitamin $B_{12}$ deficiency; vitamin A toxicity |
| | Gingivitis, swollen, spongy, bleeds easily, retracted gums | Vitamin C, niacin, folate, zinc deficiency; severe vitamin D deficiency; excessive vitamin A |
| | Sore, swollen, scarlet, raw-beefy tongue | Folate, niacin deficiency |
| | Soreness, burning tongue, purplish/magenta colored | Riboflavin deficiency |
| | Smooth, beefy-red tongue | Vitamin $B_{12}$, niacin deficiency |
| | Glossitis (sore, swollen, red and smooth tongue) | Riboflavin, niacin, vitamin $B_6$, vitamin $B_{12}$, folate deficiency; severe iron deficiency |
| Neck | Thyroid gland enlargement; goiter | Iodine deficiency |
| Skin | Slow wound healing, pressure injury | Zinc, vitamin C, protein deficiency; malnutrition; inadequate hydration |
| | Acanthosis nigracans (velvety pigmentation in body folds, around neck, etc.) | Obesity; insulin resistance |
| | Eczema | Riboflavin, zinc deficiency |
| | Follicular hyperkeratosis (goose flesh) | Vitamin A or C deficiency |
| | Seborrheic dermatitis (scaliness, waxiness, oiliness, crusty plaques on the scalp, lips, nasolabial folds) | Biotin, vitamin $B_6$, zinc, riboflavin, essential fatty acid deficiency; vitamin A excess or deficiency |
| | Petechiae (purple or red spots due to bleeding under skin) | Vitamin C or K deficiency |
| Skin | Xerosis (abnormal dryness) | Vitamin A, essential fatty acid deficiency |
| | Pellegra (thick, dry, scaly, pigmented skin on sun-exposed areas) | Niacin, tryptophan, vitamin $B_6$ deficiency |
| | Pallor (pale skin) | Iron, vitamin $B_{12}$, folate deficiency; anemia |
| | Poor skin turgor | Dehydration |
| Nails | Beau's lines (transverse ridges, horizontal grooves on the nail) | Severe zinc deficiency, protein deficiency, hypocalcemia |
| | Muehrcke's lines (transverse white lines) | Malnutrition; hypoalbuminemia |
| | Kolonychia (spoon-shaped, concave) | Iron, protein deficiency; anemia |
| | Splinter hemorrhage | Vitamin C deficiency |
| | Brittle, soft, dry, weak or thin; splits easily | Magnesium deficiency; severe malnutrition; vitamin A and selenium toxicity |
| | Central ridges | Iron, folate, protein deficiency |
| Skeletal and Muscular System | Demineralization of bone | Calcium, phosphorous, vitamin D deficiency; excessive vitamin A |
| | Epiphyseal enlargement of wrists, legs, and knees; bowed legs, rickets or osteomalacia, frontal bossing (prominent forehead) | Vitamin D deficiency |
| | Bone tenderness/pain | Vitamin D deficiency |
| | Calf tenderness, absent deep tendon reflexes; foot and wrist drop | Thiamin deficiency |
| | Peripheral neuropathy, tingling, "pins and needles" | Folate, vitamin $B_6$, pantothenic acid, phosphate, thiamin, vitamin $B_{12}$ deficiency; vitamin $B_6$ toxicity |
| | Muscle cramps | Chloride, sodium, potassium, magnesium, calcium, vitamin D deficiency; dehydration |

Adapted from Mordarski, B, Wolff, J. *Nutrition Focused Physical Exam Pocket Guide*. Academy of Nutrition and Dietetics, 2015.

hypothyroidism. The presence of fine, silky hair is associated with hyperthyroidism. If a patient has fine, silky hair and has had recent weight loss, this could indicate that the thyroid is overactive and the patient may need to be evaluated by the physician for hyperthyroidism. Another abnormality would be hair that is sparse, thin, and easily plucked without pain, which could indicate a potential protein deficiency.[79]

Irregularities of the hair can also be seen on other areas of the body with hair. Lanugo—very fine soft hair all over the body—can indicate caloric deficiency and is seen in some patients with **anorexia nervosa (AN)**. Corkscrew hairs or unemerged coiled hairs can be seen with a vitamin C deficiency or with Menkes syndrome (a genetic syndrome that leads to copper deficiency, deterioration of the nervous system, and the presence of brittle, kinky hair).[79]

The eyes can also show indications of nutritional deficiencies and overall nutritional status. Eyes that appear "hollow" can indicate loss of subcutaneous fat as well as dehydration.[80] Vitamin deficiencies, especially vitamin A, can be observed in the eyes. Night blindness, dry membranes, dull or soft corneas, infection, or ulceration in the eyes can indicate a vitamin A deficiency, which can lead to keratomalacia. As a vitamin A deficiency advances, Bitot's spots may appear (foamy, silver-gray spots) on the membranes that cover the white of the eyes. Angular palpebritis (redness and fissures of the eyelid corners) can indicate niacin, riboflavin, iron, and vitamin $B_6$ deficiency. A condition called angular blepharitis (inflammation of eyelids or "grittiness" under the eyelids) can indicated riboflavin, biotin, vitamin $B_6$, or zinc deficiency. Angular blepharitis can also be caused by poor eye hygiene and must be ruled out if a vitamin deficiency is suspected. Pale conjunctiva may indicate that a vitamin $B_6$, vitamin $B_{12}$, folate, iron, or copper deficiency anemia may be present. Note that anemias are not always nutrition related, and the presence of non-nutritional anemia, as in the case of anemia of chronic disease, should be ruled out. The eye can also provide a window to the impaired lipid levels in the patient because xanthelasma (small, yellowish lumps around eyes) or white rings around the iris in both eyes can indicate hyperlipidemia.[79]

## Oral Cavity: Mouth, Lips, and Tongue

Healthy oral status is critical in the maintenance of good nutritional status because the mouth is the entry point into the body for adequate nutrition and hydration. Abnormalities in the oral area can affect chewing or swallowing, which can contribute directly to malnutrition. Soreness and pale and burning lips and mouth can indicate riboflavin deficiency. Angular stomatitis or cheilitis

(swelling or fissures at the corners of the mouth) can also indicate riboflavin deficiency as well as niacin, iron, vitamin $B_6$, and vitamin $B_{12}$ deficiencies. Angular stomatitis can also be present in vitamin A toxicity. The tongue can also reflect the presence of nutrient deficiencies. A sore, swollen, beefy-red tongue can be caused by a folate or niacin deficiency. A burning, purplish, or magenta tongue may indicate lack of adequate riboflavin. Glossitis of the tongue (a sore, swollen, red, and smooth tongue) may reflect a deficiency of a number of B vitamins or iron. Gum health can also show signs and symptoms of vitamin deficiency. The presence of gingivitis and swollen, spongy, reddened gums can indicate a vitamin C, niacin, folate, zinc, or vitamin D deficiency.[79]

The oral exam should also evaluate the teeth. Missing teeth not only indicate generally poor nutrition but also inadequate dental care. Dental caries can indicate excessive sugar intake, a vitamin D or vitamin $B_6$ deficiency, or inadequate fluoride consumption. Excessive fluoride intake can present as gray-brown spots or mottling on the teeth. The patient or individual should be asked to open his or her mouth as wide as possible, and the opening should be the width of three fingers. This ensures that the patient can open his or her mouth wide enough to accommodate eating utensils and food intake. The presence of any lesions should be noted. An observation of the hard palate can be accomplished by asking the patient to tilt his or her head back. Look for any abnormal nodules, redness, or inflammation.[78] Does the patient have any clicking in the jaw? The presence of a temporal-mandibular joint problem can create soreness in this area and affect chewing.

## Neck

The neck should be inspected for the presence of swollen or hard lymph nodes on either side of the neck, under the jaw, and behind the ears. Swollen lymph nodes can indicate recent infection, and hard and fixed lymph nodes can indicate a possible tumor. In the healthy state, lymph nodes should not be palpable. The thyroid also can be assessed for enlargement, which can indicate a goiter possibly caused by an iodine deficiency.[78]

## Nails

The nails can indicate a variety of nutrient deficiencies and medical conditions. Beau's lines (transverse ridges, horizontal grooves on nails) can indicate a severe zinc or protein deficiency but can also be present after a severe illness such as a myocardial infarction or high fever. Muehrcke's lines (transverse white lines) may be present with malnutrition or hypoalbuminemia but also be present with chronic liver or renal disease. Spoon-shaped nails (koilonychia) may be present with iron or protein deficiency but can also be seen in patients with diabetes, systemic lupus, Raynaud's disease, and hypothyroidism.[79]

## Abdomen

In general, a full abdominal evaluation is not completed for a routine NFPE, but it can be part of the exam if there is any indication of gastrointestinal abnormalities. The abdominal skin area should be observed first for color and surface characteristics. Color should be similar to the other areas of the body and show no signs of jaundice, cyanosis, redness, or bruising. A shiny and firm abdomen can indicate ascites caused by cirrhosis of the liver, heart failure, or malignancy. Symmetrical distention of the abdomen that is symmetrical may indicate obesity, enlarged organs, fluid retention, or gas. If the distention is not symmetrical, this could indicate a bowel obstruction, hernia, or cysts, among other conditions. Bowel sounds can be assessed by listening for clicks and gurgles with a stethoscope; a range of five to 35 per minute are noted to be normal. This should be completed for all four quadrants of the abdomen. Increased bowel sounds can indicate hunger, gastroenteritis, or early stages of intestinal obstruction. Decreased bowel sounds can occur with peritonitis and ileus.[75]

## Bones and Muscles

Bone tenderness and pain may be related to a vitamin D deficiency, but medical causes such as fractures, arthritis, and cancer should be evaluated as possible sources of pain. Calf tenderness and foot and wrist drop may indicate a thiamine deficiency, and muscle twitching may be related to a magnesium or vitamin $B_6$ excess or deficiency, or a calcium or vitamin D deficiency.[75,79] If a medical examination has ruled out other causes of pain and tenderness in the bones and muscles, then nutrition could be reviewed for possible deficiencies or excesses.

**Recap** An NFPE is an important aspect of the nutritional assessment process to ensure that an accurate nutrition problem is identified. A nutrition-focused oral examination may provide important information as to the cause of inadequate intake, weight loss, or possible nutrient deficiencies. Remember to consider the population that is being examined because findings will vary based on age, gender, and medical conditions. Review YouTube videos for NFPEs; these offer more-thorough details about how to conduct an exam.

# ▶ Malnutrition

**Preview** Simply defined, malnutrition is any nutritional imbalance.[81] Recent advances in the understanding of cytokine-driven inflammatory responses and greater knowledge about how inflammation can affect nutritional assessment and intervention has warranted further review of the criteria to define malnutrition syndromes.[82]

## Nutrition and Inflammation

By itself, nutrition supplementation is not effective in preventing or reversing protein loss when the body is experiencing an active inflammatory state. Inflammation itself causes anorexia, and so further loss of LBM will occur. Adequate nutrition, however, can help limit additional protein losses and improve outcomes in the critically ill patient.[83] Acute inflammation also affects nutritional status by increasing the resting metabolic rate and energy requirements. Protein requirements are also greater because of inefficient protein utilization when compared to healthy adults. Expansion of the extracellular fluid compartment occurs as does the production of positive acute-phase reactants that are needed for the immune response and tissue repair. This prevents the production of albumin and skeletal muscle proteins.

Previous definitions of malnutrition were based on pediatric malnutrition syndromes in underdeveloped countries. Malnutrition that occurs in a critically ill adult in a developed nation, however, is often related to an inflammatory state and not inadequate intake initially. Use of serum albumin as a prognostic indicator of nutritional status has been challenged, and although albumin is low in hospitalized patients, it is caused by cytokine-mediated **inflammatory responses** caused by injury, inflammatory conditions, or infection.[52] Serum albumin can be drastically reduced by acute injury within 24 hours. Inflammation causes even greater changes in serum albumin than does protein-energy malnutrition (PEM). We use PED protein-energy deficiency in other chapters. does even when calorie and protein intakes are adequate. These factors all suggest that non-nutrition factors are more important determinants of serum albumin levels than either protein intake or nutrition status. Although it has a shorter half-life than albumin, prealbumin is also affected by inflammation, so its use in assessing nutritional status is also limited.[84]

## Cachexia

Another malnutrition syndrome of some controversy among practitioners is the definition of cachexia. Many medical references define **cachexia** as wasting of both adipose tissue and skeletal muscle. The syndrome can be seen in a variety of conditions, including cancer and AIDS.[85] However, with the increased recognition of inflammation's impact on nutritional status, the European Society for Clinical Nutrition and Metabolism (ESPEN) has defined cachexia as a systemic proinflammatory condition with metabolic aberrations that include insulin resistance, increased lipolysis, increased lipid oxidation, increased protein turnover, and loss of both body fat and muscle.[86] Despite the mild to moderate intensity of cytokine-mediated inflammation, nutrition support alone is not effective without successfully treating the underlying condition. Modern medicine has been able to keep individuals alive in this proinflammatory state, although body cell mass erodes and muscle weakness increases.

## Kwashiorkor

**Kwashiorkor** also has been defined as a pediatric PEM syndrome occurring in underdeveloped countries and is characterized by edema in underweight children who were thought to have inadequate protein intake but adequate caloric intake. Further review of the literature shows that some studies found no difference in the macronutrient intake of children who developed kwashiorkor compared to those who did not.[87] Edema reportedly resolved in these children before improvements in serum albumin and while they were still consuming a low-protein diet. Infection and other stressors may have contributed to the development of kwashiorkor syndrome in these children. Based on these factors, the diagnosis of kwashiorkor should not be routinely used for adult patients in developed countries because there appear to be additional factors responsible for pediatric kwashiorkor in underdeveloped nations. Malnutrition caused by inadequate protein intake is generally unusual in modern medicine because critically ill patients generally have inadequate intake of both protein and energy. Current nutrition-support interventions, when provided, contain balanced macronutrients, including protein, and adequate energy and essential micronutrients.[88]

Adult PEM, sometimes referred to as *marasmic kwashiorkor*, results from a systemic inflammatory response from infection, injury, or some other inflammatory condition that continues beyond several days. Although the classic Wellcome criteria for PEM in children is the presence or absence of edema and a body weight above or below 60% of the standard for that age, the weight limits are different for adults.[89] In adult PEM, weight at approximately 80% per standard weight for height is indicative of PEM. When albumin or prealbumin was considered a valid marker of protein status, patients were often given the PEM diagnosis; however, reduced protein levels are now known to be principal manifestations of systemic inflammatory responses and not of inadequate nutritional intake. Although patients with lowered albumin or prealbumin are at nutritional risk because of inflammation, they may not be malnourished. Malnutrition may ensue, as in a critically ill patient who has not had adequate intake for 10 to 14 days.[90] Early feeding in the most severe forms of systemic inflammation, including severe sepsis, multiple trauma, severe burns, and closed head injuries, can improve outcomes before PEM develops.[91,92,93]

## Sarcopenia

**Sarcopenia**, another syndrome associated with malnutrition, may also be affected by inflammatory factors. Defined as a loss of skeletal muscle mass and strength with aging, sarcopenia includes a loss of α-motor neuron input, changes in anabolic hormones, decreased intake of dietary protein, and a decline in physical activity.[94] Loss of muscle mass can begin as early as the fourth decade of life, with evidence suggesting that skeletal muscle mass and skeletal muscle strength decline in a linear fashion, with as much as 50% of mass being lost by the eighth decade of life.[95] For diagnostic purposes, sarcopenia has been defined as appendicular skeletal muscle mass/height$^2$ (($m^2$)) that is less than two standard deviations below the mean for young and healthy reference populations.[96] Research on sarcopenia has suggested that it is a "smoldering" inflammatory state propelled by both cytokines and oxidative stress.[53] Sarcopenia may be described as a condition of both cachexia and failure to thrive. Some evidence suggests that chronic disease triggers hormonal changes, and inadequate nutritional intake and declining activity levels may be multifactorial causes for sarcopenia.[97]

Although clinicians generally think of patients with sarcopenia as frail older adults, sarcopenia can occur in obese patients as well. Dubbed **sarcopenic obesity**, these patients also exhibit decreased muscle mass or strength and are characterized as having excess energy intake, limited physical activity, low-grade inflammation, insulin resistance, and changes in hormonal milieu. Muscle strength has been determined to be more important that muscle mass, so muscle "quality" is affected, which leads to a decrease in fiber size and number and a reduction in the contractility of the intact muscle fibers.[98] These manifestations can lead to functional limitations, increased morbidity, and a potential for increased mortality. In

# HIGHLIGHT

## Sarcopenia

Because sarcopenia can have adverse outcomes such as immobility, falls, disability, and death in older adults, a rapid screen has been developed to increase the recognition and treatment of sarcopenia. Although the methodology to assess for sarcopenia can be ultrasound, BIA, computed tomography, or magnetic resonance imaging, a questionnaire has been validated to rapidly diagnose sarcopenia. The SARC-F was developed and found to have excellent specificity in identifying persons with sarcopenia. Evidence shows that sarcopenia can be alleviated by resistance exercise, leucine-enriched amino acids, and vitamin D. The screen takes less than 15 seconds to complete and is thus a cost-effective and quick evaluation to screen for sarcopenia. See **TABLE A**.

### TABLE A

| Component | Question | Scoring |
|---|---|---|
| Strength | How much difficulty do you have lifting and carrying 10 lbs? | None = 0<br>Some = 1<br>A lot or unable = 2 |
| Assistance in walking | How much difficulty do you have walking across a room? | None = 0<br>Some = 1<br>A lot, uses aids, or unable = 2 |
| Rise from a chair | How much difficulty do you have transferring from a chair or bed? | None = 0<br>Some = 1<br>A lot or unable without help = 2 |
| Climb stairs | How much difficulty do you have climbing a flight of 10 stairs? | None = 0<br>Some = 1<br>A lot or unable = 2 |
| Falls | How many times have you fallen in the last year? | None = 0<br>1–3 falls = 1<br>4 or more falls = 2 |

A SARC-F score of ≥ 4 indicates a high risk for sarcopenia.

Modified from Morley, JE, Cao, L. Rapid screening for sarcopenia. *J Cachexia Sarcopenia Muscle.* 2015;6:312-314. Malmstrom, TK, Miller, DK, Simonsick, EM, Ferruci, L, Morley, JE. SARC-F: a symptom score to predict persons with sarcopenia at risk for poor functional outcomes. *J Cachexia Sarcopenia Muscle.* 2016;7(1):28-36.

a study of 4,652 adults 60 years of age and older, the prevalence of sarcopenic obesity was 18.1% in women and 42.9% in men. Although sarcopenic obesity was higher in men, mortality risk was greater in women with sarcopenic obesity.[99]

The presence of inflammation helps to rule out nutrition intake as a causative factor of adult malnutrition. Once nutrition risk is identified due to compromised intake and/or loss of body mass (weight loss), the clinician determines whether inflammation is present. Inflammation is believed to be a causative factor for malnutrition if the individual has an active infection, presence of injury, the person has edema or low serum albumin, or altered C-reactive protein levels, among others. If inflammation is absent, starvation-related malnutrition (or malnutrition in the context of social or environmental circumstances including pure chronic starvation or anorexia nervosa) is suspected. If inflammation is of mild to moderate intensity and is sustained, this is suggestive of chronic disease-related malnutrition (as in organ failure, pancreatic cancer, rheumatoid arthritis, and sarcopenic obesity). If there is a marked inflammatory response, this is suggestive of acute disease or injury-related malnutrition (as in major infection, burns, trauma, and closed head injury).[88,100]

## Adult Malnutrition

The Academy and ASPEN have developed a consensus statement for the identification and documentation of adult malnutrition (undernutrition).[101] This consensus statement will help determine the prevalence of malnutrition in various healthcare settings, especially in acute care where the Center for Medicare and Medicaid has voiced concerns about which malnutrition code is used and the wide variation in the prevalence and incidence within the same geographic area or populations with similar demographics.[102]

## Diagnosis of Adult Malnutrition

The presence of malnutrition in the hospital setting was first portrayed in the 1974 article "The Skeleton in the Hospital Closet" in which the importance of adequate nutritional care could help reduce length of stay (LOS) and healthcare costs.[103] Current statistics on adult malnutrition range from 15% to 60%, depending on the patient population and the characteristics used to identify its occurrence.[104] Some medical conditions have higher rates of malnutrition than others, including pancreatic cancer (85%), lung cancer (13% to 50%), head and neck cancers (24% to 88%), gastrointestinal cancer (55% to 80%), cerebrovascular accident (16% to 49%), and chronic obstructive pulmonary disease (25%).[105] Nutrition deficits in hospital patients can lead to muscle loss and weakness, which can increase the risk for falls, pressure injuries, infections, delays in wound healing, and hospital readmission rates. Malnutrition as a comorbid condition can increase the LOS and time spent in rehabilitation.[106] As a result of all possible comorbidities and hospital LOS, identifying, diagnosing, and treating malnutrition in addition to the primary illness are critical processes.

Appropriate documentation and care of the malnourished hospitalized patient can lead to reimbursement for the additional care provided. With the transition to the 10th edition of the *International Classification of Disease* (ICD-10) in 2015, modifications have been made in coding. See **TABLE 9.6** for the ICD-9 and ICD-10 codes, which are available at www.cms .gov.icd10. Severe protein-calorie malnutrition can be considered a major complication or comorbidity (MCC) based on the primary diagnosis. Mild or moderate protein-calorie nutrition is considered a complication or comorbidity (CC).

Characteristics for the diagnosis of adult malnutrition have been defined so that the condition can be consistently detected and diagnosed. The Academy and ASPEN workgroups determined that the presence of two or more of the following characteristics are needed to further assess the individual for a diagnosis of malnutrition:[101]

- Insufficient energy intake
- Weight loss
- Loss of muscle mass
- Loss of subcutaneous fat
- Localized or generalized fluid accumulation that may sometimes mask weight loss and
- Diminished functional status as measured by handgrip strength

Patients should be assessed at admission and at frequent intervals throughout their stays based on screenings and assessment standards for various types of healthcare settings—acute, transitional, or long term. The clinician should share the data with all members of the healthcare team, including the physician, because the clinician is responsible for documenting a diagnosis of malnutrition.[100]

In addition to insufficient energy intake and weight loss, an NFPE specific to malnutrition can be conducted to assess for physical characteristics. Muscle mass loss can be assessed in the upper body because this area is more prone to muscle loss, independent of functional status. Assessment via inspection of the temporal area (depression at the temples), as well as the shoulders, clavicles, deltoids, pectoralis muscles, and interosseous muscles in the hands will reveal signs of muscle loss in the presence of malnutrition. Loss of subcutaneous fat can be best assessed in the orbital (eye), triceps (upper arm), and ribs and chest areas. The presence of pitting edema or fluid accumulation can be local (usually in the lower extremities) or generalized, and the clinician must consider other causes of fluid retention, including heart failure, liver and kidney disease, stomach cancer (ascites), lymphedema, and hyperthyroidism.[107] Muscle function reacts early to nutritional deprivation, and handgrip strength can be assessed using a dynamometer, a simple noninvasive marker of muscle strength in the upper extremities.[108] Clinical signs of inflammation may also be revealed with the NFPE, including fever or hypothermia as well as other nonspecific signs of systemic inflammatory response (e.g., tachycardia, and hyperglycemia).[100]

The diagnosis of malnutrition may not be appropriate for certain patients based on age or disease process. For example, a diagnosis of malnutrition should not be considered for the older adult who consistently consumes less than recommended calories but maintains a stable but lower than recommended weight and is able to function well in the

**TABLE 9.6** ICD-9 and ICD-10 codes for malnutrition

| ICD-9 Code | ICD-10 Code | ICD-9 Title | ICD-10 Title | Criteria/Description | MCC/CC |
|---|---|---|---|---|---|
| 260 | E40 | Kwashiorkor should rarely be used in the United States. | Kwashiorkor should rarely be used in the United States. | Nutritional edema with dyspigmentation of skin and hair | MCC |
| 260 | E42 | Kwashiorkor should rarely be used in the United States. | Marasmic kwashiorkor should rarely be used in the United States. | | |
| 261 | E41 | Nutritional marasmus should rarely be used in the United States. | Nutritional marasmus should rarely be used in the United States. | Nutritional atrophy; severe malnutrition otherwise stated; severe energy deficiency | MCC |
| 262 | E43 | Other severe protein-calorie malnutrition | Unspecified severe protein-calorie malnutrition | Nutritional edema without mention of dyspigmentation of skin and hair | MCC |
| 263 | *E44 | Malnutrition of moderate degree | Moderate protein-calorie malnutrition | No definition given (use criteria from the Academy or ASPEN) | CC |
| 263.1 | E44.1 | Malnutrition of mild degree | Mild protein-calorie malnutrition | No definition given (use criteria from the Academy or ASPEN) | CC |
| 263.2 | E45 | Arrested development following protein-calorie malnutrition | Retarded development following protein-calorie malnutrition | | CC |
| 263.8/9 | E46 | Other protein-calorie malnutrition | Unspecified protein-calorie malnutrition | A disorder caused by lack of proper nutrition or an inability to absorb nutrients from food. An imbalanced nutritional status resulting from insufficient intake of nutrients to meet normal physiological requirements. | CC |
| 263.9 | E64 | Unspecified protein-calorie malnutrition | Sequelae of protein-calorie malnutrition | | CC |

MCC = major complications or comorbidities; CC = complications or comorbidities.

Adapted from: Phillips, W. Coding for malnutrition in the adult patient: what the physician needs to know. Practical Gastroenterol., September 2014. Retrieved January 2, 2017.

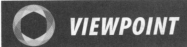

## VIEWPOINT

### Predatory Publishing

*J. Scott Thomson, MS, MLIS, AHIP*

It could happen to you!

- You receive an email inviting you to submit an article to an impressive-sounding journal and think, "That's strange. . . . I've never heard of this publisher."
- You receive an invitation to serve as editor or reviewer for a journal and think, "I've never heard of any of these people. How did they get my name?"
- Or you simply stumble onto a journal's website and something doesn't seem quite right.

If any of the above examples sound familiar, you may have had a brush with the less-reputable side of the scholarly publishing world: predatory publishing.

*Predatory publishing* is an emerging term used to describe any form of scholarly communication that exploits scholars or the peer-review system itself. The Internet has removed many of the traditional barriers to publishing, and this has led to a proliferation of new online publishers, many of whom use an open-access (OA) model of publication. Unlike traditional publications for which users have to pay to access content, OA publications are freely available online, and the costs associated with publication are recouped in other ways. One common method is to rely on the authors to pay the costs associated with publishing and editing their publications. Many OA publishers are legitimate, and some are even quite prestigious, but others have exploited the model, usually by creating predatory open-access journals.

Predatory OA journals are probably the most common form of predatory publishing encountered today. The exact details of how they work varies from instance to instance, but here's a typical example. An article is submitted to a journal and is quickly accepted for publication. Despite assurances of a traditional editorial and review process, the article receives little if any copy editing and is rushed into publication. The author never receives any notes, comments, or editing requests that would typically come from an established and scientific peer-review process. At some point in the process, the author may be presented with a substantial and often unexpected invoice for the costs associated with the publication and review of the paper.

Publishers of this type come in many shapes and sizes, and they use many different models to achieve their goals, which can make them difficult to spot. However, there is help. Many universities and organizations maintain guides with information to help you identify and avoid predatory publishers. Here are a few examples to help you get started.

- Rosalind Franklin University. Predatory Publishing. http://guides.rosalindfranklin.edu /predatorypublishing.
  This guide provides an overview of predatory publishing along with a list of red flags to look out for when evaluating a publisher.
- Think–Check–Submit. http://thinkchecksubmit.org/.
  This guide was created and maintained by a consortia of publishers and scholarly societies to help you pick the right journal for your research—and avoid the wrong ones!

Remember, this type of fraudulent activity isn't limited to journals. There are scams involving books and conferences, so when in doubt, check it out!

---

community environment. Other individuals for whom this criterion would not apply include patients with a muscle-loss condition related to a spinal cord injury but who consume adequate calories and protein, or terminally ill individuals for whom nutrition interventions would not be effective.[100]

A careful review of the patient's primary complaint, review of systems, medical, nutrition and psychosocial histories, physical exam results, laboratory markers of inflammation, anthropometric measures, food intake, and functional status should be reviewed to make the initial diagnosis of malnutrition. Based on the findings, a nutritional plan of care can be developed and should be reassessed frequently to ensure that the interventions put into place help to the patient to achieve optimal nutritional health.

Determining calorie, protein, and fluid needs for the individual is the next important step in the nutrition-assessment process and will be discussed in the next several sections.

**Recap**    Most of the body's protein is contained in the skeletal muscle, which is the body compartment most affected by protein malnutrition. Cytokines have a significant effect on muscle regulation when inflammation is present, including promoting muscle catabolism, preventing protein synthesis and repair, affecting contractility and function, and triggering cell death. All of the effects of cytokines on muscle tissue contribute to the development of protein-energy undernutrition or malnutrition.[88]

# ▶ Estimating Energy Requirements

> **Preview** The gold standard for measuring caloric needs is the use of indirect calorimetry. In the absence of the resources needed to conduct indirect calorimetry studies, predictive equations are used to define caloric needs.

## Indirect Calorimetry

To complete a nutritional assessment and determine the effectiveness of planned nutrition interventions, an accurate determination of energy needs is required. Although the Academy's Evidence Analysis Library (EAL) has determined that the gold standard for determining energy needs or **resting metabolic rate (RMR)** is indirect calorimetry, this method is unrealistic for most clinical practice settings.[109] **Indirect calorimetry** is the measurement of pulmonary gas exchange; it measures the consumption of oxygen and the production of carbon dioxide. The amount and mixture of macronutrients (carbohydrate, fat, and protein) oxidized by the body produces a specific amount of heat and carbon dioxide and the consumption of a specific amount of oxygen. A ratio of carbon dioxide production to oxygen consumption, known as the *respiratory quotient* (RQ), is used to calculate metabolic rate.[110] The use of indirect calorimetry is costly because of equipment needs, requires more time to complete, and requires trained personnel to run the test. In addition, the condition of the patient must be considered; critically ill or cognitively impaired patients may not be able to participate in the measurement.[111] Portable indirect calorimeters, which measure gas exchange and RMR, have been around since the 1970s and are accurate to within 5%.[112] As a result of the challenges of using indirect calorimetry, several **predictive equations for estimating energy needs** have been developed to estimate energy requirements. These equations have been compared to indirect calorimetry, and the accuracy of each has been substantiated.[113] The equations recommended for assessing energy needs vary based on the type and health status of the individual being assessed. Intra-individual variations in energy needs of 7.5% to 17.9% also exist between individuals matched for age, gender, height, and weight.[114,115] Therefore, the determination of energy needs for an individual will be an estimate and may need to be adjusted based on changes in weight status and nutritional intake.

## Predictive Equations for Estimating Energy Needs

In 2005, the EAL's Working Group determined the Mifflin–St. Jeor equation to be the most reliable equation for estimating resting energy requirement (REE). Equation results are within 10% in both non-obese and obese individuals when compared to other equations reviewed (Harris-Benedict, Owen, and the World Health Organization, Food and Agriculture Organization, and United Nations University, or WHO–FAO–UNO).[116,117,118,119] Estimates using the Mifflin–St. Jeor were found to be 82% accurate in the nonobese adult and 70% accurate in the obese adult (BMI >30). The Mifflin–St. Jeor in nonobese adults was noted to underestimate energy needs as much as 18% and overestimate needs by as much as 15% because of individual variability. In obese adults, errors in estimation tend to be underestimates, with maximal underestimation by 20% and maximal overestimation by 15%. For older adults, accuracy within 10% is not available because of limited research in this population group; the equation may underestimate needs by 18% in older men and 31% in older women.

The Harris-Benedict equation (HBE) was also evaluated by the EAL 2005 Working Group. Developed in 1919, this is the oldest tool for estimating energy needs.[120] This equation is only found to be 45% to 81% accurate in nonobese adults and tends to overestimate energy needs. Similarly, in obese individuals, only 38% to 64% of the estimates are accurate, with most errors tending to be overestimates. In older adults, accuracy within 10% is not possible and can both underestimate and overestimate needs in men and women because of individual variation. The Owen equation is, a lesser-known and seldom-used equation is 73% accurate in nonobese adults and 51% in obese adults.[121] As with the other equations, the data in older adults are limited and exist only for older white females with an underestimation of 27% and an overestimation of 12%. Accuracy of the WHO–FAO–UNO equation developed by Schofield is not reported for nonobese or obese adults in any of the evaluated studies. For older adults, the accuracy of this equation is unknown.[119,122]

Although the Mifflin–St. Jeor and Harris-Benedict equations for estimating energy needs are generally recommended for healthy adults, several equations have been developed specifically for critically ill patients. The Critical Illness Workgroup of the Academy's EAL

## TABLE 9.7  Validated predictive equations for estimating energy needs

| Healthy | Harris-Benedict (1919) | Men: Wt(13.75) + Ht(5) − age(6.8) + 66<br>Women: Wt(9.6) + Ht(1.8) − age(4.7) + 655 |
| --- | --- | --- |
| | Owen (1986, 1987) | Men: Wt(10.2) + 879<br>Women: Wt(7.2) + 795 |
| | Mifflin–St. Jeor (1990) | Men: Wt(10) + Ht(6.25) − age(5) + 5<br>Women: Wt(10) + Ht(6.25) − age(5) − 161 |
| | Livingston (2005) | Men: 293 × Wt(0.4430) − age(5.92)<br>Women: 248 × Wt(0.4356) − age(5.09) |
| Critically ill | Swinanmer (1990) | BSA(941) − age(6.3) + T(104) + RR(24) + Vt(804) − 4243 |
| | Ireton-Jones (1992) | Wt(5) − age(10) + Male(281) + Trauma(292) + Burns(851) |
| | Brandl (1999) | HBE(0.96) + HR(7) + Ve(32) + T(48) − 702 |
| | Faisy (2003) | 8(wt) + 14(ht) + 42(Ve) + 94(T) − 4834 |
| | Penn State (1998, 2004, 2010) | Age ≥ 60 with BMI ≥ 30 kg/m²: Mifflin(0.71) + Tmax(85) + Ve(64) − 3085<br>All others: Mifflin(0.96) + Tmax(167) + Ve(31) − 6212 |

Wt = weight (kg); Ht = height (cm); age in years; BMI = body mass index; BSA = body surface area in m²; T = temperature in °C; RR = respiratory rate in breaths/min; Vt = tidal volume in L/breath; HBE = Harris-Benedict in kcal/day; HR = heart rate in beats/min; Tmax = maximum body temperature previous 24 hours in °C; Ve = minute ventilation in L/min.

Adapted from Frankenfield, DC, Ashcraft, CM. Estimating energy needs in nutrition support patients. Tutorial. *J Parenter Enteral Nutr*. 2011;35(5):564.

project evaluated the accuracy of the predictive equations for energy expenditure and concluded that the Ireton-Jones and Penn State equations were the most accurate in assessing critically ill obese patients.[119,123,124] Several other predictive equations have been developed for critically ill patients, including the Fick method and the HBE with stress factors.[125] The Critical Illness Workgroup concluded that these equations consistently underestimate patient needs and should not be used. The Swinamer equation was also evaluated in the critically ill, and it was determined that additional validation study is needed because there was insufficient evidence to reject this formula.[126]

The Ireton-Jones equation has been studied in both spontaneously breathing and ventilator-dependent patients.[123] The EAL Critical Illness Workgroup concluded that there was insufficient evidence to reject the equation and that further validation studies were needed to confirm its accuracy. The equation was revised in 1997 but did not perform as well as the 1992 version and is not recommended for use.[127] The Penn State equations are specific to ventilator-dependent patients.[124,128] The equations include the Harris-Benedict (HBE) equation and add max body temperature in the previous 24 hours, and ventilation in L/min. to determine estimated energy needs. Although only one study was evaluated by the EAL, both equations were unbiased and precise. The equation was accurate 79% of the time in nonobese patients and can be used for critically ill patients on ventilators. Additional validation was recommended because of the limited data available. **TABLE 9.7** lists equations that have been developed for both healthy and critically ill adult patients.

**Recap**  The use of indirect calorimetry is costly because of equipment needs and both time and trained personnel requirements. In addition, a patient's condition must be considered critically ill, and cognitively impaired patients may not be able to participate in the measurement.[111] As a result of the challenges of using indirect calorimetry, several predictive equations have been developed to estimate energy requirements.

# ▶ Estimating Protein Requirements

> **Preview**  Protein is needed for buildup and repair functions in the body. Protein is the only macronutrient that contains nitrogen.

Protein is the major building block in the body and is present in enzymes, membrane carriers, blood-transport molecules, the intracellular matrices, hair, fingernails, serum albumin, keratin, collagen, and hormones. Because of demand by every cell in the human body, a constant source of protein is needed to maintain the structural integrity and function of all cells. The major difference between proteins and the other macronutrients, (carbohydrates and fats) is that protein contains an amino or nitrogen group.[129]

## Protein Requirements in Healthy Adults

Protein requirements are based on whether the body is in a healthy state or if disease status dictates that added or decreased protein is warranted by the medical condition. For healthy adults, the Recommended Daily Allowance (RDA) is 0.8 g/kg body weight per day of good-quality protein. The RDA for adult men is 56 g/day; for adult females, 46 g/day. At this level of intake, this amount of protein meets the needs of 97% to 98% of all healthy individuals in a group. Requirements for protein during pregnancy and lactation are higher because of fetal growth and the production of breast milk, with the Dietary Reference Intakes (DRIs) recommending 0.88 g/kg body weight during pregnancy and 1.05 g/kg during lactation; the RDA is set at 71 g protein for both pregnancy and lactation.[130]

Several studies have suggested that older adults may benefit from higher protein intakes to preserve bone and muscle mass. Osteoporosis and sarcopenia are morbidities frequently associated with aging. Evidence exists that the anabolic response of muscle to dietary protein is decreased in older adults. In addition, an increase in dietary protein increases circulating insulin growth factor, which has anabolic effects on both muscle and bone and increases calcium absorption, which is also beneficial to bone health.[131] Short-term studies in older individuals have reported positive outcomes on muscle mass at protein intakes of 1.6 to 1.8 g/kg per day; however, longer-duration studies are necessary to determine safety and efficacy.[132] It has been suggested that increasing the RDA for older individuals to 1.0 to 1.2 g/kg per day would be beneficial for bone and muscle health without compromising renal function, until long-term protein supplementation trials have been completed.[131]

## Protein Needs in Critical Illness

Needs for dietary protein are increased for certain conditions in which catabolism is occurring in the body, such as in critical illnesses where the patient requires treatment in the intensive-care unit (ICU). These illnesses include sepsis and systemic inflammatory-response syndrome, trauma, neurological injuries such as traumatic brain injury or stroke, pancreatitis, respiratory failure, multiorgan failure, and surgery. There is limited evidence on defining the protein needs in patients who are critically ill. The 2007 Academy EAL work group on protein needs in critical illness concluded that there are not enough adequately powered studies to determine protein requirements in critically ill adults.[133] A study in which critically ill patients undergoing continuous renal-replacement therapy were provided with more than 2 g protein/kg/day reported that the probability of survival increased by 21% for every daily 1-g increase in nitrogen balance. After multivariate analyses controlled for age, gender, diagnosis, and Acute Physiology and Chronic Health Evaluation (APACHE) II score, no significant results connected protein intake with mortality.[134] Similarly, a review of protein needs in critically ill patients suggests that, although there are limited and poor-quality studies, 2.0 g to 2.5 g protein/kg normal body weight is safe and could be an optimal level for patients who are critically ill. In addition, it has been noted that most critically ill patients receive less than half of this level for the first week or longer in the ICU.[135] Patients who have sustained burns over at least 20% of total body surface area (TBSA) require 20% to 25% of energy intake in the form of protein, equivalent to 1.5 g/kg to 2.0 g/kg body weight.[136] For patients with burns covering of less than 10% of TBSA or obese patients, the recommendation for protein is 1.2g/kg body weight. Protein needs decrease as healing occurs, and adequacy of protein intake can be determined by wound healing of burns and donor sites, the adherence of skin grafts, and nitrogen-balance measurements.

The following is a summary of recommendations for protein needs in critical illness:[137]

- 20% to 25% of total calories for stressed patients, including those with burns
- 1.2 to 2.0 g/kg actual body weight if BMI is < 30 (may be higher in burn or trauma patients)
- 2.5 g/kg/day in early postop burn patients and as much as 4 g/kg/day during flow period

- 2.0 to 2.5 g/kg/day for continuous renal-replacement therapy
- ≥ 2.0 g/kg ideal body weight if BMI is 30 to 40 and hypocaloric feeding is used
- ≥ 2.5 g/kg ideal body weight if BMI is > 40 and hypocaloric is feeding used

## Protein Needs for Pressure Injuries

Protein requirements are increased for patients with pressure injuries to promote healing. The National Pressure Ulcer Advisory Panel, the European Pressure Ulcer Advisory Panel, and the Pan Pacific Pressure Injury Alliance joined together to develop the most current guidelines for the prevention and treatment of pressure injuries, including nutrition recommendations.[138] The seven recommendations regarding protein requirements are as follow:

1. Provide adequate protein for positive nitrogen balance for adults assessed to be at risk of a pressure injury.
2. Offer 1.25 g to 1.5 g protein/kg body weight daily for adults at risk of a pressure injury who are assessed to be at risk of malnutrition, when compatible with goals of care; reassess as conditions change.
3. Provide adequate protein for positive nitrogen balance for adults with pressure injuries.
4. Offer 1.25 grams to 1.5 grams protein/kg body weight daily for adults with current pressure injuries who are assessed to be at risk of malnutrition, when compatible with goals of care; reassess as conditions change.
5. Offer high-calorie, high-protein nutritional supplements in addition to the usual diet to adults with nutritional risk and pressure-injury risk if nutritional requirements cannot be achieved by dietary intake.
6. Assess renal function to ensure that high levels of protein are appropriate for the individual. (Clinical judgment is needed to determine the level of protein required for each individual based on the number of pressure injuries present, current overall nutritional status, comorbidities, and tolerance to nutritional interventions.)
7. Supplement with high protein, arginine, and micronutrients for adults with pressure injuries at stage III or IV or multiple pressure ulcers when nutritional requirements cannot be met with traditional high-calorie and protein supplements.[138]

## Protein Needs for Chronic Kidney Disease

Adjustments in protein intake are necessary for patients with chronic kidney disease (CKD), depending on the stage of renal disease and whether the patient is receiving dialysis. Dietary intake of protein for individuals not receiving dialysis with a glomerular filtration rate of <25 mL/min (stage IV CKD) are advised to consume a diet providing 0.60 g protein/kg body weight/day, which will limit toxic nitrogenous metabolites, the development of uremic symptoms, and the occurrence of other metabolic consequences. Evidence-based guidelines support that a low-protein diet may slow the progression of renal failure and delay the need for dialysis. Approximately 50% of the protein should be of high biological value.[139] For individuals already receiving dialysis therapy, protein intake depends on the type of dialysis, maintenance hemodialysis (MHD), or chronic peritoneal dialysis (CPD), requiring 1.2 g protein/kg body weight/day and 1.2 g to 1.3 g protein/kg body weight/day, respectively. For both MHD and CPD, 50% of protein should be of high biological value. For patients in the earlier stages (I to II) of CKD, protein intake at the DRI level is recommended with 12% to 15% of calories from protein (0.8 g protein/kg body weight/day) to slow the progression of the disease. At stage III CKD, reducing protein intake to 10% of calories is recommended.[140] The nutrition professional should consider the overall nutritional status of the patient when estimating protein needs to prevent excessive or inadequate protein intakes. If a patient with CKD has a pressure injury as a comorbidity, protein needs may need to be adjusted to meet healing requirements as well as address the current stage of CKD.

**Recap**    Protein requirements are based on whether the body is in a healthy state or if disease status dictates added or decreased protein. For healthy adults, the RDA is 0.8 g/kg body weight per day of good-quality protein. Needs for dietary protein are increased for certain conditions in which catabolism is occurring in the body.

## ▶ Estimating Fluid Requirements

**Preview**    Adequate fluid intake is needed to sustain life because the amount of water in the average adult's body is must be from 50% to 65%, depending on gender and age. Fluids are needed for almost all body functions, including digestion, and metabolism, excretion of waste products, as a medium for biochemical reactions, as a regulator of body temperature, as a conductor of electrical messages to muscles and nerves, and to lubricate joints.

## Equations for Estimating Fluid Needs

For adults, several equations are used to calculate fluid needs as part of a nutritional assessment. The body surface area (BSA) method allows for 1,500 mL/m² × BSA = mL fluid required daily. This method is not routinely used to estimate fluid needs.[141] The Adolph method, which is also known as the Recommended Dietary Allowance method, uses 1 ml of fluid per calorie of intake. The fluid-balance method is urine output + 500 ml per day, and the Holiday-Segar method is based on body weight with 100 mL/kg for the first 10 kg body weight, + 50 mL/kg for the second 10 kg body weight + 20 mL/kg for the remaining kg body weight (< 50 years of age), or + 15mL for remaining kg body weight (> 50 years of age).[142,143,144] Generally, most nutrition clinicians use the single-calculation equations for estimating fluid needs for normal-weight adults as follows: 25 mL/kg for patients with congestive heart disease or renal failure; 30 mL/kg for average adults; and 35 mL/kg for patients with infection or draining wounds.[145,146] For obese adults, the following equation has been suggested:[145]

$$[(\text{kg body weight} - 20) \times 15] + 1500$$

Despite the different methods available to calculate fluid needs, the Academy's EAL concluded that there is no evidence supporting either clinical or biochemical measurements as a gold standard for addressing hydration status in individuals.[147]

## Factors That Can Impact Fluid Needs

The nutrition professional must be aware of factors that can alter fluid requirements so that adjustments to the assessment can be made. If a patient is exhibiting conditions such as anabolism, burns, constipation, dehydration, diarrhea, emesis, fever, fistulas or drains, hemorrhage, hot or dry environments, hyperventilation, hypotension, medications, nasogastric suctioning, and polyuria, the individual's fluid intake must reflect increased needs. Fluid needs are also estimated to show a 7% increase for each degree Fahrenheit above normal body temperature in individuals with increased body temperature. Polyuria can results from poor glucose control, excess alcohol, excess caffeine,

**Recap** Despite the importance of fluid in the body, the Academy's EAL concluded there is no evidence, either clinical or biochemical measurements, that are available to best assess hydration status in individuals, although several methods have been described.

and osmotic diuresis. The following conditions may decrease fluid requirements: cardiac disease (especially heart failure), edema, fluid overload, hepatic failure with ascites, medications, renal failure, syndrome of antidiuretic hormone, significant hypertension, and "third spacing" of fluids.[148]

# ▶ Nutritional Assessment and Management of Eating Disorders

**Preview**   Conditions such as eating disorders require special nutrition considerations. Eating disorders (EDs) encompass many different conditions, including anorexia nervosa, bulimia nervosa, and binge eating.[149]

The *Diagnostic and Statistics Manual of Mental Disorders*, 5th edition (DSM-V), defines anorexia nervosa as a restriction of energy intake relative to required needs that leads to a significantly low body weight in the context of age, developmental trajectory, and physical health.[150] **Bulimia nervosa (BN)** is characterized by episodes of binge eating, or consuming a large amount of food quickly followed by vomiting or purging. **Binge-eating disorder (BED)** is described as recurrent eating of large quantities of food to the point of feeling uncomfortably full and not regularly vomiting or purging the excess intake. In addition to the three main eating disorders, a category of other feeding and eating disorders or eating disorders not otherwise specified includes the following:

- Atypical anorexia nervosa (weight is not below normal)
- Bulimia nervosa (with less-frequent behaviors)
- Binge-eating disorder (with less-frequent occurrences)
- Purging disorder (purging without binge eating)
- Night eating syndrome (excessive nighttime food consumption)
- Avoidant–restrictive food-intake disorder (failure to consume adequate amounts of food, with serious nutritional consequences but without the psychological features of anorexia nervosa)
- Pica (eating things that are not food and do not provide nutritional value) and
- Rumination disorder (regurgitation of food that has already been swallowed; the regurgitated food is often reswallowed or spit out)

## Prevalence of Eating Disorders

In a study of the prevalence of eating disorders in a nationally representative sample of 10,123 adolescents aged 13 to 18 years, the current rates of five eating disorders were similar to previous studies: AN 0.3%, BN 0.9%, BED 1.6%, subthreshold anorexia nervosa 0.8%, and subthreshold binge-eating disorder 2.5%.[151] Additional findings indicated there was no female preponderance for AN or BN and only 3% to 28% had specifically discussed eating or weight problems with a healthcare professional.

Because of the complex psychodynamics of EDs, treatment is a collaborative effort that involves medical, psychiatric, psychosocial, and nutritional interventions. Nutrition professionals who work with patients with EDs should receive initial and ongoing training on the management of psychiatric disorders as well as in working with specific population groups such as adolescents, athletes, and obese patients who exhibit BEDs.[152] The nutrition professional may be the first person to recognize an individual's symptoms of an ED, or this professional may be the initial health practitioner who is consulted by the patient for his or her condition.

## Management of Eating Disorders

Despite the prevalence of EDs, evidence-based practice guidelines on nutrition management are lacking. A review of nutrition practice management of EDs concluded that few studies have addressed the effectiveness of the nutrition interventions prescribed for this category of disease.[153] The guidance supports the importance of nutrition and establishes that the goals of initial treatment for anorexia nervosa are to restore weight, improve nutrition status, and aim for a return to normal eating. However, limited information exists on how to achieve these goals.[154,155,156,157,158] It has been suggested that nutrition interventions are at times neglected as effective behavioral therapy will restore normal eating behaviors. One study noted that nutritional professionals who work with EDs have the best nutritional knowledge when compared to other healthcare professionals who work with these patients, so it is important to have an RDN on the healthcare team in the management of EDs.[159] One key missing factor in the nutrition treatment of these individuals is a working definition of what "normal eating patterns" actually encompass.[153]

## Nutrition Guidelines for Eating Disorders

The American Psychiatric Association's nutritional rehabilitation guidelines for AN include goals such as restoring weight, normalizing eating patterns, achieving normal perceptions of hunger and satiety, and correct biological and psychological sequelae of malnutrition. Starting calorie needs should be estimated at 30–40 kcals/kg per day or approximately 1,000–1,600 kcals/day. During the weight-gain phase, intake amounts are increased to as high as 70-100 kcals/kg per day as some male patients require a large number of calories to gain weight. Established expected rates of controlled weight gain are 2–3 lb/week for hospitalized patients and 0.5–1 lb/week for outpatients. Patients gaining excessive amounts of weight should be monitored for refeeding syndrome and fluid retention, especially for those weighing < 70% of healthy body weight. In addition to increased calorie intake, patients may benefit from vitamin and mineral supplementation. Serum potassium should be monitored in patients who are persistently vomiting.[157]

Goals for individuals with BN are to help the patient develop a structured meal pattern that helps reduce the episodes of dietary restriction and the urge to binge and purge. Adequate caloric intake can help prevent craving and promote satiety. Nutrition restoration is not a central focus of treatment, because most BN patients are of normal weight. Note that although these individuals maintain a normal weight, this does not equate to a healthy nutritional status.[157]

Although the American Psychiatric Association provides treatment regimens and goals for EDs, specific nutrition interventions have been recommended for the nutrition professional based on review of 41 topic papers, studies, and guidelines on EDs.[153] See **TABLE 9.8** for a list of nutrition interventions.

## Eating Disorders in Special Populations

The nutrition professional should be aware of eating disorders in special population groups, including athletes and adolescents. Athletes may initially diet to reduce body weight for enhanced performance, but this behavior can lead to true eating disorders. These disorders are more prevalent in sports that promote LBM, including running, wrestling, gymnastics, and dance.[160] Female athletes who do not consume adequate caloric intake may experience changes in bone-mineral density typical of osteoporosis and amenorrhea in addition to low body weight. Healthcare professionals who work with adolescents should be aware that this age period has increased vulnerability to EDs because of peer pressure and biological changes in the body that are specific to that age group. A developing trend in EDs includes adolescents with type 1 diabetes mellitus who omit taking insulin as a means of controlling their weight. This has been referred to as *diabulimia*.[152]

**TABLE 9.8** Nutrition interventions recommended by the American Psychiatric Association

| Topic | Intervention |
|---|---|
| Provide education on meal planning | Focus on "when" rather than "what" the patient eats and aid with the establishment of a regular pattern of meals and snacks. Plan the introduction of a variety of foods including "binge foods "and "forbidden foods." Use food exchange lists, food models, and portion-controlled foods to ensure a variety of food choices. Make changes in steps rather than at one time. Include fats from dressings, butter, nuts, seeds, avocado, and olive oil. Provide an outline of several model intake days based on calorie needs. Have patients help develop eating plans that will give them confidence to succeed. Help families develop healthy guidelines for family meals. |
| Provide accurate nutrition information to patient including on the following topics | Metabolism, energy requirements, determinants of body weight Nutrition myths and misinformation Normal calorie and fat intake Dental health and gut function Calcium intake and osteoporosis Fluid intake Reading nutrition labels |
| Provide advice on normal eating | Eat for enjoyment and health and aim for flexible and spontaneous eating behaviors. Focus on what others eat and what normal eating really means rather than aiming for a perfect diet. Restrict eating to one room in the house. Sit down when eating and do not engage in other activities while eating. Develop sensitivity to cues for eating: presence of appetite, time of day, social situation, and visual appeal. Use appropriate utensils and eat at a moderate pace. Avoid measuring food. Eat with others when possible. |
| Review psychological education topics. | Biological and psychological effects of starvation. List consequences of binge eating and purging. Help overcome guilt associated with eating fattening or high calorically dense foods. Provide education on disadvantages of avoiding food and food groups and encourage increasing food choices and food experiences. |
| Provide advice on stopping weight-loss behaviors. | Help patient refrain from restrictive dieting, break the binge–purge cycle in BN, and restore a healthy weight in AN. Avoid excessive exercise. Comment on stability of weight even when eating behaviors have improved. Support patients to accept and maintain a healthy body weight. |
| Develop rapport and therapeutic alliance when providing nutrition counseling. | Engage client: show genuine concern; aim for trusting and open relationship, which will help patients share fears and abnormal eating behaviors. This promotes trust in the nutrition professional and increases openness to change. Establish supportive rather than confrontational relationship. Remain nonjudgmental with nonadherence and manipulative behaviors. Show empathy; acknowledge how difficult it is to make changes in food behaviors. Collaborate with the patient by involving patient in food planning and decision making. |

*(continues)*

**TABLE 9.8** *(continued)*

| Topic | Intervention |
|---|---|
| | Use motivational strategies; discuss barriers to change and examine pros and cons of change. Use goal setting by having patient leave each session with a goal he or she can accomplish. Identify how the goal will benefit the person. Demonstrate skills, including maintaining a sense of humor, being firm and consistent, remaining calm, refraining from power struggles, being persuasive and curious, establishing credibility, and being warm, open, patient, and encouraging. |
| Use behavioral strategies. | Avoiding weighing between sessions. Develop a hierarchy of food and eating situations and start with the easiest to change. Explain self-monitoring to identify links between emotions and food. To reduce binge eating: limit access to food that encourages binge eating; after episode of binge eating, encourage person to return to usual eating pattern for the next scheduled meal; limit the amount of food available at the meal and discard leftovers; avoid missing snacks or meals; avoid eating from large packages and containers; teach healthy coping behaviors to promote self-control. |
| Promote practical and social eating skills. | Practice going to a restaurant and eating in a group and for special occasions. Provide advice on shopping, meal preparation, cooking, and meal plans. Discuss the relationship between food and culture to explain eating in social context. |
| Discuss appetite regulation. | Encourage increased attention to normal hunger and satiety cues. Explain how appetite generally reflects biological needs. |
| Dietary guidelines during inpatient treatment | Promote a food environment that is planned and secure for consistency and control. Place limitations on foods that patients may refuse to eat; allow three to five dislikes. Discourage the use of caffeinated beverages. Encourage the consumption of a varied diet that includes energy-dense foods; avoid energy-dilute foods and chewing gum. |
| Refeeding | Introduce food gradually with small frequent feedings to reduce sensations of bloating. Reduce the use of raw fruits and vegetables because of their filling effects. These foods are not calorically dense and delay gastric emptying. Use whole grains and bran to aid in constipation. Advise patients that they will have feelings on being overly full for 2–3 weeks as the body adjusts to food and encourage eating regardless of fullness. Yogurt may help improve immunological markers independently of weight gain. Avoid excessive sodium to reduce the risk of fluid and electrolyte overexpansion. Provide a structured, low-stress environment with support and encouragement. |
| Meal supervision | Patients should be supervised for one hour after each meal. Set expectations about the amount of food that should be eaten in a set time period. The reintroduction of food can be facilitated by therapist modeling and clinicians' own healthy attitudes about eating and weight. Encouragement from other patients and staff members can help overcome initial resistance to eating. Provide both empathy and understanding of patient's struggle while encouraging consumption of food. |

Modified from American Psychiatric Association. American Psychiatric Association; treatment of patients with eating disorders, 3rd ed. *Am J Psychiatry*. 2006;163(7):1-54. Hart, S, Russell, J, Abraham, S. Nutrition and dietetic practice in eating disorder management. *J Hum Nutr Diet*. 2011;24:144-153.

**Recap** Nutrition assessment and management are integral components of treatment for the ED patient. Specialized training, collaboration with the interdisciplinary team, and communication skills are needed to ensure that the nutrition practitioner is well versed not only in the nutritional care of the ED patient but also in the behavioral aspects of treatment so that nutrition interventions and nutrition counseling can be delivered effectively. There continues to be a need for evidence-based nutrition and behavior therapies for EDs to improve treatment outcomes.

# ▶ Nutritional Assessment and Management of the HIV Patient

**Preview** HIV is a retrovirus, an RNA retrovirus that inserts a DNA copy of its genome into host cells, particularly immune cells, to replicate. As a result, the immune cells (known as CD4 or T-cells) become dysfunctional, which leads to cell destruction. Other cells such as disease-fighting macrophages are also rendered dysfunctional. The condition makes it difficult for the body to fight off infections and some other diseases; these **opportunistic infections** take advantage of a weak immune system and signal that the person is suffering from acquired immunodeficiency syndrome (AIDS). As a result, the disease process itself leads to malnutrition and wasting. The infection causes an inflammatory response and can decrease lean body mass.

## Prevalence of Human Immunodeficiency Virus

The **human immunodeficiency virus (HIV)** can be passed to others via direct contact with bodily fluids. Transmission to others can occur through unprotected sex, needle sharing, or exposure to HIV-infected blood. A mother with HIV can infect her child during pregnancy, delivery, or breastfeeding.[161,162] Nearly 34 million people in the world today live with HIV infections. Although the global occurrence of AIDS has plateaued, it remains one of the leading causes of death around the world, especially in Africa.[163] In the United States, an estimated 1.1 million people over the age of 13 years live with HIV or AIDS, and infection rates are highest in groups that are the most subject to health disparities.[164] The prevalence of this disease points to the large number of individuals who could benefit from improved medical care for HIV and AIDS, including nutrition care.

## Importance of Nutrition in HIV

Nutrition is an essential component in promoting the health and quality of life of individuals living with HIV. Anorexia and inadequate intake are not the only contributors to the development of malnutrition seen in HIV and AIDS patients. Gastrointestinal disorders, including nausea, vomiting, and malabsorption; altered nutrient and metabolite use; increased energy requirements; and side effects of medications used to treat the disease are among the many causes of the impaired nutritional status seen in these individuals.[165] The nutritional complications of the disease may be caused by the HIV infection itself, opportunistic infections, or the medication regimens prescribed for disease management.[166] Nutritional assessment of the HIV patient should include evaluation of anthropometry (including estimation of body cell mass and fat distribution of lipodystrophy), biochemical tests, medication-related side effects, client history, food history, and physical examination, which would include NFPE findings that may influence nutritional status.[167,168,169,170]

## Weight Loss in HIV

Weight loss is one sign of disease progression in HIV infection and is indicative of malnutrition.[171] As little as 5% weight loss is associated with increased mortality risk.[172] Typically, weight loss in HIV infection has a disproportionately higher loss of LBM in men and a higher loss of fat in women early in the disease, and increasing LBM loss as the disease progresses.[173] The AIDS wasting syndrome, defined in 1987 by the CDC, is the unintentional weight loss of more than 10% of premorbid body weight.[174]

Medication treatments such as the use of protease inhibitors and highly active antiretroviral therapy (HAART) promote weight increase in these individuals. The weight increase promoted by medication use does not translate into LBM repletion. Medication administration has been associated with a pathologic redistribution of body fat in peripheral areas, fat atrophy, and visceral adiposity known as **lipodystrophy**.[175] This makes the anthropometric assessment of height, body weight, lean body mass, and fat distribution an important component of the nutritional assessment for individuals with HIV. In assessing weight loss, the criteria specified by the Academy and ASPEN can be used to determine whether the weight loss indicates moderate or severe malnutrition.[100] An NPFE should be used to assess for muscle wasting and fat loss, gain, or lipodystrophy, depending on the treatment regimen of the patient.[100]

## Biochemical Measurements in HIV

Biochemical measurements are also important parts of the nutritional assessment of HIV patients. **TABLE 9.9** lists the recommended biochemical measurements for baseline assessment.[165] Metabolic abnormalities associated with the disease can lead to altered use, storage, and excretion of nutrients. These include impaired immune function, side effects of medications (including antiretroviral therapies), infections, and changes in hormonal status. A fasting lipid profile can provide information on lipid metabolism and can be compared to physical assessment in patients who have fat redistribution. Individuals with HIV and evidence of lipodystrophy are known to have increased LDL cholesterol, increased triglycerides, and decreased HDL cholesterol levels. This lipid profile can increase the risk for developing cardiovascular disease.[176] Individuals with a diagnosis of HIV are also known to suffer from altered insulin sensitivity, mitochondrial toxicity, and lactic acidosis.[177,178] Abnormal plasma proteins, micronutrients, and other nutrition-related laboratory values have been associated with an increased mortality risk.[179–181] Laboratory values specifically affected by this disease include albumin, transthyretin, glucose, vitamin $B_{12}$, C-reactive protein, zinc, and serum iron, to name a few. Abnormal laboratory results are often related to the systemic inflammatory response rather than to true nutritional deficiencies. Anemia of chronic disease is often present in these individuals.[182]

## Food- and Nutrition-Related History in HIV

Client and food histories are also a vital component of an accurate nutrition assessment. The following information should be obtained when assessing a patient with HIV:[165,182]

- Current diagnoses including opportunistic infections and chronic illnesses
- Use of alcohol, tobacco, and recreational drugs (some recreational drugs may influence appetite)
- Past surgeries that may affect nutritional status (e.g., gastrointestinal surgeries)
- Current medications, medication management, and medication compliance
- Bowel habits
- Exercise level
- Weight history and changes in weight status
- Food history
- Issues that would affect nutritional intake, including difficulty chewing or swallowing, mouth pain, changes in taste, anorexia, or satiety issues
- Food allergies, intolerances, or aversions
- Vitamin or mineral supplements or herbal therapies
- Social and financial issues that affect food security, including living situation and family and friend support
- Food-preparation abilities and facilities, including food-safety techniques
- Ethnic and religious beliefs

## Food–Drug Interactions in HIV

There are many drug–nutrient interactions and medication side effects that the nutrition professional should be cognizant of when conducting a nutrition assessment. **TABLE 9.10** shows a list of medications and specific directions regarding whether the medication should be taken with or without food.[183] A component of the nutrition assessment

| **TABLE 9.9** Recommended biochemical measures for baseline assessment in HIV |
| --- |
| **Biochemical Parameter** |
| Albumin, prealbumin |
| Complete blood count with differential |
| Fasting lipid profile (total cholesterol, HDL cholesterol, LDL cholesterol, TG) |
| Fasting blood glucose |
| Renal panel (creatinine, BUN, total calcium, phosphorous, chloride, potassium, $CO_2$, and sodium) |
| Liver panel (total protein, alanine aminotransferase, aspartate aminotransferase, alkaline phosphatase, bilirubin, gamma-glutamyl transferase, lactate dehydrogenase, and prothrombin time) |
| CD4, CD8, and viral load |
| Serum testosterone |
| Serum zinc and selenium |
| Serum vitamin A, folate, and vitamin $B_{12}$ |

Adapted from: Earthman, et. Al. Evaluation of nutrition assessment parameters in the presence of human immunodeficiency virus infection. *Nutr Clin Prac*. 2004;19:330-339.

## TABLE 9.10 HIV drugs and food interactions

| Medication | Food Requirements |
| --- | --- |
| **Nucleoside/Nucleotide Reverse Transcriptase Inhibitors** | |
| Abacavir (*Ziagen*) | May be taken with or without food |
| Emtricitabine (*Emtriva*) | May be taken with or without food |
| Lamivudine (*Epivir*) | May be taken with or without food |
| Tenofovir disproxil (*Viread*) | Take with food |
| Zidovudine (*Retrovir*) | May be taken with or without food, although taking with food may reduce nausea. |
| **Combination Pills** | |
| *Atripla* (efavirenz, emtricitabine, & tenofovir disoproxil combined) | Take on empty stomach (preferably at bedtime) to reduce incidence of side effects. Avoid taking soon after a high fat meal at this increases risk of side effects. |
| Lamivudine and zidovudine (sometimes called Cobivir) | May be taken with or without food, although taking with food may reduce nausea |
| *Descovy* (tenofovir alafenamide and embtricitabine combined) | Take with or without food |
| *Eviplera* (rilpivirine, emtricitabine and tenofovir disproxil combined) | Take with food |
| *Kivexa* (lamivudine and abacavir combined | May be taken with or without food |
| *Stribild* (elvitegravir, emtricitabine, tenofovir and cobicistat, a boosting agent) | Take with food |
| *Triumeq* (dolutegravir, abacavir and lamivudine combined) | May be taken with or without food |
| *Trizivir* (zidovudine, lamivudine and abacavir combined) | May be taken with or without food |
| *Truvada* (Tenofovir disproxil and emtricitabine combined) | Take with or after food |
| **Non-Nucleoside Reverse Transcriptase Inhibitors** | |
| Efavirenz (*Sustiva*) | Take on empty stomach (preferably at bedtime) to reduce incidence of side effects. Avoid taking soon after a high fat meal at this increases risk of side effects. |
| Etravirine (*Intelence*) | Take with or after food (within two hours after a main meal or within ½ hour after a snack). |
| Nevirapine (*Viramune and Viramune prolonged-release*) | Take with or without food. |
| Rilpivirine (*Edurant*) | |

**TABLE 9.10** (*continued*)

| Protease Inhibitors | |
|---|---|
| Atazanavir (*Reyataz*) (taken with a booster dose of ritonavir or cobcistat) | Take with or after food (within two hours after a main meal or within ½ hour after a snack). |
| Darunavir (Prezista) (always taken with a booster dose of ritonavir or cobicistat | Taken with or after food (within ½ hour after a meal). |
| Fosamprenavir (*Telzir*) (usually taken with ritonavir) | May be taken with or without food. |
| Lopinavir/ritonavir (*Kaletra*) | Take with or without food |
| Ritonavir (*Norvir*) | May be taken with or without food, but taken with fatty meal minimizes risk of nausea. |
| Tipranavir (*Aptivus*) (must be taken with ritonavir) | Take with or after food to reduce the side effects. |
| **Fusion and Entry Inhibitors** | |
| Maraviroc (Celsnetri) | May be taken with or without food. |
| Enfuvirtide (*Fuzeon*) | Administered by injection. No food restrictions |
| **Integrase Inhibitors** | |
| Dolutegravir (*Tivicay*) | May be taken with or without foods. If patient has some resistance to integrase inhibitors, it should be taken with food. |
| Raltegravir (*Isentress*) | May be taken with or without food; do not chew, crush, or split tablets. |

Modified from: Interactions between drugs and food. AIDSMAP. Available at: http://www.aidsmap.com/Interactions-between-drugs-and-food/page/3080183/#item3080185nd food., Updated August 2016. Retrieved November 12, 2016.

should include a discussion on current medications and timing of medications (in relation to meals and dosing) in efforts to assist the patient in assessing the need for changes to promote medication efficacy. For instance, some medications for HIV should be taken with food; if the patient skips a meal, the medication may cause nausea, which can further interfere with promoting an optimum nutrition status and affect nutrition status. In addition, if the patient is taking medications such as isoniazid (an antitubercular medication) for opportunistic infections, this increases the requirement for pyridoxine, folate, niacin, and magnesium. For optimum effectiveness, these medications should be taken with food.

A clinical evaluation of gastrointestinal (GI) function is recommended in patients with HIV. In a study of 671 HIV-infected patients, 88% exhibited at least one abnormality of GI function.[184] Diarrhea was present in 38.9%, a history of liver disease was present in 40.3%, and 12.2% had at least one stool pathogen. Other GI complications of the disease include malabsorption, nausea and vomiting, stomatitis or odynophagia, dysgeusia, and oral or esophageal candidiasis (thrush). Many of the symptoms occur as a result of opportunistic infections or medication side effects. A summary of GI concerns in HIV patients is depicted in **TABLE 9.11**. An NFPE is useful in assessing the HIV patient for malnutrition as well as for signs of vitamin and mineral deficiencies. HIV patients may exhibit iron-deficiency anemia. This can occur as a side effect of some of the medications used to treat the disease. An NFPE may help identify pale conjunctiva and koilonychias.

**TABLE 9.11** Problems observed in HIV-infected individuals

| Problem | Possible Causes and/or Implications |
|---|---|
| Anorexia | Opportunistic infections and medications |
| Diarrhea | Opportunistic infections, including foodborne infections including *Salmonella*, *Campylobacter*, and *Cryptosporidium*; medications; or HIV-associated enteropathy (no enteric pathogen identified) |
| Malabsorption | Opportunistic infections (e.g., *Mycobacterium*, avium complex, *Cytomegalovirus*); HIV-associated enteropathy; symptoms may include steatorrhea, bloating, or diarrhea |
| Nausea and vomiting | Non-Hodgkin's and Burkett's lymphomas; medications; food-borne opportunistic infections |
| Stomatitis | Oral ulcers, oral or esophageal candidiasis can cause sore mouth or painful swallowing or both |
| Dysgeusia | Altered taste caused by medications or zinc deficiency |
| Oral or esophageal problem | Yeast infection association with sore mouth and oral or esophageal ulcers, candidiasis (thrush), pain with eating or swallowing. |

Adapted from Earthman, et. Al. Evaluation of nutrition assessment parameters in the presence of human immunodeficiency virus infection. *Nutr Clin Prac.* 2004;19:330-339.

## Importance of Food Safety in HIV

Because the HIV patient's immune function is depressed, food safety is a critical topic to review during the food- and nutrition-related history and MNT. The US Food and Drug Administration has developed online material to reduce the risk of food-borne illness. This tool describes foods that can potentially be a greater risk in persons with HIV or AIDS.[185] All foods—meats, poultry, shellfish, and eggs—should not be consumed raw, and raw milk should be avoided. Raw sprouts should be cooked; hot dogs and deli meats should be reheated to 165 °F. Soft cheeses should be avoided, and hard cheeses and processed cheeses should be chosen. All raw vegetables should be thoroughly washed or cooked. Assurance of a safe water supply is also critical in preventing opportunistic infections.

## Nutritional Management of HIV

Since the success of HAART in 1996 to treat HIV, the nutritional management of the disease has changed. In the early years of HIV treatment, the major nutritional concern was wasting or "slim disease," but with effective medical therapy, new complications of medical progress have surfaced, including insulin resistance, fat redistribution, dyslipidemia, lactic acidosis, food safety, and bone abnormalities. Even though modern HIV management requires significant expertise in dealing with these nutrition issues, there have not yet been guidelines issued that specifically target the nutritional care of HIV patients.[186] Despite the use of HAART, undernutrition or wasting continues to be a concern, especially in developing countries that do not have access to medical treatments. MNT is indicated when significant weight loss (> 5% in three months) or a significant loss of BCM (> 5% in three months) has occurred. MNT should be considered when BMI is below 18.5 kg/m². The combination of oral food and enteral nutrition is appropriate. However, if oral intake is possible, nutrition intervention should be implemented in the following steps: nutrition counseling, calorie-dense, high-protein food choices, and oral nutritional supplements. Enteral or parenteral nutrition should be used if adequate intake cannot be achieved orally. Protein intake should achieve 1.2 g/kg per day and may be increased to 1.5 g/kg per day in acute illness. Goals of nutritional support include an improved nutritional status, decreased functional impairment from undernutrition (muscular fatigue), improved tolerance to antiretroviral treatment, alleviated GI symptoms (nausea, diarrhea, bloating), and improved quality of life.[187] The nutritional management of conditions related to HAART and prolonged survival of the HIV patient, including dyslipidemia and bone abnormalities, should be based on current guidelines for these disorders.

Nutrition assessment and management of the HIV patient is critical to survival. Nutrition counseling and nutrition counseling with oral nutrition supplements have shown to positively influence health outcomes in HIV.[188,189,190]

> **Recap**   The nutrition professional is an important part of the interprofessional team who not only addresses undernutrition but also implements nutrition interventions that address the secondary complications related to medication management and the increased survival rate of patients with HIV.

# ▶ Mini Nutritional Assessment

> **Preview**   Although nutrition screens do not provide the entire clinical picture, they do help identify those at nutritional risk so that MNT can be initiated.

## Development of the Mini Nutritional Assessment

The development of the Mini Nutritional Assessment started in 1989 when researchers in geriatric practice identified the need for a nutrition screening and assessment tool to identify institutionalized, frail, and older adults. Nutrition assessments were not then routinely performed in clinical practice outside the United States. The goal was to develop a nutrition-assessment tool that would be analogous to the Mini-Mental Status Exam, a tool used to assess cognitive function. The ideal nutrition-assessment tool needed to be reliable, inexpensive, and quick to perform.[191] The MNA was initially validated in 1990–1991 and further validated in the New Mexico Aging Process Study, a longitudinal survey on nutrition and aging in 2001 by the Nestlé Research Centre in Switzerland. In 2001, an MNA short form (MNA-SF) was developed and validated.[192] Since 1994, the MNA has been translated into 24 languages. Many studies continue to evaluate the sensitivity, specificity, and reliability of the tool in different settings and different countries. In both

medical practice and clinical research, the MNA is the most widely used tool for nutritional screening and assessment in older adults.

## Completing the MNA

The MNA helps categorize older adults as well nourished, at risk of malnutrition, or malnourished. Its 18 self-reported questions were derived from the four parameters of assessment: anthropometric, general, diet and food history, and self-assessment. The screen is performed as a two-step process. **FIGURE 9.3** depicts a full MNA tool. The MNA-SF can be completed as a first-step screening tool to determine if further evaluation is needed. The first six items on the MNA makes up the MNA-SF (Part 1, Screening), which can help detect a decline in intake or appetite over the preceding three months, chewing or swallowing problems, digestive issues, weight loss in the previous three months, current mobility impairment, an acute illness or major stress in the previous three months, a neuropsychological problem (dementia or depression), and a decrease in BMI.

If the MNA-SF shows the individual to be at nutritional risk, then the full MNA (Part 2, Assessment) can be completed. The second part of the MNA assesses living arrangements, the presence of polypharmacy, pressure injuries, the number of complete meals eaten daily, the amount and frequency of specific foods and fluids, and the mode of feeding. The individual reports nutrition and health status, and the screener measures height and weight (to calculate BMI), midarm circumference, and calf circumference.[191,193] The MNA-SF takes only a few minutes to complete; if nutrition risk is noted, then completing the assessment section of the MNA takes an additional 10–15 minutes. Scores from both parts are added to determine risk of malnutrition. If cognitive impairment is present, caregiver or healthcare staff may provide the information on meal intakes and weight changes.

## The MNA in Various Clinical Settings

The MNA has been evaluated in older adults in different clinical settings, including community, home care, outpatients, hospital, and long-term care patients with good acceptability and validity. When different settings are compared for the prevalence of malnutrition, there are extremely large differences per settings. The presence of malnutrition in the community has been reported as 1%–2%;

# MNA®

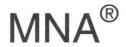

**Nestlé NutritionInstitute**

| Last name: | | First name: | | |
|---|---|---|---|---|
| Sex: | Age: | Weight, kg: | Height, cm: | Date: |

Complete the screen by filling in the boxes with the appropriate numbers. Total the numbers for the final screening score.

## Screening

**A   Has food intake declined over the past 3 months due to loss of appetite, digestive problems, chewing or swallowing difficulties?**
0 = severe decrease in food intake
1 = moderate decrease in food intake
2 = no decrease in food intake                                                                           ☐

**B   Weight loss during the last 3 months**
0 = weight loss greater than 3 kg (6.6 lbs)
1 = does not know
2 = weight loss between 1 and 3 kg (2.2 and 6.6 lbs)
3 = no weight loss                                                                                        ☐

**C   Mobility**
0 = bed or chair bound
1 = able to get out of bed / chair but does not go out
2 = goes out                                                                                              ☐

**D   Has suffered psychological stress or acute disease in the past 3 months?**
0 = yes            2 = no                                                                                  ☐

**E   Neuropsychological problems**
0 = severe dementia or depression
1 = mild dementia
2 = no psychological problems                                                                             ☐

**F1 Body Mass Index (BMI) (weight in kg) / (height in m)²**
0 = BMI less than 19
1 = BMI 19 to less than 21
2 = BMI 21 to less than 23
3 = BMI 23 or greater                                                                                     ☐

IF BMI IS NOT AVAILABLE, REPLACE QUESTION F1 WITH QUESTION F2.
DO NOT ANSWER QUESTION F2 IF QUESTION F1 IS ALREADY COMPLETED.

**F2 Calf circumference (CC) in cm**
0 = CC less than 31
3 = CC 31 or greater                                                                                      ☐

**Screening score**                                                                                    ☐☐
**(max. 14 points)**

12-14 points:  ☐   Normal nutritional status
8-11 points:   ☐   At risk of malnutrition
0-7 points:    ☐   Malnourished

**FIGURE 9.3** Mini-Nutrition Assessment.

in home care 4%–9%; in outpatients 9%; in hospitalized patients 20%–23%; and in long-term care patients 21%–37%.[194,195] In 11 studies that evaluated cognitively impaired individuals, the prevalence of malnutrition was 15% (range of 0%–62%), and the risk of malnutrition was 44% (range of 19%–87%).[191] **FIGURE 9.4** indicates how the scoring on the MNA can be used to guide nutrition interventions.

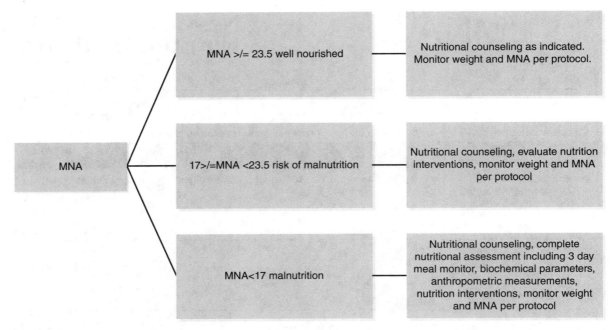

**FIGURE 9.4** The MNA diagnostic tool for malnutrition and a guide for nutritional intervention.
Data from Lim, SL, et al. *J Parenter Enteral Nutr.* 2016;40(7):966-972.

## The MNA in Nutrition Research Studies

More than 200 studies have been published that used the MNA in clinical research. The International Association of Gerontology and International Academy of Nutrition and Aging Task Force recommends the use of the MNA for nutrition studies in older adults.[191] Intervention studies have noted associations with improvements in MNA scores. Both the MNA and MNA-SF have been found to be sensitive, specific, and accurate in identifying nutritional risk in older adults.[195] The MNA is widely used in nutrition research studies focusing on older adults. Christner reported that both the MNA and the MNA-SF were useful for evaluating malnutrition risk in older hospitalized patients when compared to the Nutrition Risk Screening 2002 (NRS-2002) tool.[196] Agreement between the MNA and MNA-SF was highly significant for malnutrition and for patients at risk of malnutrition ($p < 0.001$), whereas no agreement was found between the MNA-SF and the NRS 2002. The MNA indicated that 91.1% of the older hospitalized patients were either malnourished or at risk of malnutrition; the MNA-SF indicated that 93.4% were malnourished or at risk. The NRS 2002, however, revealed that only 66.0% of patients fell into the malnourished or at-risk category, which was significantly different from the MNA and MNA-SF results.

An iteration of the MNA-SF has been developed for patients undergoing hemodialysis, because the short form was found to underestimate the risk of malnutrition. However, research comparing the results obtained using the full MNA and the subjective global assessment (SGA) tools yielded comparable outcomes. The modification to increase accuracy in identifying malnutrition in individuals receiving hemodialysis treatment is an example of a disease-specific MNA-SF nutritional screen. Dubbed the MNA-T1, this screen switched the self-reported nutritional status questions with neuropsychological problems.[197] Other derivations of the MNA and MNA-SF will probably be developed to address specific conditions and diseases.

## Limitations of the MNA

Although no specific limitations of the MNA-SF nutritional screen and the MNA nutritional assessment have been noted, the MNA is specific to older adults and is not as reliable in predicting malnutrition and risks as the MUST is for younger adults (20 to 64 years of age).[198]

**Recap** The MNA and the MNA-SF are useful and ready-to-use tools for older adults.

# ▶ Malnutrition Universal Screening Tool (MUST)

**Preview**   The MUST is a five-step tool to identify adults who are malnourished, at risk of malnutrition, or obese. This tool includes management guidelines that can be used to initiate nutrition interventions or care plans to address risk factors. It can be used in all healthcare settings as well as in the community, and by all care workers.

## Completing the MUST

The MUST screening tool was developed in 2003 by the Malnutrition Advisory Group, a standing committee of the British Association for Parenteral and Enteral Nutrition (BAPEN).[199] It is the most commonly used nutrition-screening tool in the United Kingdom and is also used in other countries. In addition to the standard screening tool, a MUST calculator, a Malnutrition Self-Screening Tool, and a mobile application are available to clinicians. The MUST is available in six languages, including English.

To use the tool, go to http://www.bapen.org.uk/pdfs/must/must_full.pdf. To complete the MUST, the clinician must complete the steps listed in **TABLE 9.12**.

## Rationale for MUST Development

BAPEN's foundation for developing the MUST has been influenced by the overall level of malnutrition in the United Kingdom. Defined by a BMI of less than 20, malnutrition is present in 10% to 40% of all hospitalized patients in the United Kingdom. An estimated one of every seven adults over age 65 years has a medium or high risk for malnutrition. This statistic is much higher when the number of individuals that reside in institutions is taken into account. The MUST also addresses obesity (BMI >30). Obesity increases the risk of chronic disease prevalence as well as healthcare costs.

## Validity of the MUST

The MUST has been validated in hospital inpatients and has been shown to predict clinical outcomes, including length of hospital stay, discharge destination from the hospital, rate of admission to the hospital, number of physician visits, and overall mortality. Patients with

**TABLE 9.12** Steps to complete the MUST screen

| Step Number | Description |
|---|---|
| Step 1 | Measure height and weight to get a BMI score using chart provided. If unable to measure height, use recently documented or self-reported height; or use other method of determining height—demispan, ulna, or knee height. If height or weight cannot be obtained, use subjective criteria to assist in judgment of nutritional risk. |
| Step 2 | Note percentage unplanned weight loss and score using tables provided. |
| Step 3 | Establish acute disease effect and score. |
| Step 4 | Add scores from steps 1, 2, and 3 to obtain overall risk of malnutrition. |
| Step 5 | Use management guidelines or local policy to develop care plan. |
| Calculating screen score | Scoring for the tool rates items as 0, 1, or 2 as follows:<br>■ BMI 20.0 kg/m² = 0 points; 18.5–20.0 kg/m² = 1 point; < 18.5 kg/m² = 2 points<br>■ Weight loss within the last 3 to 6 months less than 5% = 0 points; 5%–10% = 1 point; > 10% = 2 points<br>■ Presence of acute disease: add 2 points in the case of acutely ill patients with no nutritional intake or likelihood of no nutritional intake for more than 5 days.<br>■ A cumulative score of 0 indicates low risk of malnutrition; a score of 1 point indicates a moderate risk of malnutrition; a score of ≥ 2 points strongly suggests increased risk of malnutrition. |

Modified from Stratton RJ, Hackston A, Longmore D, et al. Malnutrition in hospital outpatients and inpatients: Prevalence, concurrent validity and ease of use of the Malnutrition Universal Screening Tool (MUST) for adults. *Br J Nutr*. 2004;92:799-808.

higher MUST scores have up to two to four longer LOS in high- than low-risk patients in elderly medical hospital wards.[200] In the community, the MUST is a predictor of rate of hospital admissions and physician visits. It has also contributed to the body of literature that supports nutrition interventions that improve patient outcomes. In a study of 150 hospital admissions for people ages 85 ± 5.5 years, the MUST screen identified 58% of patients are at nutrition risk. Although only 56% of the patients could be weighed, the authors indicated that all the patients could be screened with the MUST by using the subjective criteria for weight (see MUST tool under "Online Resources"). Those patients with no measured or reported weight had a greater risk of malnutrition and poorer clinical outcomes than those who could be weighed. Researchers concluded that the MUST screen could be used to determine nutrition risk for all patients, even those who cannot be weighed.[201]

## Evaluation of the MUST

Since the introduction of the MUST, many studies have been conducted in a variety of healthcare settings and geographic locations, and with different patient types and medical diagnoses. A study of nursing home residents attempted to determine the agreement between the MNA, the MNA-SF, the Nutrition Risk Screening (NRS-2002), and the MUST.[202] Predictive value and survival analysis were performed to compare the nutrition risk classifications measured from the different tools. The MNA was considered the reference tool in the study. Results identified 22.6% of women and 17% of men as malnourished. In addition, 56.7% of females and 61% of males were at risk of malnutrition. Agreement between the MNA, NRS-2002, and the MUST was considered to be "fair." All of the screening tools point toward a significant association between malnutrition and mortality. Since the MUST and the NRS-2002 do not assess the functional, psychological and cognitive elements that are important risk factors in older adults residing in institutions, the MNA has been identified as the most appropriate tool in this care setting.

A study focusing on nursing home residents compared the use of the MNA, the NRS-2002, and the MUST. The concluded that the MNA was the most appropriate tool for these individuals. Both the NRS-2002 and MUST identified malnutrition in 8.6% of the 200 nursing home residents, whereas the MNA identified malnutrition in 15.4% of the sample.[203] Based on these results, the MNA may be more sensitive at capturing the risk of elderly patients who may be at marginal risk of malnutrition and could benefit from nutrition interventions.

In a comparison study of the MUST and the MNA-SF in 149 older hospitalized patients (65–99 years of age), findings indicated a moderate agreement between the MUST and the MNA-SF. Both screens predicted mortality, but the LOS increased progressively as risk level increased in the MNA-SF; this was not reported with the MUST. Patients with normal risk on the MNA-SF had an average LOS of six days, those "at risk" had an average LOS of nine days, and the malnourished individuals had an average LOS of 12 days. The MNA-SF was also noted to be superior to the MUST in predicting hospital readmission rates.[204]

Disease- or condition-specific studies have been conducted comparing nutrition-screening tools, including the MUST. One study compared the adequacy of the MNA-SF, NRS-2002, and MUST nutritional screening tools in 215 post–hip repair surgical patients (71.6% female; mean age 83.5 ± 6.09 years). For this sample, the MNA identified 95 individuals at risk of malnutrition and 25 malnourished. The MUST results were different, identifying 31 individuals at low risk for malnutrition and 13 at high risk. The NRS-2002 identified 70 individuals at medium risk and 11 at high risk for malnutrition. No differences in LOS and complications were noted between the patients' nutritional statuses of each screening tool, but only the MNA-SF predicted that well-nourished patients would have lower rates of readmission over a six-month follow-up period. The MNA-SF was the most accurate tool at predicting mortality 36 months after surgery.[205]

## Malnutrition Self-Screening Tool

A Malnutrition Self-Screening Tool has been developed by BAPEN that is based on the MUST. An electronic version of this tool can be viewed at http://www.malnutritionselfscreening.org/self-screening.html. The validity of the Malnutrition Self-Screening Tool was determined in a study involving outpatient individuals with irritable bowel disease (IBD). Malnutrition is a common comorbidity affecting clinical outcomes in patients with IBD.[206] This was a prospective validation study with a total sample of 154 individuals suffering from IBD. The self-administered tool was completed by the patients and followed by a MUST screen conducted by healthcare professionals. All patients were able to complete the screen independently. There was a high level of agreement between the MUST conducted by healthcare staff and the self-assessment completed by the IBD individuals. Ninety-six percent of the patients reported that the Malnutrition

Self-Screening Tool was easy to understand and complete. Use of self-screening nutritional-risk tools can help identify patients who need additional nutrition support without increasing time for staff to conduct the evaluation. Self-screening tools are appropriate for community-living adults who are able to complete the tool with no or limited assistance. This format can help clinicians and researchers identify a greater number of patients at nutritional risk for malnutrition.[207]

## Limitations of the MUST

Although it has been determined that the MUST is a valid screening tool for the identification of malnutrition in adults, its use has several limitations. The tool requires a height and weight to determine BMI. If the height and weight cannot be obtained, then the subjective criteria outlined by the tool can be used to determine nutrition risk and the parameter that affects the final score. Several studies, especially the ones using older adults as their sample, have reported that the MNA or the MNA-SF is a more accurate indicator of nutritional risk and predictor of LOS, hospital admission, and mortality. A positive aspect of the tool is that training time for the healthcare professional is less than one hour and the self-screening tool is easy for community-living adults to complete without assistance.[200]

> **Recap**   To prevent malnutrition and identify individuals at risk, nutrition screening should be conducted for community-dwelling adults. Any of the validated nutritional screening tools discussed thus far can be used to help identify malnutrition and the chance of reducing the incidence of comorbid conditions that are exacerbated by inadequate nutritional status.

## ▶ Subjective Global Assessment

> **Preview**   Although the MNA and the MUST are nutrition-screening tools, the **subjective global assessment (SGA)** is a validated nutritional assessment tool that involves evaluating five components of a patient's medical history (weight status and dietary-intake changes, gastrointestinal symptoms, functional capacity, and metabolic stress from disease) and three components of physical examination (muscle wasting, fat depletion, and nutrition-related edema).[208–210]

## Subjective Global Assessment Seven-Point Scale

The SGA consists of a subjective summation of the eight components that classifies patients into one of three categories: A = well nourished, B = moderately malnourished, and C = severely malnourished.[208] **FIGURE 9.5** shows the conventional SGA tool. The SGA has been researched in different patient types and has been determined to be a valid assessment tool in older adults, clinical and surgical hospital patients, rehabilitation center patients, critical-care patients, and children.[211,212,213,214]

Developed almost 30 years ago, the SGA is not an efficient tool for detecting small changes in nutrition status during follow-up assessments.[215,216] To make the SGA more sensitive in detecting small changes in nutrition status, the tool was expanded to a seven-point scale. The seven-point SGA scale was tested in a study with a patient sample consisting of 680 peritoneal dialysis patients. Ratings for nutrition status range from one to seven, with ratings of one to two denoting severe malnutrition, three to five indicating moderate malnutrition, and six to seven indicating a well-nourished individual. The revisions accomplished the goal of making the tool more sensitive to detect small changes without sacrificing the original ratings of the conventional SGA.[217] The sensitivity of the seven-point SGA was further confirmed in a study of 67 adult inpatients assessed as malnourished (per the SGA) and then reassessed using both the conventional SGA and the seven-point SGA at one, three, and five months after the baseline assessment. It took a significantly shorter time to note a one-point change using the seven-point SGA than the conventional SGA tool. This tool can be used to help identify individuals needing nutrition interventions.[218] See **FIGURE 9.6** for the seven-point SGA tool.

## Patient-Generated Subjective Global Assessment

Another iteration of the SGA is the **patient-generated subjective global assessment (PG-SGA)**. This tool has been specifically developed for patients with cancer.[219] When compared to the conventional SGA, the PG-SGA includes additional questions regarding nutritional symptoms and short-term weight loss. The PG-SGA was designed so that patients could complete their medical histories using checkboxes. The physical exam is then completed by the healthcare professional, physician,

A. History
  1. Weight Change
     Maximum weight _____ Wt. 1 year ago _____ Wt. 6 months ago _____ Current Wt. _____
     Overall loss in past 6 months:              Amount = _____ lbs; % loss _____.
     Change in past 2 weeks:              _____ increase;
     _____ no change;
     _____ decrease.
     Other history: (Change in clothing size, loose fitting clothes, etc.)
     A = No significant change; B = 5-10% weight loss; C = 10% or more sustained weight loss
  2. Dietary-intake change (relative to normal)
     (Have eating patterns changed over last several weeks or months? Has amount of food eaten changes? Are certain foods they used to eat that they no longer eat? What happens if they try to eat more? How does typical breakfast, lunch, dinner compare with 6 to 12 months ago?
     A = No significant change; B = poor but improving or borderline but declining; C = starvation, unable to eat.
  3. Gastrointestinal symptoms (that persisted for > 2 weeks)
     _____ None (A); _____ Some symptoms (B) (nausea, vomiting, diarrhea); _____ Many symptoms (C)
  4. Functional capacity
     _____ No dysfunction (e. g. full capacity) (A)
     _____ Dysfunction: Mild (B); _____ Severe (C) _____ Duration = # _____ weeks.
  5. Disease and its relation to nutritional requirements
     Metabolic demand (stress): _____ No stress (A); _____ Low—moderate stress (B); _____ High stress (C)
B. Physical (for each trait specify: A = normal, B = mild-moderate, C = severe)
  # _____ loss of subcutaneous fat (triceps, chest)
  # _____ muscle wasting (quadriceps, deltoids)
  # _____ ankle edema
  # _____ sacral edema
  # _____ ascites
C. SGA rating (select one)
  _____ A = Well-nourished
  _____ B = Moderately (or suspected of being) malnourished
  _____ C = Severely malnourished

**FIGURE 9.5** Subjective global assessment.

Adapted from: Subjective Global Assessment. Covinsky, KE, Martin, GE, Beyth, RJ, et al. The relationship between clinical assessments of nutritional status and adverse outcomes in older hospitalized medical patients. *J Am Geriatr Soc.* 1999;47:532-538.

nurse, or RDN. The Scored PG-SGA is an advanced version of the PG-SGA. This version allows for a numerical score to be generated that indicates whether a patient is well nourished, moderately nourished, or severely malnourished. For each component of the Scored PG-SGA, points from zero to four are assigned to each criterion, depending on the effect of the symptom on nutritional status. The total points are calculated, and the score is used to guide the level of nutrition intervention appropriate for the risk level.[220] The Scored PG-SGA was also evaluated as an assessment tool to identify malnutrition in older adults admitted to rehabilitation centers, in efforts to address the strong evidence showing malnutrition is both underrecognized and underdiagnosed in rehabilitation settings.[221] Fifty-seven older adults admitted to a rehabilitation center were assessed for malnutrition using the Scored PG-SGA, the MNA, or the *International Statistical Classification of Diseases and Health Related Problems*, 10th revision, *Australian Modification* (ICD10-AM) to determine the validity of the tools and the prevalence of malnutrition.[211,222] The incidence of malnutrition varied, with the nutrition assessment tool used with 28% of patients noted to be malnourished with the MNA, 46% with the ICD10-AM, and 53% with the Scored PG-SGA. The Scored PG-SGA showed strong concurrent validity, whereas the MNA indicated moderate concurrent validity. The Scored PG-SGA nutrition assessment tool was determined to be suitable for nutrition assessment in the older adult population, although caution must be taken with the MNA to identify all patients at risk of malnutrition.

Point SGA tool

**Assessment criteria**

| Weight | Rating | 7 | 6 | 5 | 4 | 3 | 2 | 1 |
|---|---|---|---|---|---|---|---|---|
| Weight loss | | 0% | <3% | 3-<5% | 5-<7% | 7-<10% | 10-<15% | >/=15% |
| Weight increase trend | Add one point | | | | | | | |
| Weight loss trend- in one month | Deduct 1 point | | | | | | | |
| **Intake** (in the last 2 weeks) | | 100% | >75%-100% | 50-75%- but increasing | 50-75%-- no change or decreasing | <50% but increasing | <50%-no change or decreasing | <25% |
| **Gastrointestinal symptoms** (present for > 2 weeks): nausea, vomiting, diarrhea | | No symptoms | Very few intermittent symptoms (once/day) | Some symptoms (2-3 times/week) improving | Some symptoms (2-3 times/week) No change | Some symptoms (2-3 times/week) getting worse | Some or all symptoms >3 times/day | |
| **Functional status** (nutrition related) | | Full functional capacity | | Mid to moderate loss of stamina | | | Severe loss of functional ability (bedridden) | |
| **Disease affecting nutritional needs** | | No increase in metabolic demands | | Mild to moderate increase in metabolic demands | | | Drastic increase in metabolic demands | |
| **Muscle waste** (at least 3 areas) | | No depletion | | Mild to moderate depletion | | | Severe depletion | |
| **Fat stores** | | No depletion | | Mild to moderate depletion | | | Severe depletion | |
| **Edema** (nutrition related) | | No edema | | Mild to moderate edema | | | Severe edema | |
| **Nutritional status** | | Well nourished | | Mild to moderately malnourished | | | Severely malnourished | |
| **Overall SGA rating (select one)** | | 7 | 6 | 5 | 4 | 3 | 2 | 1 |

**FIGURE 9.6** Seven-point SGA tool.

Data from Lim SL, Lin XH, Daniels L. Seven-Point Subjective Global Assessment Is More Time Sensitive Than Conventional Subjective Global Assessment in Detecting Nutrition Changes. *J Parenter Enteral Nutr.* 2016;40(7):966-972.

# Evaluation of the Subjective Global Assessment Tool

In a systematic literature view, Fink et al. reported that several nutrition screening tools are more sensitive than the SGA in identifying nutrition risk in patients. Based on their analysis, the NRS 2002 was a better predictor of postoperative complications and the Mini Nutrition Assessment screening tool was reported to be the best suited for elderly hospitalized patients.[223] Note that this review was only based only on the conventional SGA and does not reflect the iterations of the SGA that may be more sensitive to changes in nutrition status—namely, the seven-point SGA, the PG-SGA, and the Scored PG-SGA.

**Recap** When the conventional SGA was developed in the late 1980s, the physical examination for fat loss, muscle wasting, and edema was typically performed by a physician or advanced-practice nurse; however, with the training of other healthcare professionals on nutrition-focused physical examination, however, by training other healthcare professionals to perform NFPEs, the SGA can be completed by any trained healthcare professional. RDNs trained to complete an NFPE are able to conduct an SGA and use other nutritional assessment tools to assess for malnutrition and promptly implement nutrition interventions.

# ▶ Chapter Summary

A complete and thorough nutrition assessment is based on gathering all factors that can affect nutritional status. Anthropometric and biochemical data as well as medical and food- and nutrition-related history must be assembled. This data can be used to confirm or refute nutrition-focused physical findings to determine the presence of nutritional problem(s).

Adult malnutrition has been defined by the Academy and ASPEN collaboration in recent years, and parameters have been established that will help the clinician determine the incidence of malnutrition in different healthcare settings. In addition, evidence-based formulas have been developed and validated to determine energy, protein, and fluid needs in various conditions and disease states.

Two specific nutrition-related conditions have been reviewed—HIV infection and eating disorders.

Many other conditions and diseases, however, require specialized nutrition interventions, including diabetes, kidney disease, and heart disease, among others. Anthropometric, biochemical, client, and food- and nutrition-related history as well as nutrition-focused physical findings are all important aspects to consider when completing a nutritional assessment for these and other conditions or disease states.

Several nutrition screening and assessment tools have been developed to aid clinicians in determining nutritional risk, and these tools help identify and intervene early to prevent the development of severe malnutrition. These tools have been validated in various healthcare settings to help not only nutrition professionals but also all healthcare professionals in identifying nutritional risk and promote referral to RDNs for prompt nutrition interventions.

---

 **CASE STUDY**

## Anorexia Nervosa

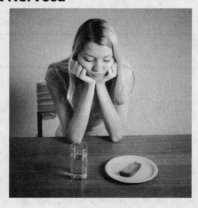

© maga/Shutterstock.

Dawna, a 26-year-old woman, was admitted to the hospital with a diagnosis of anorexia nervosa and long-standing history of restrictive-eating behavior with purging. She had lost one-third of her body weight over 6 months. On admission, Dawna was 5'6" tall and weighed 82 lbs, with a BMI of 13.2. Her resting heart rate was 50 beats per minute. She was afebrile. Laboratory values included C-reactive protein (0.7 mg/dL), white blood cell count (6,200 mm³), prealbumin (25 mg/dL), and fasting blood glucose (75 mg/dL). Dawna exhibited generalized loss of muscle and subcutaneous fat. Other

findings included lanugo hairs. Markedly underweight status was evident, with weight loss of 42 lbs over 6 months. Midarm muscle circumference measurement was below the fifth percentile.

### Questions:

1. What malnutrition syndrome would you anticipate in a patient who presents with anorexia nervosa? How would you confirm this?

   a. Severe malnutrition in the context of chronic illness

   b. Severe malnutrition in the context of environmental or social circumstances

   c. Severe malnutrition in the context of acute injury

   d. Mild or moderate malnutrition in the context of chronic illness

2. What factors indicate the type of malnutrition diagnosed?

3. Consider Dawna's history and clinical diagnosis, clinical signs and results from a physical examination, anthropometric data, laboratory indicators, dietary intake, and functional outcomes. Would you suspect reduced handgrip? Why?

Use **TABLES A** and **B**, which describe the clinical characteristics to be used to identify, document, and support a diagnosis of malnutrition.

| **TABLE A** Characteristics to support a diagnosis of malnutrition | | | | | | |
|---|---|---|---|---|---|
| **Clinical Characteristics** | **Malnutrition in Acute Illness or Injury** | | **Malnutrition in Chronic Illness** | | **Malnutrition in Social or Environmental Circumstances** | |
| | Nonsevere or moderate malnutrition | Severe malnutrition | Nonsevere or moderate malnutrition | Severe malnutrition | Nonsevere or moderate malnutrition | Severe malnutrition |
| **Intake** | <75% of estimated energy needs for >7 days | ≤50% of estimated energy needs for ≥5 days | <75% of estimated energy needs for ≥1 month | <75% of estimated energy needs for ≥1 month | <75% of estimated energy needs for ≥3 month | <50% of estimated energy needs for ≥1 month |
| **Weight Loss** | 1–2% in one week<br>5% in one month<br>7.5% in three months | >2% in one week<br>>5% in one month<br>>7.5% in three months | 5% in one month<br>7.5% in three months<br>10% in six months<br>20% in 12 months | >5% in one month<br>>7.5% in three months<br>>10% in six months<br>>20% in 12 months | 5% in one month<br>7.5% in three months<br>10% in six months<br>20% in 12 months | >5% in one month<br>>7.5% in three months<br>>10% in six months<br>>20% in 12 months |
| **Body Fat** | Mild | Moderate | Mild | Moderate | Mild | Moderate |
| **Muscle Mass** | Mild | | Mild | | Mild | |
| **Fluid Accumulation/ Edema** | Mild | Moderate to severe | Mild | Severe | Mild | Severe |
| **Reduced Handgrip** | Not applicable | Measurably reduced | Not applicable | Measurably reduced | Not applicable | Measurably reduced |

*Note:* A minimum of two of the six clinical characteristics should be present for diagnosis of either severe or nonsevere malnutrition.

1. White JV, Guenter P, Jensen G, et al. Consensus Statement: Academy of Nutrition and Dietetics and American Society for Parenteral and Enteral Nutrition: Characteristics Recommended for the Identification and Documentation of Adult Malnutrition (Undernutrition). *Journal of Parenteral and Enteral Nutrition.* 2012;36(3):275-283.
2. Kondrup J. Can food intake in hospitals be improved? *Clin Nutr.* 2001;20:153-160.
3. Blackburn GL, Bistrian BR, Maini BS, Schlamm HT, Smith MF. Nutritional and metabolic assessment of the hospitalized patient JPEN J Parenter Enteral Nutr. 1977;1:11-22.
4. Klein S, Kinney J, Jeejeebhoy K, et al. Nutrition support in clinical practice: review of published data and recommendations for future research directions. National Institutes of Health, American Society for Parenteral and Enteral Nutrition, and American Society for Clinical Nutrition. *JPEN J Parenter Enteral Nutr.* 1977;21:133-156.
5. Rosenbaum K, Wang J, Pierson RN, Kotler DP. Time-dependent variation in weight and body composition in healthy adults. *J Parenter Enteral Nutr.* 2000;24:52-55.
6. Keys A. Chronic undernutrition and starvation with notes on protein deficiency. JAMA. 1948;138:500-511.
7. Sacks GS, Dearman K, Replogle WH, Cora VL, Meeks M, Canada T. Use of subjective global assessment to identify nutritionassociated complications and death in long-term care facility residents. J Am Coll Nutr. 2000;19:570-577.
8. Norman K, Stobaus N, Gonzalez MC, Schulzke J-D, Pirlich M. Hand grip strength: outcome predictor and marker of nutritional status. *Clin Nutr.* 2011;30:135-142.
9. Hagan JC. Acute and chronic diseases. In: Mulner RM, ed. Encyclopedia of Health Services Research. Vol 1. Thousand Oaks, CA Sage; 2009:25.
10. American Dietetic Association Evidence Analysis Library. Does serum prealbumin correlate with weight loss in four models of prolonged protein-energy restriction: anorexia nervosa, non-malabsorptive gastric partitioning bariatric surgery, calorie-restricted diets or starvation. http://www.adaevidencelibrary.com/conclusion.cfm?conclusion_statement_id=251313&highlight=prealbumin& home=1. Accessed July 5, 2017.
11. American Dietetic Association Evidence Analysis Library. Does serum prealbumin correlate with nitrogen balance? http://www.adaevidencelibrary.com/conclusion.cfm?conclusion_statement_id=251315&highlight=prealbumin&home=1. Accessed July 5, 2017.
12. American Dietetic Association Evidence Analysis Library. Does serum albumin correlate with weight loss in four models of prolonged protein-energy restriction: anorexia nervosa, non-malabsorptive gastric partitioning bariatric surgery, calorie-restricted diets or starvation. http://www.adaevidencelibrary.com/conclusion.cfm?conclusion_statement_id=251263&highlight=albumin&home=1. Accessed July 5, 2017.
13. American Dietetic Association Evidence Analysis Library. Does serum albumin correlate with nitrogen balance? http://www.adaevidencelibrary.com/conclusion.cfm?conclusion_statement_id=251265&highlight=albumin&home=1. Accessed July 5, 2017.

**TABLE B** Description of clinical Characteristics

| Intake | Weight Loss | Nutrition Focused Physical Exam | Body Fat | Muscle Mass | Fluid Accumulation/Edema | Reduced Handgrip |
|--------|-------------|--------------------------------|----------|-------------|--------------------------|------------------|
| Malnutrition occurs due to insufficient food and nutrient intake or malabsorption. Recent nutrient consumption compared against estimated nutritional needs is a primary standard for defining malnutrition. | The clinician should evaluate current weight considering other clinical findings, together with the presence of under- or overhydration. | Malnutrition normally manifests in the form of physical changes that can be identified via a nutrition focused physical exam. Weigh, body fat, muscle mass, fluid accumulation, and handgrip changes should be documented as part of conducting and documenting a nutrition focused physical exam. | Loss of subcutaneous fat (as seen in orbital cavity, triceps, and fat covering the ribcage) | Muscle loss as seen in wasting of the temples, clavicles, shoulders, interosseous muscles, scapula, thigh, and calf | Evaluate the individual for generalized or localized fluid accumulation. This is usually seen in the extremities (especially the lower extremities), genital edema, or ascites. | Compare measurements to measurement standards provided by the dynamometer manufacturer. |
| The clinician should conduct or review the food and fluid intake history, calculate optimal energy needs, compare them with calculated energy consumed, and report insufficient intake as a percentage of calculated energy needs over time. | Weigh change is assessed over time and reported as a percent of weight loss from the previous weight. | | | | Weight loss is often disguised by generalized edema. Unplanned, unexplained weight increase can be seen in the presence of fluid accumulation. | |

# CASE STUDY

## Cirrhosis with Portal Hypertension and Ascites

Steven, a 52-year-old man, sees you for a follow-up clinical appointment. He has an established history of cirrhosis and portal hypertension in the setting of long-term ethanol abuse. Steven had gained 10 lbs over the prior 2 weeks and exhibits massive ascites. Additional findings included mild encephalopathy with poor concentration, asterixis, and sclera icterus. A family member reports that Steven's food intake had been severely compromised for weeks. At presentation, the patient is 5'8" tall and weighs 161 lbs (usual weight ~150 lbs). He is afebrile. Laboratories included total bilirubin (3.8 mg/dL), aspartate aminotransferase (96 IU/L) alanine aminotransferase (111 U/L), alkaline phosphatase (162 IU/L), serum albumin (1.7 g/dL), prothrombin time (18 seconds), white blood cells (3700 mm³), C-reactive protein (27 mg/L), prealbumin (6.8 mg/dL), hemoglobin (8 g/dL), hematocrit (32%), and fasting glucose (107 mg/dL). Physical findings are notable for ascites and extensive loss of muscle and subcutaneous fat.

### Questions:

1. What nutrition syndrome would you anticipate in a patient who presents with cirrhosis with portal hypertension and ascites, and how would you confirm this?
   a. Severe malnutrition in the context of chronic illness
   b. Severe malnutrition in the context of environmental or social circumstances
   c. Severe malnutrition in the context of acute injury
   d. Mild or moderate malnutrition in the context of chronic illness

2. What factors indicate the type of malnutrition diagnosed?

# CASE STUDY

## Multiple-Trauma Victim

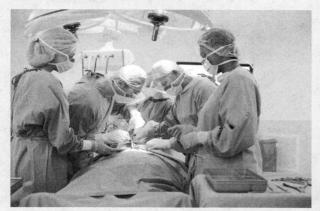

© Squaredpixels/Getty Images.

Stuart, a 38-year-old man, is suffering from multiple traumas secondary to a motor vehicle accident. His injuries include a ruptured spleen, grade III liver laceration, left femur fracture, and bilateral pulmonary contusions. His status was post damage control celiotomy, splenectonmy, and packing of the liver. He was transferred to the trauma intensive-care unit on a ventilator, where he continued to be resuscitated. Postsurgery day two of admission, Stuart had a temperature (102°F), heart rate (98 beats per minute), respiratory rate (26 breaths per minute), white blood cell count (25K/mm³), and pCO₂ (28 mm Hg). He was markedly edematous, with a weight gain of 15 lbs above his usual body weight. His open abdomen was dressed. Additional laboratory data: C-reactive protein (45 mg/dL), serum albumin (2.6 g/dL), prealbumin (11.0 mg/dL) and glucose (220 mg/dL). He has an increased metabolic rate by indirect calorimetry (REE of 3,000 kcal). Dietary intake is anticipated to be compromised for a week or more. He is reported to have been well nourished with suitable dietary intake before his injury.

### Questions:

1. What malnutrition syndrome would you anticipate in a multiple-trauma victim early in his course? How would you confirm this?
   a. Severe malnutrition in the context of chronic illness
   b. Severe malnutrition in the context of environmental or social circumstances
   c. Severe malnutrition in the context of acute injury
   d. Mild or moderate malnutrition in the context of chronic illness

2. What factors indicate the type of malnutrition diagnosed?

# Learning Portfolio

## Key Terms

Anorexia nervosa (AN)
Anthropometry
Binge-eating disorder (BED)
Body mass index (BMI)
Bulimia nervosa (BN)
Cachexia
Client history
Food- and nutrition-related history
Human immunodeficiency virus (HIV)
Indirect calorimetry
Inflammatory response
Kwashiorkor
Lipodystrophy
Malnutrition

Malnutrition Universal Screening Tool (MUST)
Mini Nutrition Assessment (MNA)
Nutritional assessment
Nutritional status
Nutrition-focused physical examination (NFPE)
Nutrition screening
Opportunistic infection
Patient-generated subjective global assessment (PG-SGA)
Predictive equations for estimating energy needs
Resting metabolic rate (RMR)
Sarcopenia
Sarcopenic obesity
Subjective global assessment (SGA)

## Study Questions

1. The height of a patient with severe muscular deformities or multiple contractures can best be measured by:
   a. Standing height.
   b. Segmental measurement.
   c. Arm span.
   d. Bioelectrical impedance analysis.

2. Effective medications for managing HIV have resulted in other metabolic abnormalities that require nutrition management. Which of the following occurs?
   a. Lipodystrophy
   b. Nutritional anemias
   c. Low blood glucose levels
   d. Elevated HDL cholesterol levels

3. What characteristic is not included in the diagnosis of adult malnutrition?
   a. Loss of subcutaneous fat
   b. Insufficient protein intake
   c. Diminished functional status
   d. Insufficient energy intake

4. Bone tenderness and pain may be present with a _____ deficiency.
   a. Vitamin A
   b. Vitamin C
   c. Vitamin D
   d. Vitamin K

5. _____ is a method of determining body composition that is generally equivalent to underwater weighing.
   a. Air-displacement plethysmography
   b. Bioelectrical impedance analysis
   c. Waist-to-hip ratio
   d. Dual-energy x-ray absorptiometry

6. Which component is generally *not* part of a client history?
   a. Medical history
   b. Surgeries
   c. Treatments
   d. Dietary supplement use

7. A major limitation of a food- and nutrition-related history may be:
   a. Interviewer questions that are too specific.
   b. Too many interview questions to answer.
   c. Clients with impaired cognition may not be able to provide accurate information.
   d. Information given by the caregiver is not the same as the client would provide.

8. The most commonly used technique for a nutrition-focused physical exam is:
   a. Inspection.
   b. Palpation.
   c. Percussion.
   d. Manipulation.

9. A limitation of the Malnutrition Universal Screening Tool is that:
   a. It requires a current height and weight to determine BMI.
   b. It can only be completed by advanced healthcare practitioners.
   c. It takes a significant amount of time to complete.
   d. It should only be used for hospitalized patients.

10. Bitot's spots may be present in which deficiency?
    a. Iron
    b. Folate
    c. Vitamin A
    d. Vitamin D

11. The prevalence of obesity in American adults is:
    a. 15.3%.
    b. 26.7%.
    c. 36.5%.
    d. 41.2%.

12. A predictive resting energy equation noted to be specific for ventilator-dependent patients is the:
    a. Mifflin–St. Jeor.
    b. Penn State.
    c. Harris-Benedict.
    d. Owen.

13. The extent to which a nutritional screen gives negative results in those who are free of the disease or condition is called:
    a. Sensitivity.
    b. Reliability.
    c. Accuracy.
    d. Specificity.

14. Spoon-shaped nails can be present in a:
    a. Vitamin A or vitamin D excess.
    b. Vitamin C deficiency.
    c. Protein or iron deficiency.
    d. Riboflavin deficiency.

15. Gray-brown spots or mottling on teeth can indicate:
    a. A vitamin C deficiency.
    b. Excessive sugar intake.
    c. A high acid intake.
    d. Excess fluoride intake.

16. Adult malnutrition is similar to pediatric:
    a. Kwashiorkor.
    b. Marasmus.
    c. Marasmic kwashiorkor.
    d. Cachexia.

17. Sarcopenia is characterized by the loss of:
    a. Lean muscle mass and body fat.
    b. Body fat.
    c. Muscle mass.
    d. Body weight.

18. Appropriate interventions for weight change or weight loss in patients are determined by:
    a. Starting with an oral nutrition supplement first.
    b. Altering the diet consistency.
    c. Liberalizing the diet.
    d. Investigating the root cause of the weight loss.

19. Malnutrition in the context of social or environmental circumstances may be present in patients with:
    a. Major infection.
    b. Cancer.
    c. Rheumatoid arthritis.
    d. Anorexia nervosa.

20. A patient with a hemoglobin A1C of 7.9% has an estimate average glucose (eAG) of approximately:
    a. 212 mg/dL.
    b. 80 mg/dL.
    c. 183 mg/dL.
    d. 97 mg/dL.

21. Muscle mass loss is *not* assessed in which one of the following areas of the body?
    a. Ribs or chest area
    b. Temporal area
    c. Clavicle area
    d. Interosseous area of the hand

22. The equation found most reliable in predicting resting energy requirements is the _____ equation.
    a. Harris-Benedict
    b. Ireton-Jones
    c. Penn State
    d. Mifflin–St. Jeor

23. Recommended protein intakes for patients at risk of malnutrition or with existing pressure injuries who are assessed to be at risk of malnutrition is:
    a. 1.0–1.2 g/kg body weight.
    b. 1.25–1.5 g/kg body weight.
    c. 1.5–1.7 g/kg body weight.
    d. ≥ 2.0 g/kg body weight.

24. A diet history tool that asks the client to recall food and beverage intake from the previous day is called a:
    a. Food-frequency questionnaire.
    b. Daily food checklist.
    c. 24-hour food recall.
    d. Direct meal observation.

25. Recommendations for protein in a patient who is in stage III CKD are:
    a. 10% of calorie intake from protein.
    b. 15% of calorie intake from protein.
    c. 0.8 g/kg body weight.
    d. 1.0 g/kg body weight.

26. Weight gain goals for hospitalized patients with anorexia nervosa are:
    a. Preventing further weight loss while in hospital.
    b. 0.5 – 1.0 lb/week
    c. 1 – 2 lb/week
    d. 2 – 3 lb/week

27. Which of the nutrition-screening and assessment tools contains both a nutrition-screening tool and a nutritional assessment?
    a. Nutrition risk screening
    b. Malnutrition Universal Screening Tool
    c. ubjective global assessment
    d. Mini Nutritional Assessment

28. The best indicator of kidney function is:
    a. Glomerular filtration rate.
    b. Serum creatinine.
    c. Blood urea nitrogen.
    d. Serum sodium level.

29. The subjective global assessment does not review which of the following?
    a. Change in body weight
    b. Gastrointestinal symptoms
    c. Biochemical measures
    d. Functional capacity

30. Coarse, dry, brittle hair can indicate:
    a. Hyperthyroidism.
    b. Hypothyroidism.
    c. Hyperparathyroidism.
    d. Protein deficiency.

## Discussion Questions

1. Discuss the difference between a nutrition screen and a nutrition assessment.
2. Compare and contrast the diagnosis of adult malnutrition in the following contexts: acute injury or illness, chronic illness, and social or environmental circumstances.
3. Discuss the positive aspects and the limitations of the MUST.

## Activities

1. Conduct a food- and nutrition-related history interview with one of your friends or family members. Use the list of questions in the section on food history to conduct the interview.
2. Review the history of a patient or client. What details of the client history are important in completing a nutritional assessment?
3. Contact a local senior center and ask the director if you can conduct a Mini Nutritional Assessment and a Malnutrition Universal Screening Tool at the center. Determine whether any individuals are at nutritional risk. Tell any individuals who are at nutritional risk to follow up with their physicians.
4. Calculate your estimated energy needs using three of the predictive equations. What were the differences in the results?
5. Calculate the protein and fluid needs for an older adult female who is 62 inches and 130 lbs with a current pressure injury who is assessed to be at risk of malnutrition.
6. Measure the height of a peer using the methods described in the chapter.
7. Once the height and weight are obtained, calculate the BMI. What does the BMI tell you about your peer?
8. View the Nestlé Nutrition Institute videos under "Online Resources" section that follows. Conduct a basic NFPE with one of your peers.
    a. What nutrient deficiency were you able to identify in your peer? What physical signs were used to determine the identified deficiency?
    b. If no nutrition deficiency was identified, what physical characteristics did you use to reach that conclusion?

## Online Resources

**Snapshot—NCP Step 1: Nutrition Assessment**

https://www.andeal.org/vault/2440/web/files/20140602-NA%20Snapshot.pdf

**Academy of Nutrition and Dietetics Critical Thinking Skills in Nutrition Assessment and Diagnosis**

http://www.eatrightpro.org/~/media/eatrightpro%20files/practice/position%20and%20practice%20papers/practice%20papers/practice%20papers/practice%20paper%20critical%20thinking%20skills%20in%20nutrition%20assessment.ashx

**Skinfold measurement technique video**

https://youtu.be/XMpifYMxHVo

**Diet History Part 1**

https://www.youtube.com/watch?v=76OfeSesBw0

**Diet History Interview**

https://www.youtube.com/watch?v=CruhCMRTpnQ

**Patient-Generated Subjective Global Assessment**

http://pt-global.org

**The Minnesota Semistarvation Experiment**

http://www.epi.umn.edu/cvdepi/video/the-minnesota-semistarvation-experiment/

**Alliance to Advance Patient Nutrition**

http://malnutrition.com

**Nutrition Focused Physical Assessment Part 1: Setting the Stage for Success**

https://www.nestlenutrition-institute.org/Resources/Online-Conferences/Pages/NutritionFocusedPhysicalAssessmentPart1SettingtheStageforSuccess.aspx

**Nutrition Focused Physical Assessment Part 2: Creating Your Malnutrition Toolbox**

https://www.nestlenutrition-institute.org/Resources/online-conferences/Pages/NutritionFocusedPhysicalAssessmentPart2CreatingYourMalnutritionToolbox.aspx

**Nutrition Focused Physical Assessment Part 3: Micronutrient Deficiencies**

https://www.nestlenutrition-institute.org/Resources/online-conferences/Pages/NutritionFocusedPhysicalAssessmentPart3MicronutrientDeficiencies.aspx

**Mini Nutrition Assessment Resources: Nestlé Nutrition institute**

http://www.mna-elderly.com/

**Malnutrition Universal Screening Tool (MUST)**

http://www.bapen.org.uk/pdfs/must/must_full.pdf

**Malnutrition Self-Screening Tool**

http://www.malnutritionselfscreening.org/self-screening.html

## References

1. Mann J, Truswell S. *Essentials of Human Nutrition*. 4th ed. New York, NY: Oxford University Press; 2012.
2. Ferguson M. Nutrition Screening Evidence Analysis Project presentation; 2009; February 10. https://www.andeal.org/topic.cfm?key=2193&cat=3853.
3. American Society of Parenteral Enteral Nutrition (ASPEN). Malnutrition Screening for Hospital Patients Widespread but Hospitals Fall Short on Nutrition Care Plans. https://www.nutritioncare.org/Press_Room/2014/Malnutrition_Screening_for_Hospital_Patients_Widespread_but_Hospitals_Fall_Short_on_Nutrition_Care_Plans/.
4. Department of Health and Human Services, Centers for Medicare & Medicaid Services. Revisions to Appendix PP: Interpretive Guidelines for Long-Term Care Facilities; 2008. https://www.cms.gov/Regulations-and-Guidance/Guidance/Transmittals/downloads/R36SOMA.pdf.
5. Academy of Nutrition and Dietetics. Nutrition Screening (NSCR) Systematic Review (2009–2010). http://www.andeal.org/topic.cfm?menu=3584.
6. Nestlé Nutrition Institute. Validity in Screening Tools. MNA Mini Nutrition Assessment. http://www.mna-elderly.com/validity_in_screening_tools.html.
7. American Dietetic Association. ADA's definitions for nutrition screening and nutrition assessment: Identifying patients at risk. *J Am Diet Assoc*. 1994; 94(8):838-839.
8. ASPEN. Board of Directors and Clinical Practice Committee. Definition of terms, style, and conventions used in ASPEN Board of Directors–approved documents; 2015. https://www.researchgate.net/publication/7557179_Definition_of_Terms_Style_and_Conventions_Used_in_ASPEN_Guidelines_and_Standards.

9. Academy of Nutrition and Dietetics. *International Dietetics and Nutrition Terminology (IDNT) Reference Manual: Standardized Language for the Nutrition Care Process.* 4th ed. Chicago, IL: Academy of Nutrition and Dietetics; 2013.

10. Duren DL, Sherwood BJ, Czerwinski SA, et al. Body composition comparisons and interpretation. *J Diab Sci Technol.* 2008; 2(6):1139–1146.

11. Chernoff R. *Geriatric Nutrition: The Health Professional's Handbook.* 4th ed. Burlington, MA: Jones & Bartlett Learning; 2014; 443.

12. Roche AF. Anthropometric variables: effectiveness and limitations. In: *Assessing the Nutritional Status of the Elderly: State of the Art Report of the Third Ross Roundtable on Medical Issues.* Columbus, OH: Ross Laboratories; 1982.

13. Collins N. Measuring height and weight. *Adv Skin Wound Care.* 2002; 15(2):91–92.

14. Centers for Disease Control and Prevention (CDC). *Anthropometric Reference Data for Children and Adults: United States, 2007–2010.* https://www.cdc.gov/nchs/data/series /sr_11/sr11_252.pdf.

15. Murphy RA, Patel KV, Kritchevsky SB. Weight change, body composition, and risk of mobility disability and mortality in older adults: A population-based cohort study. *J Am Geriatr Soc.* 2014; 62:1476–1483.

16. You JW, Seung JL, Kim YE, et al. Association between weight change and clinical outcomes in critically ill patients. *J Crit Care.* 2013;28(6):923–927.

17. Nakagawa T, Toyazaki T, Chiba N, et al. Prognostic value of body mass index and change in body weight in postoperative outcomes of lung cancer surgery. *Interact Cardiovasc Thorac Surg.* 2016; 23(4):560–566.

18. American Medical Directors Association. *Clinical Practice Guideline: Altered Nutritional Status in the Long-Term Care Setting.* Columbia, MD: American Medical Directors Association; 2010.

19. Rossman I. The anatomy of aging. In: Rossman I, ed. *Clinical Geriatrics.* Philadelphia, PA: Lippincott; 1979.

20. Mitchell MK. *Nutrition Across the Life Span.* Philadelphia, PA: WB Saunders Company; 1997: 479.

21. Estimating height in bedridden patients. http://www .rxkinetics.com/height_estimate.html.

22. Pribram V. *Nutrition and HIV.* Appendix 10. Equations to Calculate Height and Estimation of Height from Ulna Length; 2013. http://onlinelibrary.wiley.com /doi/10.1002/9781118786529.app10/pdf.

23. Auyeung TW, Lee JS, Kwok T, et al. Estimation of stature by measuring fibula and ulna bone length in 2443 older adults. *J Nutr Health Aging.* 2009; 13(10):931–936.

24. Haapala H, Peterson MD, Daunter A, Hurvitz EA. Agreement between actual height and estimated height using segmental limb lengths for individuals with cerebral palsy. *Am J Phys Med Rehabil.* 2015; 94(7): 539–546.

25. Freedman DS, Horlick M, Berenson GS. A comparison of the Slaughter skinfold-thickness equations and BMI in predicting body fatness and cardiovascular disease risk factor levels in children. *Am J Clin Nutr.* 2013; 98(6):1417–1424.

26. Wohlfahrt-Veje C, Tinggaard J, Winther K, et al. Body fat throughout childhood in 2647 healthy Danish children: Agreement of BMI, waist circumference, skinfolds with dual x-ray absorptiometry. *Eur J Clin Nutr.* 2014; 68(6):664–670.

27. National Heart Lung and Blood Institute (NHLBI). *Managing Overweight and Obesity in Adults: Systematic Evidence Review from the Obesity Expert Panel.* Washington, DC: NHLBI; 2013.

28. Bhaskaran K, Douglas I, Forbes H, dos-Santos-Silva I, Leon DA, Smeeth L. Body-mass index and risk of 22 specific cancers: A population-based cohort study of 5.24 million UK adults. *Lancet.* 2014;384(9945):755–765.

29. NCHS Data Brief No. 219. Prevalence of obesity among adults and youth: United States, 2011–2014; 2015. https://www.cdc .gov/nchs/data/databriefs/db219.pdf.

30. Winter JE, MacInnis RJ, Nowson CA. The influence of age on the BMI and all-cause mortality association: A meta-analysis. *J Nutr Health Aging;* 2016; 7:1–5.

31. Hillier SE, Beck L, Petropoulou BA, Clegg ME. A comparison of body composition measurement techniques. *J Hum Nutr Dietet.* 2014; 27:626–631.

32. Harrison GG, Buskirk ER, Carter JEL, et al. Skinfold thickness and measurement technique. In: Lohman TG, Roche AF, Martorell R, eds., *Anthropometric Standardization Reference Manual.* Champaign, IL: Human Kinetics; 1988.

33. Durnin JV, Womersley S. Body fat assessed from total body density and its estimation from skinfold thickness: Measurements of 481 men and women aged from 16-72 years. *Br J Nutr.* 1974; 32:77–79.

34. Chambers AJ, Parise E, McCrory JL, Cham R. A comparison of prediction equations for the estimation of body fat percentage in non-obese and obese older Caucasian adults in the United States. *J Nutr Health Aging.* 2014; 18(6):586–590.

35. CDC. *Anthropometric Reference Data for Children and Adults: United States, 2003–2006;* 2008. http://www.cdc.gov/nchs /data/nhsr/nhsr010.pdf.

36. de Oms M, Habicht JP. Anthropometric reference data for international use: Recommendations from a World Health Organization Expert Committee. *Am J Clin Nutr.* 1996; 64:650–658.

37. Guigoz Y, Bruno V, Garry PL. Assessing the nutritional status of the elderly: The Mini Nutritional Assessment as part of the geriatric evaluation. *Nutr Rev.* 1996; 54:S59–S65.

38. Portero-McClellan KC, Staudt C, Silva FR, et al. The use of calf circumference measurement as an anthropometric tool to monitor nutritional status in elderly inpatients. *J Nutr Health Aging.* 2010; 14(4):266–270.

39. Nutrition screening as easy as MNA. A guide to completing the Mini Nutrition Assessment (MNA). Nestle Nutrition Institute. http://www.mna-elderly.com/forms/mna_guide_english .pdf.

40. Chan JM, Rimm EB, Colditz GA, Stampfer MJ, Willett WC. Obesity, fat distribution, and weight gain as risk factors for clinical diabetes in men. *Diabetes Care.* 1994; 17:961–969.

41. Potts J, Simmons D. Sex and ethnic group differences in fat distribution in young United Kingdom South Asians and Europids. *J Clin Epidemiol.* 1994; 47:837–841.

42. Dobbelsteyn CJ, Joffres MR, MacLean DR, Flowerdew G. A comparative evaluation of waist circumference, waist-to-hip ratio and body mass index as indicators of cardiovascular risk factors. The Canadian Heart Health Surveys. *Intern J Obesity.* 2001; 25(5):652–661.

43. Czemichow S, Kengne AP, Huxley RR, et al. Comparison of waist-to-hip ratio and other obesity indices as predictors of cardiovascular disease risk in people with type 2 diabetes: A prospective cohort study from ADVANCE. *Eur J Cardiovasc Prev Rehabil.* 2011; 18(2):312–319.

44. de Koning L, Merchant AT, Pogue J, Anand SS. Waist circumference and waist-to-hip ratio as predictors of cardiovascular events: Meta-regression analysis of prospective studies. *Eur Heart J.* 2007; 28(7):850–856.

45. Dehghan M, Merchant AT. Is bioelectrical impedance accurate for use in large epidemiological studies? *Nutr J.* 2008; 7:26.

46. Kelly TL, Wilson KE, Heymsfield SB. Dual energy x-ray absorptiometry body composition reference values from NHANES, 2009. *PLoS One.* 2009; 4(9):e7038. http://journals.plos.org/plosone/article/citation?id=10.1371/journal.pone.0007038.

47. Houtkooper LB, Going SB, Sproul J, et al. Comparison of methods for assessing body composition over 1 y in postmenopausal women. *Am J Clin Nutr.* 2000; 72:401–406.

48. Gallagher D, Kovera AJ, Clay-Williams G, et al. Weight loss in postmenopausal obesity: No adverse alterations in body composition and protein metabolism. *Am J Physiol Endocrinol Metab.* 2000; 279:E124–E131.

49. How Does the BOD POD Work? http://ybefit.byu.edu/Portals/88/Documents/How%20Does%20The%20BOD%20POD%20Work.pdf.

50. Maddalozzo GF, Cardinal BJ, Snow CA. Concurrent validity of the BOD POD and dual energy x-ray absorptiometry techniques for assessing body composition in young women. *J Am Diet Assoc.* 2002; 102(11):1677–1679.

51. Fields DA, Gunatilake R, Kalaitzoglou E. Air displacement plethysmography: Cradle to grave. *Nutr Clin Prac.* 2015; 30(2):219–226.

52. Banh L. Serum proteins as markers of nutrition: What are we treating? Nutrition Issues in Gastroenterology. Series No. 43. *Prac Gastroenterol.* 2006; 30(10):46–64.

53. Jensen GL. Inflammation roles in aging and sarcopenia. *J Parenter Enteral Nutr.* 2008; 32(6):656–659.

54. Chan LN, Mike LA. The science and practice of micronutrient supplementations in nutritional anemia: An evidence-based review. *J Parenter Enteral Nutr.* 2014; 38(6):656–672.

55. Kuzuya M, Kanda S, Koike T, et al. Lack of correlation between total lymphocyte count and nutritional status in the elderly. *Clin Nutr.* 2005; 24(3):427–432.

56. Morley JE. Dehydration, hypernatremia, and hyponatremia. *Clin Geriatr Med.* 2015; 31(3):389–399.

57. National Kidney Foundation. Glomerular filtration rate (GFR). https://www.kidney.org/kidneydisease/siemens_hcp_gfr.

58. Foreback, C. Glycated hemoglobin in the diabetic patient. *Med Lab Observer.* 2015; 47(6):14–20.

59. NHLBI. What is cholesterol? https://www.nhlbi.nih.gov/health/health-topics/topics/hbc/.

60. Zarny LA, Berstein LH. Serum cholesterol: an indicator of malnutrition. *J Am Dietet Assoc.* 1995; 95(9):A25.

61. Hamada S, Gulliford MC. Mortality in individuals aged 80 and older with type 2 diabetes mellitus in relation to glycosylated hemoglobin, blood pressure, and total cholesterol. *J Am Geriatr Soc.* 2016; 64:1425-1431.

62. Bickley LS. *Bates' Guide to Physical Examination and History Taking.* 11th ed. Chapter 1, Overview: Physical Examination and History Taking. Philadelphia, PA: Wolters Kluwer Health/Lippincott Williams & Wilkins; 2013: 4–6.

63. Ternent CA, Bastawrous AL, Morin NA, Ellis CN, Hyman NH, Buie WD. Standards Practice Task Force of the American Society of Colon and Rectal Surgeons. Practice parameters for the evaluation and management of constipation. *Dis Colon Rec.* 2007; 50:2013–2022.

64. Müller-Lissner S, Kamm M, Scarpignato C, Wald A. Myths and misconceptions about chronic constipation. *Am J Gastroenterol.* 2005; 100:124–129.

65. Academy of Nutrition and Dietetics. Nutrition Care Manual. Client History Gastrointestinal Disease, Constipation. https://www.nutritioncaremanual.org/topic.cfm?ncm_toc_id=268232.

66. Burke BS. The diet history as a tool in research. *J Am Diet Assoc.* 1943; 23:1041–1046.

67. Skypala IJ, Venter C, Meyer R, et al. The development of a standardized diet history tool to support the diagnosis of food allergy. *Clin Transl Allergy.* 2015; 5(7). http://ctajournal.biomedcentral.com/articles/10.1186/s13601-015-0050-2#Abs1.

68. National Cancer Institute (NCI). 24-hour dietary recall (24HR) at a glance. https://dietassessmentprimer.cancer.gov/profiles/recall/.

69. US Department of Agriculture. Automated multiple-pass method. https://www.ars.usda.gov/northeast-area/beltsville-md/beltsville-human-nutrition-research-center/food-surveys-research-group/docs/ampm-usda-automated-multiple-pass-method/.

70. NCI. Observing protein & energy nutrition (OPEN) study. http://epi.grants.cancer.gov/past-initiatives/open/.

71. NCI. Food frequency questionnaire at a glance. https://dietassessmentprimer.cancer.gov/profiles/questionnaire/.

72. NCI. Usual Dietary Intakes: NHANES Food Frequency Questionnaire (FFQ). http://epi.grants.cancer.gov/diet/usualintakes/ffq.html?&url=/diet/usualintakes/ffq.html.

73. Bernstein M, Munoz N. Chapter 7: Nutritional Assessment for the Older Adult. In: *Nutrition for the Older Adult.* 2nd ed. Burlington, MA: Jones and Bartlett Learning; 2016:179.

74. Scollard T. Malnutrition and nutrition-focused physical assessment. Power Point presentation at Utah Academy of Nutrition and Dietetics annual meeting, March 27, 2015. http://www.eatrightutah.org/docs/AM15-Speaker2-01c.pdf.

75. Collins N, Harris C. The physical assessment revisited: Inclusion of the nutrition-focused physical exam. *Ostomy Wound Manag.* 2010. http://www.o-wm.com/files/owm/pdfs/Nutrition411_Layout%201.pdf.

76. MedlinePlus. Percussion. https://medlineplus.gov/ency/article/002281.htm.

77. Bistrain BR. Clinical nutritional assessment. In: Goldman L, Ausiello D, eds. *Cecil Medicine.* 23rd ed. Philadelphia, PA: Saunders Elsevier; 2008.

78. Seidel HM, Stewart RW, Ball JW, Dains JE, Flynn JA, Solomon BS. *Mosby's Guide to Physical Examination.* 7th ed. St. Louis, MO: Mosby; 2011.

79. Mordarski B, Wolff J. *Nutrition Focused Physical Exam Pocket Guide.* Chicago, IL: Academy of Nutrition and Dietetics; 2015.

80. Gross CR, Lindquist RD, Wooley AC, Granieri R, Allard K, Webster B. Clinical indicators of dehydration severity in elderly patients. *J Emerg Med.* 1992; 10(3):267–274.

81. *Dorland's Illustrated Medical Dictionary.* 32nd ed. New York, NY: Elsevier Health Sciences Division; 2011.

82. Jensen GL. Inflammation as the key interface of the medical and nutrition universes: A provocative examination of the future of clinical nutrition and medicine. *J Parenter Enteral Nutr.* 2006; 30:453–463.

83. Simpson F, Doig GS. Parenteral vs. enteral nutrition in the critically ill patient: A meta-analysis of trials using the intention to treat principle. *Intensive Care Med.* 2005; 31(1):12–23.

84. Lopez-Hellin J, Baena-Fustegueras JA, Schwartz-Riera S, Garcia-Arumi E. Usefulness of short-lived protein as nutritional indicators in surgical patients. *Clin Nutr.* 2002; 21:119–125.

85. Chabner BA, Thompson EC. Cachexia in cancer. Merck Manual (professional version). http://www.merckmanuals.com/professional/hematology-and-oncology/principles-of-cancer-therapy/cachexia-in-cancer.

86. Arends J, Bodoky G, Bozzetti F, et al. ESPEN guidelines on enteral nutrition: Non-surgical oncology. *Clin Nutr.* 2006; 25:245–259.

87. Lin CA, Boslaugh S, Ciliberto HM, et al. A prospective assessment of food and nutrient intake in a population of Malawian children at risk for kwashiorkor. *J Pediatr Gastroenterol Nutr.* 2007; 44(4):487–493.

88. Jensen GL, Bistrain B, Roubenoff R. Heimburger DC. Malnutrition syndromes: A conundrum vs continuum. *J Parenter Enteral Nutr.* 2009; 33(6):710–716.

89. Wellcome Trust Working Party. Classification of infantile malnutrition. *Lancet.* 1970; 2:302–303.

90. Plank LD, Connolly AB, Hill GL. Sequential changes in the metabolic response in severely septic patients during the first 23 days after the onset of peritonitis. *Ann Surg.* 1998; 228(2):146–158.

91. Lewis SJ, Egger M, Sylvester PA, Thomas S. Early enteral feeding versus "nil by mouth" after gastrointestinal surgery: Systematic review and meta-analysis of controlled trials. *Br Med J.* 2001; 323:1–5

92. Artinian V, Krayem H, DiGiovine B. Effects of early enteral feeding on the outcome of critically ill mechanically ventilated medical patients. *Chest.* 2006; 129:960–967.

93. Perel P, Yanagawa T, Bunn F, et al. Nutritional support for head-injured patients. *Cochrane Database Sys Rev.* 2006; 4:CD001530.

94. Morley JE, Baumgartner RN, Roubenoff R, et al. Sarcopenia. *J Lab Clin Med.* 2001; 137:231–243.

95. Metter EJ, Conwit R, Tobin J, Fozard JL. Age-associated loss of power and strength in the upper extremities in women and men. *J Gerontol A Biol Sci Med Sci.* 1997; 52:B267–B276.

96. Iannuzzi-Sucich M, Prestwood KM, Kenny AM. Prevalence of sarcopenia and predictors of skeletal muscle mass in healthy older men and women. *J Gerontol A Biol Sci Med Sci.* 2002; 57(12): M772–M777.

97. Walston JD. Sarcopenia in older adults. *Curr Opin Rheumatol.* 2012; 24(6): 623–627.

98. Stenholm S, Harris TB, Rantanen T, et al. Sarcopenic obesity: Definition, etiology, and consequences. *Curr Opin Clin Nutr Metab Care.* 2008; 11(6):693–700.

99. Batsus JA, Mackenzie TA, Barre LK, et al. Sarcopenia, sarcopenic obesity, and mortality in older adults: Results from the National Health and Nutrition Examination Survey III. *Euro J Clin Nutr.* 2014; 68:1001–1007.

100. White JV, Guenter P, Jensen G, et al. Consensus statement of the Academy of Nutrition and Dietetics/American Society for Parenteral and Enteral Nutrition: Characteristics recommended for the identification and documentation of adult malnutrition (undernutrition). *J Acad Nutr Diet.* 2012; 112:730–738.

101. White JV, Guenter P, Jensen G, et al. Consensus statement of the Academy of Nutrition and Dietetics/American Society for Parenteral and Enteral Nutrition: characteristics recommended for the identification and documentation of adult malnutrition (undernutrition). *J Parenter Enteral Nutr.* 2012; 36(3):275–283.

102. Bentley DV. Diagnosis coding confusion discussed at ICD-9-CM Coordination and Maintenance Meeting. Just Coding. March 29, 2011. www.justcoding.com.

103. Butterworth CE. The skeleton in the hospital closet. *Nutr Today.* 1974; 9:4–7.

104. Mueller C, Compher C, Druyan ME, et al. Nutrition screening, assessment, and intervention. *J Parenter Enteral Nutr.* 2011; 35(1):16–24.

105. National Alliance for Infusion Therapy and the American Society for Parenteral and Enteral Nutrition Public Policy Committee and Board of Directors. Disease-related malnutrition and enteral nutrition therapy: A significant problem with a cost-effective solution. *Nutr Clin Pract.* 2010; 25(5):548–554.

106. National Heart, Lung, and Blood Institute Acute Respiratory Distress Syndrome (ARDS) Clinical Trials Network, Rice TW, Wheeler AP, et al. Initial trophic vs. full enteral feeding in patients with acute lung injury: The EDEN randomized trial. *JAMA.* 2012; 307(8)795–803.

107. Dennett C. Nutrition-focused physical exam. *Todays Dietitian.* 2016; 18(2):36.

108. Norman K, Stobäus N, Gonzalez MC, Schulzke JD, Pirlich M. Hand grip strength: Outcome predictor and marker of nutritional status. *Clin Nutr.* 2011; 30:135–142.

109. Compher CW, Frankenfield DC, Roth-Yoursey L. Evidence Analysis Working Group. Best practice methods to apply to measurement of resting metabolic rate in adults: A systematic review. *J Am Diet Assoc.* 2006; 106:881–903.

110. Frankenfield DC, Ashcraft LM. Estimating energy needs in the nutrition support patient. *J Parenter Enteral Nutr.* 2011; 35(5):563–570.

111. Foltz MB, Schiller MR, Ryan AS. Nutrition screening and assessment: Current practices and dietitians' leadership roles. *J Am Diet Assoc.* 1993; 93:1388–1395.

112. Phang PT, Rich T, Ronco J. A validation and comparison study of two metabolic monitors. *J Parenter Enteral Nutr.* 1990; 14:259–264.

113. Academy of Nutrition and Dietetics. Nutrition Care Manual. Predictive equations: validation of prediction equations. https://www.nutritioncaremanual.org/topic.cfm?ncm_toc _id=144908.

114. Shetty PS, Henry CJ, Black AE, Prentice AM. Energy requirements of adults: an update on basal metabolic rates (BMRs) and physical activity levels (PALs). *Eur J Clin Nutr.* 1996; 50:S11–S23.

115. Shetty P. Energy requirements of adults. *Public Health Nutr.* 2005; 8(7A):994–1009.

116. Heymsfield SB, Harp JB, Rowell PN, Nguyen AM, Pietrobelli A. How much may I eat? Calories estimates based upon energy expenditure prediction equations. *Obes Rev.* 2006; 7:361–370.

117. Frankenfield DC, Smith JS, Cooney RN, Blosser SA, Sarson GY. Relative association of fever and injury with hypermetabolism in critically ill patients. *Injury.* 1997; 28:617–621.

118. Frankenfield D, Roth-Yousey L, Compher C. Comparison of predictive equations for resting metabolic rate in nonobese and obese adults: A systematic review. *J Am Diet Assoc.* 2005; 105(5):775–789.

119. EAL Working Group—Energy Needs. Academy of Nutrition and Dietetics Evidence Analysis Library. EE: Evidence analysis: Estimating RMR with prediction equations (2006). https://www.andeal.org/topic.cfm?menu=5299&cat=2694.

120. Harris JA, Benedict FG. A biometric study of human basal metabolism. *Proc Natl Acad Sci USA.* 1918; 4(12):370–373.

121. Owen OE, Holup JL, D'Alessio DA, et al. A reappraisal of the caloric requirements of men. *Am J Clin Nutr.* 1987; 46(6):875–885.

122. Schofield WN. Predicting basal metabolic rate, new standards and review of previous work. *Hum Nutr Clin Nutr.* 1985; 39(Suppl 1): 5–41.

123. Ireton-Jones CS, Turner WW Jr, Liepa GU, Baxter CR. Equations for the estimation of energy expenditures in patients with burns with special reference to ventilatory status. *J Burn Care Rehabil.* 1992; 13(3):330–333.

124. Frankenfield DC. Energy Dynamics. In: Matarese LE, Gottschlich MM, eds. *Contemporary Nutrition Support Practice: A Clinical Guide.* Philadelphia, PA: WB Saunders; 1998:79–98.

125. Frankenfield D, Hise M, Malone A, Russell M, Gradwell E, Compher C. Evidence Analysis Working Group. Prediction of resting metabolic rate in critically ill adult patients: Results of a systematic review of the evidence. *J Am Diet Assoc.* 2007; 107(9):1552–1561.

126. Swinamer DL, Grace MG, Hamilton SM, Jones R, Roberts P, King EG. Predictive equation for assessing energy expenditure in mechanically ventilated critically ill patients. *Crit Care Med.* 1990; 18:657–661.

127. Ireton-Jones CS, Jones JD. Why use predictive equations for energy expenditure assessment? *J Am Diet Assoc.* 1997; 97:A44.

128. Frankenfield D, Smith S, Cooney RN. Validation of 2 approaches to predicting resting metabolic rate in critically ill patients. *J Parenter Enteral Nutr.* 2004; 28(4):259–264.

129. National Academies of Science, Engineering, and Medicine. Chapter 10: Protein and Amino Acids. In: *Dietary Reference Intakes for Energy, Carbohydrate, Fiber, Fat, Fatty Acids, Cholesterol, Protein, and Amino Acids (Macronutrients).* Washington, DC: National Academies Press; 2005. https:// www.nap.edu/read/10490/chapter/12.

130. Dietary Reference Intakes (DRIs): Recommended Dietary Allowances and Adequate Intakes, Total Water and Macronutrients. https://fnic.nal.usda.gov/sites/fnic.nal.usda .gov/files/uploads/DRI_RDAs_Adequate_Intakes_Total _Water_Macronutrients.pdf.

131. Gaffney-Stomberg E, Insogna KL, Rodriguez NR, Kerstetter JE. Increasing dietary protein requirements in elderly people for optimal muscle and bone health. *J Am Geriatr Soc.* 2009; 57:1073–1079.

132. Wolfe RR. The underappreciated role of muscle in health and disease. *Am J Clin Nutr.* 2006; 84:475–482.

133. Academy of Nutrition and Dietetics Evidence Analysis Library. Critical Illness (2006-2007): Protein needs. "What level of protein intake or what protein delivery is associated with improvements in mortality?" http://www.andeal.org /topic.cfm?menu=3369&cat=3369.

134. Scheinkestel CD, Kar L, Marshall K, et al. Prospective randomized trial to assess caloric and protein needs of critically ill, anuric, ventilated patients requiring continuous renal replacement therapy. *Nutrition.* 2003; 19(11-12):909-916.

135. Hoffer LJ, Bistrian BR. Appropriate protein provision in critical illness: A systematic and narrative review. *Am J Clin Nutr.* 2012; 96:591–600.

136. Mayes T, Gottschlich MM. Burns. In: Matarese LE, Gottschlich MM, eds. *Contemporary Nutrition Support Practice.* 2nd ed. Philadelphia, PA: WB Saunders Co; 2003: 595–615.

137. Academy of Nutrition and Dietetics. Nutrition Care Manual. Critical illness: Comparative standards. https://www .nutritioncaremanual.org/topic.cfm?ncm_toc_id=269153.

138. National Pressure Ulcer Advisory Panel, European Pressure Ulcer Advisory Panel, and Pan Pacific Pressure Injury Alliance. *Prevention and Treatment of Pressure Ulcers: Quick Reference Guide.* 2nd ed.; 2014. http://www.npuap .org/wp-content/uploads/2014/08/Quick-Reference-Guide -DIGITAL-NPUAP-EPUAP-PPPIA-Jan2016.pdf.

139. National Kidney Foundation Kidney Disease Outcomes Quality Initiative (KDOQI). KDOQI Clinical Practice Guidelines for Nutrition in Chronic Renal Failure. http:// www2.kidney.org/professionals/KDOQI/guidelines _nutrition/doqi_nut.html.

140. Stall S. Protein recommendations for individuals with CKD stages 1–4. *Nephrol Nurs J.* 2008; 35(3):279–282.

141. Snively WD. Body surface area as a dosage criterion in fluid therapy: Theory and application. *Metabolism.* 1957; 6(1):70–87.

142. Adolph EF. The metabolism and distribution of water in body and tissues. *Physiol Rev.* 1933; 13(3):336–371.

143. American Dietetic Association. Chapter 1, Nutrition Assessment of Adults. In: *Manual of Clinical Dietetics.* 6th ed. Chicago, IL: American Dietetic Association; 2000: 33.

144. Holliday MA, Segar WE. The maintenance need for water in parenteral fluid therapy. *Pediatrics.* 1957; 19(5):823–832.

145. Brummit P. Clinical Dietitians in Healthcare Facilities. *Dietary Documentation Pocket Guide.* 2nd ed. Chicago, IL: American Dietetic Association; 2002.

146. Kobriger AM. *Hydration: Maintenance: Dehydration, Laboratory Values, and Clinical Alterations.* Chilton, WI: Kobriger Presents; 2005.

147. Academy of Nutrition and Dietetics. Evidence Analysis Library. *Hydration: Estimating Fluid Needs*; 2007. http:// www.andeal.org/topic.cfm?menu=2820&cat=3217.

148. Dietetics in Health Care Communities. *Pocket Resource for Nutrition Assessment.* 8th ed. Chicago, IL: Academy of Nutrition and Dietetics; 2013.

149. National Eating Disorder Association. Types and Symptoms of Eating Disorders. http://www.nationaleatingdisorders .org/general-information.

150. The Center for Eating Disorders at Sheppard Pratt. *Anorexia Nervosa.* http://www.eatingdisorder.org/eating-disorder -information/anorexia-nervosa/.

151. Swanson S, Crow S, Le Grange D, Swendsen J, Merikangas K. Prevalence and correlates of eating disorders in adolescents. Results from the National Comorbidity Survey Replication Adolescent Supplement. *Arch Gen Psychiatr.* 2011; 68(7):714–723.

152. American Dietetic Association: Standards of Practice and Standards of Professional Performance for registered dietitians (competent, proficient, and expert) in disordered eating and eating disorders (DE and ED). *J Am Diet Assoc.* 2011; 111:1242-1249.e37.

153. Hart S, Russell J, Abraham S. Nutrition and dietetic practice in eating disorder management. *J Hum Nutr Diet.* 2011; 24:144-153.

154. Gowers S, Pilling S, Treasure J, et al. Eating disorders. In: *Core Interventions in the Treatment and Management of Anorexia Nervosa and Related Eating Disorders.* London: National Institute for Clinical Excellence; 2004: 1–261.

155. Winston AP, Gowers S, Jackson AA, et al. *Guidelines for the Nutritional Management of Anorexia Nervosa.* London: Royal College of Psychiatrists; 2005: 42.

156. Ozier AD, Henry BW. Position of the American Dietetic Association: Nutrition intervention in the treatment of eating disorders. *J Am Diet Assoc.* 2011; 111:1236–1241.

157. American Psychiatric Association. American Psychiatric Association; treatment of patients with eating disorders, 3rd ed. *Am J Psychiatry.* 2006; 163(7):1–54.

158. Wakefield A, Williams H. *Practice Recommendations for the Nutritional Management of Anorexia Nervosa in Adults*; 2009: 1–45. http://cedd.org.au/wordpress/wp-content/uploads/2014/09/Practice-Recommendations-for-the-Nutritional-Assessment-of-Anorexia-Nervosa-in-Adults.pdf.

159. Cordery H, Waller G. Nutritional knowledge of health care professionals working in the eating disorders. *Eur Eat Disord Rev.* 2006; 14:462–467.

160. Rosen DS. Identification and management of eating disorders in children and adolescents. *Pediatrics.* 2010; 126:1240–1253.

161. Meyer RR, Alder R. Human immunodeficiency virus (HIV). *Magill's Medical Guide* (online edition); 2016. http://www.cengage.com/search/productOverview.do?N=197+4294891683&Ntk=P_EPI&Ntt=20284504821069771651498819252478625389&Ntx=mode%2Bmatchallpartial.

162. HIV in the United States: At a Glance. http://www.cdc.gov/hiv/pdf/statistics_basics_factsheet.pdf.

163. UNAIDS. *Global Report: UNAIDS Report on the Global AIDS Epidemic*; 2013. http://files.unaids.org/en/media/unaids/contentassets/documents/epidemiology/2013/gr2013/UNAIDS_Global_Report_2013_en.pdf.

164. CDC. About HIV/AIDS. http://www.cdc.gov/hiv/basics/whatishiv.html.

165. Earthman CP. Evaluation of nutrition assessment parameters in the presence of human immunodeficiency virus infection. *Nutr Clin Prac.* 2004; 19:330–339.

166. Nerad J, Romeyn M, Silverman E, et al. General nutrition management in patients infected with human immunodeficiency virus. *Clin Infect Dis.* 2003; 36(Suppl):S52–S62.

167. Grinspoon S, Mulligan K. Weight loss and wasting in patients with human immunodeficiency virus. *Clin Infect Dis.* 2003; 36(Suppl):S69–S78.

168. American Dietetic Association and Dietitians of Canada. Position of the American Dietetic Association and Dietitians of Canada: Nutrition intervention in the care of persons with human immunodeficiency virus infection. *J Am Diet Assoc.* 2000; 100:708–717.

169. Shevitz AH, Knox TA. Nutrition in the era of highly active antiretroviral therapy. *Clin Infect Dis.* 2001; 32:1769–1775.

170. Polsky B, Kotler D, Steinhart C. HIV-associated wasting in the HAART era: Guidelines for assessment, diagnosis, and treatment. *AIDS Patient Care STD.* 2001;15:411–423.

171. Palenicek JP, Graham NM, He YD, et al. Multicenter AIDS Cohort Study Investigators: weight loss prior to clinical AIDS as a predictor of survival. *J Acquir Immune Defic Sydr.* 1995; 10:366–373.

172. Tang A, Forrester J, Spiegelman D, Knox TA, Tchetgen E, Gorbach SL. Weight loss and survival in HIV positive patients in the era of highly active antiretroviral therapy. *J Acquir Immune Defic Syndr.* 2002; 31(2):230–236.

173. Kotler DP. Nutritional alterations associated with HIV infection. *J Acquir Immune Defic Syndr.* 2000; 25(Suppl):S81–S87.

174. Council of State and Territorial Epidemiologists, AIDS Program, Center for Infectious Diseases. Revision of the CDC surveillance case definition for acquired immunodeficiency syndrome. *Morb Mortal Wkly Rep.* 1987; 36(Suppl 1):1S-15S.

175. McDermott AY, Shevitz A, Knox T, Moen K, Johansen D, Paton N. Effect of highly active antiretroviral therapy on fat, lean, and bone mass in HIV-seropositive men and women. *Am J Clin Nutr.* 2001; 74:679–686.

176. Hadigan C, Meigs JB, Corcoran C, et al. Metabolic abnormalities and cardiovascular disease risk factors in adults with human immunodeficiency virus infection and lipodystrophy. *Clin Infect Dis.* 2001; 32:130–139.

177. Nolan D, Hammond E, Martin A, et al. Mitochondrial DNA depletion and morphologic changes in adipocytes associated with nucleoside reverse transcriptase inhibitor therapy. *AIDS.* 2003; 17:1329–1338.

178. Gelato MC. Insulin and carbohydrate dys-regulation. *Clin Infect Dis.* 2003; 36(suppl 2):91–95.

179. Jones CY, Tang AM, Forrester JE, et al. Micronutrient levels and HIV disease status in HIV-infected patients on highly active antiretroviral therapy in the Nutrition for Healthy Living cohort. *J Acquir Immune Defic Syndr.* 2006; 43:475–482.

180. Papathakis PC, Rollins NC, Chantry CJ, Bennish ML, Brown KH. Micronutrient status during lactation in HIV-infected and HIV-uninfected South African women during the first 6 months after delivery. *Am J Clin Nutr.* 2007; 85:182–192.

181. Drain PK, Baeten JM, Overbaugh J, et al. Low serum albumin and the acute phase response predict low serum selenium in HIV-1 infected women. *BMC Infect Dis.* 2006; 6:85.

182. Fields-Gardner C, Campa A. Position of the American Dietetic Association: Nutrition intervention and human immunodeficiency virus infection. *J Am Diet Assoc.* 2010; 110:1105–1119.

183. NAM AIDSMAP. Interactions Between Drugs and Food. http://www.aidsmap.com/Interactions-between-drugs-and-food/page/3080183/#item3080185nd food.

184. Knox T, Speigelman D, Skinner SG, Gorbach S. Diarrhea and abnormalities of gastrointestinal function in a cohort of men and women with HIV infection. *Am J Gastroenterol.* 2000; 95:3482–3489.

185. US Food and Drug Administration. Food Safety for People with HIV/AIDS. http://www.fda.gov/Food/FoodborneIllnessContaminants/PeopleAtRisk/ucm312669.htm#Transport.

186. Bartlett JG. Integrating nutrition therapy into medical management of human immunodeficiency virus. *Clin Infect Dis.* 2003; 36(Suppl 2):551.

187. Ockengaa J, Grimbleb R, Jonkers-Schuitemac C, et al. ESPEN guidelines on enteral nutrition: Wasting in HIV and other chronic infectious diseases. *Clin Nutr.* 2006; 25:319–329.

188. Rabeneck L, Palmer A, Knowles JB, et al. A randomized controlled trial evaluating nutrition counseling with and without oral supplementations in malnourished HIV-infected patients. *J Am Diet Assoc.* 1998; 98:434–438.

189. Burger B, Schwenk A, Junger H, et al. Oral supplements in HIV infected patients with chronic wasting: A prospective trial. *Med Klin.* 1994; 89:579–581, 633.

190. Berneis K, Battegay M, Bassetti R, et al. Nutritional supplements combined with dietary counseling diminish whole body protein catabolism in HIV-infected patients. *Eur J Clin Invest.* 2000; 30:87–94.

191. Secher M, Soto ME, Villars H, Abellan van Kan G, Vellas B. The Mini Nutritional Assessment (MNA) after 20 years of research and clinical practice. *Rev in Clin Gerontol.* 2007; 17:293–310.

192. Rubenstein LZ, Harker JO, Salvá A, Guigoz Y, Vellas B. Screening for undernutrition in geriatric practice: Developing the short-form mini-nutritional assessment (MNA-SF). *J Gerontol A Biol Med Sci.* 2001; 56:366-372.

193. Nestlé Nutrition Institute. MNA Mini Nutritional Assessment. http://www.mna-elderly.com/default.html.

194. Guigoz Y, Laque S, Vellas B. Identifying the elderly at risk for malnutrition: The Mini Nutritional Assessment. *Clin Geriatr Med.* 2002; 18:737–757.

195. Guigoz Y. The Mini Nutritional Assessment (MNA) review of the literature. What does it tell us? *J Nutr Health Aging.* 2006; 10:466–486.

196. Christner S, Ritt M, Volkert D, et al. Evaluation of the nutritional status of older hospitalized geriatric patients: A comparative analysis of a Mini Nutritional Assessment (MNA) version and the Nutritional Risk Screening (NRS 2002). *J Human Nutr Diet.* 2016; 29(6):704–713.

197. Tsai AC, Chang TL, Chang MZ. An alternative short-form Mini-Nutritional Assessment for rating the risk of malnutrition in persons on hemodialysis. *J Clin Nurs.* 2013; 22:2830–2837.

198. van Bokhorst-de van der Schueren MA, Guaitoli PR, Jansma EP, de Vet HC. Nutrition screening tools: Does one size fit all? A systematic review of screening tools for the hospital setting. *Clin Nutr.* 2014; 33(1):39–58.

199. British Association of Parenteral and Enteral Nutrition (BAPEN). Malnutrition Universal Screening Tool (MUST). http://www.bapen.org.uk/pdfs/must/must_full.pdf.

200. Elia M. The "MUST" report; nutritional screening of adults—A multidisciplinary responsibility: Development and use of the "Malnutrition Universal Screening Tool" ("MUST") for adults. Redditch: BAPEN; 2003.

201. Stratton RJ, King CL, Stroud MA, Jackson AA, Elia M. "Malnutrition Universal Screening Tool" predicts mortality and length of hospital stay in acutely ill elderly. *Br J Nutr.* 2006; 95:325–330.

202. Donini LM, Poggiogalle E, Molfino A, et al. Mini-Nutritional Assessment, Malnutrition Universal Screening Tool, and Nutrition Risk Screening tool for the nutritional evaluation of older nursing home residents. *J Am Med Direc Assoc.* 2016; 17:959.e11–959.e18.

203. Diekmann R, Winning K, Uter W, et al. Screening for malnutrition among nursing home residents—a comparative analysis of the Mini Nutritional Assessment, the nutritional risk screening, and the Malnutrition Universal Screening Tool. *J Nutr Health Aging.* 2013; 17(4):326–331.

204. Rasheed S, Woods RT. Predictive validity of "Malnutrition Universal Screening Tool" ("MUST") and short form Mini Nutrition Assessment (MNA-SF) in terms of survival and length of hospital stay. *e-ESPEN Journal.* 2013; 8:e44–e50.

205. Koren-Hakin T, Weiss A, Hershkovitz A, et al. Comparing the adequacy of the MNA-SF, NRS-2002 and MUST nutritional tools in assessing malnutrition in hip fracture operated elderly patients. *Clin Nutr.* 2016; 35:1053–1058.

206. Valentini L, Schulzke J. Mundane, yet challenging: The assessment of malnutrition in inflammatory bowel disease. *Eur J Intern Med.* 2011; 22(1):13–15.

207. Sandhu A, Mosli M, Yan B, et al. Self-screening for malnutrition risk in outpatient inflammatory bowel disease patients using the Malnutrition Universal Screening Tool (MUST). *J Parenter Enteral Nutr.* 2015; 40(4):507–510.

208. Detsky AS, McLaughlin JR, Baker JP, et al. What is subjective global assessment of nutritional status? *J Parenter Enteral Nutr.* 1987; 11:8–13.

209. Baker JP, Detsky AS, Wesson DE, et al. Nutritional assessment; a comparison of clinical judgment and objective measurements. *N Engl J Med.* 1982; 306:969–972.

210. Hirsch S, Obaldia N, Petermann M, et al. Subjective global assessment of nutritional status: Further validation. *Nutrition.* 1991; 7:35–37.

211. Marshall S, Young A, Bauer J, Isenring E. Malnutrition in geriatric rehabilitation: Prevalence, patient outcomes, and criterion validity of the scored Patient-Generated Subjective Global Assessment and the Mini Nutritional Assessment. *J Acad Nutr Diet.* 2016; 116:785–794.

212. Raslan M, Gonzalez MC, Torrinhas RS, Ravacci GR, Pereira JC, Waitzberg DL. Complementarity of subjective global assessment (SGA) and nutritional risk screening 2002 (NRS 2002) for predicting poor clinical outcomes in hospitalized patients. *Clin Nutr.* 2011; 30(1):49–53.

213. Bector S, Vagianos K, Suh M, Duerksen DR. Does the Subjective Global Assessment predict outcomes in critically ill medical patients? *J Intens Care Med.* 2016; 31(7):485–489.

214. Secker DJ, Jeejeebhoy KN. Subjective Global Nutrition Assessment for children. *Am J Clin Nutr.* 2007; 85(4):1083–1089.

215. Visser R, Dekker FW, Boeschoten EW, Stevens P, Krediet RT. Reliability of the 7-point subjective global assessment scale in assessing nutritional status of dialysis patients. *Adv Perit Dial.* 1999; 15:222–225.

216. Kalantar-Zadeh K, Kleiner M, Dunne E, Lee G, Luft F. A modified quantitative subjective global assessment of nutrition for dialysis patients. *Nephrol Dial Transplant.* 1999; 14(7):1732–1738.

217. Churchill DN, Taylor DW, Keshaviah PR. Adequacy of dialysis and nutrition in continuous peritoneal dialysis: association with clinical outcomes. Canada-USA (CANUSA) Peritoneal Dialysis Study Group. *J Am Soc Nephrol.* 1996; 7:198–207.

218. Lim SL, Lin XH, Daniels L. Seven-point Subjective Global Assessment is more time sensitive than conventional Subjective Global Assessment in detecting nutrition changes. *J Parenter Enteral Nutr.*2016; 40:966–972.

219. Ottery FD. Rethinking nutritional support of the cancer patient: The new field of nutritional oncology. *Sem Oncol.* 1994; 21:770–778.

220. Ottery FD. Patient-Generated Subjective Global Assessment. In: McCallum PD, Polisena CG, eds. *The Clinical Guide to Oncology Nutrition*, Chicago, IL: American Dietetic Association; 2000: 11–23.

221. Watterson C, Fraser A, Banks M, et al. Evidence based practice guidelines for the nutritional management of malnutrition in patients across the continuum of care. *Nutr Diet.* 2009; 66(Suppl 3):S1–S34.

222. National Centre for Classification in Health. Australian Coding Standards for I.C.D.-10-AM. Sydney, Australia: National Centre for Classification in Health; 2008.

223. Da Silva Fink J, Daniel de Mello P, Daniel de Mello E. Subjective global assessment: A systematic review of the literature. *Clin Nutr.* 2015; 34:785–792.

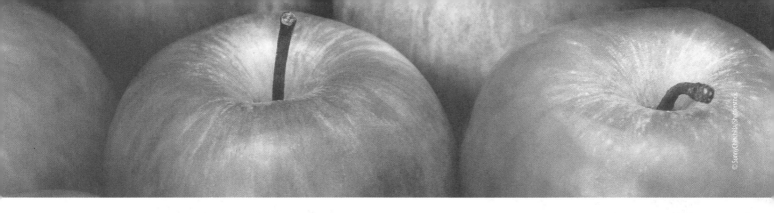

# CHAPTER 10

# Nutritional Assessment in Health Promotion, Disease Prevention, and Treatment

**Chimene Castor**, EdD, RDN, LDN, FAND, CHES
**Oyonumo E. Ntekim**, PhD, MD, MDSA

## CHAPTER OUTLINE

- Introduction
- Cardiovascular Disease
- Obesity
- Diabetes
- Nutrition Interventions in the Treatment of Chronic Diseases
- Chapter Summary

## LEARNING OBJECTIVES

After reading this chapter, the learner will be able to:

1. Define and describe the role of nutrition to address cardiovascular disease.
2. Identify the nutrition-related diseases and the role of diet and lifestyle changes in managing each disease.
3. Explain the effects of diet and other lifestyle factors such as sleep, smoking, and physical activity on the heart.
4. Discuss the specific role of lifestyle changes in the management of coronary artery disease and cardiovascular disease.
5. Explain the role of diet in the management of obesity.
6. Explain the role of diet in the management of diabetes.
7. Summarize the key features of nutrition interventions for the treatment of chronic diseases.

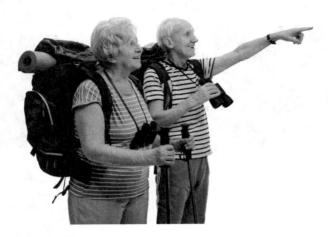

© Ljupco Smokovski/Shutterstock.

## ▶ Introduction

The term **cardiovascular disease (CVD)** encompasses several disorders of the cardiovascular system, including coronary heart disease, cerebrovascular disease (stroke), peripheral arterial disease, rheumatic heart disease, congenital heart disease, and deep vein thrombosis.[1] CVD is the leading cause of death in industrialized nations. Atherosclerosis, a primary cause of CVD, is caused by factors that include hypertension, **hypercholesterolemia**, chronic inflammation, **obesity**, and **diabetes mellitus (DM)**, specifically type 2 diabetes mellitus (T2DM).[2] **Atherosclerosis** is the pathology of plaque building up in cardiac vessels that subsequently leads to hardening and narrowing of the arteries.[3,4] The pathophysiology of atherosclerosis is a slow process that starts at a young age. Poor dietary habits and high levels of cholesterol in the blood increases circulating lipoproteins in the blood, leading to hypercholesterolemia. CVD is associated with a chronic inflammatory process.[5] Because Western diets are consistent with high fat consumption, many people consuming this type of diet suffer from obesity. A body mass index that is greater than 30 kg/m² is considered obese.[6]

Although obesity is the leading risk factor for many chronic diseases, CVD and T2DM are among those that have the most morbid outcomes. Like all physiologic systems, the cardiovascular system is subject to disease from many causes, including congenital, acquired, and induced forms. According to the Centers for Disease Control and Prevention (CDC), half of all adults with chronic health conditions such as heart disease, stroke, cancer, diabetes, and arthritis are reported to be obese.[7] Fighting obesity in our society has been a challenge because of little emphasis on the behavioral and emotional factors contributing to the obesity epidemic. Obesity, physical inactivity, and poor eating habits are synergistic risk factors for CVD in Western populations.[8,9] Segregating nutrition from the larger picture when evaluating the health status of any individual can be difficult. Many factors beyond diet affect nutritional status, which are often not considered. Environment, psychology, stress, finances, and day-to-day lifestyle choices cannot easily be separated from nutrition and other health-related choices because they are all interconnected to influence health and well-being.

## ▶ Cardiovascular Disease

**Preview** Cardiovascular diseases are leading cause of death worldwide, especially in the United States and Canada.

### An Overview

Cardiovascular disease includes hypertension, coronary artery disease (CAD), heart failure (HF), congenital heart disease (CHD), and cerebrovascular accidents (CVAs), or strokes. CVD accounts for 17.7 million deaths annually and is expected to exceed 23.6 million by 2030.[10,11] According to the American Heart Association, CVD accounts for 30% of all global death, with 80% of those deaths found in low- and middle-income countries.[12] In the United States, the mortality rate in 2015 from heart disease, stroke, and other CVD associated illnesses was 787,000. CVD is responsible for one out of every three deaths in the America, which amounts to one life every 40 second. Among the cardiovascular diseases, stroke is the main cause of death, contributing to 31% of all deaths in worldwide.[1,10] **FIGURE 10.1** shows what happens when plaque builds up inside the endometrium of a blood vessel and blocks blood flow.

### Overview of Cardiovascular Disease

In 2014, CVD—including hypertension, CAD, HF, CHD, and CVA were responsible for 31% of deaths globally. Approximately 80,100 Americans die from heart disease each year—or one in every three deaths.

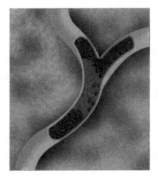

**FIGURE 10.1** As an arterial plaque builds up inside the endometrium of a blood vessel, it increasingly blocks blood flow.

Death rates in the United States from heart attack are shown in **FIGURE 10.2**.

Heart disease remains the leading cause of death in the United States. More than 82 million Americans suffer from some form of CVD, and approximately 1 million people die each year from CVD complications.[13] In the United States, someone has a heart attack every 42 seconds, and someone dies from a heart disease-related event every minute. Although a historical gender gap in CVD deaths remains, it has narrowed significantly especially among postmenopausal women.[14]

## The Cardiovascular System

The cardiovascular system is subject to pathologies like any other body system. Some of the pathologies are associated with lifestyle, which means they can be modified, unlike other pathologies that are unmodifiable such as genetics, age, and gender. An infrequent cause of CVD is the infection of the arteries and veins that feed the heart muscle and the rest of the circulating system. The root cause of most cardiovascular diseases is atherosclerosis,[10,14] or the hardening of arteries. Athersclerosis is a common process in humans, although the extent of the hardening determines whether or not the disease manifests itself. Onset of atherosclerosis is the accumulation of soft, fatty streaks in the intima of the arterial walls. The accrued streaks harden over time into fibrous plaques and compromise the elasticity of the arterial walls as well as narrow the luminal diameter of the affected vessels. Thus, the branch points of arteries have predilections for plaque accumulation.[4,15,16] The accumulation of soft fatty streaks in arterial walls is injurious. As a result, the body naturally reacts to this accumulation by attracting immune cells such as tissue macrophages and leukocytes that scavenge the deposits. This immune reaction

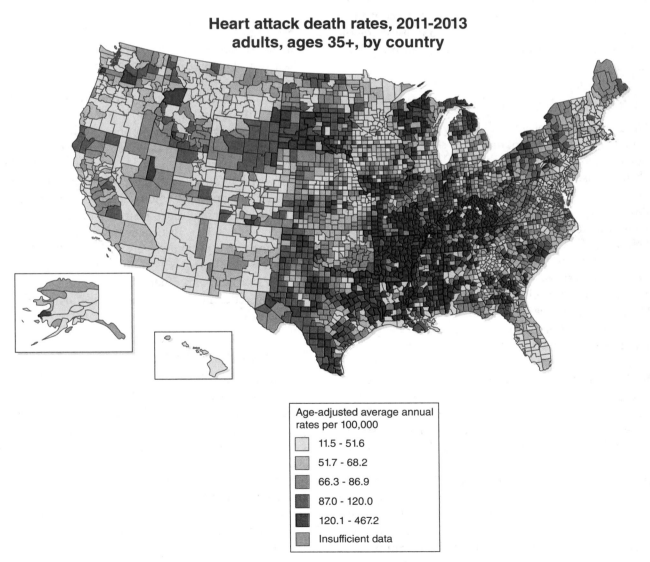

**Heart attack death rates, 2011-2013
adults, ages 35+, by country**

Age-adjusted average annual
rates per 100,000

☐ 11.5 - 51.6
☐ 51.7 - 68.2
☐ 66.3 - 86.9
☐ 87.0 - 120.0
☐ 120.1 - 467.2
☐ Insufficient data

**FIGURE 10.2** 2011–2013 heart attack death rates in US adults.

results in local inflammation, which is a typical cellular response to injuries. The chronic inflammation associated with the immune response results in fibrosis of the injured vessels. The immune cells, which imbibe the accumulated low density lipoproteins (LDLs) and lipids called *foam cells*, trigger new cycles of inflammation and more scavenging immune cells rush to the injured site. The foam cells eventually die and mix with the necrotic muscle cells to form plaques. The plaques undergo mineralization by reacting with calcium and thereby harden even further.[5]

## Risk for Cardiovascular Disease

The risks for CVD can be divided into two distinct types—namely, nonmodifiable and modifiable. The nonmodifiable factors include age, ethnicity, and family history. The modifiable factors include obesity, unhealthy diet patterns, hypercholesterolemia, sedentary life, diabetes mellitus, tobacco consumption, excessive alcohol consumption, and uncontrolled hypertension.[16,17,18] The worldwide obesity epidemic has made it the leading cause among all modifiable factors for CVD.[19,20]

## Risk Factors Associated with CVD

Food-intake patterns and lifestyle behavior (e.g. **physical activity**, smoking, poor sleep patterns, and body weight) are associated with the development of chronic diseases. Adults who eat the recommended portions of vegetables, for example have fewer cardiovascular events than those who consume less than recommended amounts and who have sedentary behaviors.[24]

Quantity and quality of sleep are important for normal physiological functions. Sleep disorders affects 50 to 70 million people in the United States. Sleep disorders are associated with increased mortality. Furthermore, chronic sleep disturbances are reportedly associated with health problems such as increased body mass index (BMI), poor physical health, substance abuse, depression, and negative alteration in metabolic and endocrine functions.[21] Lack of sleep is associated with overeating; a preference for foods high in sodium and fat; frequent snacking; and increased alcohol consumption. This pattern of eating was found to lead to excess energy intake, increasing the risk for obesity and obesity-associated diseases.[22] These factors may be contributors to the high incidence of CVD in these subpopulations. With more people adopting busier lifestyles, it is becoming increasingly more difficult to get the recommended amount of sleep. Adequate sleep has been associated

with lower CVD risk and symptoms. It is plausible that the circadian preference has interactive effects on sleeping homeostasis.[23] In addition, obstructive sleep apnea increased the risk for hypertension and CVD as well as obesity. Inclusively, these data suggest that total lifestyle and nutrition play a vital role in the overall cardiovascular health.[24,25,26]

Smoking is one of the leading preventable causes of premature death in the United States.[27] According to the 2014 US Surgeon General's report on the consequences of smoking, tobacco use is a major cause of mortality and is associated with heart disease, stroke, multiple cancers, respiratory diseases, and other costly illnesses.[28] Smoking leads to poor health conditions and therefore decreased productivity and increased absenteeism from smoking-related illness.[4,29] Some racial and ethnic minorities have higher rates of tobacco use and alcohol consumption placing that at a disproportionate risk for associated health consequences.

## Gut Microbiome

Gut microbiome plays an important role in chronic diseases that include inflammatory bowel disease, obesity, T2DM, CVD, and cancer.[30] The introduction of dietary microbes into the intestine could potentiate a beneficial outcomes over time. The incorporation of several common dietary components can affect intestinal microbiota that can potentially cause shifts in favor of beneficial bacteria genera. Significant weight reduction has been found to reduce cardiovascular episodes and T2DM symptoms when subjects were introduced to energy-restricted diets, resulting in 95% improved conventional CVD risk factors such as decreased low-density lipoproteins levels.[31,32,33,34] **FIGURE 10.3** lists key interventions that will improve the management of the CVD. RDNs and other healthcare providers must focus on reducing factors that would further worsen the cardiovascular health of individuals.

## Coronary Heart Disease

Cardiovascular diseases are pathologies of the heart and the vessels linked to the heart. Among the many causes of cardiovascular diseases are poor nutrition, genetics, gender, age, behavioral, and psychological determinants. Coronary heart disease is a condition in which there is a buildup of plaque inside the coronary arteries called *atherosclerosis* that over time narrows the arteries, limits the blood flow to the heart, and increases the risk of heart attack. Hypertension is a known risk factor for the development of heart disease and stroke. **FIGURE 10.4** shows the anatomy of the heart and how the blood supplies oxygen to cardiac muscles.

## Lifestyle Interventions

- Limit intake of foods high in saturated food and foods high in sodium.
- Promote adequate sleep: between 7 and 9.5 hours.
- Consume adequate amounts of monosaturated and polysaturated fats.
- Encourage adherence to medication prescriptions and discuss with primary caregivers the interactive effects of medications and herbal supplements.
- Reduce or eliminate smoking.

## Food and Nutrition Interventions

- Follow a healthy diet of whole grains, fruits, and vegetables.
- Increase foods high in fiber.
- Omega-3 fatty acids may help reduce inflammation.
- Consume a balanced diet with good sources of vitamins E, B$_6$, B$_{12}$, riboflavin, and niacin, or use a multiple vitamin supplement.

**FIGURE 10.3** Lifestyle and nutrition interventions.

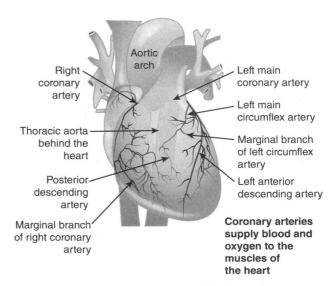

**FIGURE 10.4** Diagram of anatomy of the heart showing how the blood supplies oxygen to the cardiac muscles.

## VIEWPOINT

### Easy Targets: Marketing Junk Food to Children

*Robin B. Dahm, RDN, LDN*

#### Introduction

The incidence of childhood obesity in the United States continues to rise. Research shows that children are easily swayed by advertising and that advertising on TV and in schools affects children's food choices.[1,2] As one way to address childhood obesity, government agencies—primarily the Division of Advertising Practices (DAP) of the Federal Trade Commission (FTC)—are looking more closely at how food is marketed to this demographic.[1]

The answer is not as straightforward as globally banning the marketing of nutrient-poor, calorically dense foods to children. How should the government balance corporate commercial speech and First Amendment protections against protections for children?[1] What advertising methods should be regulated?

#### Junk-Food Ads Are Everywhere That Children Are

New mainstream technologies are constantly entering our lives. They offer the food industry a variety of ways to market products to children: game-filled websites, Internet-based prizes, interactive video games, and product placements targeted to children.[1] Although fast-food companies have pledged to reduce this kind

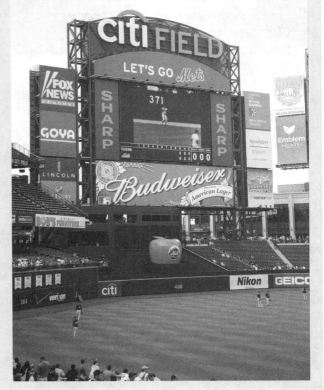

© Frank Romeo/Shutterstock.

of marketing to children, today's youths are seeing more fast-food advertisements than they did only in 2015.[1] In addition, kids' meals are falling far short of the nutritional standards for calories and sodium.[1]

Schools are fertile ground for food companies to market their products directly to children.[2] Their junk-food ads are announced over PA systems, posted on buses, printed in school newspapers, and aired over in-school television channels and radio stations. Even for schools following current USDA guidelines for making campus-available foods more healthful, companies can still advertise food products not sold on school property.[2]

### The DAP Combats Deceptive Food Advertising

The DAP regulates marketing practices that may be unsafe or unhealthful such as deceptive advertising to children. This organization does so in several ways, including the following:[1]

- limiting the number of minutes for child-directed marketing on television;
- evaluating a broadcaster's history of "[serving] the educational and informational needs of children through the licensee's overall programming, including programming specifically designed to serve such needs" when a broadcast license is up for renewal; and
- declaring specific marketing practices unfair or deceptive and creating prohibitions against them.

### Big Bucks Spent to Market Junk Foods to Children

In 2006, the FTC found that the food industry spent some $870 million marketing products to children younger than 11 years of age and more than $1 billion to adolescents.[1] **FIGURE A** shows how the majority of these expenditures were for unhealthful foods (such as carbonated beverages, cereals, fast foods, and candy) and fast-food restaurants. Note that no part of the chart

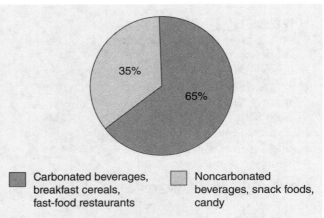

Carbonated beverages, breakfast cereals, fast-food restaurants

Noncarbonated beverages, snack foods, candy

**FIGURE A** Food industry marketing to children; 2006.

Data from Centers for Disease Control and Prevention. STLT Gateway. https://www.cdc.gov/phlp/winnable/advertising _children.html. Accessed May 20, 2017.

represents healthful foods. The food industry also spent more than $116 million to market carbonated beverages to students in schools.[1]

### Conclusion

Childhood obesity continues to be an ongoing problem in the United States, one fueled in part by the large amount of junk-food marketing to children. Government agencies must continue to monitor and enforce a delicate balance: a company's right to advertise its product versus children's rights not to be overexposed to the unfair marketing of junk foods.

### References

1. Centers for Disease Control and Prevention. STLT Gateway. https://www.cdc.gov/phlp/publications/ winnable/advertising_children.html.
2. Food marketing to children in school: Reading, writing, and a candy ad? https://cspinet.org/sites/ default/files/attachment/schoolmarketing_0.pdf.

---

Coronary artery disease can affect the two main coronary arteries or any of their branches. The mechanisms for heart disease and related diseases is narrowing of vascular lumen or the occlusion of the lumen in more severe cases (Figure 10.1). Contributing events can be chronic as in the case of arteriosclerosis and atherosclerosis or acute as in the case of thrombosis.

Deposition of arteriosclerotic plaques in the intima of the arteries overtime narrows the lumen of the involved vessel. Over time, the disease can progress and cause progressive narrowing of the coronary arteries. If the oxygen demand of the heart increases during exertion, chest pain may ensue, creating a condition called *stable angina pectoralis*. When pain is experienced at rest because of restricted blood flow to the heart muscle caused by narrowing of the native coronary arteries, it is referred to as *unstable angina pectoralis*. The latter can progress to *myocardial infarction*, an injury to the heart muscle from complete occlusion of the blood supply to portions of the myocardium. The extent and severity of heart muscle damage depends on the location and duration of the occlusion. It is not uncommon for sudden cardiac death to occur from plaque rupture causing an occlusion downstream in a coronary artery.

## Risk Factors for CVD

CVD has both modifiable and non-modifiable risk factors. Genetics and age are risk factors associated with CVD that cannot be modified. Having the genetic predisposition to CVD, however, does not condemn someone to becoming diseased; lifestyle, nutrition, and the environment can interact in ways that prevent, delay, or promote the onset of CVD. Studies have demonstrated that a healthy diet, moderate physical activity, and alcohol in moderation can prevent cardiovascular disease. The risk factors for coronary heart disease (also known as *ischemic heart disease*) are similar to those of the other CVDs. Smoking, uncontrolled hypertension, family history, homocysteinuria, hyper-cholesterolemia, diabetes, and age—including postmenopausal women who are not on estrogen therapy—are risk factors. Other rare conditions can also contribute to CVD, including vasculitis, pulmonae, and chronic thrombosis. This segment focuses on the common causes of CVD, including ischemic heart disease in general.

## Hypertension

Blood pressure (BP) is defined as the force of blood pushing against the walls of the arteries carrying blood from the heart to other parts of the body. Blood pressure normally rises and falls throughout the day. But if it stays high for a long time, it can damage the heart and lead to health problems (**FIGURE 10.5**). High blood pressure increases the risk for heart disease and stroke, which we now know are leading causes of death in the United States. Approximately 600 million people worldwide and about one in three adult Americans have **hypertension**.[35,36] Hypertension (HTN) or high blood pressure is defined as having a sustained systolic and diastolic BP ≥140 mm Hg and ≥90 mm Hg, respectively.[37,38] Hypertension is a known risk for heart disease and stroke: two leading causes of death in the United States. High BP alone was responsible for 1100 deaths in the United States per day in 2014.[39] According to the CDC's National Center for Health Statistics survey for 2011–2012, the prevalence of hypertension among men was 29.7% and among women 28.5% in the United States. Chronic elevated blood pressure worsens arteriosclerosis, and atherosclerosis later in turn exacerbates hypertension. Arteries that may already harden from atheromatous plaques can weaken, rupture, and bleed when subjected to high pressure. In instances where the narrowing of renal afferent arteries occurs through atherosclerosis, the renal macular dense cells will intervene by activating the renin–aldosterone–angiotensin system to raise blood pressure because of perceived reduced blood flow and pressure to the kidney, which may result in increased blood pressure or exacerbation of existing hypertension. Categories of BP values in adults are listed in **TABLE 10.1**. Figure 10.5 shows how blood exerts pressure on the walls and creates blood pressure as it travels through a vascular lumen.

## Lipids and Lipoproteins

Among the known risk factors for heart disease are low blood levels of high-density lipoproteins (HDLs), elevated blood low-density lipoproteins (LDLs), high blood triglycerides (TGs), diabetes mellitus, hypertension, and central obesity.[40] LDLs are the most atherogenic lipids mentioned, primarily

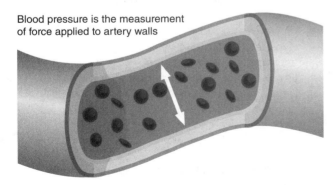

Blood pressure is the measurement of force applied to artery walls

**FIGURE 10.5** Blood pressure is caused by the force exerted by the blood on the inside of the vascular lumen.

Data from Centers for Disease Control and Prevention. High Blood Pressure Frequently Asked Questions (FAQs). Centers for Disease Control and Prevention Web site. https://www.cdc.gov/bloodpressure/about.htm. Updated November 30, 2016.

**TABLE 10.1** Blood pressure categories*

| Category | Systolic Blood Pressure (mm Hg) | Diastolic Blood Pressure (mm Hg) |
|---|---|---|
| Normal | <120 | <80 |
| Prehypertension | 120–139 | 80–89 |
| Stage 1 hypertension | 140–159 | 90–99 |
| Stage 1 hypertension | ≥160 | ≥100 |

*For those 18 years and older who are not on medicine for hypertension or do not have short-term illness or chronic illnesses such as kidney disease and diabetes mellitus.
Data from Centers for Disease Control and Prevention. QuickStats: Percentage Distribution of Blood Pressure Categories Among Adults Aged >18 Years, by Race/Ethnicity—National Health and Nutrition Examination Survey, United States, 1999–2004. *MMWR-Morbid Mortal W.* 2007;56(24):611. https://www.cdc.gov/mmwr/preview/mmwrhtml/mm5624a6.htm.

delivering cholesterol to cells, including those of the arterial endothelium. Existing evidence suggests a strong relationship between elevated LDL cholesterol and high blood pressure from increased formation of atherosclerotic plaques within the vascular internal, narrowing, and reduced pliability of vessels. LDLs vary in size, and smaller sized and denser LDL particles carry higher risks for heart diseases. On the other hand, elevated HDLs have been shown to be protective. One of many roles of HDL is to convey cholesterol away from cells to the liver for degradation. The profiles of the lipids—LDL, HDL, and TG—that are considered to be healthy or may pose cardiovascular risks have been established and are listed in **TABLES 10.2**.[40,41]

## Elevated Triglycerides

High TGs are seen in certain pathologies such as diabetes mellitus, metabolic syndrome, obesity, and heart disease. Elevated TGs are indirectly *atherogenic*, so they are not an independent risk factor in heart disease.[41] TGs are important in the assembly of lipoproteins such as very low-density lipoproteins (VLDLs), which contain 55% to 60% triglycerides. It is logical that VLDL remnants increase in circulation under moderate to high TG levels.

The Adult Treatment Panel III (ATP III) recommendation for treatment of hypertriglyceridemia (TG ≥150 mg/dL) is linked to LDL's therapeutic goal. The aim is to reach the LDL goal by increasing physical activity and managing weight. Pharmacological therapy is recommended for the management of TG if they are still elevated after LDL goals are reached. For TGs ≥500 mg/dL, lowering the level to prevent onset of pancreatitis is paramount, followed by lowering total daily energy intake from fat to ≤15%, implementing weight management, and instituting a physical activity regime.[40,41]

## Treatment of Low HDL Cholesterol

Similarly, the treatment of low HDL (< 40 mg/dL) is linked to achieving LDL cholesterol goals. Upon attaining the LDL goal, weight management and increased physical activity are recommended in the ATP III guidelines. TG levels are integrally linked to HDL management in two ways. First, TG levels between 200mg/dL and 499 mg/dL requires the reduction of the non-HDL cholesterol 30 mg/dL above the LDL level.[16,42] Second, TG isolated low HDL with TG < 200mg/dL requires an appropriate pharmacotherapy.

Three risk categories were established in the ATP III recommendations to guide practitioners in the management of CHD. **TABLES 10.3** shows LDL

| **TABLE 10.2** LDL cholesterol: Primary target of therapy | |
|---|---|
| **Step 1** ATP III classification of LDL, total, and HDL cholesterol. Determine lipoprotein levels: obtain complete lipoprotein profile after 9- to 12-hour fast. | |
| < 100 mg/dL | Optimal |
| 100–129 mg/dL | Near optimal/above optimal |
| 130–159 mg/dL | Borderline high |
| 160–189 mg/dL | High |
| ≥ 190 mg/dL | Very high |
| **Total Cholesterol** | |
| < 200 mg/dL | Desirable |
| 200–239 mg/dL | Borderline high |
| ≥ 240 mg/dL | High |
| **HDL Cholesterol** | |
| < 40 mg/dL | Low |
| ≥ 60 mg/dL | High |

**Step 2** Identify presence of clinical atherosclerotic disease that confers high risk for coronary heart disease (CHD) events (CHD risk equivalent):
- Clinical CHD
- Symptomatic carotid artery disease
- Peripheral arterial disease
- Abdominal aortic aneurysm

**Step 3** Determine presence of major risk factors (other than LDL):
Major risk factors (exclusive of LDL cholesterol) that modify LDL goals
- Cigarette smoking
- Hypertension (BP ≥ 140/90 mm Hg or on antihypertensive medication)
- Low HDL cholesterol (< 40 mg/dL)*
- Family history of premature CHD (CHD in male first degree relative < 55 years; CHD in female first degree relative < 65 years)
- Age (men ≥ 45 years; women ≥ 55 years)

*HDL cholesterol ≥60 mg/dL counts as a "negative" risk factor; its presence removes one risk factor from the total count.

Note: In ATP III, diabetes is regarded as a CHD risk equivalent.

Reproduced from Management of Blood Cholesterol in Adults: Systematic Evidence Review from the Cholesterol Expert Panel. National Heart, Lung, and Blood Institute. https://www.nhlbi.nih.gov/health-pro/guidelines/current/cholesterol-guidelines/quick-desk-reference-html.

**TABLE 10.3** LDL cholesterol goals and endpoints for therapeutic lifestyle changes and drug treatment in various risk classifications

| Risk Category | LDL Goals (mg/dL) | Therapeutic Lifestyle Changes are Initiated at This LDL Level (mg/dL) | Drug Therapy Is Considered at This LDL Level (mg/dL) |
|---|---|---|---|
| CHD or CHD risk equivalents (10-year risk > 20%) | < 100 | ≥ 100 | ≥ 130 (100–129 optimal) |
| Two-plus risk factors (10-year risk 20%) | < 130 | ≥ 130 | 10-year risk 10–20%: ≥ 130 10-year risk < 10%: ≥ 160 |
| Zero to one risk factor** | < 160 | ≥ 160 | ≥ 190 (160–189: LDL-lowering drug optional) |

Reproduced from Expert Panel on Detection, Evaluation, and Treatment of High Blood Cholesterol in Adults (Adults Treatment Panel III), Third Report of the National Cholesterol Education Program (NCEP), NIH publication no 02-5215 (Bethesda, MD. National Heart, Lung, and Blood Institute, (2002), pp. 11-15-11-20.

cholesterol goals, endpoints for therapeutic lifestyle changes, and drug treatments in various risk classifications. Once the risk category is established, the type and management goals can be established.

## Dyslipidemia: The Role of Medical Nutrition Therapy Intervention

**TABLE 10.4** describes the key to the management of dyslipidemia and the key objectives for health practitioners.

Anthropometric measurements, clinical and past medical histories, laboratory values, thorough food and diet histories, genetics factors, evaluation of food and knowledge, psychosocial history, and weight

**TABLE 10.4** Management of dyslipidemia

| Medical Practitioners | Dietitians |
|---|---|
| Reduce inflammation and promote increased blood flow. | Limit intake of saturated food and foods high in sodium. |
| Promote adequate sleep: > 7hrs but < 9.5 hours. Consume adequate intake of monounsaturated and polyunsaturated fat. Reduce smoking. | Encourage adherence to medication prescriptions as well address the effects of misused medications and herbal products with primary caregivers. |

Data from Health Topics. National Heart, Lung, and Blood Institute Web site. https://www.nhlbi.nih.gov/health-topics. Date unknown; Haffner SM, American Diabetes Association. Management of dyslipidemia in adults with diabetes. *Diabetes Care*. 2003;26:S83; Evert AB, Boucher JL, Cypress M, Dunbar SA, Franz MJ, Mayer-Davis EJ, et al. Nutrition therapy recommendations for the management of adults with diabetes. *Diabetes Care*. 2013;36(11):3821-3842.

history are the key features to examine when assessing dyslipidemia. Evaluation of inappropriate intake of dietary fats and nutrition-related knowledge deficits as well as daily consumption of food with high levels of fat and sodium and large amounts of processed foods are also areas that require nutrition investigation and targeting for intervention.

The following list shows food and nutrition interventions to address dyslipidemia:

- Follow healthy diet of whole grains, fruits and vegetables
- Omega 3 fatty acid may be beneficial to reduce inflammation
- Increase foods high in fiber

For those who are overweight or obese, dietary goals should include weight loss of one to two pounds per week, education about healthy food choices, eating foods with lower amounts of sodium and fat, and lifestyle changes including increasing physical activity and quitting smoking. Barriers to positive health changes should be identified and the readiness of individuals to make behavioral changes involving nutrition or lifestyle should be addressed. Dietary and lifestyle interventions should include nutrition education and counseling, and they should address behavioral and social factors. Motivational interviewing (MI) can help provide comprehensive guidance for age and activity level, and it can also encourage gradual increases in physical activity.

**Recap**    Cardiovascular disease is the leading cause of death worldwide. Risk factors for CVD include hypertension and elevated plasma lipids. Elevated plasma lipids, hypertension, type 2 diabetes, metabolic syndrome, and cardiovascular diseases are among the constellation of pathologies that stem from obesity. Lifestyle changes that include a healthy diet and moderate physical activity, can lower the risk of cardiovascular disease.

# ▶ Obesity

**Preview**    Obesity and overweight have emerged as troubling global health threats. According to the World Health Organization (WHO), an estimated 500 million adults are obese worldwide. The problem is most notable in the United States, where the prevalence of obesity is a chief contributing factor to preventable deaths.

## Overview of Obesity

Obesity is a chronic disease that affects and exacerbates health problems such as hypertension, diabetes mellitus type 2, dyslipidemia, cardiovascular disease, osteoarthritis of large and small joints, some cancers, respiratory distress, obstructive sleep apnea, and sleep.[43] Obesity's behavioral and psychosocial complications often hinder effective treatment and management of obesity. According to the WHO, approximately 500 million adults worldwide are obese. The prevalence of obesity makes it the leading cause of preventable death in the United States and poses a major public-health challenge.[44,45,46] The association between obesity and other chronic diseases is a public-health concern that calls for aggressive nutritional preventative intervention and treatment.

Obesity is a significant contributing factor to preventable deaths in the United States and poses a major public-health challenge globally. An estimated 93 million Americans are affected by obesity. These individuals are at higher risk of impaired mobility and experience negative social stigma. The multifactorial pathology of obesity results in the accumulation of excessive body fat. Regardless of the cause of obesity, the principal physiologic mechanism is *anabolism*. Succinctly, the amount of energy exceeds what the body requires to perform both basal metabolic functions and physical activities.

## Obesity and Metabolic Syndrome

Obesity is the accumulation of excess body fat from the dysregulation of the body's weight-control system, which is typified by a BMI equal to or more than 29.5 kg/m². There are exceptions such as persons who have large lean muscle mass, typically athletes. Sedentary lifestyles and an abundant variety of energy-dense processed foods have contributed significantly to the worldwide obesity epidemic. In fact, prolonged excessive caloric intake is the key contributor to obesity. The excess energy consumed is converted to triglycerides and stored in fat cells (adipocytes). Fat cells can divide like other cells and so can increase both in size and number to accommodate excess calories. When their storage capacity is exhausted, excess fats will accumulate in the surrounding tissues— so-called ectopic fat—which is strongly associated with insulin resistance.

Obesity increases the risk for the development of cardiovascular disease, type 2 diabetes mellitus, hypertension, arthritis, and cancer among other illnesses. It also carries an increased risk for morbidity and mortality. The anatomic fat distribution in obesity is an important health risk factor. In men, fat accumulation around the core of the body—known as an *android* shape—is more common. A pear-shaped accumulation of fat around the hips and buttocks that is predominant women is termed a *gynoid* shape (**FIGURE 10.6**).

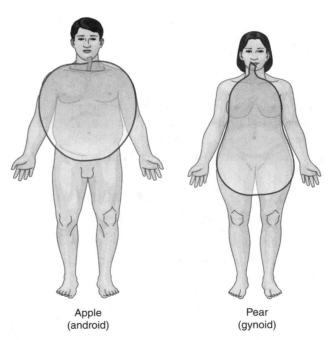

Apple
(android)

Pear
(gynoid)

**FIGURE 10.6** Accumulations of body fat in the abdomen (android) versus in the hips and thighs (gynoid).

The android form carries a greater disease risk. The increased risk in the android type deposit comes from the fact that the visceral and subcutaneous fat stores in the abdominal region are more easily mobilized into circulation than those stored in the gluteal-femoral region.

The increased mobilization of the free fatty acids (FFAs) from the central obese fat tissues is accompanied by the release of inflammatory cytokines such as interleukin-6. These cytokines gain proximal access to the liver, where their metabolic actions include promoting insulin resistance and increased liver synthesis of the triglycerides used in VLDL synthesis. This is one reason why hypertriglyceridemia is seen in obesity (**FIGURE 10.7**).

A Genetic mutation that causes derangements in leptin and adiponectin secretion by adipocytes can also result in obesity. Leptin is an appetite-suppressing hormone, and adiponectin reduces the release of FFAs into the blood. Conversely, any increase in levels of another hormone, ghrelin, will stimulate hunger and lead to overnutrition. An individual's genes interact with the environment and can contribute to whether he becomes obese or maintains normal body weight.

Obesity is a complex disorder involving an excessive amount of body fat associated with high triglycerides and low levels of HDL cholesterol, type 2 diabetes, high blood pressure, metabolic syndrome (a combination of high blood sugar, high blood pressure, high triglycerides, and low HDL cholesterol), heart disease, and stroke (**FIGURE 10.8**).[47] Maintaining an energy balance in which input equals output is therefore the most important principle in preventing obesity (**FIGURE 10.9**).

> **Recap** Obesity is a significant cause of preventable deaths in the United States. Obese individuals are at higher risk of many other chronic conditions such as diabetes, heart disease, and cancer.

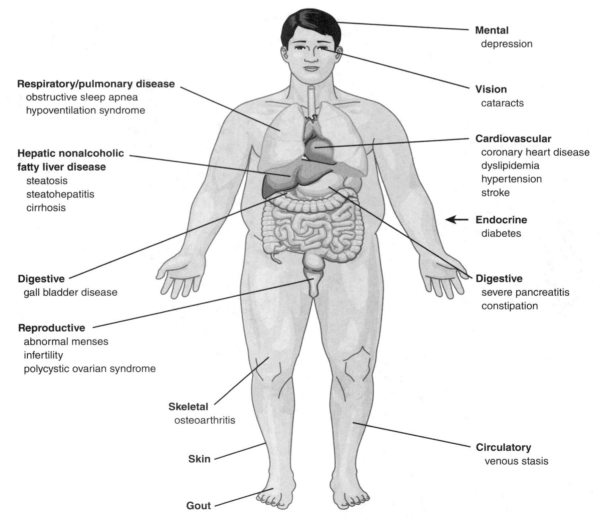

**Mental**
depression

**Vision**
cataracts

**Respiratory/pulmonary disease**
obstructive sleep apnea
hypoventilation syndrome

**Cardiovascular**
coronary heart disease
dyslipidemia
hypertension
stroke

**Hepatic nonalcoholic fatty liver disease**
steatosis
steatohepatitis
cirrhosis

**Endocrine**
diabetes

**Digestive**
gall bladder disease

**Digestive**
severe pancreatitis
constipation

**Reproductive**
abnormal menses
infertility
polycystic ovarian syndrome

**Skeletal**
osteoarthritis

**Skin**

**Circulatory**
venous stasis

**Gout**

**FIGURE 10.7** The Physiological Impact of Obesity

Data from Physiological Impact of Obesity. Obesity Society Website. http://www.obesity.org/home. Date unknown.

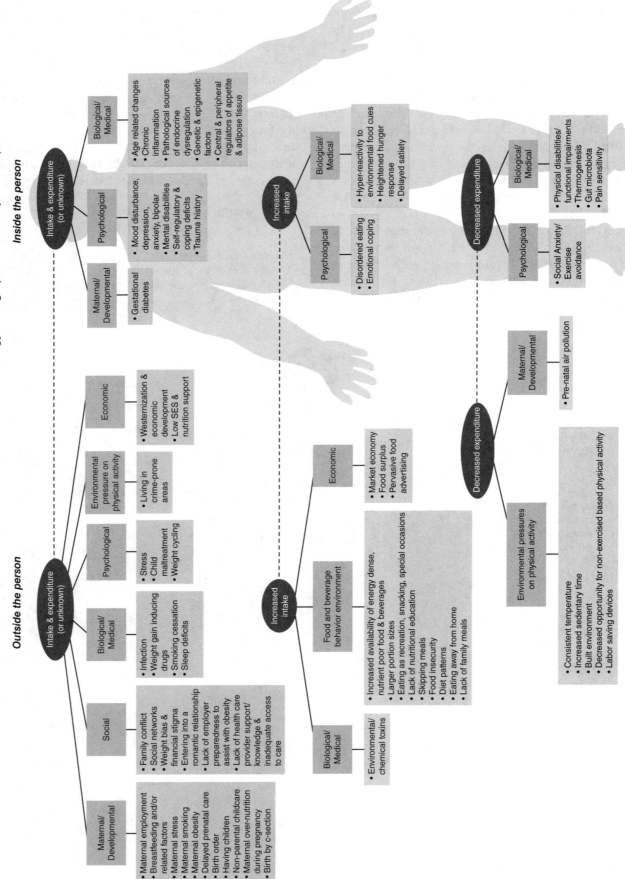

**FIGURE 10.8** The potential contributors to obesity.

Modified from The Obesity Society: Potential Contributors to Obesity Infographic. http://www.obesity.org/obesity/resources/facts-about-obesity/infographics/potential-contributors-to-obesity. Accessed 7/27/17.

*Potential contribution indicate anything that has been put forth in the research literature as a question of investigation and is not intended to be a verification of whether or not; or the extent to which, each may or may not contribute.

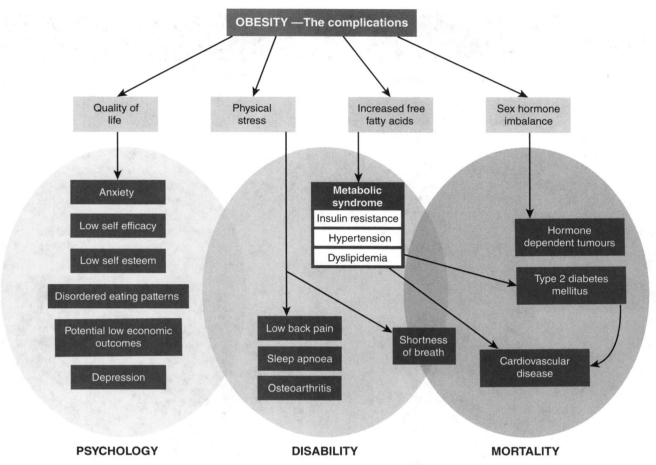

**FIGURE 10.9** The complications of obesity.

# ▶ Diabetes

**Preview**    Diabetes mellitus is a derangement of glucose homeostasis. Approximately 30.3 million Americans have diabetes and more than 84 million have prediabetes. Diabetes can lead to increased risk of other conditions such as heart disease, stroke and kidney disease. Dietary and lifestyle changes can improve blood glucose control.

## Overview of Diabetes

Diabetes mellitus is a derangement of glucose homeostasis. According to the CDC, 9.4% of the US population—approximately 30.3 million people—had diabetes in 2017.[10,44] In addition, 84.1 million adults ages 18 and older have prediabetes; this is approximately 34% of the adult US population. In adults 65 and older, 23.1 million have prediabetes.[10]

Type 2 diabetes mellitus (T2DM) accounts for some 90% to 95% of all diagnosed cases of diabetes, and type 1 diabetes mellitus (T1DM) accounts for approximately 5% of diabetes cases. The health and economic costs for both types of diabetes are enormous, with diabetes now the seventh leading cause of death in the United States. According to the CDC, people with T1DM do not make enough insulin; in comparison, those with T2DM cannot use insulin properly. Insulin allows blood sugar (glucose) to enter cells, where it can be used for energy. When the body does not have enough insulin or cannot use it effectively, glucose builds up in the blood. High blood glucose levels can lead to heart disease, stroke, blindness, kidney failure, and the amputation of toes, feet, or legs.[48] In the long term, uncontrolled blood glucose can result in pathologies including hyperlipidemia, CHD, atherosclerosis, neuropathy, retinopathy, and renal disease.

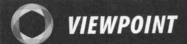

## VIEWPOINT

### Nutrition Policies and Politics

*Robin Rood, RD, LD, MEd, MA*

Before the major industrialization of the food industry in the 1950s and the invention of heavily processed frozen food, many families grew their own food in their own gardens. In fact, "Victory Gardens" allowed citizens to contribute to the national war efforts by growing their own vegetables during World War I (1916 to 1918) and World War II (1941 to1945).[1]

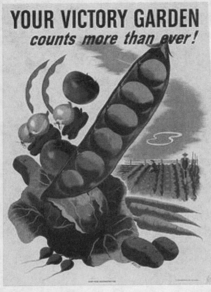

Reproduced from U.S. Agriculture Department. War Food Administration.

Today we have reinvented our past by calling it the "farm to table movement"—that is, by shopping at farmer markets and buying locally sourced food. It is also common today to join a community-supported agriculture or CSA venture. In these ventures, consumers purchase shares of a farmer's crops and then receive weekly shipments of garden fruits and vegetables for the length of the growing season. This arrangement provides fresh and nutritious foods to customers as well as steady income to farmers.

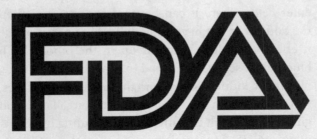

Reproduced from FDA.gov.

In the meantime, politics has played an important role in making sure our food supply is healthy and safe. It was not always this way. In the 1800s, anyone could put anything in the food market and sell it with almost no regulation at all. Basic food purity and inspection acts were passed in the first few decades of the 20th century. More information about these laws can be found on the Food and Drug Administration's history page at FDA.gov.[2]

A variety of toxic substances, including narcotics, were legal ingredients in baby food, beverages, and medicines until the federal government created laws to prohibit manufacturers from putting them in foods.

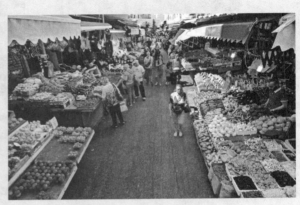

© ChameleonsEye/Shutterstock.

It was not until 1929 that were laws firmly established to control ingredients in food. By the 1930s, insecticides and weed killers were under attack and regulated for poisoning people in the foods they consumed. In the 1940s and 1950s, food manufacturing standards were written; around the same time, the cosmetic industry was forced to eliminate harmful and injurious ingredients in their products sold to consumers. All of these regulations were reactions to harms to consumers caused by manufacturers.

By the late 1950s through the 1980s, an approach to food and chemical production became friendlier to consumers with the formation of a list of 200 foods and chemicals—the "Generally Recognized as Safe" (GRAS list)—in 1958.[3] This list contains food additives most of us take for granted such as acetic acid, caffeine, and sweeteners. In 2015, trans fats were removed from the GRAS list because they were determined to be unsafe for consumption.

Other laws were passed such as the Consumer Protection Act, Child Protection Act, and Food Additive Act as well as sanitation programs for food factories and distribution centers. These were early policies for many other food-related laws and were created because federal inspectors found infected cows on dairy farms, rats in factories, and tapeworms advertised for use as diet aids.

These were just a few examples of the freewheeling business atmosphere of unscrupulous manufacturers preying on customers for profit during this time. It still happens today as food recalls in the news can attest.

As of 1990, the Nutrition Labeling Act required all packaged foods to include a Nutrition Facts Panel and list the standard serving size.[4] This label has been updated over the years to include more nutrition information to consumers on protein, carbohydrates, fats, vitamins, and minerals. The latest update was in May 2016 when the label was reorganized and items such as serving size and calories per serving were highlighted so consumers could educate themselves at a glance about the types of ingredients in the products. **FIGURE A** shows the old and new Nutrition Facts Labels.

### References

1. Wikipedia. Victory garden. https://en.wikipedia.org/wiki/Victory_garden, n.d.
2. US Food and Drug Administration (FDA). History; 2015. http://www.fda.gov/AboutFDA/WhatWeDo/History.
3. FDA. Guidance for industry: Frequently asked questions about GRAS for substances intended for use in human or animal food; 2016. http://www.fda.gov/Food/GuidanceRegulation/GuidanceDocumentsRegulatoryInformation/IngredientsAdditivesGRASPackaging/ucm061846.htm.

(A)                                    (B)

**FIGURE A** The (A) old and (B) new Nutrition Facts labels.

Reproduced from FDA. Changes to the Nutrition Facts Label. Retrieved from: http://www.fda.gov/Food/GuidanceRegulation/GuidanceDocumentsRegulatoryInformation/LabelingNutrition/ucm385663.htm.

4. FDA. Food labeling guide; 2016. http://www.fda.gov/Food/GuidanceRegulation/GuidanceDocumentsRegulatoryInformation/LabelingNutrition/ucm2006828.htm.

## The Role of Medical Nutrition Therapy in Prediabetes and Diabetes

Of the more than 30 million US adults with diabetes, almost 34% of adults are not aware of their condition. Another 84.1 million US adults—more than one-third of the adult population—have prediabetes; an estimated 90% are not aware of their condition.[10,43,44] People with prediabetes who take part in a structured lifestyle change program can cut their risk of developing type 2 diabetes by as much as 58%.[10] There is a strong need for use of medical nutrition therapy to slow the progression of diabetes and reduce related consequences. According to the Academy of Nutrition of Dietetics, medical nutrition therapy is critical for the development of nutrition interventions for DM, CVD, obesity, and other nutrition-related diseases. Diabetes mellitus is considered a risk factor for CHD according to the ATP III's recommendations.[49] In addition, the presence of diabetes increases the risk of death from CVD. There is ample evidence that shows acceleration of atherosclerosis in diabetes because of reduced blood circulation through narrowed vessels.

Several complications can arise from diabetes, including the following.

- Heart disease and stroke: People with diabetes are twice as likely to have heart disease or a stroke as people without diabetes—and at an earlier age.
- Blindness and other eye problems: Diabetic retinopathy (damage to blood vessels in the retina), cataracts (clouding of the lens), and glaucoma (increased fluid pressure in the eye) can all result in vision loss.
- Kidney disease: High blood sugar levels can damage the kidneys long before a person has symptoms. Kidney damage can cause chronic kidney disease, which can lead to kidney failure.

In the Nutrition Care Process (NCP), the Academy of Nutrition and Dietetics, specifies intervention when T2DM and overweight status (BMI 26 to 29.5) are both present. **FIGURE 10.10** shows an example of the Nutrition Care Process that can be used for T2DM and overweight patients.

- *Assessment Data*: Anthropometrics measurements, clinical history, laboratory values, food and diet history, genetics factors, food and knowledge history, psychosocial history
- *Nutritional Diagnoses (PES)*: Overweight related to poor food choice and food and knowledge deficit as evidenced by BMI of 27 and limited physical activities
- *Goal*: To lose 1–2lbs per week and to become educated about healthy food choices
- *Barrier and address behavior*: Stage of changes (precontemplation, contemplation, preparation, action, maintenance, and replacement)
- *Intervention*: Nutrition education and counseling and addressing behavioral and social factors. Using motivational interviewing (MI) to provide comprehensive coursing for age, activity level and ways to gradually increase physical activities BMI closer to desirable, behavior change such as increased consumption of fruits and vegetables and whole grains and increased physical activities.

**FIGURE 10.10** Nutrition Care Process for type 2 diabetes mellitus coupled with overweight (BMI 26–29.5).

Modified from Nelms MN, Sucher K, Lacey K, Roth SL, Habash D, Nelms RG, et al. *Nutrition Therapy and Pathophysiology*. 2nd ed. 2015. Belmont, CA: Brooks/Cole Cengage Learning.

Some of the recommended strategies to reduce the incidence of T2DM include providing nutrition education to promote lifestyle and environmental changes. Healthy eating and active living to most effectively achieve weight loss and regular physical activity are the cornerstones for the prevention and treatment of many chronic conditions. (**FIGURE 10.11**). Also important is addressing the

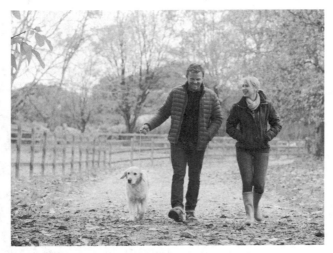

**FIGURE 10.11** Physical activity is a critical component for improving health.

© Monkey Business Images/Shutterstock.

existing barriers to intervention such as health literacy and food insecurity and imparting information about ways to effectively use available resources to help reduce chronic health conditions.

**Recap**  In 2017, T2DM was the seventh-leading cause of death in the United States. Type 2 diabetes accounts for almost 95% of all diagnosed cases of diabetes, and type 1 accounts for approximately 5%. The health and economic burden for diabetes is tremendous, so dietary and lifestyle modifications are essential to both preventing and treating this disease.

# ▶ Nutrition Interventions in the Treatment of Chronic Diseases

**Preview**  The Nutrition Care Process is a comprehensive approach that incorporates behavioral and emotional models in preventing, diagnosing, and treating nutrition-related diseases.

Nutrition plays a vital role in the management of chronic diseases. The goal of nutrition care is to restore a state of nutritional balance by positively influencing factors that are contributing to the imbalance or altered state of health.[49] This section provides an evidence-based framework approach to address nutritional problems of some chronic diseases.

## The Nutrition Care Process

The Nutrition Care Process (NCP) is a comprehensive approach that incorporates behavioral and emotional models in to the prevention, diagnosis, and treatment of nutrition-related diseases. Recent advances in basic science research have generated new capabilities and techniques to largely prevent nutrition-associated diseases. For instance, today an evidenced-based framework is essential to clinical dietetics professionals when using NCP (see **FIGURE 10.12**). The process requires that dietitians gather and consider all necessary nutrition-related information so they can conduct comprehensive nutritional assessments.

The NCP is a systematic problem-solving method that includes defined steps relevant to disease management.[50] Using a system of standardized nutrition language, the four steps (shown in **FIGURE 10.13**) are (1) nutrition assessment, (2) nutrition diagnosis, (3) nutrition intervention,

**Steps in the Nutrition Care Process**

**1** Nutrition assessment → Food/Nutrient-related history (FH)
Anthropometric measurements (AD)
Biochemical data, medical tests, and procedures (BD)
Client history (CH)
Comparative standards (CS)

**2** Nutrition diagnosis → Intake (NI)
Clinical (NC)
Behavioral-environmental (NB)
Other (NO)

**3** Nutrition intervention → Food and/or Nutrient delivery (ND)
Nutrition education (E)
Nutrition counseling (C)
Coordination of nutrition care (RC)

**4** Nutrition monitoring and evaluation → Food/Nutrient-related history (FH)
Anthropometric measurements (AD)
Biochemical data, medical tests, and procedures (BD)
Client history (CH)
Comparative standards (CS)

**FIGURE 10.12** The Nutrition Care Process.

Modified from Nelms MN, Sucher K, Lacey K, Roth SL, Habash D, Nelms RG, et al. *Nutrition Therapy and Pathophysiology*. 2nd ed. 2015. Belmont, CA: Brooks/Cole Cengage Learning.

and (4) nutrition monitoring and evaluation. **FIGURE 10.14** describes one example of nutritional intervention for addressing CVD, and **FIGURE 10.15** shows the four key nutritional goals to managing CVD. Registered dietitian nutritionists must be comprehensive in their assessments to ensure that objectives and interventions are effective in managing CVD and associated diseases.

## Factors that Influence Health Status

### Race and Ethnicity

Race and ethnicity may influence the rate and severity of chronic health conditions. The burden of diabetes, for example, may be higher among both ethnic minority groups and those who are uninsured.[51] African-American women bear among the highest burdens, with 12.6% of that population affected by diabetes.[23,52] The high number of individuals affected means increased mortality rates, high economic costs, reduced quality of life, and more complicated health problems.[53,54] The prevalence of overweight and obesity is approximately 58% among non-Hispanic black women. Furthermore, studies report that African Americans, Hispanics and Latinos, American Indians,

Pacific Islanders, and some Asian Americans are at higher risk than whites.[6]

### Smoking

All forms of tobacco generate toxins that damage the vascular endothelium lining and promote systemic atherosclerosis. Smoking causes hypoxia in all tissues, including cardiac tissues. Tissue demand for oxygen increases the heart rate and cardiac muscle workload as the heart works to meet tissue requirements. Tobacco toxins damage the membranes of blood cells, including platelets, and thus elevates the risk for blood clot formation or thrombus. Smoking cessation has been shown to reduce the risk for CVD by 50% after 18 months; the risk drops to that of nonsmokers after 15 years.[55]

### Diet

Dietary patterns affect the risk of chronic degenerative diseases and conditions. Atherogenic diets significantly increase CVD risk. Diets that are high in cholesterol, saturated fats, and trans fats also promote atherosclerosis. Elevated levels of these dietary lipids increase the

- *Nutrition assessment*: Nutrition assessment is a systematic process of obtaining, verifying and interpreting data in order to make informed decisions about the nature and cause of nutrition-related problems.
- *Nutrition diagnosis*: This is the identification and descriptive labeling of an actual occurrence of nutrition problems that dietetics practitioners are responsible for treating independently. PES—problem, etiology, signs, and symptoms—statements are used in this step. It is the format used in the Nutrition Care Process to write a nutrition diagnosis.
- *Nutrition Interventions*: These include a specific set of activities and associated materials used to address a (nutrition-related problem). It is a client-driven process and should be logically linked to the cause of the problems. The intent of the intervention is to change a nutrition-related behavior, risk factor, environmental condition, or aspect of health status for an individual or larger group. This includes the establishment of ideal goals and expected outcomes.
- *Nutrition Monitoring and Evaluation*: This process is an active commitment to measuring and recording the appropriate outcome indicators relevant to a nutrition diagnosis to determine how much progress is being made and whether or not the client's goals are being met. Progress is monitored, measured, and evaluated on a planned schedule.

**FIGURE 10.13** The four domains to assessing nutritional status.

Republished with permission of Cengage Learning, Nelson Education from Nelms MN, Sucher K, Lacey K, Roth SL, Habash D, Nelms RG, et al. *Nutrition Therapy and Pathophysiology*. 2nd ed. 2015. Belmont, CA: Brooks/Cole Cengage Learning.; Permission conveyed through Copyright Clearance Center, Inc.

production of LDL as well as lower HDL production in the liver.[53] Well-designed diets rich in fruits, vegetables, vitamins, minerals, omega-3 fatty acids, phytochemicals, and fibers can help lower blood lipids and confer protective effects against chronic diseases.

## Physical Activity

Regular physical activity has many advantages, including strengthening the heart muscle, promoting angiogenesis, increasing insulin sensitivity, raising of HDL cholesterol levels, lowering blood pressure, circulating inflammatory cytokines, and reducing LDL cholesterol. In the absence of routine physical activity, the heart and vascular system capacities subside, which leads to the heart muscle having reduced pumping ability. As little as 15 to 30 minutes of moderate exercise, five days per week is likely to increase heart health and reduce risks for chronic diseases.

- *Assessment Data*: Food-frequency recall and intake records, computer nutrient analysis, anthropometrics measurements, clinical history, laboratory values, food and diet history, genetics factors, food and knowledge history, psychosocial history, and weight history
- *Nutritional Diagnoses (PES)*: Food- and nutrition-knowledge deficit food choice
- *Goal*: To lose 1 to 2 lbs per week and educated about healthy food choices
- *Barrier and address behavior*: Stage of changes—precontemplation, contemplation, preparation, action, maintenance, and replacement
- *Intervention*: Nutrition education and counseling to address behavioral and social factors. Use motivational interviewing (MI) to provide comprehensive coursing for age and activity level and find ways to gradually increase physical activities. BMI closer to desirable, behavior change such as an increase consumption of fruits and vegetables and whole grains. Increase physical activities.
- *Monitoring and Evaluation*: Repeat lab values after three to six months; dietary recall. Goals: TC, HDL, and LDL within normal limits.

**FIGURE 10.14** NCP nutritional intervention: CVD.

Modified from Nelms MN, Sucher K, Lacey K, Roth SL, Habash D, Nelms RG, et al. *Nutrition Therapy and Pathophysiology*. 2nd ed. 2015. Belmont, CA: Brooks/Cole Cengage Learning.

**Food and Nutrition Goals for CVD Management.**
- Follow a healthy diet with lots of whole grains, fruits, and vegetables.
- Increase intake of folic acid and vitamins $B_6$ and $B_{12}$ to reduce elevated plasma total homocysteine concentrations.
- Omega-3 fatty acid may be beneficial in reducing inflammation.
- Consume a balanced diet with good sources of vitamins E, $B_6$, and $B_{12}$ and riboflavin.

**FIGURE 10.15** The role of nutrition in the management of CVD: the four key nutritional goals to manage CVD.

Modified from Nelms MN, Sucher K, Lacey K, Roth SL, Habash D, Nelms RG, et al. *Nutrition Therapy and Pathophysiology*. 2nd ed. 2015. Belmont, CA: Brooks/Cole Cengage Learning.

## The Transtheoretical Model and Stages of Change

The transtheoretical model (TTM) is an integrative, biopsychosocial model to conceptualize the process of intentional behavior change. Inherent in the TTM, change involves progress through a series of six stages over time.

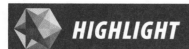

### Good Nutrition Improves Health

*Did you know that good nutrition can help improve your health?* According to the Society of Obesity, obesity is a large problem in the United States, encompassing more than one-third of adults. These staggering numbers reveal an overall health problem and contribute to high medical costs. At its core, obesity is an individual problem, one detrimental to individual health and self-esteem. Individuals should actively seek solutions to minimize their weight gain, including adopting a healthy, well-balanced diet and getting enough exercise. In addition to grave personal effects, the high medical costs of dealing with obesity affect individuals, employers, and insurance providers.

Growing bellies increase the risk of various cancers, cardiovascular disease, and diabetes, all leading causes of death. The medical bills associated with these high price-tag diseases, among many other medical complications associated with obesity, total $147 billion, and employers wind up with a $73.1 billion bill. To reduce this burden, employers should take action by implementing healthy living programs, offering gym memberships, and even catering healthy meals.

According to Prochaska and DiClemente's stages of change (SOC) model, the TTM (**FIGURE 10.16**) uses stages of change to integrate processes and principles of change from across major theories of intervention. TTM construes change as a process involving progress through a series of six stages. When in precontemplation, people do not intend to take action in the foreseeable future or within the next six months. At this stage, they tend to avoid reading, talking, or thinking about their high-risk behaviors. In the stage of contemplation, people are aware of the benefits of changing their behavior within the next six months and are aware that their ambivalence can keep them stuck in this stage. In the preparation stage, people intend to take action in the immediate future within the next six months. Individuals have a plan of action such as joining a health education class, consulting a counselor, or taking their medications. In maintenance, people strive to prevent relapse, are less tempted to relapse, and are more confident they can continue their changes. The continuous success at this stage requires self-efficacy to address temptation and maintenance of abstinence from behavior. In the termination stage, individuals are no longer likely to succumb to temptation and have total self-efficacy. Termination, however, may not be practical for a majority of people.

## Motivational Interviewing

Motivational interviewing is a counseling intervention that is effective in bringing about long-term changes in health-related factors and behaviors associated with CVD risk.[56,57] MI is defined as a client-centered directive method that enhances an individual's intrinsic motivation to change by exploring and resolving ambivalence. MI techniques will help patients adopt the nutritional treatments needed to address their nutritional diagnoses through nutrition education, counseling, and intervention.[58] MI focuses on individual clients' needs and concerns. Its goal is not to focus or concentrate on current interests, concerns, and needs but to resolve ambivalence and move a person through change by counteracting resistance with the individuals to make behavior change.

## Reinforcing and Encouraging Change Talk

The method of reinforcing and encouraging change talk relies on communication, not manipulation, as a way to convince individuals to evoke change rather than trick them into it. The focus of MI is on eliciting a person's intrinsic motivation for change in a noncoercive way, allowing the individual to become concerned about problem behavior. In this way, MI is concerned with the motivational processes inherent in the individual that will facilitate that change.[59] In addition to the use of MI, individuals will be assessed to determine their self-efficacy.[57,58] MI has become a widely adopted and effective approach to change behaviors and has the potential to improve cardiovascular health status.[58]

## Self-Efficacy

Albert Bandura[59] defined *self-efficacy* as one of the constructs of social cognitive theory. It is the perception of an individual's level of confidence to

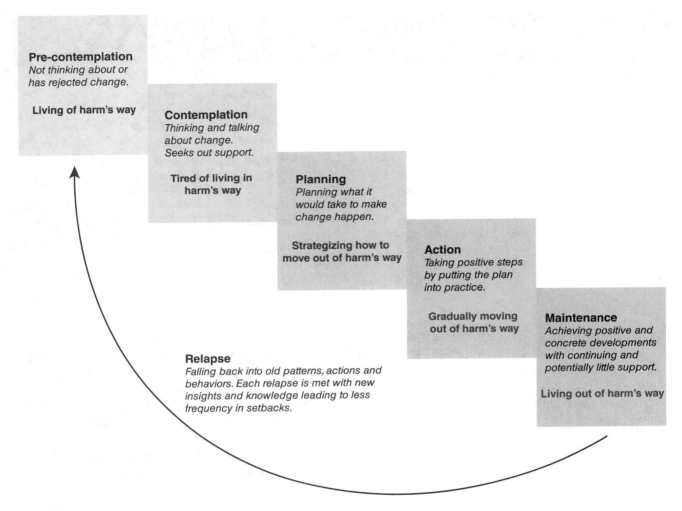

**FIGURE 10.16** The transtheoretical model and stages of change.

Data from The Transtheoretical Model. Pro-Change Behavior Systems Web site. https://www.prochange.com/transtheoretical-model-of-behavior-change. Date uknown. Accessed August 16, 2017.

perform a specific behavior in a specified situation.[58] In addition, it is an individual's level of confidence to change a behavior or cognition. The components of the model include interactions with a positive coping response and increased self-efficacy. These components can decrease the probability of engaging in eating behavior. When applying the theory with individuals engaged in poor health decisions, it may be suitable to determine how participants perceive their self-efficacy to engage in specific desirable behaviors.[60]

## Activity Guidelines for Americans

Regular physical activity helps improve a person's overall health and fitness and reduces the risk of many chronic diseases. Fitting regular exercise into a daily schedule may seem difficult at first. To address this challenge, the *2008 Physical Activity Guidelines for Americans* (**TABLE 10.5**) are more flexible than ever, giving people the freedom to reach their physical activity goals through different types and amounts of activities each week.[61]

The *Physical Activity Guidelines for Americans* do not include guidelines for children younger than 6 years old. Physical activity in infants and young children is, of course, necessary for healthy growth and development. Children younger than 6 can be physically active in ways that are appropriate for their age and stage of development. Children should participate in about 60 or more minutes of physical activity. Physical activity guidelines for children younger than six that are specific to the early care and education setting are included in *Caring for Our Children: National Health and Safety Performance Standards; Guidelines for Early Care and Education Programs* (3rd ed.). **FIGURE 10.17** lists the key guidelines for adults'

**TABLE 10.5** Physical activity guidelines

| Moderate Intensity | |
|---|---|
| Walking briskly (3 miles per hour or faster but not racewalking) | Water aerobics |
| Bicycling slower than 10 miles per hour | Tennis (doubles) |
| Ballroom dancing | General gardening |
| **Vigorous Intensity** | |
| Racewalking, jogging, or running | Swimming laps |
| Tennis (singles) | Aerobic dancing |
| Bicycling 10 miles per hour or faster | Jumping rope |
| Heavy gardening (continuous digging or hoeing) | Hiking uphill or with a heavy backpack |

Modified from Centers for Disease Control and Prevention. Physical Activity. https://www.cdc.gov/physicalactivity/index.html Accessed 7.27.17 and Office of Disease Prevention and Health Promotion. Chapter 2. Physical Activity has Many Benefits. Available at https://health.gov/paguidelines/guidelines/chapter2.aspx accessed July 18, 2017.

physical activity to improve their health and the key points in managing chronic medical conditions.

## Bone Strengthening

The CDC recommends that adults perform two hours and 30 minutes (150 minutes total) of moderate-intensity aerobic activity (e.g., brisk walking) every week.

> **Recap**  NCP is used to address the nutritional needs of individuals with chronic conditions that require dietary modifications and intervention. Lifestyle choices such as a healthy diet, smoking cessation and regular physical activity are important the the prevention and management of chronic diseases.

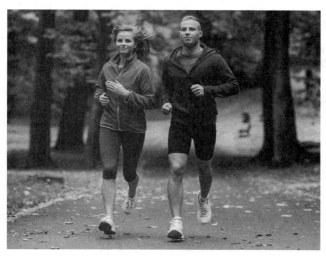
© Jacek Chabraszewski/Shutterstock.

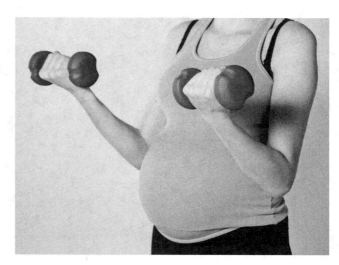
© Elina Manninen/Shutterstock.

### Key Activity Guidelines for Adults

- All adults should avoid inactivity. Some physical activity is better than none, and adults who participate in any amount of physical activity gain some health benefits.
- For substantial health benefits, adults should have at least 150 minutes (2 hours and 30 minutes) a week of moderate intensity aerobic physical activity or 75 minutes (1 hour and 15 minutes) a week of vigorous intensity aerobic activity, or an equivalent combination of moderate and vigorous intensity aerobic activity. Aerobic activity should be performed in episodes of at least 10 minutes and preferably should be spread throughout the week.

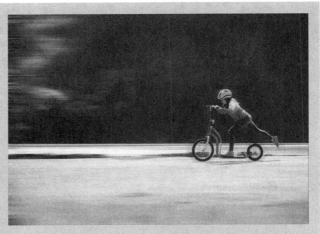

© Here/Shutterstock.

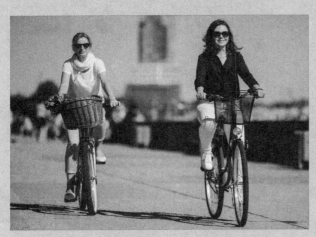

© Jacek Chabraszewski/Shutterstock.

- For additional and more extensive health benefits, adults should increase their aerobic physical activity to 300 minutes (5 hours) a week of moderate intensity or 150 minutes a week of vigorous intensity aerobic physical activity, or an equivalent combination of moderate and vigorous

intensity activity. Additional health benefits are gained by engaging in physical activity beyond this amount.

- Adults should also do muscle-strengthening activities that are moderate or high intensity and involve all major muscle groups at least twice a week because these activities provide additional health benefits.

### Key Messages for People with Chronic Medical Conditions

- Adults with chronic conditions obtain important health benefits from regular physical activity.
- When adults with chronic conditions do activity according to their abilities, physical activity is safe.
- Adults with chronic conditions should be under the care of a healthcare provider. People with chronic conditions and symptoms should consult their healthcare provider about the types and amounts of activity appropriate for them.

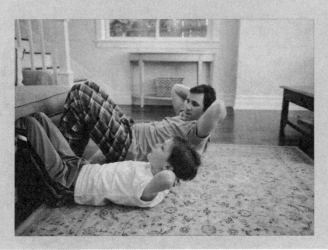

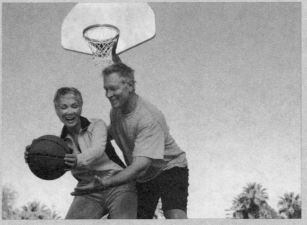

**FIGURE 10.17** Key guidelines for physical activity.

# ▶ Chapter Summary

Along with evidence-based and translational approaches to addressing nutritional problems, this chapter provides an overview of prevention and intervention for chronic diseases, especially cardiovascular diseases. A comprehensive approach is vital for the successful implementation of a nutritional intervention. The NCP provides RDNs with a framework for MNT and provides a systematic approach for delivering a comprehensive nutritional assessment to prevent and treat nutrition-related diseases.

## CASE STUDY

In order to address the risk factors associated with cardiovascular disease, nutritional education usually focuses on hypertension, hyperglycemia, weight loss, and decreasing triglycerides. The goals for this particular case are as follows:

1. To improve a patient's nutritional status
2. To provide education and counseling on nutrition-related recommendations
3. To improve diet adherence
4. To improve nutrition-related laboratory values.

Mary is a 56-year-old female with five children. Originally from Jamaica, she has been living in the United States for over 20 years. During that time, she has worked as a night nurse as well as a consultant health educator for the health department of the District of Columbia. Mary is currently retired and is working as a volunteer at the local hospital, traveling all over the world. She recently started feeling tired and out of breath, and she has not been able to walk for one week. Mary thought that it was a "bug" from her recent trip to Kenya. During her weekly lunch outing with her girlfriends, she started having chest pain and was taken to the hospital. She was admitted on September 19th with chest pain and an elevated BP of 200/110. She has an elevated hemoglobin A1C level (10.6), which indicates that her type 2 diabetes has been uncontrolled for the past three months. She also has a history of heart failure and vitamin D deficiency. Mary thinks that she has sleep apnea and has not been sleeping well, but she believed that it was because she used to work at night and never adjusted to sleeping through the night.

During her interview visit, it was determined that Mary has gained 15 lbs. in one week and has had difficulty in walking and breathing for the past one week. When admitted to the hospital, she had a poor appetite and ate only 25% of her meals over three days. Before this, she had eaten well and used to go out with her girlfriends twice a week to the Golden Corral for its all-you-can-eat buffet, even though she mostly ate salad and fruits.

Mary walks with her friends three miles per day, five days a week; swims twice a week; and does yoga for 30 minutes a day. Mary has always tried to take good care of herself because she knows her family had a history of heart disease, obesity, and dyslipidemia. Both parents and two sisters have heart problems.

- *Anthropometric Data*
  - Current weight = 160 lbs.; height = 5'7"; usual body weight = 140 lbs. × 2 months
- *Medications include*
  - Current medications: Bumex, Diovan, thiamine, Lasix, MVI, vitamin D, Lipitor, fish oil, niacin
  - Previous medications: Metformin, MVI, vitamin D, flaxseed
- *Laboratory Data*
  - Hs-CRP: 0.630 mg/L
  - Cholesterol: 207mg/dL
  - HDL cholesterol: 56 mg/dL
  - LDL cholesterol: 140 mg/dL
  - Triglyceride: 304 mg/dL
  - BUN: 10
  - Creatinine: 1.0
  - Na: 128
  - BNP: 2400
  - GFR: > 60
  - Glucose: 220
  - HbA1C: 5.3%
  - Vitamin D: 25-OH; total: 7 ng/mL
  - NRBC: 0.2
  - EOS: 0.0
  - BASO: 0.0
  - NRBC: 0.01
- *Nutrition Diagnostic Statement: Example*
  - Unplanned weight gain related to CHF as evidence by (aeb) 15lbs x 1 week and difficulty walking
  - Inadequate food intake r/t reported difficulty breaking AEB intake less than 75%
- *Food and Nutrition*
  - Avoid excesses of calories, sodium, fluids, if weight loss in this case, add extra calories and snacks to return to a more desirable body weight

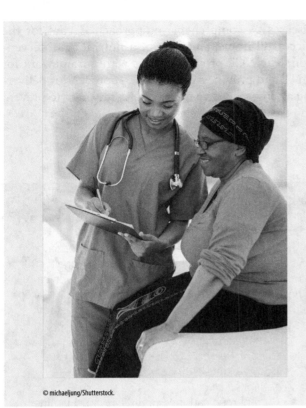

© michaeljung/Shutterstock.

- Evidence supports the se of the DASH diet. This diet includes the consumption of foods containing flavonoids such as chocolate, pomegranate, apples, and onions. Flavonoids may help to reduce blood-clot formation
- Ensure adequate intake of omega-3 fatty acids
- Nutrition Education, Counseling, Care Management: Consider behavioral or cognitive approach to counseling and nutritional education.
  - Use patient-centered approach; incorporate patient's nutritional preferences, likes, and dislikes in the developing the menu.
  - Reduce the consumption of sodium and processed foods that may impact fluid shifts.

### Questions:

1. What other nutrition assessment information do you need before you conduct the interview with Mary?
2. Are there any food-drug interactions that are a concern for Mary? Why?
3. What recommendations would you make about Mary's diet?
4. How would you counsel Mary? Would you consider a coordination of care?

 ## CASE STUDY

Mark is a 52-year-old single man with hypertension (BP 200/93), high total cholesterol (310 mg/dL) and high HDL cholesterol (32 mg/dL). Mark has recently become divorced. He is an IT manager and works 12-hour days. He eats in his car from fast-food restaurants. His breakfast is from McDonald's or Burger King: cheese, eggs, biscuit sausages, an 8-oz orange juice, and a 16-oz coffee with five creamers and ten sugars. He does not have the time to exercise on a daily basis, and he has gained 28 lbs in

180 days (he is currently 179 lbs and 5'6"). Mark walks twice a week and plays basketball every Saturday.

### Questions:

1. Using the Nutrition Care Process, what are Mark's nutritional diagnoses?
2. What interventions would be most beneficial for Mark?
3. What signs and symptoms would you want to monitor and evaluate?

# Learning Portfolio

## Key Terms

Atherosclerosis
Cardiovascular disease (CVD)
Diabetes mellitus (DM)
Hypercholesterolemia

Hypertension
Obesity
Physical activity

## Study Questions

1. Omega-3 fatty acids are associated with:
   a. Reduced blood urea nitrogen
   b. Reduced high-density lipoprotein cholesterol
   c. Reduced systemic inflammation
   d. Reduced risk of iron-deficiency anemia
2. Leptin has what function in the body?
   a. It suppresses appetite.
   b. It reduces the release of FFAs into the blood.
   c. It stimulates appetite.
   d. It leads to overnutrition.
3. Adiponectin has what function in the body?
   a. It suppresses appetite.
   b. It reduces the release of FFAs into the blood.
   c. It stimulates appetite.
   d. It leads to overnutrition.
4. Ghrelin has what function in the body?
   a. It suppresses appetite
   b. It stimulates appetite
   c. It leads to overnutrition
   d. B and C
5. During what life stage does atherosclerosis begin?
   a. Childhood
   b. Young adulthood
   c. Middle age
   d. Old age
6. The genesis of atherosclerosis is triggered by:
   a. Poor dietary habits that lead to elevated cholesterol
   b. Poor dietary habits that lead to elevated triglycerides
   c. CVD
   d. Elevated HDL cholesterol
7. The risks for CVD can be divided into which two categories?
   a. Genetic and modifiable
   b. Diet and physical activity
   c. Modifiable and nonmodifiable
   d. Diseases and lifestyle choices
8. Modifiable factors for CVD include:
   a. Age, ethnicity, and family history
   b. Age, family history, and obesity
   c. Family history, obesity, and tobacco consumption
   d. Obesity, tobacco consumption, and hypercholesterolemia
9. Nonmodifiable factors for CVD include:
   a. Age, ethnicity, and family history
   b. Age, gender, and obesity
   c. Family history, obesity, and tobacco consumption
   d. Obesity, tobacco consumption, and hypercholesterolemia
10. Android fat accumulation is:
    a. Located in the trunk of the body
    b. Located in the hips
    c. Located in the trunk and the hips
    d. Also known as the "pear shape" accumulation
11. Gynoid fat accumulation is:
    a. Located in the trunk of the body
    b. Located in the hips
    c. Also known as the "apple shape" fat accumulation
    d. Also known as the "fruit shape" accumulation
12. Which of the following does not correctly describe a stage in the transtheoretical module of change?
    a. In precontemplation, people intend to act in the foreseeable future or within the next six months. At this stage, they begin reading reading, talking, or thinking about their high-risk behaviors and seek guidance for taking the first steps even though they are not yet ready to change behavior.
    b. In the stage of contemplation, people are aware of the benefits of changing their behavior within the next 6 months and are aware that their ambivalence can keep them stuck in this stage.
    c. In preparation, people intend to act in the immediate future within the next 6 months. Individuals have a plan of action such as joining a health education class, consulting a counselor, or taking their medications.
    d. In maintenance, people strive to prevent relapse, are less tempted to relapse, and are more confident they can continue their changes.

## Discussion Questions

1. By making healthy choices, you can lower your risk for heart disease. Discuss how sleep and physical activities may help lower your risk for heart disease.
2. Discuss the role of behavioral changes in improving nutritional health and overall wellbeing.
3. How can assessment of readiness to change and motivational interviewing be used to help patients and clients manage chronic conditions and improve health?

## Activities

1. Describe a body system that is affected by obesity and determine the role of healthy eating and comprehensive nutritional intervention in managing obesity. Provide key samples of healthy meals.
   a. How does obesity affect the system?
   b. Provide key nutritional intervention for the selected system.

2. Using Figure 10.8, provide three ways to address and improve the health of individuals. Discuss the role of the registered dietitian nutritionist (RDN) in addressing these contributing factors. Now consider the following.
   a. Name three contributing factors to obesity.
   b. Discuss how an interdisciplinary approach can support patients or customers in improving their nutritional health.

## Online Resources

American Heart Association: http://www.heart.org/HEARTORG/

American Diabetes association: http://www.diabetes.org/?referrer=https://www.google.com/

Office of Disease prevention and health promotion, physical activity guidelines: https://health.gov/paguidelines/

NIH National Institute for Diabetes and Digestive and Kidney Diseases: https://www.niddk.nih.gov/

## References

1. World Health Organization (WHO). Cardiovascular disease. Geneva, Switzerland: WHO; 2016. http://www.who.int/topics/cardiovascular_diseases/en/. Accessed December 1, 2016.
2. Matthews AT, Ross MK. Oxyradical stress, endocannabinoids and atherosclerosis. *Toxics.* 2015; 3(4):481–498. doi:10.3390/toxics3040481.
3. Kumar V, Abbas AK, Fausto N. Eds. *Robbins and Cotran: Pathologic Basis of Disease.* 7th ed. Philadelphia, PA: Elsevier Saunders; 2005.
4. Tomaselli GF. Prevention of cardiovascular disease and stroke: Meeting the challenge. *JAMA.* 2011; 306:2147–2148.
5. Acute and chronic inflammation. In: Kumar V, Abbas AK, Fausto N. Eds. *Robbins and Cotran: Pathologic Basis of Disease.* 7th ed. Philadelphia, PA: Elsevier Saunders; 2005.
6. Ogden CL, Carroll MD, Fryar CD, Flegal KM. Prevalence of obesity among adults and youth: United States, 2011–2014. NCHS Data Brief No. 219; 2015; November. https://www.cdc.gov/nchs/data/databriefs/db219.pdf. Accessed August 16, 2017.
7. National Center for Chronic Disease Prevention and Health Promotion. National Diabetes Statistics Report, 2017: Estimates of Diabetes and Its Burden in the United States. Atlanta, GA: Centers for Disease Control and Prevention (CDC). https://www.cdc.gov/diabetes/pdfs/data/statistics/national-diabetes-statistics-report.pdf. Accessed August 16, 2017.
8. WHO. Cardiovascular disease. Geneva, Switzerland: WHO; 2016. http://www.who.int/topics/cardiovascular_diseases/en/. Accessed December 1, 2016.
9. Centers for Disease Control and Prevention (CDC). Heart Disease Fact Sheet https://www.cdc.gov/dhdsp/data_statistics/fact_sheets/fs_heart_disease.htm. Accessed August 16, 2017.
10. National Center for Chronic Disease Prevention and Health Promotion: Estimates of Diabetes and Its Burden in the United States. Atlanta, GA: CDC; 2017.
11. Mozaffarian D, et al. Heart disease and stroke statistics—2016 Update. A report from the American Heart Association. *Circulation*; 2016; 132. doi.10.1161/CIR.0000000000000350.
12. American Heart Association. Heart disease and stroke statistics—2015 update. http://news.heart.org/american-heart-association-statistical-report-tracks-global-figures-first-time.
13. Centers for Disease Control and Prevention (CDC). Heart Disease Fact Sheet https://www.cdc.gov/dhdsp/data_statistics/fact_sheets/fs_heart_disease.htm. Accessed August 16, 2017.
14. Roger VL, Go AS, Lloyd DM, et al. Heart disease and stroke statistics—2011 update A Report from the American Heart Association. *Circulation.* 2011; Feb 1;123(4):e18–e209. Accessed August 16, 2017. https://www.ncbi.nlm.nih.gov/pmc/articles/PMC4418670/.
15. Kumar V, Abbas AK, Fausto N. Eds. *Robbins and Cotran: Pathologic Basis of Disease.* 7th ed. Philadelphia, PA: Elsevier Saunders; 2005.
16. National Heart, Lung, and Blood Institute. ATP III at-a-glance: Quick desk reference.. http://www.nhlbi.nih.gov/health-pro/guidelines/current/cholesterol-guidelines/quick-desk-reference-html. Accessed October 10, 2016.
17. Keenan NL, Rosendorf KA. Prevalence of hypertension and controlled hypertension—United States, 2005–2008. *Morb Mortal Wkly Rep.* 2011; 60(Suppl):94–97. https://www.cdc.gov/nchs/products/databriefs/db133.htm.
18. CDC. Division for Heart Disease and Stroke Prevention. Blood pressure fact sheet https://www.cdc.gov/dhdsp/data_statistics/fact_sheets/fs_bloodpressure.htm. Accessed October 10, 2016.
19. WHO. Cardiovascular diseases; 2016. http://www.who.int/topics/cardiovascular_diseases/en/. Accessed December 1, 2016.
20. NIH National Institute for Diabetes and Digestive and Kidney Diseases. Overweight and obesity statics. https://www.niddk

.nih.gov/health-information/health-statistics/overweight -obesity. Accessed August 16, 2017.

21. Yaggi HK, Araujo AB, McKinlay JB. Sleep duration as a risk factor for the development of type 2 diabetes. *Diabetes Care.* 2006; Mar;29(3):657–661. World Heart Federation. Risk factors fact sheet: Hypertension. http://www.world-heart -federation.org/cardiovascular-health/cardiovascular-disease -risk-factors/. Accessed August 16, 2017.

22. Auslander W, Haire-Joshu D, Houston C, Rhee CW, Williams JH. A controlled evaluation of staging dietary patterns to reduce the risk of diabetes in African-American women. *Diabetes Care.* 2002; 25(5):809–814.

23. Knutson, Kristen L. "Does inadequate sleep play a role in vulnerability to obesity?." *American Journal of Human Biology* 24.3 (2012): 361–371.

24. Tilghman J. Obesity and diabetes in African American women. *ABNF.* 2003; May-Jun;14(3):66–68.

25. Moore PJ, Adler NE, Williams DR, Jackson JS. Socioeconomic status and health: The role of sleep. *Psychosom Med.* 2002; 64(2):337–344.

26. Nishiura C, Noguchi J, Hashimoto H. Dietary patterns only partially explain the effect of short sleep duration on the incidence of obesity. *Sleep.* 2010; 33(6):753–757.

27. CDC. Smoking and tobacco use: Tobacco-related mortality. https://www.cdc.gov/tobacco/data_statistics/fact_sheets /health_effects/tobacco_related_mortality/index.htm. Accessed August 16, 2017.

28. CDC. 2014 Surgeon General's report: The health consequences of smoking—50 years of progress. Atlanta, GA: US Department of Health and Human Services. Accessed August 17, 2015.

29. WHO. Cardiovascular diseases: CVD prevention and control— Missed opportunities. 2016. http://www.who.int/cardiovascular_ diseases/prevention_control/en/. Accessed December 1, 2016.

30. Shukla SD, Budden KF, Neal R, Hansbro PM. Microbiome effects on immunity, health and disease in the lung. *Clin Transl Immunology.* 2017; 6(3):e133. https://www.ncbi.nlm.nih.gov /pmc/articles/PMC5382435/. doi:10.1038/cti.2017.6.

31. Chung H, Kasper DL. Microbiota-stimulated immune mechanisms to maintain gut homeostasis. *Curr Opin Immunol.* 2010; 22(4):455–460. doi:10.1016/j.coi.2010.06.008.

32. Clemente JC, Ursell LK, Parfrey LW, Knight R. The impact of the gut microbiota on human health: An integrative view. *Cell.* 2012; 16;148(6):1258–1270. doi:10.1016/j.cell.2012.01.035.

33. Org E, Mehrabian M, Lusis A. Unraveling the environmental and genetic interactions in atherosclerosis: Central role of the gut microbiota. *Atherosclerosis.* 2015; 241(2):387–399. doi:10.1016/j.atherosclerosis.2015.05.035.

34. Marchesi JR, Adams DH, Fava F, Hermes GDA, et al. The gut microbiota and host health: A new clinical frontier. *Gut.* 2015; 65:330–339. doi:10.1136/gutjnl-2015-309990.

35. WHO. Cardiovascular disease. 2016. http://www.who.int /cardiovascular_diseases/en/. Accessed December 1, 2016.

36. CDC. High blood pressure fact sheet. https://www.cdc.gov /dhdsp/data_statistics/fact_sheets/fs_bloodpressure.htm Accessed August 16, 2017.

37. National Heart, Lung, and Blood Institute. ATP III at-a-glance: Quick desk reference.. http://www.nhlbi.nih.gov/health-pro /guidelines/current/cholesterol-guidelines/quick-desk -reference-html. Accessed October 10, 2016.

38. Keenan NL, Rosendorf KA. Prevalence of hypertension and controlled hypertension—United States, 2005–2008. *Morb Mortal Wkly Rep.* 2011; 60(Suppl):94–97. https://www.cdc .gov/mmwr/preview/mmwrhtml/su6001a21.htm.

39. CDC. Division for Heart Disease and Stroke Prevention. Blood pressure fact sheet https://www.cdc.gov/dhdsp/data_statistics /fact_sheets/fs_bloodpressure.htm. Accessed October 10, 2016.

40. National Cholesterol Education Program (NCEP). Third report of the National Cholesterol Education Program (NCEP) expert panel on detection, evaluation, and treatment of high blood cholesterol in adults (Adult Treatment Panel III) final report. *Circulation.* 2002; 106:3143–421.

41. Fedder DO, Koro CE, L'Italien GJ. New National Cholesterol Education Program III guidelines for primary prevention lipid-lowering drug therapy projected impact on the size, sex, and age distribution of the treatment-eligible population. *Circulation.* 2002; 105:152–156.

42. Expert Panel on Detection, Evaluation, and Treatment of High Blood Cholesterol in Adults (Adults Treatment Panel III). Third report of the National Cholesterol Education Program (NCEP). NIH publication no 02-5215. Bethesda, MD; National Heart, Lung, and Blood Institute; 2002; 11-15–11-20.

43. Ogden CL, Carroll MD, Fryar CD, Flegal, KM. Prevalence of Obesity Among Adults and Youth: United States, 2011–2014. National Center for Health Statistics; 2011. https://www.cdc .gov/nchs/data/databriefs/db219.pdf.

44. Ogden CL, Carroll MD, Fryar CD, Flegal, KM. Prevalence of Obesity Among Adults and Youth: United States, 2011–2014. National Center for Health Statistics; 2011. https://www.cdc .gov/nchs/data/databriefs/db219.pdf.

45. WHO. Obesity and overweight. 2016. http://www.who.int /mediacentre/factsheets/fs311/en/.

46. National Heart, Lung, and Blood Institute. Health Information for the Public. https://www.nhlbi.nih.gov/health/. Accessed August 16, 2017.

47. Mayo Clinic. https://www.mayoclinic.org/. Accessed November 1, 2016.

48. Kochanek KD, Xu JQ, Murphy SL, Miniño AM, Kung HC. Deaths: Final data for 2009. *Nat Vital Stat Rep.* 2011; 60(3). National Heart, Lung, and Blood Institute. What Are Coronary Heart Disease Risk Factors? https://www.nhlbi.nih.gov/health /health-topics/topics/hd. Accessed October 10, 2016.

49. The Nutrition Care Process (NCP). In: Nelms M, Sucher KP. Eds. *Nutrition Therapy and Pathophysiology.* 3rd ed. Pacific Grove, CA: Brooks/Cole; 2015.

50. Nelms M, Sucher K. Eds. *Nutrition Therapy and Pathophysiology.* 3rd ed. Pacific Grove, CA: Brooks/Cole; 2015.

51. Depner CM, Stothard ER, Wright KP Jr. Metabolic consequences of sleep and circadian disorders. *Curr Diabetes Reports.* 2014; 14(7):1–9.

52. Mottillo S, Filion KB, Genest J, et al. The metabolic syndrome and cardiovascular disease risk. *J Am Coll Cardiology.* 2012; 56:1113–1132.

53. Dincer S, Altan M, Terzioglu D, Uslu E, Karsidag K, Batu S, Metin G. Effects of a regular exercise program on biochemical parameters of type 2 diabetes mellitus patients. *J Sports Med Phys Fitness.* 2015; Nov;56(11):1384–1391.

54. Duclos M, Dejager S, Postel-Vinay N, di Nicola S, Quéré S, Fiquet B. Physical activity in patients with type 2 diabetes and hypertension—Insights into motivations and barriers from the MOBILE study. *Vasc Health Risk Manage.* 2015; 11:361.

55. CDC. Quitting smoking. 2017. https://www.cdc.gov/tobacco /data_statistics/fact_sheets/cessation/quitting/index.htm.

56. Markland D, Ryan RM, Tobin VJ, Rollnick S. Motivational interviewing and self- determination theory. *J Soc Clin Psych.* 2005; 24(6):811–831.

57. Thompson DR, Chair SY, Chan SW, Astin F, Davidson PM, Ski CF. Motivational Interviewing: A useful approach to improving cardiovascular health? *J Clin Nurs.* 2011; 20(9–10):1236–1244.

58. Miller WR, Rollnick S. Meeting in the middle: Motivational interviewing and self-determination theory. *Inter J Behav Nutr Phys Act.* 2012;9:5.

59. Bandura A. Self-efficacy: Toward a unifying theory of behavioral change. *Psych Rev.* 1977; 84:191–215.

60. Ogedegbe G, Mancuso CA, Allegrante JP, Charlson ME. Development and evaluation of a medication adherence self-efficacy scale in hypertensive African-American patients. *J Clin Epidemiol.* 2003; 56(6):520–529.

61. Office of Disease Prevention and Health Promotion. Health.gov. Physical activity guidelines for Americans. 2017. https://health .gov/paguidelines/guidelines/. Accessed August 16, 2017.

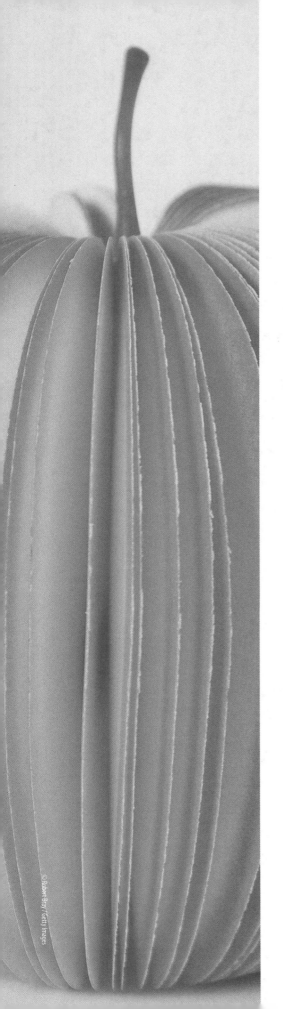

# Application: Nutrition Coaching and International Nutrition

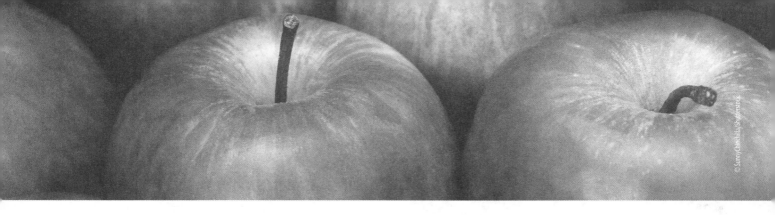

# CHAPTER 11

# Counseling and Health Coaching Theory and Approaches

**Karen Chapman-Novakofski**, PhD, RDN
**Diane Rigassio Radler**, PhD, RD

## LEARNING OBJECTIVES

After completing this chapter, the reader should be able to:
1. Identify communication skills needed for the nutrition education researcher.
2. Identify key counseling skills needed for providing medical nutrition therapy.
3. Describe counseling theories and techniques.
4. List the components and rationale for motivational interviewing.
5. Describe how health coaching has been used successfully.

## ▶ Introduction

Health **coaching** is not disease treatment, although it may be considered disease management. Health coaching is primarily health promotion with a **client-centered approach** or **learner-centered approach**. Like other forms of education, coaching may be individual, face to face, group, asynchronous, or remotely through modern technology. These different strategies are explored in the description of successful implementation of lifestyle changes.

The health coach may use **behavior theories**, behavior models, or motivational interviews, but whichever techniques are used, the learner is the one

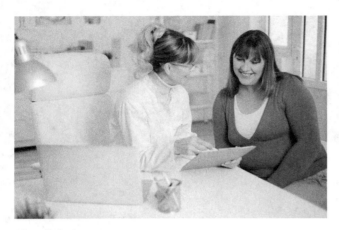

© M_a_y_a/E+/Getty Images.

who sets the goals and agendas. The health coach should have a good understanding of why behavior occurs so that strategies to help change patients' or clients' behavior can be effective and individualized.

Effective communication is central to health coaching, regardless of the methods employed. Communication for the researcher as well as the clinician is described. Although some of the techniques may be used in both areas, some communication techniques are unique to each. This chapter begins with basic communication and interviewing skills as a foundation for the focus on health coaching. The practice paper from the Academy of Nutrition and Dietetics on communication concludes with reminders that nutrition educators need to hone basic communication skills and strive to become skillful at new strategies and through nontraditional methods.[1]

## ▶ Basic Communication and Interviewing Skills for the Nutrition Researcher

**Preview** Oral and written communication skills that are essential for the effective nutrition researcher will also be an asset to practical and research-related health coaching.

In many ways, basic communication and interviewing skills are similar for the nutrition researcher and the clinician. Yet each practice setting has a unique set of terms that practitioners must be fluent in. In addition, the focus and aims of the researcher and clinician are different, and this should be addressed in communication and interviewing styles. For the researcher,

the focus of communication changes, depending on whether the researcher is communicating with a potential granting agency, a compliance officer, research participants, the editorial office of a scientific journal, or the general public.

## Basic Communication: Written

We learned the basics of writing in grade school, but writing well is difficult for most people and requires concerted effort. For the nutrition researcher, technical or scientific writing is required by granting agencies, compliance officers, and editorial offices. For the nutrition researcher, writing often begins with a research proposal, then writing for the compliance officers who usually constitute an institutional review board (IRB), and finally a report to the funding agency and a research article for a scientific journal.

The **research proposal** will usually have a specific goal, objectives, and hypotheses. The specific goal is the broad view. For instance, "To decrease childhood obesity rates in the Mississippi Delta region." The objectives are specific and measurable. For instance, "To decrease the intake of sugar-sweetened beverages of children aged 6 to 9 years." The hypothesis is often written as a null hypothesis. A null hypothesis states the statistical statement of the objective in the negative. For instance, "There will be no statistical difference in sugar-sweetened beverage intake between the intervention group and control group of children aged 6 to 9 years."

The methods part of a research proposal provides step-by-step procedures for how the intervention or project will be conducted. This often includes who the participants will be as defined by inclusion and exclusion criteria, as well as recruitment procedures. Just writing that "participants will be recruited" is not a procedure. An example of a procedure for recruitment: "A flyer will be sent to all parents of children

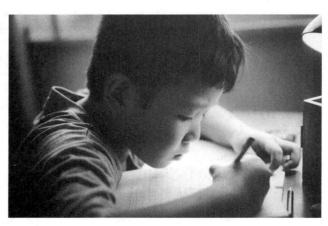

© ndquang/Shutterstock.

in first, second, and third grades at the Yellow School through regular mail by the school's main office."

Documentation of the intervention or program itself must be clear. How outcomes will be evaluated should include details about any questionnaires, measurements, and thresholds for results to be compared against. In the example of childhood obesity, the body mass index *Z*-scores might be used. There are growth standards from the World Health Organization as well as the Centers for Disease Control and Prevention.[2] All measurements should have references supporting the quality of the evaluations or the procedure described to be sure they are of high quality. Finally, potential limitations and how the researcher might address these should be discussed.[3,4]

Many of these document components are also included when writing to the IRB for approval of the project. Primarily, this writing has to be clear about any risks to the participants, ways to minimize those risks, and all procedures to be sure the participants understand and agree to be in the study. Often a consent form has to be included with the IRB protocol submissions. The consent form will need to include certain items specific to each university or research setting, but in general it will include the purpose of the study, an explanation of what participants will be expected to do and how long the study take, any risks involved, any benefits, and any incentives; as well as how confidentiality will be maintained. This consent form should be at a lower reading level than the rest of the IRB proposal.[5]

Writing a research paper and submitting it to a scientific journal requires a slightly different writing skill set and is reflective of each individual journal. Each journal will have its own guidelines for authors (GFA), which will specify how many pages, what subheadings are allowed, and other specifics to the journal. For instance, some journals want authors to include implications for practice or research, whereas others want a concluding statement about the potential impact of the results. Along with the main part of the research article, the references will need to be included according to the GFA, as well any tables or figures, a title page with all authors listed, and a cover letter to the editor. The cover letter should include the article title, address ethical concerns of not having published the research elsewhere, and that all authors contributed to and read the paper, as well as how the paper fits with the mission or scope of the journal.[6]

Writing for the public is a form of technical writing, but for a layperson audience, the writer must assume the readers are not familiar with the topic. The reading level should be lower, at least at the sixth-grade level.

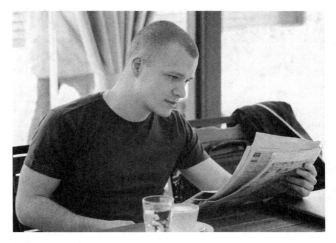

© Jovica Varga/Shutterstock.

Microsoft Word will provide the **Flesch-Kincaid grade reading level**.[7] Where this feature is located in the software depends on the software version. Simple and direct words should be used (**TABLE 11.1**). Care must be taken to ensure that the meaning of the message is not distorted by simplifying the language.

## Basic Communication: Oral

Oral communications for the nutrition researcher generally include presenting research to professional audiences or being interviewed by members of the news media. Research presentations to professional audiences may be considered easier because no one knows the research as well as the presenter does. However, other experts will be in the room and may ask challenging questions. This sometimes creates anxiety for the speaker. A clear plan for the presentation can help reduce that anxiety.[8]

After determining how long the presentation will be, the presenter should consider what content will be included in the presentation. An introductory slide and a concluding or key-points slide will be the beginning and end, respectively. The introductory slide will provide some background to the problem and explain the objectives of the research to be presented. Citations should be included to substantiate the background and information provided. Presenters should remember that they are telling a story, even if it is about their own research. If data can be presented visually, then appealing graphs or charts should be used. In some presentations, a few slides before the concluding remarks may compare and contrast the results with the literature. Citations should be provided here as well. Concluding remarks should summarize approximately three key messages for the audience to remember.[8]

**TABLE 11.1**  Simple and direct words

| This Word(s) is Simpler | Than This Word(s) |
|---|---|
| Activity | Exercise |
| Bone loss | Osteoporosis |
| Doctor | Physician |
| Eat | Consume |
| Hard time breathing | Dyspnea |
| Hard time swallowing | Dysphagia |
| Heart disease | Cardiovascular disease |
| High blood pressure | Hypertension |
| Hunger | Appetite |
| Itchy skin | Pruritus |
| Kidney disease | Renal disease |
| Numbness | Paresthesias |
| Sick feeling | Nauseous |
| Sickness | Malady |
| Skin condition | Dermatitis |
| Stomach | Gastrointestinal tract |
| Taste changes | Dysguesia |
| Tired | Fatigued |
| Weakness | Frailty |
| What you usually do | Routine |

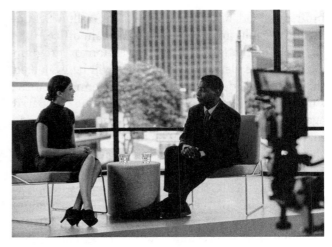

© Monkey Business Images/Shutterstock.

minimal amount while the interviewee has a lot to say. However, some dialogue will make the interview more interesting for the listener. The interviewee should not rush to fill every pause, staying focused on the response and not wandering off topic. At the end of the interview, one or two key points should be made about the topic. Interviewees should think about how they sound before the interview and practice modulating their voices to avoid sounding monotonic. More people will listen to an excited speaker.[9]

## Basic Communication: Body Language

Whether speaking to a professional or a layperson audience, the speaker should try to make body language both professional and engaging. Body language will often provide part of the first impression that will either make the person a frequently invited speaker or create a feeling of hostility, egotism, nervousness, or dullness. The speaker should first think of how he or she stands. A professional will stand straight with shoulders somewhat relaxed, chin slightly tipped up, and feet slightly apart. During the talk, the speaker should be cognizant of hand gestures or nervous gestures. Hand gestures can be used to emphasize a point but should not be used continuously. Nervous gestures such as tucking hair behind the ear or rubbing the chin can be distracting. If the speaker cannot control these actions, he or she should try joining the hands lightly in front of the body until needing to emphasize a point. A good speaker will have a neutral or positive facial expression, and change the expression as needed during the presentation. Visually recording oneself can provide good feedback.[10]

In the same way some people feel anxiety when giving an oral presentation, being interviewed can also be stressful. Whether the interview is for television, radio, or print media, being prepared can help lessen anxiety. The interviewee should ask for the interview questions in advance when possible. If the interviewer has no specific questions to offer, the interviewee should provide some of his or her own. The interviewer should only be speaking a

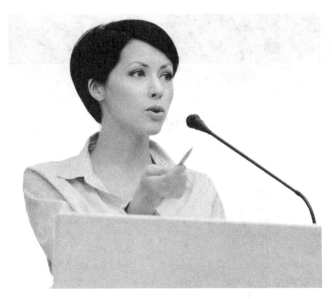

© Karramba Production/Shutterstock.

## Interviewing Skills

Developing interviewing skills for the nutrition researcher begins with defining the goal of the interview and creating the interview guide. These are both "preinterview" skills. Skills during the interview reflect personal skills as well as data-collection skills. Finally, knowing how to analyze and interpret interview data is important.

Those who conduct nutrition research-related interview should be trained. Goodell et al. have developed a five-step training protocol for interviewers that includes ethics training, a review of basic qualitative research methods and data-collection procedures, mock interviews with a previously recorded interview, mock interviews within the research team, and mock interviews within the participant or closely related population.[11] Ethics training is required for any research that involves people. This is available through the university, the Collaborative Institutional Training Initiative (www.citiprogram.org), or the National Institutes of Health Office of Extramural Research: Protecting Human Research Participants (phrp.nihtraining.com). A protocol for conducting the interview and analyzing the data should be submitted to the IRB and will require a consent form, a method of obtaining oral consent, or the submission of a waiver of written consent by the researcher.[5]

A developing rapport with the participants is essential, as is active listening and being comfortable with conversational pauses. Mock interviews provide a forum for training, practice, and developing **self-efficacy** as a nutrition research interviewer.

Defining the interview questions is related to the research objectives. The first set of questions may be brainstormed within the research team. Next, the questions generally are sent to an expert panel for review and suggestions. Note that this step also requires IRB approval at many institutions. Have a questionnaire for your expert panel to complete about the interview content and process items such as length and complexity of questions.

## Cognitive Interviewing to Refine Questions

**Cognitive interviewing** is formative work completed to be sure the questions and answers are understood by the target interviewee population. Although cognitive interviewing has its roots in police questioning, it is now often used to conduct "face validation" of questionnaires.[12,13] This type of pilot testing is also considered human research and will require IRB approval at most universities.[14]

The cognitive interviewing approach begins with an explanation of the process to the interviewee, as in the following example:

> Our goal today is to get a better idea of how the questions are being interpreted by different people and if the current wording is understandable and make sense. To do this, I would like you to "think aloud" as you answer the questions. By "think aloud," I mean to please say out loud what you are thinking when I read the question or as you try to answer the question.
>
> At times, I'll stop to ask you questions about specific words, your interpretation of a question, your interpretation of the possible answers, or to repeat things back to me in your own words.
>
> Please keep in mind that I want to hear all of your opinions and reactions. Don't hesitate to speak up whenever something seems unclear, is hard to answer, or doesn't seem to apply to you. There are no wrong or right answers, and all of your thoughts or questions will have value to me.

Before conducting a cognitive interview, you need the questionnaire including any closed-end responses, a set of prompts for areas where you want more information in particular, and to practice asking the questions. Practice with a colleague and digitally record the session. Listen to the session yourself, and ask a third party to also provide feedback on what you the interviewer did well, what may need more practice, and any

**VIEWPOINT**

## Health and Nutrition Blogs

*Robin Rood, RD, LD, MED, MA*

Nutrition blogs are the latest source of information available to consumers who are trying to make changes to their diets. Easy-to-find nutrition and diet-related answers are available among the hundreds of blogs found on the Internet. Some Internet sites even review nutrition blogs. A quick review of many of the personal nutrition blogs out there shows a few things they have in common.

First, they all have clever names or titles that often reflect the author's personal story or philosophy about diet and nutrition.

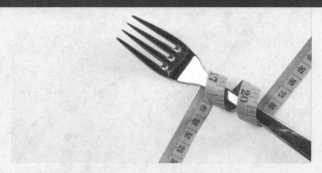
© Kenishirotie/Shutterstock.

Also, the nutritional blogosphere includes dedicated sites from national organizations such as the American Heart Association (www.heart.org).

The Academy of Nutrition and Dietetics blog called Stone Soup (www.foodandnutrition.org/Stone-Soup/) is connected to the Academy's *Food and Nutrition* magazine. Stone Soup is written by RDNs and includes information and recipes on all topics of nutrition, including discussions of paleo and vegan diets, two of the most popular topics in the personal nutrition genre.

Robin's paleo lifestyle

Next, the photography of the food items they promote are beautiful.

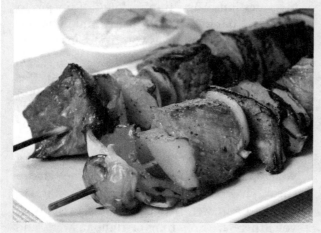
© David P. Smith/Shutterstock.

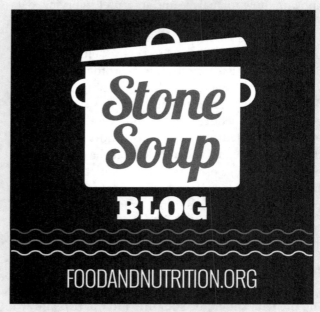
Stone Soup BLOG

FOODANDNUTRITION.ORG

Courtesy of Academy of Nutrition and Dietetics.

There are often recipes to follow or videos to watch that impress the viewer with how simple it is to follow their food plan or lifestyle.

Even the best-written opinion should not be confused with evidence. Although personal testimonials are helpful, they are no substitute for scientific, evidence-based nutrition information or medical recommendations, and they definitely do not replace a visit to an RDN or physician if there is a real medical concern.

The federal government also offers current discussions on healthy nutrition plans, agriculture, and food-labeling laws on the Food and Drug Administration (www.fda.gov) and US Department of Agriculture (www.usda.gov) websites.

Frequently, blogs offer free advice but without includ-ing any way of fact-checking their information— even

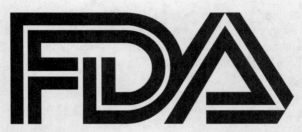

Reproduced from FDA.gov.

when presenting readers the option to purchase items such as supplements, books, or cooking tools. Finally, many blogs may be legitimate sites, but some may be scams with information that is inaccurate or even dangerous. Extreme dieting and leaving out major food groups for no good reason is no way to stay healthy no matter how many followers a nutrition blogger has

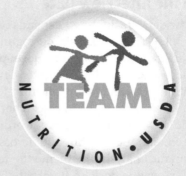

Reproduced from USDA.

acquired. Ask questions and keep doing research to find the answers you are looking for to achieve good health. The Internet is a powerful tool for finding good nutrition information.

areas of concern. It is important that the interviewer be very relaxed and comfortable with the questionnaire, the probes, and the process of cognitive interviewing.[13]

Between five and 15 interviewees should be scheduled for cognitive interviewing, depending on the diversity of the population the questionnaire will be assessing. Demographics that may affect the responses should be represented in those participating in cognitive interviewing. For instance, if the questionnaire is about snack choices, then age, income, occupation, dietary concerns, medical conditions, and other demographics would be important. However, if the questionnaire was to be used with male adults with type 2 diabetes between ages 45 and 60 years, some of these would not be important, but having a meal plan, their self-efficacy to follow a meal plan, and medications may be important.[13]

Once a round of interviews is completed, the group developing the questionnaire should discuss the responses and decide what to change. The cognitive interviews resume with any participants in the first round whose responses resulted in a change. The entire questionnaire can be reviewed or just those sections that required changing. Through this iterative process, the questionnaire is developed with relevance and understanding by the target group.[13]

## Personal Skills in Interviewing

Successful interviewing does not come easily to everyone. The successful interviewer will be able to quickly develop rapport with the interviewee. Having a neutral or slightly positive affect and body position is important. Being too encouraging can compromise data if the interviewee tries to please the interviewer to gain

acceptance. Practicing interpersonal nonverbal skills with a colleague, videotapes, or self-assessment can help.

Nonverbal communication includes facial expressions, gestures, and body positions. The amount of eye contact can depend on the interviewee's status relative to the interviewer and cultural background. Too much eye contact can be intimidating; zero eye contact can show distrust or lack of interest. Nodding slightly once in a while can be encouraging, but enthusiastic agreement can sway the interviewee's responses. Nervous or subconscious gestures or movements can convey impatience. These might include biting the lip, looking at a watch or phone, or tapping the foot.

At the beginning of the interview, the interviewer should explain the nature of the research to engage the interviewee's interest and "buy in" and increase the chance of getting quality data. Developing a common ground and empathy for the research can help establish an open and positive relationship during the interview. If the interviewee trusts the interviewer and sincerely wants to provide quality information, then he or she will think about the questions and provide robust responses. The interviewer has to actively listen and allow pauses without rushing the interviewee.[15]

Research interviews involve fewer numbers of participants than do **quantitative** research efforts that collect numbers such as demographics, surveys, and biochemical data. The purpose of the research interviews is to probe more deeply into people's thoughts and feelings than might be achievable in a survey. Interviews are a type of **qualitative research** in which the interviews are data and are continued to be collected until **saturation** occurs, which means no additional or new themes or thoughts are being offered by the interviewees.

## Analyzing the Interview Data

How interview data are analyzed depends on the purpose of the interviews. Analysis of cognitive interviewing is targeted at refining the questionnaire as previously described. Analysis of interview data to answer qualitative research questions may follow several formats. In content analysis, researchers look for how often and in what context certain words, phrases, or themes are mentioned within and across all interviews. In thematic analysis, the theme the researchers are looking for may be decided before the interviews or as a result of reading the interviews. In general, a code book is developed to inform the coders or researchers as they analyze the interviews. The code book describes phrases or words that allow researchers to compare and synthesize the data.

More than one coder should always be used so that interpretation is not biased. Coders should first become familiar with all the data. After interviews are coded and disagreements resolved, themes among the data are usually extracted to provide meaning and interpretation of the interviews. This is often described as an inductive approach using content analysis. However, **qualitative data** analysis is much more complex than already briefly described, and resources for further reading or training are provided (**TABLE 11.2**).

---

**TABLE 11.2** Qualitative methods resources

**Articles**

Swift JA, Tischler V. Qualitative research in nutrition and dietetics: getting started. *J Hum Nutr Diet*. 2010; Dec;23(6):559–566.

Draper A, Swift JA. Qualitative research in nutrition and dietetics: data collection issues. *J Hum Nutr Diet*. 2011; Feb;24(1):3–12.

Goodell LS, Stage VC, Cooke NK. Practical qualitative research strategies: Training interviewers and coders. *J Nutr Educ Behav*. 2016; Sep;48(8):578–585.

**Webinars**

Society for Nutrition Education. What is qualitative research? https://vimeo.com/32724104.

Sage Publishing. Successful qualitative research. http://connection.sagepub.com/blog/sage-connection/2015/06/02/successful-qualitative-research-webinar-recording-with-extended-qa/.

---

**Recap** Basic communication skills for the nutrition researcher involve written, oral, and body language. The targeted audiences for nutrition researchers vary, from institutional compliance offices to the layperson audience to the science community and also news media. Communication skills learned as a researcher will provide a robust framework for health coaching skills.

# ▶ Nutrition Counseling Skills for Providing Medical Nutrition Therapy

**Preview** Effective communication skills are paramount in counseling clients regarding health promotion and disease management. Nutrition education and counseling rely on establishing good rapport, assessing health literacy, and determining motivation and readiness to implement new knowledge.

Nutrition counseling is an opportunity to combine science and art—applying the scientific concepts of nutrition and physiology with the art of counseling for behavior change. This section presents the skills and strategies for successful counseling when providing **medical nutrition therapy (MNT)**. The registered dietitian nutritionist (RDN) should have a toolbox full of options to tackle the range of clients and situations. The skills and strategies discussed here should be practiced; this may be in a "safe" role-play environment, then implemented in the counseling situation, and revisited as needed to hone the skills.

## Counseling Spectrum: Client Focused

Successful counseling for behavior change and implementation of MNT involves a client-centered (or patient-centered) approach. This individualized model may apply evidence-based treatment guidelines with the focus on the client at that time; the role of the counselor is to help the client become independent and move to self-management. Clients who are empowered will find **internal motivation** to change and implement health behaviors for disease prevention or disease management. Client-focused counseling puts the client and the healthcare team members on an even level. The client should be an informed and active participant in the treatment options and care plan, whereas the healthcare team works in a proactive and interprofessional manner to bring in community resources and navigate the health system.[16,17] For example, to control dyslipidemia, the National Lipid Association recommends a patient-centered approach with the first-line treatment being lifestyle interventions related to dietary intake and physical activity. The clinician and the patient should discuss the alternatives, including lipid-lowering drugs for their potential benefits and side effects. The informed patient can then set goals with all the treatment options based on his or her readiness to change. More details on counseling based on stages of change are discussed later in this chapter. Ideally, patients would try diet and physical activity interventions and move to pharmaceutical treatments if those lifestyle changes fail to produce the intended effect.[18,19]

## Establishing Rapport

Establishing good rapport is one key to successful nutrition counseling. Effective counselors form a bond with their clients while maintaining a professional relationship. Good first impressions are critical for good rapport; both the counselor and the client will observe each other and form an opinion at first sight. The counselor must be perceived as professional, knowledgeable, approachable, unbiased, and nonjudgmental. Counselors do not have the tools or the wisdom to know which clients will be successful and which will require long durations of counseling over time or revising goals that are not achievable.[20,21]

To establish rapport, greet the client with a smile and a friendly tone of voice. A handshake is customary in most circumstances in the United States. Consider the situation of the ambulatory clinic setting versus a home care setting or an in-patient acute-care or rehabilitation setting; each may warrant its own modified greeting. A handshake, for example, may be appropriate in an ambulatory setting but may not be possible in an acute-care setting. After the friendly greeting, most rapport is built with small talk about the weather or the time of the year and current events. The counselor can ask about the client's plans for summer vacation or talk about last night's baseball game.[22]

In a counseling atmosphere in which the counselor will interact with clients repeatedly over time, good rapport can build at each encounter. Writing or recording notes about what is important to a client for follow-up at subsequent appointments can be useful. For example, if client Sue mentions she is going to visit her daughter Fiona in Boston for the holidays, it will resonate with her if the counselor asks about the trip at the next appointment with Sue. Most people like to talk about themselves and what is important to them; they will respond favorably to a counselor who remembers and cares. However, set boundaries to maintain the professional counselor–client relationship. Sharing too much personal information can sabotage counseling progress and detract from the current agenda.[23]

## Nutrition and Health Literacy

Before counseling and education, the counselor must establish the client's **health literacy**, or "the degree to which individuals have the capacity to obtain, process, and understand basic health information and services needed to make appropriate health decisions."[24] The prevalence of poor health literacy nationwide is unknown. However, one study of an academic hospital in Vermont found 605 of the inpatients had poor health literacy.[25] The 2003 National Assessment of Adult Literacy included a health literacy section, and researchers concluded that 12% of adults did not even have basic health literacy, 53% had intermediate literacy, and just 12% had proficient health literacy.[26]

Health literacy varies for each individual based on his or her own knowledge and skill and that of the healthcare system and situation. Achieving and maintaining

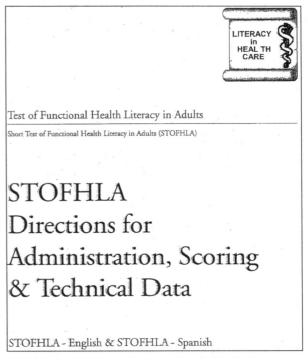

health literacy is essential to navigating healthcare resources, asking the right questions to understand treatment options, and obtaining referrals for appropriate healthcare providers. Health literacy is also critical to treatment success and managing chronic disease, for example, managing good blood sugar control at and in between meal times, and long term for understanding and achieving optimal glycosylated hemoglobin.[27,28,29,30,31] Without being health literate, clients may not appreciate the relationship between dietary intake and health promotion and disease outcomes.

There are several measures of health and **nutrition literacy**, including the Shortened Test of Functional Health Literacy in Adults (S-TOFHL),[32,33] the Newest Vital Sign (NVS),[34] the Rapid Estimate of Adult Literacy Measure (REALM),[35] and the Nutrition Literacy Assessment (NLA).[36]

The S-TOFHL measures reading comprehension and numeracy and requires seven or so minutes to complete. It is available in English, four other languages, and electronically. The test uses a cloze format in which clients complete multiple-choice sentences. The passage topics reflect preparation for an upper gastrointestinal test and patient rights and responsibilities on a Medicaid form.

The NVS measures literacy and numeracy using a Nutrition Facts Label and six questions in English and Spanish. This tool has been validated against the TOFHLA, and has been shown to take about three minutes to administer.

NVS questionnaire

| Question | Answer | Points: for every correct answer- allow 1 point |
|---|---|---|
| Read to participant: this information is on the back of a container of a pint of ice cream. | | |
| 1. If you eat the entire container, how many calories will you eat? | 1,000 | |
| 2. If you are allowed to eat 60 grams of carbohydrates as a snack, how much ice cream could you have? | Possible answers: 1 cup (or any variation up to 1 cup), half the container. | |
| 3. Your doctor advises you to reduce the amount of saturated fat in your diet. You usually have 42 g of saturated fat each day, which includes one serving of ice cream. If you stop eating ice cream, how many grams of saturated fat would you be consuming each day? | 33 | |
| 4. If you usually eat 2,500 calories in a day, what percentage of your daily value of calories will you be eating if you eat one serving? | 10% | |
| Read to participant: pretend that you are allergic to the following substance: penicillin, peanuts, latex gloves, and bee stings. | | |
| 5. Is it safe for you to eat this ice cream? | No | |
| 6. If the answer t question 5 is no, ask: why not? | Due to the presence of peanut oil | |

| Score |
|---|
| 0-1= high likelihood (50% or more) of limited literacy |
| 2-3= the possibility of limited literacy |
| 4-6= adequate literacy |

The REALM consists of 66 words that the client reads aloud and is available in English and Spanish. A short form includes 18 words and their relationships with two additional words each.

The NLA, now referred to as NLit, includes sections on nutrition and health (10 items), energy sources in food (10 items), household food measurement (nine items), food labels and numeracy (10 items), consumer skills (nine items), and food groups (16 items). It has also been adapted for use by

| List 1 | List 2 | List 3 |
| --- | --- | --- |
| fat | fatigue | allergic |
| flu | pelvic | menstrual |
| pill | jaundice | testicle |
| dose | infection | colitis |
| eye | exercise | emergency |
| stress | behavior | medication |
| smear | prescription | occupation |
| nerves | notify | sexually |
| germs | gallbladder | alcoholism |
| meals | calories | irritation |
| disease | depression | constipation |
| cancer | miscarriage | gonorrhea |
| caffeine | pregnancy | inflammatory |
| attack | arthritis | diabetes |
| kidney | nutrition | hepatitis |
| hormones | menopause | antibiotics |
| herpes | appendix | diagnosis |
| seizure | abnormal | potassium |
| bowel | syphilis | anemia |
| asthma | hemorrhoids | obesity |
| rectal | nausea | osteoporosis |
| incest | directed | impetigo |

patients with breast cancer[37] and for parents of children receiving nutritional counseling.[38] The measure is not yet available publicly but can be obtained from the author on request.

A listing and PDF versions of several health literacy tools are available through the National Library of Medicine (http://healthliteracy.bu.edu/).

## Readiness to Change

After building rapport and assessing health literacy, the counselor may assess the client's readiness to change. The transtheoretical model applies constructs from several theories on change and is depicted in five steps in the **stages of change** representation in **TABLE 11.3**.[39] Clients may progress through the stages in a linear manner, and they may also recycle through the stages until the new behavior is a habit.[39]

## Setting an Agenda

Once the counselor has assessed the client's readiness to change and determined that the client is in the action phase, the counselor should establish a plan for the session. Setting an agenda for the counseling session is a useful tool for starting MNT in a client-centered manner. Depending on the counselor's practice setting, the agenda may be dictated by the constraints of time and environment. In an acute setting, for example, extensive counseling may not be appropriate based on the stage of change, the time available for discussion, and the hospital setting. In this case, a client-centered agenda informs the counselor of the most important topics to discuss before the client is discharged; additional counseling can then be part of the coordination of care when the client is stable and has more time to focus and learn. Alternatively, in the ambulatory clinic setting or home care with an hour appointment and opportunities for follow-up, the counselor may ask the client to set an agenda with a broader scope. This reveals the client's priorities to the counselor, which is helpful in understanding what is important to address in the session. The counselor may augment the agenda based on what he or she feels the client must know and to set goals before the session ends. The agenda may be consulted on subsequent appointments, with agenda items used to reinforce prior concepts and then be revised as necessary.[23]

## Approach to Intervention

With the agenda set, the counselor can work with the client and approach the behavior change with intervention strategies. Behavioral counseling interventions may be done in one or more interactions, but

**TABLE 11.3** Stages of change in the transtheoretical model

| Stages of Change | Characteristics | Counseling Approach |
|---|---|---|
| Precontemplation | The client does not intend to make changes in the next six months; may be characterized as resistant or not ready. | The client may not be motivated, which may be the result of a knowledge deficit. |
| Contemplation | The client intends to make changes in the next six months, is aware of the pros and cons of changing, and may be contemplating the costs and benefits of change. | The client may be receptive to learning facts but is not expected to act immediately. |
| Preparation | The client is ready to make changes within the month; he or she may have made some decisions or have taken some action to plan to change. | The counselor should use appropriate skills and techniques to discuss behavior change. |
| Action | The client is taking action to change. | The counselor should use appropriate skills and techniques to help the client change behavior. |
| Maintenance | The client has made changes and works to prevent relapse; the client is confident he or she can continue healthy behavior. | The counselor may have less-frequent contact with the client and may serve a supportive role as needed. |

Adapted from Prochaska J, DiClemente C. Stages and processes of self-change of smoking: Toward an integrative model of change. *Clin Psychol.* 1983;51(3):390-395.

the intent is to engage the client in self-management practices that are aimed at health promotion and disease prevention. **TABLE 11.4** lists the **Five A's** that can help the counselor work through intervention steps to help the client adopt healthier behaviors.[40,41]

The first step is to *assess* or *ask*; the counselor inquires about the behavior. To ascertain if a client meets the guidelines for physical activity (PA), the counselor would ask what type of PA, including its frequency, intensity, and duration. If the client does not meet the guidelines for PA, then the counselor's second step is to *advise* on the recommendations for PA. Then in a client-centered approach to behavior change, the counselor and the client *agree* on a goal; in this third step, the counselor is *assisting* the client to make a reasonable goal. The final step is to *arrange* a plan for follow-up.

## Establishing and Prioritizing Goals

Working with an agenda and an intervention approach, the client can develop goals with the guidance of the counselor. Goals should be client centered and attainable. **TABLE 11.5** describes **SMART goals**. Each letter of the acronym describes a goal that is reasonable and achievable within a practical time frame.[42]

**TABLE 11.4** Five major steps to intervention (The five A's)

| Step | Intervention |
|---|---|
| Assess (Ask) | Identify the behavior (e.g., tobacco use). |
| Advise | Encourage the client to stop the unhealthy behavior (e.g., quit tobacco use) or promote the healthy behavior (e.g., choose a physical activity). |
| Agree | In a client-centered approach, the client agrees to attempt to change a behavior. |
| Assist | The counselor helps the patient with a plan for behavior change. |
| Arrange | The counselor and client agree to a follow-up plan. |

Adapted from Whitlock EP, Orleans CT, Pender N, Allan J. Evaluating primary care behavioral counseling interventions: an evidence-based approach. *Am J Prev Med.* 2002;22(4):267-84 and Agency for Healthcare Research and Quality. Five Major Steps to Intervention (The 5A's"). 2012. Available at http://www.ahrq.gov/professional/clinicians-providers/guidelines-recommendations/tobacco/5steps.html.

**TABLE 11.5** Setting SMART goals

| Term | Attribute | Example |
|------|-----------|---------|
| **S**pecific | The more specific, the better (who, what, where, when, why, how) | John decides to lose 10 pounds in the next three months. |
| **M**easurable | How will the goal attainment be measured? | John will weigh himself weekly on Wednesday mornings. |
| **A**ttainable | Is the goal achievable? Is it possible? | John will work with the RDN to change his dietary intake to reduce 500 calories a day. |
| **R**ealistic | Is the goal reasonable within a timeline? | On a 500-calorie day deficit, John could lose a pound a week. |
| **T**imely | Set a realistic timeline for accountability. | John will communicate with the RDN every two weeks by email and provide updates on his progress. |

Data from Bowman J, Mogensen L, Marsland E, Lannin N. The development, content validity and inter-rater reliability of the SMART-goal evaluation method: A standardised method for evaluating clinical goals. *Aust Occup Ther J.* 2015; 62(6):420–427.

## Strategies to Facilitate Behavior Change

Once goals are set, the counselor can help the client stay on track with self-monitoring techniques. The counselor may have many strategies in his or her coaching toolbox, so it is important to offer a few strategies and help the client choose what might work best and understand that he or she can employ various strategies in different circumstances because behavior change is fluid. Self-monitoring techniques are rooted in cognitive behavior theory; these will be addressed later in this chapter but are summarized in this section and in **TABLE 11.6**.

Setting goals is usually the first step in promoting behavior change. SMART goals are a good way to ensure the goals are reasonable and attainable. Long-range goals may need to be developed over time using more-proximal goals so that the client realizes success and does not get frustrated at the apparent lack of progress. In addition, goals should be related to a behavior rather than a physiological outcome because the client is in control of the behavior. For example, if a long-term goal is to reduce total cholesterol and improve HDL cholesterol, then behavior-change goals may be related to changing dietary intake and increasing aerobic exercise.

Self-monitoring is an important strategy in achieving goals and desirable behaviors. It can make the client accountable to the steps needed to bring about change. Examples are a food diary that can track calories, fat, or carbohydrates or an activity log that tracks steps taken or heart rate.

Frequent contact between client and counselor can help keep the client more committed to continuing positive behavioral change. Frequent contact may also be in the form of peer support and can be done in person or using **telehealth**.

The counselor who provides feedback and reinforcement helps facilitate behavior change by showing clients how their choices create progress toward their goals. Feedback can also be used to revise goals or make new goals based on a client's success.

*Self-efficacy* refers to a client's perception of his or her ability to make behavior change. This perception may be enhanced in four ways.[43] First, *mastery of a skill* refers to the client making simple behavior changes such as choosing to drink water instead of a sugar-sweetened beverage. Second, *modeling a behavior* can be as simple as watching someone engaged in a healthy behavior. Third, *verbal persuasion* can take the form of coaching or peer support groups. Fourth, *physiological feedback* comes when the body responds to the behavioral change.

External incentives may be another strategy for implementing behavior change as a reward for attaining a goal. Financial incentives may be used by an employer or health insurance company. Tangible incentives may also be arranged such as getting a manicure or a new pair of pants for accomplishing a goal.

The modeling strategy involves the client being able to observe or speak with someone who has successfully implemented change. The model should be credible and similar to the client looking to make the change. A single mom of three young children, for example, may not relate to a model of an older retired man but may relate to a mom who has managed to include her children in the process of changing her behavior.

Problem solving has five components: (1) identify the problem, (2) identify solutions, (3) evaluate the positive and negative attributes of the solutions, (4) implement a solution, and (5) measure its success in achieving behavior change. Problem solving may be

**TABLE 11.6** Strategies for behavior change

| Strategy | Principle | Example of Client Behavior |
|---|---|---|
| Goal setting | Set SMART goals (see previous section). | Cut up an apple before leaving the house and eat it on the commute to work at least three days a week to increase fruit intake. |
| Self-monitoring | Identify cues to behaviors and obtain progress to goal. | Use a food log to track saturated fat intake. |
| Frequent contact | Establish trust with a counselor and develop accountability; may include peer support or group contact. | Connect with a counselor using telehealth to monitor body weight every Wednesday morning. |
| Feedback and reinforcement | Provide data on progress to goal; supports behavior change. | Receive advice on the food log; encourage good behaviors. |
| Self-efficacy enhancement | Highlight how a client perceives his or her ability to make behavioral change. | Walk a mile to the store rather than use the car for a short errand. |
| Incentives | Set tangible rewards for goal attainment. | Get a manicure when 5 pounds have been lost. |
| Modeling | Observe another person who has been successful at change. | Attend a fitness class to observe the instructor's technique. |
| Problem solving | Explore client's barriers to success and brainstorm strategies to overcome them. | Rain may interfere with walking, so client opts to walk briskly through the mall. |
| Relapse prevention | Deviations from goals may be brief relapses in behavior change; client identifies possible relapse. | Identify healthy food choices for an anticipated holiday meal. |

Modified from Artinian NT, Fletcher GF, Mozaffarian D, Kris-Etherton P, Van Horn L, Lichtenstein AH, et al. Interventions to Promote Physical Activity and Dietary Lifestyle Changes for Cardiovascular Risk Factor Reduction in Adults: A Scientific Statement From the American Heart Association. *Circulation*. 2010;122(4):406-441.

used when a barrier to change is anticipated such as bad weather that may interfere with outdoor physical activity or an office party that may stymie efforts at calorie control.

Counselors may discuss relapse prevention as a strategy to successful behavior change; in doing so, they teach the client that relapse may happen but that it can be a normal part of change. Recognizing that relapse may occur, the client may feel less failure and better prepared to resume the desired behaviors. Some of the aforementioned strategies can be useful in relapse prevention such as modeling, feedback and reinforcement, self-efficacy enhancement, and problem solving.

## Management of Roadblocks to Success

Counselors need to recognize that changing behavior is difficult. First, the client must buy into the need for change before making the actual behavioral change. Promoting change may mean a change in habits and a change in the antecedents or cues for the current behavior. For example, if a client has a current behavior of buying a coffee and breakfast pastry from the coffee shop in the lobby of his office building, the counselor and client must recognize that it may be impossible to enter the building from another door to avoid the cue (coffee shop), so the approach to change may be for the client to bring healthy breakfast foods to the office to have on hand.

## HIGHLIGHT

A recent survey study of dietitians in Australia, New Zealand, and Great Britain found that smartphone health applications (apps) were being used by more than half of respondents, primarily to provide information and patient self-monitoring.[1] Systematic reviews of the efficacy of health apps in achieving behavior goals are promising but inconclusive.[2]

Health apps might be more effective if professionals were involved in the development of these apps. A survey of more than 100,000 apps found that only 17 had been developed with identifiable nutrition professional input.[3] An evaluation of features in diet-tracking apps found that all used food-item entry or barcode scanning. The authors suggested that voice recognition, image scanning, and artificial intelligence were emerging features for app improvements.[4] Culturally appropriate apps in language other than English and at varying levels of health literacy are also needed.[5]

### References

1. Chen J, Lieffers J, Bauman A, Hanning R, Allman-Farinelli M. The use of smartphone health apps and other mobile health (mHealth) technologies in dietetic practice: A three country study. *J Hum Nutr Diet*. 2017. https://www.ncbi.nlm.nih.gov/pubmed/28116773.

2. Schoeppe S, Alley S, Lippevelde W, et al. Efficacy of interventions that use apps to improve diet, physical activity and sedentary behaviour: A systematic review. *Int Nutr Phys Act*. 2016; 13(1):127.

3. Nikolaou CK, Lean ME. Mobile applications for obesity and weight management: Current market characteristics. *Int Lond*. 2017; 41(1):200–202.

4. Franco RZ, Fallaize R, Lovegrove JA, Hwang F. Popular nutrition-related mobile apps: Assessment. *JMIR Mhealth Uhealth*. 2016; 4(3).

5. Coughlin SS, Hardy D, Caplan LS. The need for culturally tailored smartphone applications for weight control. *J Ga Public Health Assoc*. 2016; Winter;5(3):228–232.

Another roadblock to success may involve the client's social circle and subjective norms, which may be personal interactions at work, in social circumstances, or at home with significant others. For example, a norm at the office may be going out to lunch every Friday. If the behaviors of the office workers are to choose less-healthy options, the client trying to change behavior may feel the pressure to conform and then abandon the strategies to attain the SMART goals. Another example may be that significant others in the home environment are not supportive of the clients' goals and behaviors. Counselors can coach clients to be aware of putative roadblocks and discuss potential obstacles with significant others. Raising awareness may be a way to mitigate the roadblocks. The section titled "Social Cognitive Theory" in this chapter elaborates on expectancies and beliefs, evaluative standards, and self-efficacy.

**Recap** In a successful counseling session, the health coach or clinician assesses the client's readiness to change, nutrition, and health literacy. The coach or clinician helps set client-centered SMART goals and strategizes on plans to manage roadblocks to success. Clients should feel empowered to implement behavior change and skills for goal attainment.

## ▶ Counseling Theories and Techniques

**Preview** Counseling theories and techniques help the health coach address issues that are important to achieving behavior change.

### Cognitive Behavior Therapy

**Cognitive behavior therapy (CBT)** is a psychotherapy approach to helping clients improve their perception of self, situations, and environments as a way to changing their behavior. After identifying erroneous or deleterious beliefs and perceptions, the client or patient is guided in examining these in terms of the validity or reasonableness of the beliefs or perceptions, ultimately making plans and setting goals to modify thoughts and behaviors.[49]

Within the field of nutrition and dietetics, CBT is often used with weight management and eating disorders,[51] with the dietitian or nutritionist working as part of an interprofessional multidisciplinary team.[50,51] The psychologist or psychiatrist who is trained in CBT would engage the team to provide a holistic approach to the client relative to the client's weight management or eating disorders. Training in CBT is available for dietitians and nutritionists so they can also assist a client in identifying and addressing erroneous perceptions about body image, food and food intake, food environment, and triggers for overeating or restrictive eating.

Cognitive approaches have outcomes of changing or restructuring how people think or perceive themselves and their situations. Identification of negative thoughts or perceived barriers allows for goal setting, situational planning, and "self-talk" to restructure negativity. Cognitive therapy will target attitudes and perceptions. Behavioral therapy approaches have outcomes targeting specific behavioral change such as physical activity or meal plans. Behavioral therapy provides information and skills development. Although some people will refer to CBT as one specific approach, others view it as including multiple approaches. CBT is often included when the term *lifestyle management* or *lifestyle therapy* is used.[52] Indeed, many of the behavior change theories described in this section include both cognitive and behavioral aspects.

## Behavior Change Theories

Behavior change theories have been developed in psychology and the social sciences and adopted by nutrition scientists and practitioners to explain behavior as well as develop interventions and programs. A particular theory or model is used in its entirety when the theory itself is being tested for effectiveness in predicting outcomes. However, parts of theories may be used within an educational program or an intervention to change behavior.[53] The parts of theories are usually referred to as *constructs*, which means they are conceptually similar ideas. For instance, *self-efficacy* refers to believing in one's ability to complete a task or achieve a goal. For example, the construct of self-efficacy may include several perspectives on the behavior of providing a healthy meal for one's children: the ability to plan a meal, to shop for the meal, and to cook the meal.

## Health Belief Model

The **Health Belief Model (HBM)** is a health behavior change and psychological model that began with the work of Godfrey Hochbaum in the 1950s. It was developed by Irwin Rosenstock in the 1960s, and furthered by Marshal Becker and colleagues (**FIGURE 11.1**) in the US Public Health Service in the 1970s and 1980s. Researchers may extend

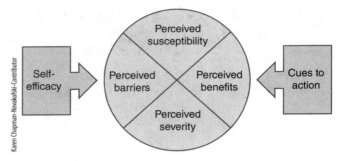

**FIGURE 11.1** The Health Belief Model.

Adapted from Becker MH (Ed.) The health belief model and personal health behavior, *Health Education Monographs* 2:324–473, 1974.

the HBM to suit their specific research questions. However, the basic HBM includes the constructs in **TABLE 11.7**.

Self-efficacy was added to the HBM, as was Cues to Action. Self-efficacy is the belief in one's abilities and Cues to Action are those occurrences that might move a person to change. In the case of calcium intake and osteoporosis, self-efficacy would be related to belief in one's ability to purchase and consume higher-calcium foods; a Cue to Action might be a relative fracturing a hip, realizing one's height has decreased, or learning how to shop and read labels to select higher-calcium foods.

The HBM is always related to a health condition, and as such, it may be used for weight reduction, diabetes, or other chronic illnesses. The HBM cannot be easily used for general health promotion, as in increased whole-grain intake, unless that behavior is associated with a disease (e.g., cancer). The HBM does not account for attitudes, beliefs, economics, or environmental factors, except as related to the six constructs as cited above.

## Theory of Reasoned Action

The **theory of reasoned action (TRA)** holds that the construct of intention is the most important determinant of behavior—that is, if a person intends to adopt a behavior, then this person is somewhat likely to do so.[54,55] The strength of the intention also helps determine the likelihood the behavior will be adopted.

Intentions and their strengths are influenced by the constructs of attitudes and subjective norms. Attitudes are favorable or unfavorable judgments about a given behavior. They can be categorized as cognitive–evaluative or affective. "Eating fruit would be good/bad, healthy/unhealthy" is an example of a cognitive–evaluative attitude. "If I ate fruit, I would

| **TABLE 11.7** Health belief model | | |
|---|---|---|
| **Perceived Susceptibility** | An individual's assessment of his or her risk of getting a condition | People may be more likely to increase their calcium intakes if they believe they are susceptible to developing osteoporosis—for instance, if relatives have osteoporosis. |
| **Perceived Severity** | An individual's assessment of the seriousness of the condition and its potential consequences | People may be more likely to increase their calcium intake if they believe that osteoporosis could cause them pain and reduce their quality of life. |
| **Perceived Barriers** | An individual's assessment of the influences that discourage adoption of the promoted behavior | People may be less likely to increase their calcium intake if they believe that high-calcium foods cost more, tastes bad, take extra time to prepare, or cause gastrointestinal disturbances. |
| **Perceived Benefits** | An individual's assessment of the positive consequences of adopting the behavior | People may be more likely to increase their calcium intake if they believe that foods high in calcium taste good, strengthen their bones, or provide good role modeling for children. |

Adapted from Becker MH (Ed.) The health belief model and personal health behavior, *Health Education Monographs* 2:324–473, 1974.

feel good/bad" is an example of an affective attitude. Subjective norms are the surrounding people who may approve or disapprove of a behavior. There could be different subjective norms for different behaviors. For instance, subjective norms for a young mother and behaviors about breastfeeding may include her spouse, mother, other relatives, friends, and health-care providers. Behaviors about physical activity may not include the mother and other relatives. If they do include the mother and other relatives, they may not be weighted similarly. That is, for some behaviors, some of our subjective norms have more influence than others. Sometimes this relative influence is described as motivation to comply with the individual subjective norm.

In the 1980s, the construct of perceived behavioral control was added to the theory of reasoned action, and the theory's name was modified to the *theory of planned behavior*.[56] *Perceived* behavioral control refers to a person's perception of control over external factors such as food costs. More recently, the theory was modified to include self-efficacy as a form of perceived control and some expansion of subjective norms to include concepts of what people *ought* to do.[56,57] See **FIGURE 11.2**.

When this theory is used in research, measurements through questionnaires of attitudes, norms, and intentions are used to predict behavior. An example is a study examining mothers' decisions to give their preschoolers a healthy diet.[58] The researchers found that attitudes, subjective norms, and perceived behavioral control predicted intention to provide a

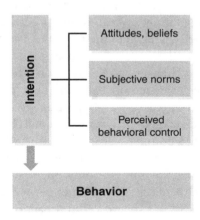

**FIGURE 11.2** Theory of planned behavior.

Adapted from Fishbein M, Ajzen I. *Belief, Attitude, Intention and Behavior: An Introduction to Theory and Research.* Reading, MA: Addison Wesley, 1975.

healthy diet. Intention and perceived behavioral control, however, predicted the behavior of providing the healthy diet.

## Social Cognitive Theory

**Social cognitive theory (SCT)** was initially developed by Albert Bandura in the 1970s.[59] The SCT focuses on four areas: (1) competencies and skills, (2) expectancies and beliefs, (3) evaluative standards, and (4) personal goals. Competencies include both declarative knowledge and procedural knowledge—that is, what needs to be in order to accomplish a task and how to do it. An example of declarative knowledge would be knowing the sodium content in food. The associated procedural knowledge would be knowing how to plan a day's food intake, shop, and cook the foods so that sodium intake is below 2,300 mg. Having both declarative and procedural knowledge prepares a person for developing the related skill.

**Outcome expectancies** and beliefs include what a person expects will occur following a particular action or behavior. Several beliefs are associated with SCT, but self-efficacy is used most often.[59] Self-efficacy is usually situational and can be influenced by mastery experiences, watching others complete tasks,[48] encouragement and support of others, time-related events, and physiological states. For instance, a person may feel she can eat five fruits and vegetables on most days because she have done this in the past (mastery) and her friend also does this. However, she may not feel able to achieve this when an upsetting personal event has occurred or when she has the flu.

Evaluative standards are those mental views of what people should do. Many parents, for example, have the evaluative standard that family members should eat their evening meals together. Because of this evaluative standard, they may have a goal of eating with the family several evenings per week. Goals help people self-regulate their behavior and organize their time and efforts.[60] Proximal goals—those that we hope to achieve in a relatively short time frame—have more influence on behavior than do distal or long-distance goals. Several proximal goals may lead to a more distal goal. An example would be a weight-loss goal of 19 pounds in six months (distal) that could be achieved by having only one sugar-sweetened beverage per week, eating out only once per week, and going to a fitness center four times per week.

Within SCT is the procedural part of the theory asserting that behavior, personal factors, and the environment interact and influence one another over time.[48] This relationship is called *reciprocal determinism*.

For example, a person may observe people at his office bring fresh fruit and vegetables for snacks (environment), self-reflect about what would happen if he also did this or if he could do this (personal factors), and then bring his own fresh fruit and vegetable snacks the next week (behavior). Over time, he may notice that some of the snacks have not been eaten or begin to rot (environment); he self-reflects to bring a smaller amount (personal) and begins to bring more realistic servings (behavior) and share with his coworkers.

> **Recap** CBT and theories of behavior change can help both the health coach and client identify strategies for behavior change. Understanding thought processes and motivators or detractors for an individual provides a framework for successful behavior change.

## ▶ Motivational Interviewing

> **Preview** Another resource in the counselor's toolbox for promoting behavior change is an approach called **motivational interviewing (MI)**. In this client-centered approach, the counselor or coach guides the conversation with the client to explore ambivalence or indecision about making healthy behavioral changes.

In health coaching, the counselor may use MI principles to help identify the client's ambivalence or indecision about making changes. In ambivalence, clients feel torn about making behavioral changes and find reasons why they cannot make those changes. A natural reaction from a healthcare provider may be to tell or dictate the healthy behaviors for health promotion and disease prevention. This reaction is referred to as the *righting reflex*.[61] This approach may backfire, however, as clients may talk themselves out of a healthy behavior in self-defense against the counselor's suggestions or directions about what they should do. This results in the so-called expert trap, in which the counselor thinks he or she can state the solutions to the client's behaviors and decisions.[61] Instead, the counselor should treat clients with "unconditional positive regard," which will allow clients to feel empowered and responsible for her own behaviors.[62] In MI, the counselor is in a partnership with clients and guides them to develop their own reasons and ways to resolve ambivalence and be successful at behavior change.

The spirit of MI is collaborative, evocative, and honors client autonomy. It is collaborative because it is seen as a partnership between the counselor and the client, rather than a coercive plan handed out from the "expert" RDN. The dietitian or nutritionist is the expect agent of change, but even so, clients have unique knowledge about themselves and are also ultimately responsible for making final decisions. In this way, MI is evocative in that the clinician coaches clients to verbalize their own motivations for change and respects that the that clients are autonomous and make their own decisions.

MI is rooted in four principles: (1) express empathy to build rapport, (2) develop discrepancy to identify the pros and cons of change, (3) roll with resistance to respect autonomy, and (4) support self-efficacy to enable change.[63] The counselor uses the MI skills of OARS: open-ended questions, affirming and supporting, reflective listening, and summarizing.

The MI approach to counseling uses questions to assess readiness to change according to the client's desire, ability, reasons, and need—which is easily remembered with the acronym DARN.[63] The counselor can assess desire, or what the client wants or likes about change; ability, or what is possible for the client to change; reasons, or why make changes; and need, or how important or urgent change might be. All of the questioning from the counselor is intended to help clients to develop their own agendas on how to make changes. This client-centered approach evokes internal motivation from within the client, which is the driver in realizing change. An example of MI in coaching follows:

Coach:  You have told me that you want to talk about carbohydrate counting; why might you want to plan your meals with carb counting? [Elicit client desire with open-ended question.]

Client:  I want to be able to have better control of my blood sugar, and I think carb counting is a way for me to stay on track in planning healthy meals.

Coach:  OK, great. How do you see carb counting fitting into your family meals? [Explore client ability to implement.]

Client:  Well, I think I can learn to make the choices for appropriate portion sizes if I understand carb counting and how it affects my blood sugar goals. [Reason.] I'm just not sure if I

| **TABLE 11.8**  Motivational interviewing resources |
|---|
| Motivational Interviewing, an MI learning resource: www.motivationalinterviewing.org |
| Molly Kellogg, RD, LCSW, for Nutrition and Health Professionals: www.mollykellogg.com |
| Rollnick S, Miller WR, Butler CC. *Motivational Interviewing in Health Care: Helping Patients Change Behavior*. New York, NY: The Guilford Press; 2008. |
| Clifford D, Curtis L. *Motivational Interviewing in Nutrition and Fitness*. New York, NY: The Guilford Press; 2016. |

can stop myself from going back for seconds! [Ambivalence.]

Coach:  So it sounds like you have the desire for better blood sugar control, but you are not sure that you can successfully follow carb counting. [Reflective.] How important is it for you? [Need.]

Client:  Good blood sugar control is important for my long-term health. I do not want to suffer complications of high blood sugar. I think carb counting will help me, and I have to think of my future and my health for my family. Maybe I can have seconds on the low-carb foods that we have for dinner.

Coach:  Okay, so we will review carb counting and make a plan for you to choose the appropriate amount of carbohydrates per meal and allow for some additional foods that will not adversely affect your blood sugar. Eating healthy can improve your glucose control over the long term to prevent complications. [Summarize.]

The details of the process of MI are beyond the scope of this chapter, but numerous resources are available to counselors. See **TABLE 11.8** for a list of print and online resources as well as training options.

**Recap**  Clinicians engaged in health coaching can use principles of MI to help clients identify their internal motivations to engage in behavior change. MI is especially useful if clients are reluctant or ambivalent about implementing healthy behaviors.

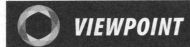
## VIEWPOINT

### Building Motivational Interviewing Skills

*Deidra Devereaux, MS, RDN*

Counseling techniques in the nutrition field have been refined, with growing empirical evidence of their effectiveness over more than two decades.[1] Motivational interviewing (MI) is now a preferred technique and critical skill for dietitians and other health-related counselors. Founders Miller and Rollnick most recently define MI as a collaborative, person-centered form of guiding to elicit and strengthen motivation for change.[2] We will reference a case study of one memorable patient in long-term care who was preretirement and immobile, with weight approaching 400 pounds. She has been my most ambivalent client, and I will reference our experience as we progress through MI's key components.

The "spirit of MI" includes three fundamental components.

1. *Collaboration.* There is a dual expert role between client and counselor, allowing the person to be an expert in their own health care based on change talk, values and beliefs.

2. *Evocation.* Conversations should lead to evoking "change talk", where the person opens up about his or her desire, ability, and need to change.

3. *Autonomy.* Respect for the person and their ultimate desire or lack thereof establishes a framework of trust and a safe space to explore ambivalence to change.

In practice, after you acquire the technical knowledge needed to facilitate improved health behaviors, in your capacity as counselor you will guide patients and build on their personal motivation to change. Because it can be faster and easier to provide education without considering a patient's values or readiness to change, success in MI requires consistent focus on motivational techniques to refine skills needed to generate positive outcomes for the patient's nutrition goals.[3] As seen with the case study, it was her experience that all dietitians are food police. I had to reassess the need to control her food intake through diet restriction (as the physician desired) because she had a wealth of nutrition knowledge from prior experience but was unmotivated. Once her diet was liberalized, trust was building in partnership with autonomy. Although MI takes time and commitment, gradually applying some or all of the principles and interventions within the context of the "spirit of MI" can help patients achieve success in changing their behavior. See **FIGURE A**.

To start, dietitians working with patients and clients should review and practice the following MI principles:

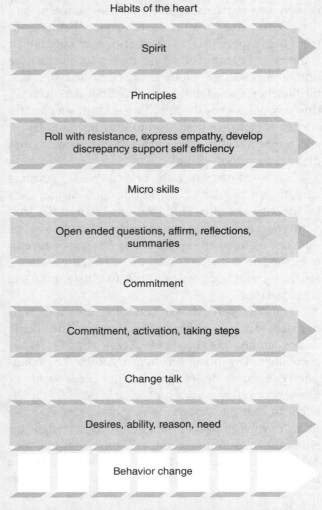

**FIGURE A** The Framework of Motivational Interviewing.

Data from Messina J. Overview of Motivational Interviewing. Coping.us. http://coping.us/motivationalinterviewing/overviewofmi.html. Date unknown.

*Roll with resistance.* Avoid potential confrontations with clients by allowing them to freely voice their apprehensions about change.

*Support self-efficacy.* Recognize the strengths presented by clients and emphasize skills they demonstrate that will contribute to their success.

*Express empathy.* Provide clients the opportunity to see the understanding of their perspective to increase authentic exchanges.

*Develop discrepancy.* Gradually guide clients to realize the gap between their goal and their current behaviors.

In our case study counseling sessions—informal meetings in a patient room—the client was most concerned about being hungry, recognizing her caloric needs were greater than her "thinner" neighbors.

I concurred that enjoying meals and feeling full were important (empathy). So we set our collaborative plan that gave her the ability to select her meals independently. The core skills that were used to motivate this patient were the open questions, affirmation, reflective listening, and summary reflections (OARS) of MI.

To be successful with clients using MI, healthcare providers should review and practice MI micro skills (or OARS), including:

*Open-ended questions.* Receive more information by asking more why and how questions or, when presented with short responses, "Tell me more about that."

*Affirmations.* Draw attention to character strengths and skills to build client confidence.

*Reflections.* Paraphrase frequently; to work toward goal setting, reword to provide understanding of the client's feelings.

*Summaries.* Reviewing each topic or discussion builds positive repetition, displays active listening, and reflects on the client's perspective.

For most nutrition professionals who work outside the outpatient setting, lengthy counseling sessions are rare.[3] In these instances, techniques can be practiced in microsessions. All nutrition counseling should allow for demonstrated effective listening, open-ended questions, and time to address change talk and move toward providing client-centered education. With time limitations, focus on MI principles: express empathy and reflect with clients, support self-efficacy by guiding with their knowledge, and work through resistance.[4] This could mean a daily visit to your patient during in a short 15-minute stay to listen and support patient nonconformity to previous diet recommendations.

Regardless of limitations in implementing MI in counseling, training and practice will improve counseling skills and can lead to behavior change.[5–7] In the case of the morbidly obese patient, after weeks of microcounseling to understand and support her knowledge and beliefs, I learned that her goal was to eventually walk again if she lost enough weight. Indeed, she gained the confidence needed to lose 50 pounds during my "MI-based nutrition care" and continued on a self-motivated journey toward her goals.

### References

1. Lundahl BW, Kunz C, Brownell C, Tollefson D, Burke BL. A meta-analysis of motivational interviewing: Twenty-five years of empirical studies. *Res Social Work Pract.* 2010; 20(2):137-160. doi: 10.1177/1049731509347850.

2. Miller WR, Rollnick S. Ten things that motivational interviewing is not. *Behav Cogn Psychother.* 2009; 37,129-140. doi: 10.1017/S1352465809005128.

3. Lu AH, Dollahite J. Assessment of dietitians' nutrition counselling self-efficacy and its positive relationship to reported skill usage. *J Hum Nutr Diet.* 2010; 23(2):144-153. doi: 10.1111/j.1365-277X.2009.01024.x.

4. Miller WR, Rollnick S. *Motivational Interviewing: Helping People Change.* 3rd ed. New York, NY: Guilford Press; 2012.

5. Van Wormer JJ, Boucher JL. Motivational interviewing and diet modification: A review of the evidence. *Diabetes Ed.* 2004; 30(3):404-419.

6. Madson MB, Loignon AC, Lane C. Training in motivational interviewing: A systematic review. *J Subst Abuse Treat.* 2009; 36(1):101-109.

7. Armstrong MJ, Mottershead TA, Ronksley PE, Sigal RJ, Campbell TS, Hemmelgarn BR. Motivational interviewing to improve weight loss in overweight and/or obese patients: A systematic review and meta-analysis of randomized controlled trials. *Obes Rev.* 2011; 12(9):709-723. doi: 10.1111/j.1467-789X.2011.00892.x.

# ▶ Successful Implementation of Lifestyle Changes

**Preview** Health coaching has brought positive outcomes for a variety of professionals and their peers. Training for health coaching varies and is unregulated. Research evaluating health coaching has found goal setting and individualization to be important components of success.

Successful implementation of lifestyle changes can be supported by a health coach, nutritionist, or healthcare provider. A review of health coaches for type 2 diabetes reported that physicians, nurses, dental professionals, medical assistants, dietetic students, and dietitians involved in health coaching interventions were mostly face-to-face and some included technology.[64,65] Peer health coaches have also achieved positive results, although their training needs careful attention, and adherence to coaching techniques might be challenging.[66,67]

Training people for health coaching includes both formal and informal approaches. In one study of medical assistants as health coaches, the assistants were trained for 40 hours over six weeks using a curriculum developed by the research team.[68] Smith et al.[69] described a university-based training certificate program designed to be completed within 12 to 18 months. Those who are accepted for enrolment must have a bachelor's or advanced degree or at least three years' experience in an allied health field.

A systematic review of health coaching for adults with type 2 diabetes found that goal setting was an important strategy, along with knowledge acquisition and individualization.[65] Patients who were followed for longer than six months had more significant improvements in hemoglobin A1C levels.[65] An earlier review of health coaching in interventions reported that significant improvements in targeted outcomes were achieved in six of 15 studies.[70] Those outcomes included one or more of the following categories: nutrition, physical activity, weight management, or medication adherence. More than 70% of these programs used goal setting, with 27% using MI.[70] At least one study reported that improvement in outcomes persisted even one year after coaching.[71]

One program, lifestyle health coaching (LHC), is one-on-one coaching with a nonphysician coach and is supported primarily by telephone and Internet-based resources for self-help. In addition to reducing disease risk factors through lifestyle change, the LHC also supports medication adherence.[72] A qualitative study of the perception of health coaches in pediatric obesity treatment reported that individualization, nutritional guidance, and links to resources were identified as most important to the families in the study.[73]

Health coaching by telephone or the Internet is a form of telehealth and is regulated by licensure laws for RDNs. Health coaching, the use of MI and behavior theory, and skill in oral and written communication can lead to successful careers for many RDNs.[74]

# ▶ Chapter Summary

A primary objective of this chapter is to identify key communication skills needed for the nutrition education researcher. Skills needed include being able

> **Recap** Creating a partnership with clients to identify problem areas and set goals in a supportive environment can lead to growth and development for both the coach and the client.

to set clear goals within the message to be communicated, and incorporating a speaking or writing style that is appropriate for the audience. These skills are similar to those needed in counseling, although counseling skills require more interaction with clients. These interactions allow a partnership to develop so that each client's stage of change is met, the counselor is supportive in a client-centered manner, and SMART goals are mutually developed.

CBT and motivational interviewing are counseling techniques that use the aforementioned skills. They require training and practice but can be useful to the health coach once learned. Effective health coaching has been shown to include goal setting and individualization.

Within research or practice, several behavior theories can provide a framework, including the Health Belief Model, theory of reasoned action, and social cognitive theory. Constructs within these theories will help the practitioner or researcher focus on the program or individual counseling in areas of need. Attitudes, self-efficacy, subjective norms, perceived barriers and benefits, and outcome expectancies are constructs within social and cognitive domains that can provide a communication framework to achieve behavioral change.

# ◆ CASE STUDY

Beth gained weight during each of her three pregnancies. By the time her third child was 2 years old, Beth weighed an additional 35 lbs compared to her weight before her first pregnancy. Beth works part-time and has been married to Ed for 10 years. Ed still plays basketball with friends at least once a week and runs most mornings. While Ed has gained only 5 lbs since their marriage. Beth has tried many types of diets but ends up feeling frustrated, tired, and guilty about not being able to lose weight.

During one of the children's well baby visits, Beth notices that her clinic has a new program called

"Healthy Weight, Healthy Me." She decides to enroll. There is a general meeting at a convenient time for her, and Ed agrees to miss basketball and care for the children.

At the meeting, Beth learns that the program is tailored to each individual's needs. There are general skill-building sessions for making menus, shopping, and cooking. Support groups are available online, and a health coach is also available for each participant. Beth makes an appointment with her health coach, Lisa, for the following week.

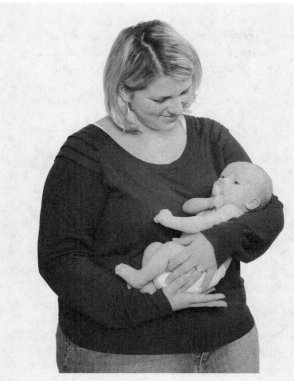

© Kletr/Shutterstock.

Lisa: Hi, my name is Lisa, and I am happy to meet you. I'm looking forward to working with you to meet your goals. First, I want to share a little about myself, as we get to know one another. Professionally, I'm a registered and licensed dietitian nutritionist, and I've been practicing for a little over 12 years. I love my job because it is so rewarding. I also love food and cooking! On a personal front, I'm married and have one daughter who is 10 years old. Although I don't have a lot of spare time, I like to garden in the summer and take occasional hikes with my family.

Beth: It's nice to meet you. I'm a little nervous because all my other attempts to lose weight have failed. I just can't seem to get the weight off, even when I eat almost nothing.

Lisa: Losing weight is not easy, but I bet you do a lot of things that aren't easy. And you are here, which means you are prepared mentally to try again. We'll review your diet and activity routines, and then I'd like to suggest that you think of one goal that you'd like to achieve before we meet again.

Before the end of this session, with Lisa's help, Beth has identified one specific, achievable, measurable goal: Beth will drink no more than two cans of sugar-sweetened beverages per week. She has been drinking two per day, with the idea that they were convenient and would provide energy. They discuss this belief and the barriers to achieving her goal. They also discuss strategies to overcome those barriers and some of the benefits of not drinking so many sugar-sweetened beverages. Finally, they discuss Beth's outcome expectancies, both positive and negative, related to achieving this goal.

### Questions:

1. Why does Lisa share her personal information with Beth?
2. Why is it important to tell Beth that losing weight is not easy?
3. Decreasing sugar-sweetened beverages is probably just one part of Beth's eating pattern that needs to be changed. Shouldn't the whole pattern be discussed?

 **CASE STUDY**

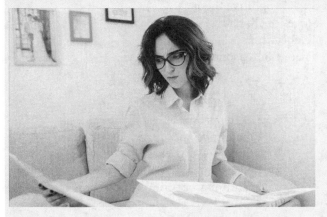

© Look Studio/Shutterstock.

Marie is a health coach and a researcher who was recently contacted by a health news reporter about the results of a study that she and her colleagues have published. The multisite study evaluated the effectiveness of in-person health coaches versus online coaches for clients trying to adopt the Dietary Approaches to Stop Hypertension, or the DASH, dietary program. They found that clients in both groups achieved personal SMART goals, but the in-person coaches' clients had a statistically significant better dietary modification. The online coaches had scripted messages to send, so they were less personalized than the in-person coaches, who had the script but were more spontaneous and individualized. Researchers could not definitely say, however, that this was the reason for the better outcome with in-person coaches.

Marie asked the health news reporter for the interview questions the day before the interview. After reviewing the questions, she sent two additional questions that she wanted the reporter to ask. Those two questions tied directly to her two main points.

Reporter: If both groups achieved their goals, does it matter if one group was statistically better than the other?

Marie: From the client perspective, it does not matter if the coaching is in-person or online, because both groups achieved their goals. From the research perspective, it matters because we want to develop coaching strategies and techniques that will be the most effective. In our next study, we plan to facilitate a more spontaneous and targeted online coaching strategy that is more similar to the in-person coaching.

Reporter: What is a SMART goal, and do you think this influenced your outcomes?

Marie: SMART goals have specific attributes. They are specific, measurable, realistic, and timely. These qualities make them more achievable. Our study did not compare those with SMART goals to those without SMART goals, so we can't say that the SMART goals were critical to the outcomes. Future studies will look at this to determine if SMART goals are a critical component. We used SMART goals because other studies have shown them to be effective.

**Questions:**

1. Why did Marie ask for the questions beforehand and then add her own questions to be asked?
2. Why did Marie provide an answer from both the client and the researcher's perspective? Shouldn't she focus on her research only?
3. The SMART goals likely influenced the outcomes because we know they work. Why didn't Marie just say that?

# Learning Portfolio

## Key Terms

Behavior theories
Client-centered approach
Coaching
Cognitive Behavior Therapy (CBT)
Cognitive interviewing
Five A's
Flesch-Kincaid grade reading level
Health Belief Model (HBM)
Health literacy
Internal motivation
Learner-centered approach
Medical nutrition therapy (MNT)
Motivational interviewing (MI)

Nutrition literacy
Outcome expectancies
Qualitative data
Qualitative research
Quantitative
Research proposal
Saturation
Self-efficacy
SMART goals
Social cognitive theory (SCT)
Stages of change
Telehealth
Theory of reasoned action (TRA)

## Study Questions

1. Communication skills for the nutrition researcher:
   a. Must comply with guidelines from the National Institutes of Health.
   b. Usually vary in tone and scope, depending on the audience.
   c. Always uses a written format.
   d. Should include several languages.

2. A research proposal usually includes:
   a. Qualitative and quantitative results.
   b. Outcomes and plans for future research.
   c. Specific goals, hypotheses, and methodology.
   d. A summary of community outreach goals.

3. In research, a consent form is intended to:
   a. Communicate the details of the study with risks and benefits.
   b. Inform a parent of a child's risk in participating in research.
   c. Request research funding.
   d. Get permission to reveal results.

4. Cognitive interviewing may be used to:
   a. Develop a research protocol.
   b. Develop a study questionnaire.
   c. Update a literature search.
   d. Update a website.

5. When writing for the public, the reading level should:
   a. Not be a concern because people can use Internet sources for definitions.
   b. Be extremely technical so people are impressed with the writer and the topic.
   c. Be written at a third-grade level or below.
   d. Be written at a sixth-grade level or below.

6. Counseling for behavior change should be:
   a. Direct.
   b. Vague.
   c. Prescriptive.

7. Client centered. When establishing rapport, the counselor should:
   a. Share detailed personal information with the client.
   b. "Friend" the client on Facebook.
   c. Be friendly and nonjudgmental.
   d. Always shake the client's hand.

8. *Health literacy* refers to:
   a. The client's capacity to understand health information.
   b. The readability of the educational handouts.
   c. The counselor's level of health education.
   d. The referral process to other health providers.

9. In the transtheoretical model of change, a client who does not intend to make changes in the near future is considered to be in what stage?
   a. Action
   b. Maintenance
   c. Preparation
   d. Precontemplation

10. In the stages of change model of behavior:
    a. Clients always progress in a linear direction to maintenance of habits.
    b. Clients progress in a linear direction but may recycle or relapse.
    c. Clients may be in more than one stage at a time.
    d. Clients maintain habits in the action stage.

11. An effective way to begin a counseling session is to:
    a. Provide a menu of counseling fees.
    b. Establish disclosure limits.
    c. Set an agenda.
    d. Offer goals.

12. The five major steps to intervention (the "Five A's") in the order they occur are:
    a. Assess, advise, agree, assist, arrange
    b. Agree, assess, arrange, advise, assist
    c. Arrange, agree, assess, assist, advise
    d. Advise, arrange, assist, agree, assess

13. Strategies to facilitate behavior change include:
    a. Goal setting and achievement.
    b. Goal setting and self-monitoring.
    c. Impediments and roadblocks.
    d. Impediments and incentives.

14. SMART goals are:
    a. Simple, Measurable, Appropriate, Realistic, Timely.
    b. Specific, Measurable, Attainable, Realistic, Timely.
    c. Specific, Movable, Appropriate, Reasonable, Thoughtful.
    d. Simple, Movable, Attainable, Reasonable, Thoughtful.

15. Within the client–counselor partnership, sharing of personal interests:
    a. Should occur if the counselor and client really have a lot in common.
    b. Is not appropriate regardless of how often counseling sessions occur.
    c. Is appropriate if the counseling sessions last at least one year.
    d. Can help establish rapport, but professional boundaries should be set.

16. When a client knows the pros and cons of changing a behavior but has done nothing to move forward, the client is in the stage of change called:
    a. Precontemplation.
    b. Contemplation.
    c. Preparation.
    d. Maintenance.

17. An agenda should be developed by the counselor when the client is in the:
    a. Contemplation stage.
    b. Preparation stage.
    c. Action stage.
    d. Maintenance stage.

18. The goal of cognitive behavior theory is:
    a. To develop a plan and establish goals to change one's thoughts and behaviors.
    b. To identify flaws in a client's beliefs or self-perceptions.
    c. To assign one individual of the healthcare team to create goals for the client.
    d. To develop both declarative and procedural knowledge.

19. Social cognitive theory is described by all of the four focus areas *except*:
    a. Personal goals.
    b. Perceived behavioral control.
    c. Evaluative standards.
    d. Competencies and skills.

20. According to the Health Belief Model, the influences that discourage an individual from adopting a promotional behavior can be categorized as perceived:
    a. Susceptibility.
    b. Severity.
    c. Barriers.
    d. Benefits.

21. As defined by the theory of reasoned action, the most important determinant of behavior is:
    a. The belief in one's abilities.
    b. The construct of intention.
    c. One's attitude toward a given behavior.
    d. A person's perceived behavioral control.

22. The motivational interviewing (MI) approach is geared toward:
    a. Discussing methods by which a counselor can dictate how the client should change his or her health behavior.
    b. Having the client provide questions to the counselor on how the counselor should help guide the client toward healthy lifestyle changes.
    c. Instructing the client to discontinue his or her health behavior.
    d. Exploring reasons behind a client's ambivalence or indecision about making healthy behavioral changes.

23. Through the MI approach, *ambivalence* is defined as:
    a. Fearing change to set habits.
    b. Having a defined mindset of goals and planning ways to achieve them.
    c. Having mixed feelings about making behavioral change and finding reasons why one cannot implement change.
    d. Being optimistic toward adapting healthy lifestyle changes without reservation.

24. The *righting reflex* is described as:
    a. The client adopting a healthier lifestyle.
    b. The counselor telling the client what to do.
    c. The client talking him- or herself out of adopting any new health behaviors.
    d. The desired goal of MI.

25. The "expert trap" is a result of:
    a. Guiding the client to identify underlying causes to behavioral change barriers.
    b. The counselor dictating what the solution is for the client and creating opposition.
    c. Using "unconditional positive regard."
    d. Partnering with the client to resolve ambivalence.

26. To easily remember the four areas of assessment within MI, the acronym DARN stands for:
    a. Direction, aim, reason, necessity.
    b. Doubt, ambivalence, reaction, new.
    c. Desire, ability, reasons, need.
    d. Determination, action, results, nuance.

27. Providing incentives or rewards is a way of:
    a. Providing external motivation.
    b. Providing internal motivation.
    c. Increasing rapport.
    d. Increasing dependency.

28. Two important components of success are:
    a. Goal setting and individualization.
    b. Action and persistence.
    c. Formal coaching and synergism.
    d. Strategy and education.

29. An area of challenge to training peer health coaches can include:
    a. Providing careful attention and adherence to coaching techniques for their specific training needs.
    b. Achieving positive results from them.
    c. Deciding whether training should be all formal or all informal.
    d. Identifying one individual profession to act as the peer health coach.

30. Health coaching can be guided by:
    a. Individuals not related to the health field.
    b. A variety of trained health peers and professionals.
    c. Heavily regulated training processes.
    d. An outside professional entity.

31. Forms of telehealth include:
    a. Health coaching by telephone or Internet.
    b. Face-to-face heath coaching.
    c. Unlicensed practice of instructing clients.
    d. Visits to the client's home for coaching.

## Discussion Questions

1. Research presentations should include an introduction, objectives, methodology, results, and discussion and then end with three primary points. Select one presentation you have delivered or a recent presentation that you attended. Did the presentation follow the guidelines listed? List the missing component and explain how each components helps to strengthen the message to be delivered.

2. Visually recording yourself can provide good feedback before you make a presentation, yet many people do not do this. From the tips and strategies presented in this chapter, which ones do you incorporate in your presentations? Which undesirable habits do you normally portray? Why are these habit hard to change?

3. Using the readiness-to-change framework, within your group, create a scenario of a person in each of the stages of change. Discuss the approaches of counseling that need to be utilized for each case.

4. Goals should be client centered and attainable. Sometimes the counselor may feel goals other than identified by the client should be addressed first. As a counselor, how should the change in goal priority should be managed?

5. Within the HBM, students may not relate to perceived susceptibility. Discuss who and when individuals may feel susceptible to diabetes, cardiovascular disease, poor pregnancy outcomes, and osteoporosis.

6. Time and money are common barriers to any lifestyle change. What strategies should the head of the household use to provide family meals at least three times per week,

7. Motivational interviewing is a collaborative effort that is similar to a coach and team members. What experiences have you had as a member of a team that relate to motivational interviewing?

8. Proximal goals are more achievable than distal goals. Please write a short essay on a situation in which proximal goals can lead to distal goal achievement (not using the text example).

## Activities

### Individual Activities

1. Students will write one SMART goal and have it approved by the instructor. After approval, students will self-monitor their progress on achieving this goal for two weeks. At the end of two weeks, students will write a reflection on the barriers and benefits of working toward this goal and their attitudes about working toward this goal. Have the students write comments about their subjective norms for this behavior.

2. Students will experience self-monitoring of their own behavior by completing a pen-and-paper food diary for one week and then using an app for one week. At the end, students will write a reflection on the pros and cons of each method of self-monitoring food-intake behavior.

### Group Activity

Motivational interviewing includes using open-ended questions, affirming and supporting the client, reflective listening, and summarizing. Have students form small groups of three. One student in each group will assume the role of health coach, one will assume the role of a client, and one will critique the health coach's style of interaction.

The client will be seeing the health coach because he has high blood lipids and wants to lower these values through diet and exercise rather than start immediately on a lipid-lowering medication. In a previous coaching session, the client and coach had mutually developed two SMART goals that were to "only eat whole grain bread, except when unavailable when eating out or at friends' homes" and to "switch from butter or margarine to olive or canola oil at home." These dietary changes are part of the Mediterranean dietary pattern. At this session, the coach and client will discuss how well the goals were achieved and what problems might have been encountered. The instructor will visit each group and make suggestions. One or two groups may present to the class as time allows. Students could also share their insights from this activity through an online learning community or platform if the class is using one of these venues.

## Online Resources

### Qualitative Methods

#### Webinars

Society for Nutrition Education. Qualitative Research: What the Journal of Nutrition Education and Behavior Looks For.
https://vimeo.com/32724104.

Successful Qualitative Research:
http://connection.sagepub.com/blog/sage-connection/2015/06/02/successful-qualitative-research-webinar-recording-with-extended-qa/

#### Health Literacy Resources

S-TOFHL:
https://www.reginfo.gov/public/do/PRAViewIC?ref_nbr=201210-0935-001&icID=204408.

NVS:
https://www.pfizer.com/files/health/nvs_flipbook_english_final.pdf.

REALM:
https://www.ahrq.gov/professionals/quality-patient-safety/quality-resources/tools/literacy/index.html

National Library of Medicine Health Literacy Toolbox:
http://healthliteracy.bu.edu/

#### Five A's Webinar

Hypertension Update: Nutritional Guidelines and Strategies:
https://learn.extension.org/events/2122

#### Communication

Developing Effective Communications by the University of Missouri Extension Service:
http://extension.missouri.edu/p/CM109

This site provides an overview of several models of communication, noting that people have many interpretations of the word *communication*. The author concludes by noting that if the receiver does not understand the message, then the communication has failed.

#### Behavior

Cognitive Behavioral Therapy by the US National Library of Medicine:
https://www.ncbi.nlm.nih.gov/pubmedhealth/PMH0072481/

Providing a thorough definition of and some detail on CBT, this site also provides examples of harmful and neutral thought patterns and what might be expected as outcomes.

Social and Behavioral Theories, by Karen Glanz, PhD, for the Department of Social and Behavioral Sciences, DHHS, NIH:
https://obssr.od.nih.gov/wp-content/uploads/2016/05/Social-and-Behavioral-Theories.pdf

Key constructs of four theories that are often used in community and public health interventions are described: the Health Belief Model, the transtheoretical model and stages of change, social cognitive theory, and the social ecological model (not discussed in this chapter). This site also covers when one theory might be used instead of another.

#### Motivational Interviewing

Introduction to Motivational Interviewing:
https://www.youtube.com/watch?v=s3MCJZ7OGRk

Motivational Interviewing:
http://www.motivationalinterviewing.org/

American Society of Addiction Medicine:
http://www.asam.org/education/live-online-cme/fundamentals-of-addiction-medicine/additional-resources/motivational-interviewing

Motivational Interviewing—Integrating the Total Diet Approach:
http://www.healthyeating.org/Health-Wellness-Providers/Professional-Development/Continuing-Education-Courses/Motivational-Interviewing.aspx

Motivational Interviewing: Obesity:
https://youtu.be/24NV35rKl5I

American Society for Nutrition:
https://www.nutrition.org/asn-blog/2015/12/motivational-interviewing-techniques-to-encourage-lifestyle-changesweight-loss/

Motivational Interviewing—A client-centered approach to healthcare behavior change:
http://www.veteransmemorialhospital.com/diabetes/MotivationalInterviewing.pdf

Health Behavior change using motivational interviewing:
http://www.adph.org/NUTRITION/index.asp?ID=1152

Shared Decision Making and Motivational Interviewing—Achieving Patient-Centered Care Across the Spectrum of Healthcare Problems:
http://www.annfammed.org/content/12/3/270.full

Motivational Interviewing—An Emerging Trend in Medical Management:
http://www.patientadvocatetraining.com/wp-content/themes/patientadvocate/static/pdf/ppai_specialreport_mi.pdf

**Motivational Interviewing by Three Federal Agencies**

Substance Abuse and Mental Health Services Administration and Health Resources Services Administration of the Department of Health and

Human Services provide an overview of MI as well as sources for training:

http://www.integration.samhsa.gov/clinical-practice/motivational-interviewing.

# References

1. Quagliani D, Herman M. Communicating accurate food and nutrition information. Practice paper of the Academy of Nutrition and Dietetic. 2012; 112(5). http://www.sciencedirect.com/science/article/pii/S221226721200322X.
2. Centers for Disease Control and Prevention. Use of World Health Organization and CDC growth charts for children aged 0–59 months in the United States. *Morb Mort Wkly Rep.* 2010; 59(No. RR-9):1–15. https://www.cdc.gov/mmwr/pdf/rr/rr5909.pdf.
3. Al-Riyami A. How to prepare a research proposal. *Oman Med J.* 2008; 23(2):66–69.
4. World Health Organization. Recommended format for a Research Protocol. 2011. http://www.who.int/rpc/research_ethics/format_rp/en/.
5. US Department of Health and Human Services, Office for Human Research Protections. Informed Consent Tips. 1993; reviewed 2016. https://www.hhs.gov/ohrp/regulations-and-policy/guidance/informed-consent-tips/index.html.
6. Elsevier. Elsevier. Journal Authors. Available at https://www.elsevier.com/authors/journal-authors. 2016.
7. Kincaid JP, Fishburne RP, Rogers RL, et al. Derivation of new readability formulas (Automated Readability and Flesch Reading Ease Formula) for Navy-enlisted personnel. Research Branch Report 8–75. Millington, TN: Naval Technical Training, US Naval Air Station; Memphis, TN. 1975: 8–75. http://www.dtic.mil/dtic/tr/fulltext/u2/a006655.pdf.
8. Alley M. *The Craft of Scientific Presentations.* 2nd ed. New York, NY: Springer Link; 2013.
9. Levy R, Lichtman F, Hu DL. The scientist-reporter collaboration: A guide to working with the press. *SIAM News.* 2014. http://scholarship.claremont.edu/cgi/viewcontent.cgi?article=2028&context=hmc_fac_pub.
10. Guo RX. The use of video recordings as an effective tool to improve presentation skills. *Polyglossia.* 2013; March; 24; 92–101. http://jairo.nii.ac.jp/0026/00004222/en.
11. Goodell LS, Stage VC, Cooke NK. Practical qualitative research strategies: Training interviewers and coders. *Educ Behav.* 2016; 48(8):578–585.
12. Geiselman RE, Fisher RP, MacKinnon DP, Holland HL. Eyewitness memory enhancement in the police interview: Cognitive retrieval mnemonics versus hypnosis. *Psychol.* 1985;70:401–412.
13. Willis GB. *Cognitive Interviewing. A Tool for Improving Questionnaire Design.* Newbury Park, CA: Sage Publications; 2005.
14. US Department of Health and Human Services. Office for Human Research Protections Human Subject Regulations Decision Charts; 2016. https://www.hhs.gov/ohrp/regulations-and-policy/decision-charts/index.html.
15. Ryan P, Dundon T. Case research interviews: Eliciting superior quality data. *Int J Case Meth Res App.* 2008: 443–450. http://www.wacra.org/PublicDomain/IJCRA xx_iv_IJCRA pg443–450 Ryan.pdf.
16. Jortberg BT, Fleming MO. Registered dietitian nutritionists bring value to emerging health care delivery models. *Nutr Diet.* 2014; 114(12):2017–2022.
17. Powers MA, Bardsley J, Cypress M, et.al. Diabetes self-management education and support in type 2 diabetes: A joint position statement of the American Diabetes Association, the American Association of Diabetes Educators, and the Academy of Nutrition and Dietetics. *Diabetes Care.* 2015; 38(7): 1372–1382. doi: 10.2337/dc15-0730.
18. Jacobson TA, Ito MK, Maki KC, et al. National Lipid Association recommendations for patient-centered management of dyslipidemia: Part 1. *J Clin Lipidol.* 2015; 9:129–169.
19. Jacobson TA, Ito MK, Maki KC, et al. National Lipid Association recommendations for patient-centered management of dyslipidemia: Part 2. *J Clin Lipidol.* 2015; 9(6):S1–S122.
20. Hancock R, Bonner G, Hollingdale R, Madden A. "If you listen to me properly, I feel good": A qualitative examination of patient experiences of dietetic consultations. *J Hum Nutri Diet.* 2012; 25(3):275–284.
21. Klawitter B. Counseling the adult learner. In: King K, Klawitter B, eds. *Nutrition Therapy Advanced Counseling Skills.* 3rd ed. Baltimore, MD: Lippincott Williams & Wilkins; 2007.
22. Bickley LS, Szilagyi PG. *Bates' Guide to Physical Examination and History Taking.* 11th ed. Baltimore, MD: Lippincott Williams & Wilkins; 2008.
23. Kellogg M. *Counseling Tips for Nutrition Therapists Practice Workbook, Volume 1.* Philadelphia, PA: Kg Press; 2006.
24. US Department of Health and Human Services. Quick Guide to health literacy fact sheet. 2010. https://health.gov/communication/literacy/quickguide/.
25. Morris NS, Grant S, Repp A, Maclean C, Littenberg B. Prevalence of limited health literacy and compensatory strategies used by hospitalized patients. *Nurs Res.* 2011; 60(5):361–366. doi: 10.1097/NNR.0b013e31822c68a6.
26. US Department of Health and Human Services. Americas Health Literacy Why We Need Accessible Health Information. 2008. https://health.gov/communication/literacy/issuebrief/.
27. Mbaezue N, Mayberry R, Gazmararian J, Quarshie A, Ivonye C, Heisler M. The impact of health literacy on self-monitoring of blood glucose in patients with diabetes receiving care in an inner-city hospital. *Med Assoc.* 2010; 102(1):5–9.
28. Powell CK, Hill EG, Clancy DE. The relationship between health literacy and diabetes knowledge and readiness to take health actions. *Diabetes Educ.* 2007; 33(1):144–151.
29. Rothman R, Malone R, Bryant B, Horlen C, DeWalt D, Pignone M. The relationship between literacy and glycemic control in a diabetes disease-management program. *Diabetes Educ.* 2004; 30:263–273.
30. Rothman R, Pignone M, Malone R, Bryant B, Horlen C, Padgett P. The relationship between health literacy and diabetes related measures for patients with type 2 diabetes. *Intern Med.* 2002; 17(Suppl):1167.
31. Schillinger D, Grumbach K, Piette J. Association of health literacy with diabetes outcomes. *JAMA.* 2002; 288:475–482.
32. Parker RM, Baker DW, Williams MV, Nurss JR. The test of functional health literacy in adults: A new instrument for measuring patients' literacy skills. *Intern Med.* 1995; 10(10):537–541.

33. Baker DW, Williams MV, Parker RM, Gazamararian JA, Nurss JR. Development of a brief test to measure functional health literacy. *Patient Educ Couns*. 1999;38(1):33–42.

34. Weiss BD, Mays MZ, Martz W. Quick assessment of literacy in primary care: The newest vital sign. *Ann Fam Med*. 2005; 3:514–522.

35. Davis TC, Crouch MA, Long SW, et al. Rapid assessment of literacy levels of adult primary care patients. *Fam Med*. 1991; 23:433–435. doi: 10.1097/NNR.0b013e31822c68a6.

36. Gibbs H, Chapman-Novakofski K. Establishing content validity for the Nutrition Literacy Assessment Instrument. *Prev Chronic Dis*. 2013;10 :120267. DOI: http://dx.doi.org/10.5888 /pcd10.120267.

37. Gibbs HD, Ellerbeck EF, Befort C, et al. Measuring nutrition literacy in breast cancer patients: Development of a novel instrument. *J Cancer Ed*. 2016; 31(3):493–499.

38. Gibbs HD, Kennett AR, Kerling EH, et al. Assessing the nutrition literacy of parents and its relationship with child diet quality. *Educ Behav*. 2016; 48(7):505–509.

39. Prochaska J, DiClemente C. Stages and processes of self-change of smoking: Toward an integrative model of change. *Clin Psychol*. 1983;51(3):390–395.

40. Whitlock EP, Orleans CT, Pender N, Allan J. Evaluating primary care behavioral counseling interventions: An evidence-based approach. *Am Med*. 2002; 22(4):267–284.

41. Agency for Healthcare Research and Quality. Five Major Steps to Intervention (The 5A's). 2012. https://www. ahrq.gov/professionals/clinicians-providers/guidelines -recommendations/tobacco/5steps.html.

42. Bowman J, Mogensen L, Marsland E, Lannin N. The development, content validity and inter-rater reliability of the SMART-Goal evaluation method: A standardised method for evaluating clinical goals. *Aust Occup Ther J*. 2015; 62(6):420–427.

43. Bandura A. Observational learning. In: Bandura A, Ed. *Social Foundations of Thought and Action: A Social Cognitive Theory*. Englewood Cliffs, NJ: Prentice-Hall; 1986.

44. Beck AT. Cognitive therapy: Nature and relation to behavior therapy [republished article]. *Behav Ther*. 2016; 47(6):776–784.

45. Calugi S, Ghoch ME, Dalle Grave R. Body checking behaviors in anorexia nervosa. *Int J Eat Disord*. 2017; 50(4):437–441. https://www.ncbi.nlm.nih.gov/labs/articles/28117905/.

46. Ozier AD, Henry BW. Position of the American Dietetic Association Nutrition intervention in the treatment of eating disorders. *JADA*. 2011; 111(8):1236–1241.

47. Fabricatore AN. Behavior therapy and cognitive-behavioral therapy of obesity: Is there a difference? *J Am Diet Assoc*. 2007; 107(1):92–99.

48. Achterberg C, Miller C. Is one theory better than another in nutrition education? A viewpoint: More is better. *J Nutr Educ Behav*. 2004; 36(1):40–42.

49. Fishbein M, Ajzen I, Reading MA. *Belief, Attitude, Intention and Behavior: An Introduction to Theory and Research*. Reading, MA: Addison Wesley; 1975.

50. Fishbein MA, Steiner ID, Fishbein M. A consideration of beliefs, attitudes, and their relationship. In: Steiner ID, Fishbein M, eds., *Current Studies in Social Psychology*. New York, NY: Holt Reinhart & Winston; 1965.

51. Ajzen I. From intentions to actions: A theory of planned behavior. In: Kuhl J, Beckmann J., eds., *Action Control: From Cognition to Behavior*. New York, NY: Springer-Verlag; 1985.

52. Fishbein M, Ajzen I. *Predicting and Changing Behavior: The Reasoned Action Approach*. New York, NY: Taylor & Francis; 2010.

53. Spinks T, Hamilton K. Investigating mothers' decisions to give their 2- to 3-year-old child a nutritionally balanced. *Diet J Nutr Educ Behav*. 2016; 48(4):250–257. https://www.ncbi.nlm.nih .gov/pubmed/27059313.

54. Bandura A. Self-efficacy: Toward a unifying theory of behavioral change. *Psych Rev*. 1977; 84:191–215. https://www .uky.edu/~eushe2/Bandura/Bandura1977PR.pdf.

55. Bandura A. Social cognitive theory of self-regulation. *Organiz Behav Hum Dec Proc*. 1991;50:248–287.

56. Miller WR, Rollnick S. *Motivational Interviewing: Helping People Change*. 3rd ed. New York, NY: Guilford Press; 2013.

57. Rogers C. What understanding and acceptance mean to me. *Psychol*. 1995; 35:7–22.

58. Rollnick S, Miller WR, Butler CC. *Motivational Interviewing in Health Care*. New York, NY: Guilford Press; 2008.

59. Shahnazari M, Ceresa C, Foley S, et al. Nutrition-focused wellness coaching promotes a reduction in body weight in overweight US veterans. *Nutr Diet*. 2013; 113:928–935.

60. Sherifali D, Viscardi V, Bai JW, Ali R, Muhammad UR. Evaluating the effect of a diabetes health coach in individuals with type 2 diabetes. *Can J Diabetes*. 2015; 40(1):84–94.

61. Vivian EM, Colbert LH, Remington PL. Lessons learned from a community based lifestyle intervention for youth at risk for type 2 diabetes. *J Obes Weight Loss Ther*. 2013; 13(1).

62. Goldman ML, Ghorob A, Hessler D, Yamamoto R, Thom DH, Bodenheimer T. Are low-income peer health coaches able to master and utilize evidence-based health coaching? *Ann Fam Med*. 2015; 1(13 Suppl):S36–41.

63. Wagner TH, Willard-Grace R, Chen E, Bodenheimer T, Thom DH. Costs for a health coaching intervention for chronic care management. *Am J Manag Care*. 2016; 22(4):e141–146. http://www.ajmc.com/journals/issue/2016/2016-vol22-n4 /costs-for-a-health-coaching-intervention-for-chronic-care -management.

64. Smith LL, Lake NH, Simmons LA, Perlman A, Wroth S, Wolever RQ. Integrative health coach training: A model for shifting the paradigm toward patient-centricity and meeting new national prevention goals. *Global Adv Health Med*. 2013; 2(3):66–74. https://www.ncbi.nlm.nih.gov/pmc/ articles/PMC3833534/.

65. Olsen JM, Nesbitt BJ. Health coaching to improve healthy lifestyle behaviors: an integrative review. *Am J Health Promot*. 2010; 25(1):e1–e12. https://www.ncbi.nlm.nih.gov /pubmed/20809820.

66. Sharma AE, Willard-Grace R, Hessler D, Bodenheimer T, Thom DH. What happens after health coaching? Observational study 1 year following a randomized controlled trial. *Ann Fam Med*. 2016; 14(3):200–207. http://www.annfammed.org /content/14/3/200.full.

67. Gordon NF, Salmon RD, Wright BS, Faircloth GC, Reid KS, Gordon TL. Clinical effectiveness of lifestyle health coaching: case study of an evidence-based program. *Am J Lifestyle Med*. 2015; 11(2):153–166. http://journals.sagepub.com/doi /abs/10.1177/1559827615592351.

68. Rice KG, Jumamil RB, Jabour SM, Cheng JK. Role of health coaches in pediatric weight management: Patient and parent perspectives. *Clin Pediatr Phila*. 2016; 56(2). https://www.ncbi .nlm.nih.gov/pubmed/27169713.

69. Kohn JB. How can registered dietitian nutritionists use health coaching techniques? *J Acad Nutri Dietet*. 2014; 114(5):824. http://jandonline.org/article/S2212–2672(14)00236-6/pdf.

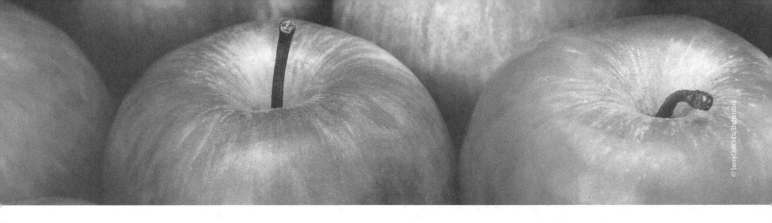

# CHAPTER 12

# International Nutrition Assessment and Research

**Mary Beth Arensberg**, PhD, RDN, LDN, FAND
**Johanna T. Dwyer**, DSc, RD
**Francisco José Rosales Herrera**, MD, DSc
*With help from **Ashley Bronston**, MS, RDN, LD in preparing the Highlight sections*

## CHAPTER OUTLINE

- Introduction
- What is on the Global Nutrition Agenda?
- Who is Supporting the Global Nutrition Agenda?
- How is an International Nutrition-Research Problem Defined?
- What is Different About the International Nutrition-Research Process?
- What Solutions Have Been Developed to Address International Nutrition Problems?
- Chapter Summary

## LEARNING OBJECTIVES

After reading this chapter, the learner will be able to:

1. List three major areas influencing the global nutrition agenda.
2. Differentiate between the five different types of organizations that may be involved in international nutrition-related research.
3. Describe how global health and development goals and resources are linked to international nutrition-research problems.
4. Explain the basis for the ethical, legal, and regulatory framework for international nutrition research.
5. List key questions that are important to answer in designing a nutrition assessment for international nutrition research and differentiate between types of international nutrition interventions and solutions using the social ecological model.

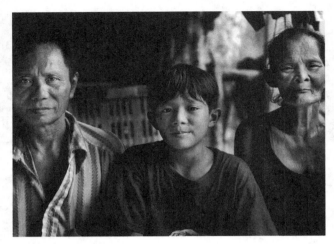

© xPACIFICA/The Image Bank/Getty Images.

# ▶ Introduction

Nutrition is a process of selecting, acquiring, or providing food that is needed for health and growth. Based on this simple definition, human nutrition can be conceptualized as a scientific and multidisciplinary approach that emphasizes the application of knowledge on human physiology, food availability, and public health to the improvement of the health of populations. Human physiology determines the essentiality of nutrients and understanding of the metabolic pathways that support human life throughout the life cycle as well as an understanding of disease processes. This is important because it is not only food availability and governmental action that determine the nutritional status of individuals and populations but also the metabolic processes that turn food into energy and the building blocks for growth and development.

Nutrition is a foundation for the development of populations and nations; as such, adequate or preferably good nutrition is a human right. This right was declared by the **United Nations (UN) Standing Committee on Nutrition (UNSCN)** from the UN System's Forum on Nutrition in 1999 (**FIGURE 12.1**).

The UNSCN also emphasized the health and social benefits associated with nutrition. In addition, the UNSCN provided guidance on the globalization of markets, as this can negatively affect vulnerable populations. The initiative sought the development and application of food and nutrition in these populations as human rights indicators, for the monitoring of how well nations govern their people. Further, the initiative explained that from a geopolitical perspective, the nutrition situation of populations were the results of many factors including socio-economic, and civil/political actions among others. If these actions were not appropriate, they could have disastrous

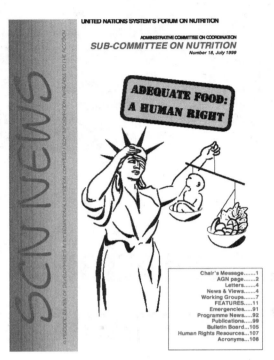

**FIGURE 12.1**  UN Sub-Committee on Nutrition declares food a human right in 1999

Reproduced from: United Nations System's Forum on Nutrition Administrative Committee on Coordination Sub-Committee on Nutrition. SCN News. 1999;18. http://www.unscn.org/layout/modules/resources/files/scnnews18.pdf.

effects on the well-being of populations. There were positive correlations seen between democracy and avoidance of undernutrition, suggesting a plausible relationship between civil and political rights and good nutrition.[1]

UN estimates at the time indicated that approximately 841 million people in developing countries, mostly women and children, did not have enough food to meet their basic nutritional needs, which infringed on their fundamental human rights.[1] Indeed, the **UN Millennium Development Goals**, derived from the United Nations Millennium Declaration signed in September 2000, emphasized the world's commitment since 2000 to meeting basic nutritional needs and fulfilling these rights (**FIGURE 12.2**).

A common focus of international nutrition research is the problems that influence the health, survival, and developmental capacity of populations in lower-income countries. It helps prioritize the conditions that impair or disrupt growth and developmental processes by examining the impact of nutrition at both macro- and microlevels. The concentration is primarily on lower-income countries because the majority of people in most of these countries remain food insecure and nutritionally deprived with respect to both energy-yielding macronutrients and most micronutrients. However, these conditions may also be present in subpopulations within

The United Nations Millennium Development Goals were derived from the UN Millennium Declaration signed in 2000. All UN member states agreed to try to achieve these goals by 2015. The Millennium Development Goals are interdependent, with all the goals influencing health and health influencing all the goals. For example, reducing poverty, hunger, and environmental degradation positively influences and depends on better health.

The eight Millennium Development Goals are:

1. to eradicate extreme poverty and hunger
2. to achieve universal primary education
3. to promote gender equality and empower women
4. to reduce child mortality
5. to improve maternal health
6. to combat HIV/AIDS, malaria, and other diseases
7. to ensure environmental sustainability
8. to develop a global partnership for development.

The Millennium Development Goals have since been replaced by 17 Sustainable Development Goals that are to be completed by 2030.

**FIGURE 12.2** UN Millennium Development Goals

Reprinted from World Health Organization, Millennium Development Goals, © 2017.

# ▶ What is on the Global Nutrition Agenda?

**Preview**   The nutritional threats to the world's population are shifting. Although undernutrition remains a significant problem, obesity and other diet-related diseases are also affecting the health, survival, and developmental capacity of countries around the globe, especially with increasingly older populations.

higher-income countries. Thus, the broader aim of international nutrition research is to assess the nutritional inadequacies that influence the developmental and sustainability capacity of populations. Once assessed, these problems can be addressed by nutrition-intervention programs.

The goal of this chapter is to address assessment and research; it does this by considering nutritional status and its determinants across various disadvantaged populations around the world. The chapter highlights the global nutrition agenda and some of the major nutrition problems that have been identified worldwide. It also examines the various types of organizations engaged in addressing these problems, discusses how global development goals are related to malnutrition, and provides resources that may be beneficial in defining an international research problem for investigation.

The chapter discusses ethical and regulatory considerations, guiding principles, adaptations of nutrition assessment methods and tools, and internationally related standards and sources to inform the research process. Finally, the chapter identifies important issues to consider in designing a nutrition assessment for international research and concludes by describing some of the global nutrition interventions that have resulted.

Malnutrition is associated with poor survival from infancy through adulthood, and it threatens quality of life. Malnutrition falls on either end of a "continuum" of nutritional status in populations and ranges from severe undernutrition and milder degrees of deprivation to being mildly overweight through to obesity. It is important to draw a distinction between undernutrition and overweight and obesity that goes beyond their physical appearances. Hunger, infection, and inadequate food supplies are still the hallmarks of undernutrition, whereas in overweight and obesity, changes to a sedentary lifestyle, lack of knowledge in food selection, and food quality and quantity are common denominators. The rate of overweight or obesity is surging in many lower-income countries, and a rising tide of obesity is affecting certain regions of the world—Latin America, Southeast Asia, China, and North Africa, for example. These populations are experiencing a "nutrition transition" that may be giving rise in part to an increasing trend of noncommunicable disease as a primary cause of death rather than infectious disease.

## An International Focus on Undernutrition

The UNSCN has been a forum for the relevant UN agencies to align their nutrition policies and programs. One of the first comprehensive world nutrition reports was produced by the UNSCN in 1987.[2] From that time to today, there have been six reports. The first report brought together nutrition information and data scattered across various UN agencies. The second report was published in October 1992, the third in December 1997, and the fourth in January 2000. The fifth report, subtitled *Nutrition for Improved Development Outcomes*, was released in March 2004, and it is recognized as the UNSCN's most analytical report to date. The sixth report focused on important nutrition-related knowledge for policy and decision makers and provided future perspectives on the world food and nutrition situation through 2015. It emphasized the implications that this situation would have on achieving the international development goals; in recognizing the right to adequate food, it articulated ways in which situations could be improved.[3]

The first UNSCN report highlighted the fact that hunger and malnutrition in lower-income countries were the most widespread causes of human suffering in the world. **FIGURE 12.3** shows the regional prevalence of underweight in children from 1980 to 1984.

Note the contrasting trends in malnutrition among the geographical regions. In Africa, the majority of countries showed an increase in child malnutrition compared to other global regions. Food quality and availability had been severely affected by poor economic development and devastating droughts. In Latin America, pervasive economic recession and an ongoing debt crisis led to high levels of undernutrition among children younger than five years old.

The report also highlighted specific micronutrient deficiencies affecting these regions. Lack of vitamin A was identified as the largest single cause of blindness among 40 million people in the world, and the deficiency contributes to child morbidity and mortality. Mineral deficiencies such as iron-deficiency anemia affected nearly half the women of reproductive age in lower-income countries and affected many of the world's children, causing poor psychological development and limiting their future work capacity. Widespread iodine deficiencies affected at least 190 million people. During pregnancy and early life, an iodine deficiency causes mental retardation, **stunted growth**, and other developmental abnormalities that are largely irreversible.[2]

More recent data on the world's nutrition status continue to show a high prevalence of children younger than five who are stunted.[4]

Stunting is defined based on the anthropometric index of height and length for age. It represents the distribution of children whose height and length for age is two Z-scores below the median of the child growth standards set by the **World Health Organization (WHO)**. The distribution of stunting among children younger than five is considered a reliable indicator of severe undernutrition. Stunted growth reflects a failure in reaching linear growth potential as a result of suboptimal health or nutritional conditions. In countries with high levels of undernutrition, stunting is often seen in more than 40% of children younger than five, and the risk of children dying from common infections is higher. In addition, stunting is associated with an increase in the rates and severity of infections and with delays in recovering from infections. The majority of countries with high rates of underweight are still found in Central and West Africa. Unfortunately, Africa has seen slow progress in reducing stunting.[4]

The importance of using the prevalence of undernutrition among children under five years of age as a statistic resides in its use as a good measure of the impact

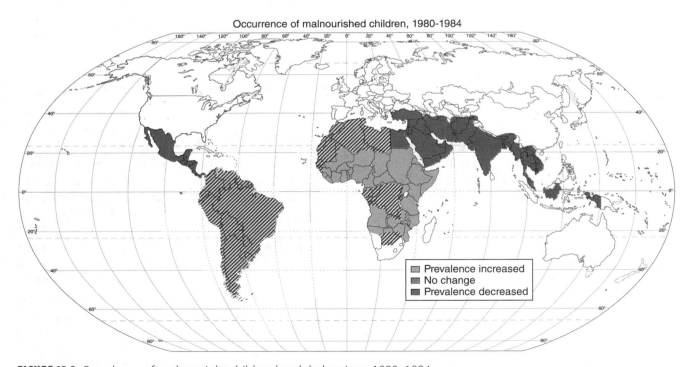

Occurrence of malnourished children, 1980-1984

Prevalence increased
No change
Prevalence decreased

**FIGURE 12.3** Prevalence of underweight children by global regions, 1980–1984

Data from: United Nations Administrative Committee on Coordination Sub-Committee on Nutrition. Changes in prevalence of underweight children by groups of countries from 1980 to 1984. SCN News. 1988;2. http://www.unsystem.org /scn/archives/scnnews02/p01.jpg.

of poor nutrition. On a population basis, high levels of stunting are associated with poor socioeconomic conditions and an increased risk of early exposure to adverse conditions. Similarly, a decrease in the national stunting rate is usually indicative of improvements in overall socioeconomic conditions of a country. Nearly half of all deaths in children under five are attributable to undernutrition. This translates into the unnecessary loss of approximately three million young lives a year.[4]

The **first 1000 days**—the period from the beginning of pregnancy until a child's second birthday—has been identified as an especially critical window of opportunity to break the intergenerational cycle of malnutrition. Approximately one-third of stunting presents as small for gestational age (<10th percentile for infants of the same gestational age) and preterm infants.[5] Undernutrition during the first 1000 days can irreversibly damage a child's physical growth and brain development, thus significantly affecting a child's ability to grow, learn, and rise out of poverty. In 2013, the WHO published *Essential Nutrition Actions: Improving Maternal, Newborn, Infant and Young Child Health and Nutrition*, providing a "compact of WHO guidance on nutrition interventions targeting the first 1000 days of life" and underscoring that the deficits acquired by age two are difficult to reverse later.[6] The first 1000 days is an important focus of the United Nations' **Scaling Up Nutrition (SUN)** movement, which is a global push for action and investment to improve maternal and child nutrition.[7]

Another condition affecting early child malnutrition is HIV and AIDS, which remain a global epidemic. Nearly 37 million people are living with HIV or AIDS; of these, more than 2 million are children, most of who were infected by their HIV-positive mothers during pregnancy, childbirth, or breastfeeding. The majority of the people living with HIV or AIDS are in low- to middle-income countries, particularly in sub-Saharan Africa.[8] Malnutrition can contribute to and result from HIV disease progression. Thus, recognizing the critical role of nutrition in HIV treatment, care and support, the **US Agency for International Development (USAID)** in coordination with the US President's Emergency Plan for AIDS Relief (PEPFAR) is working with global partners and governments to provide nutrition services as a routine part of national healthcare systems. USAID focuses on three priority areas to achieve this goal: (1) implementation of a nutrition assessment, (2) nutrition counseling, and (3) provision of a supportive framework to help prevent mother-to-child HIV transmission and improve other critical aspects of maternal health and child survival.[9]

Undoubtedly, chronic hunger and malnutrition are most prevalent in lower-income countries. The reductions in hunger and the improvement in nutrition can support productivity gains among individuals as well as nations. Indeed, the establishment of nutrition-intervention programs in poorly nourished populations can ultimately save money that otherwise would be used for the care of malnourished people. Although reducing malnutrition is often justified based on the grounds of human rights, it is these potential gains in productivity and reductions in economic costs that provide the pragmatic and moral focus for international nutrition.

## An International Focus on Diet and Noncommunicable Disease

Maternal and child undernutrition was the subject of a series in the medical journal *The Lancet* in 2008.[10] In 2013, *The Lancet* reevaluated the problem and programs addressing it. It also examined the growing issue of overweight and obesity for women and children and the consequences for lower- and middle-income countries.[11] Overweight and obesity are surging in many lower-income countries just as in higher-income countries. Although many people view this as a more recent phenomenon, the trend has been evident for more than a decade. In its 2002 report *Globalization, Diets and Noncommunicable Diseases*, the WHO stated:

> Noncommunicable diseases have become a major health problem not just in developed countries but also in developing countries. Already 79% of the deaths attributed to the noncommunicable diseases occur in developing countries. Examples from several countries show that changing these determinants is possible and can have a strong effect on the trends in noncommunicable diseases.[12]

In 2004, the **World Health Assembly (WHA)** endorsed WHO's Global Strategy on Diet, Physical

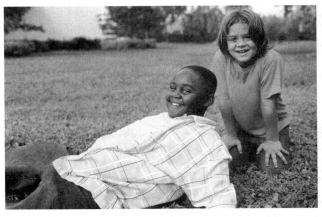

© Stockbyte/Getty Images.

In 2015, UN member states adopted a set of goals to end poverty, protect the planet, and ensure prosperity for all as part of a new sustainable development agenda.

The following 17 goals have specific targets to be achieved by 2030.

1. End poverty in all its forms everywhere.
2. End hunger, achieve food security and improved nutrition, and promote sustainable agriculture.
3. Ensure healthy lives and promote well-being for all at all ages.
4. Ensure inclusive and equitable quality education and promote lifelong learning opportunities for all.
5. Achieve gender equality and empower all women and girls.
6. Ensure availability and sustainable management of water and sanitation for all.
7. Ensure access to affordable, reliable, sustainable, and modern energy for all.
8. Promote sustained, inclusive, and sustainable economic growth, full and productive employment, and decent work for all.
9. Build resilient infrastructure and promote inclusive and sustainable industrialization and foster innovation.
10. Reduce inequality within and among countries.
11. Make cities and human settlements inclusive, safe, resilient, and sustainable.
12. Ensure sustainable consumption and production patterns.
13. Take urgent action to combat climate change and its impacts (in line with the UN Framework Convention on Climate Change).
14. Conserve and sustainably use the oceans, seas, and marine resources for sustainable development.
15. Protect, restore, and promote sustainable use of terrestrial ecosystems; sustainably manage forests; combat desertification; halt and reverse land degradation; and halt biodiversity loss.
16. Promote peaceful and inclusive societies for sustainable development; provide access to justice for all and build effective, accountable, and inclusive institutions at all levels.
17. Strengthen the means of implementation and revitalize the global partnership for sustainable development.

**FIGURE 12.4** UN sustainable development goals

Modified from UN. Sustainable Development Goals. 17 Goals to transform our world. http://www.un.org/sustainabledevelopment/sustainable-development-goals/. Accessed 12/1/16.

Activity, and Health. One of the four main objectives of the strategy was specific to research, identifying the need "to monitor scientific data and key influences on diet and physical activity; to support research in a broad spectrum of relevant areas, including evaluation of interventions; and to strengthen the human resources needed in this domain to enhance and sustain health."[13]

In 2012, the United Nations passed a resolution to adopt the Political Declaration of the High-Level Meeting of the General Assembly on the Prevention and Control of Non-Communicable Diseases.[14] The declaration called for population-based policies, multisectoral action, cross-agency work and monitoring, and the evaluation and identification of common noncommunicable disease risk factors, including an unhealthy diet and harmful use of alcohol. In response, the WHO has taken the lead in developing a *Global Action Plan for Prevention and Control of Non-Communicable Disease 2013–2020.* Efforts include recommendations on population-based actions such as promoting a healthy diet and monitoring frameworks with specific targets and indicators. The global action plan provides a road map for UN member states, WHO, other UN organizations, and additional groups to achieve the goal of a 25%

relative reduction in premature mortality from noncommunicable diseases by 2025.[15]

Although there is still a need for increased coordination and buy-in to fully implement this road map, recent years has seen more global recognition of and focus on addressing noncommunicable disease. It is included in the latest UN global goals, the **UN Sustainable Development Goals (FIGURE 12.4)**, and it is a core element of the United Nations Global Nutrition Agenda. These goals outline UN agencies' efforts to support the achievement of nutrition goals worldwide and describe specific links between nutrition and the sustainable development goals.[16] Noncommunicable disease is also part of the **UN Decade of Action on Nutrition** declared in 2016 (**FIGURES 12.5**).[17]

The UN Decade of Action on Nutrition endorses the results of the Second International Conference on Nutrition (ICN2), which was held in 2012 and produced the ***Rome Declaration on Nutrition*** and an accompanying *Framework for Action* to guide its implementation.[18,19] The first International Conference on Nutrition was held in 1992, and although many of the subsequent goals and recommendations from both conferences were similar, the ICN2 also included a clear call to action on reversing the trend in obesity (**FIGURE 12.6**).

In April 2016, the UN General Assembly passed a resolution proclaiming the UN Decade of Action on Nutrition from 2016 to 2025. The resolution aimed to "trigger intensified action to end hunger and eradicate malnutrition worldwide, and ensure universal access to healthier and more sustainable diets—for all people, whoever they are and wherever they live." It specifically called on governments to set national nutrition targets and milestones for 2025 based on internationally agreed-on indicators.

The WHO and FAO will lead the implementation of the Decade of Action on Nutrition in collaboration with the WFP, the International Fund for Agricultural Development (IFAD), and UNICEF and in coordination with the United Nations System Standing Committee on Nutrition and multiple stakeholder platforms such as the Committee on World Food Security.

The Decade of Action on Nutrition further endorses the Rome Declaration on Nutrition and its accompanying technical Framework for Action.

**FIGURE 12.5** UN decade of action on nutrition (2016–2025)

Reproduced from Food and Agriculture Organization of the United Nations. The Rome Declaration on Nutrition. Infographics. http://www.fao.org/resources/infographics/infographics-details/en/c/266118/ . 2014. Accessed 12/1/16.

Obesity has significant effects on health and healthcare costs, with an estimated 20% of global health budgets spent on obesity and associated diseases (**FIGURE 12.7**).

Worldwide, obesity has more than doubled since 1980. In 2014, more than 1.9 billion adults 18 and older were overweight; of these, more than 600 million were obese.

Most of the world's population now live in countries where overweight and obesity kill more people than underweight.[20]

The WHO has nine global targets for noncommunicable disease, including that by 2025 there will be no increase in obesity or diabetes beyond the levels of 2010.[21] Yet with the ever-increasing number of people becoming obese or overweight, it is now projected

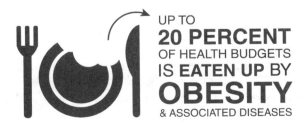

**FIGURE 12.7** Impact of obesity on global healthcare costs

Reproduced from Shelton P. Up to 20 percent of health budgets eaten away by obesity and related diseases. Global Nutrition Report 2015. September 21, 2015. http://globalnutritionreport.org/category/infographics/. Accessed 12/1/16. http://globalnutritionreport.org/2015/09/21/up-to-20-percent-of-health-budgets-eaten-away-by-obesity-and-related-diseases/.

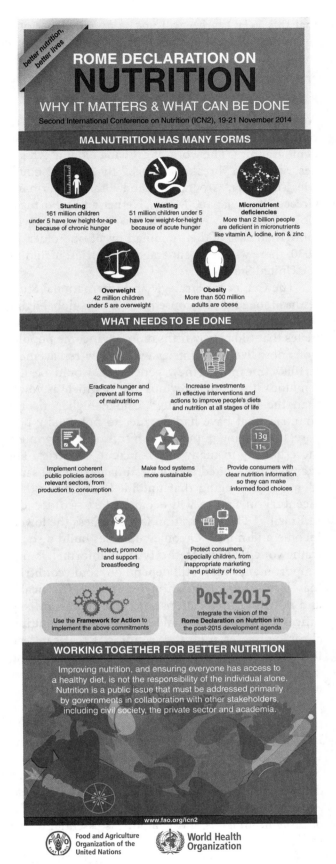

**FIGURE 12.6** The Rome Declaration on Nutrition

Reprinted from World Health Organization, General Assembly proclaims Decade of Action on Nutrition. Nutrition, © 2016Reproduced from The Rome Declaration on Nutrition. Food and Agriculture Organization of the United Nations. http://www.fao.org/resources/infographics/infographics-details/en/c/266118.

that this WHO target will *not* be met and that one-fifth of the global population and almost 1 billion of the world's adults will be obese by 2025.

## An International Focus on Older Adults

An important factor influencing the global nutrition agenda is the world population's changing age demographics. The world is growing older at what is described as a "breakneck pace." By 2020, 13 countries (Bulgaria, Croatia, Finland, France, Germany, Greece, Italy, Japan, Malta, Netherlands, Portugal, Slovenia, and Sweden) will be "superaged," with more than 20% of their populations 65 and older. By 2030, there will be 34 superaged countries, including the United States.[22]

The Center for Strategic and International Studies has looked at the consequences of a global aging population through its Global Aging Initiative. It estimates that today two-fifths of lower-income populations now live in countries with below-replacement fertility (meaning a new generation would be less populous than the previous one), which is lower than the US fertility rate.[23] Unlike higher-income countries that have had decades to potentially prepare, the graying population shift is occurring much more quickly in many lower-income countries. For example, the United Nations estimates that the same "demographic aging that unfolded over more than a century in France will occur in just two decades in Brazil."[24] The implication is that unless the lower-income and middle-income countries build a social framework to provide the type of informal family support many elders still depend on, some countries may face a humanitarian aging crisis.[23] The health and nutrition implications for these trends are significant because many older adults have multiple chronic diseases and other conditions that can lead to increased disability, frailty, and poor health and compound their changing nutrition needs and access to a nutritious diet.

The United Nations has had targeted goals related to nutrition and older adults since the early 1980s. Indeed, the 1982 World Assembly on Aging led to the 1983 release of the *Vienna International Plan of Action on Aging*, which included many nutrition recommendations in the belief that "[a]dequate, appropriate, and sufficient nutrition, particularly the adequate intake of protein, minerals and vitamins, is essential to the well-being of the elderly."[25]

In its 2016 report to the UN Secretariat, *Multisectoral Action for a Life Course Approach to Healthy Ageing: Draft Global Strategy and Plan of Action on Ageing and Health*, WHO researchers stated that "even

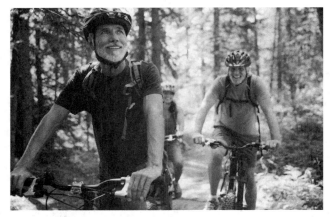

© Hero Images/Getty Images.

in very advanced years, physical activity, and good nutrition can have powerful benefits on health and well-being."[26] In the newest UN Sustainable Development Goals (Figure 12.4), aging and nutrition are relevant to many of the goals. Older adult nutrition is specifically addressed in the target for the second goal:

> Target 2.2: By 2030, end all forms of malnutrition, including achieving, by 2025, the internationally agreed targets on stunting and wasting in children under five years of age, and address the nutritional needs of adolescent girls, pregnant and lactating women and older persons.[27]

When considering international nutrition research on problems that influence the health, survival, and developmental capacity of populations, addressing the nutritional needs of older adults remains paramount. However, to date UN agencies have developed very few international nutrition programs specifically targeting older adults and their unique nutritional needs. Events such as International Day of Older Persons 2017 highlight the connection between taking advantage of the talents and contributions of older persons and implementing the 2030 Agenda and the Madrid International Plan of Action on Ageing, which is currently undergoing its third review and appraisal process.

> **Recap**   Malnutrition is associated with poor survival from infancy through adulthood and into old age, and it also threatens quality of life. Increasingly, lower-income populations are experiencing a "nutrition transition," that may be giving rise in part to an increasing trend of noncommunicable disease as a primary cause of death rather than infectious disease, and this is influencing international health and nutrition goals.

# ▶ Who is Supporting the Global Nutrition Agenda?

**Preview** Whether an organization chooses to become involved in a specific international nutrition-research project can be influenced by its mission, vision, and values.

When considering international nutrition assessment and research, it is important to understand who is supporting or funding the research. An organization's mission, vision, and values can significantly affect how and even if the organization becomes engaged in a specific research project. Five different types of organizations may be involved in international nutrition-related research: (1) multilateral organizations, (2) bilateral organizations, (3) nongovernmental organizations, (4) **partnership organizations and collaborations**, and (5) private-sector organizations. These organizations and examples of those who are engaged in nutrition research are discussed in the following sections.

One important consideration in international nutrition assessment and research is that successful collaboration across multiple types of organizations usually achieve the most meaningful nutrition and public-health outcomes.

## Multilateral Organizations

**Multilateral organizations** are funded by multiple governments and provide support to many different countries. Multilateral organizations often receive funding from both governmental and nongovernmental groups. Most of the world's major multilateral organizations are part of the United Nations, which was founded in 1945 and currently has some 190 member states, including the United States. The purposes and principles in the United Nation's founding charter still guide the mission and work of its multilateral organizations today.

As previously discussed, one of the groups that has been active in setting the UN nutrition agenda is the UN Standing Committee on Nutrition. The UNSCN has been made up of representatives from many UN groups **(TABLE 12.1)** and groups that collaborate with the United Nations.

**TABLE 12.1** Examples of multilateral organizations

| Organization | Abbreviation | Description | Website |
|---|---|---|---|
| Member Organizations of the United Nations System Standing Committee on Nutrition (UNSCN) | | | |
| Chief Executives Board for Coordination | CEB | Focuses on harmonizing efforts between organizations to address emerging issues that require policy coherence. | http://www .unsceb.org/ |
| Department of Economic and Social Affairs | DESA | Works with governments and stakeholders to help them meet their economic, social, environmental goals; guided by UN development agenda. | https://www .un.org /development /desa/en/ |
| Food and Agriculture Organization | FAO | Works with governments to achieve food security and ensure people have regular access to enough high-quality food to lead active, healthy lives. Goals include eradication of hunger, food insecurity, and malnutrition; elimination of poverty; driving economic and social progress, sustainable management, and utilization of natural resources. Includes Committee on World Food Security (CFS), which provides platform for all stakeholders to work together to ensure food security and nutrition for all. | http://www.fao .org/home/en/ |
| International Atomic Energy Agency | IAEA | Works to promote safe, secure, and peaceful use of nuclear technologies. | https://www.iaea .org/ |

*(continues)*

**TABLE 12.1** (*continued*)

| Organization | Abbreviation | Description | Website |
|---|---|---|---|
| International Fund of Agriculture Development | IFAD | Focuses on rural poverty reduction to eliminate hunger and malnutrition, raise productivity and incomes, and improve the quality of lives. | https://www.ifad.org/ |
| United Nations Children's Fund | UNICEF | Works to bring attention to and mobilize resources to address challenges facing children. | http://www.unicef.org/ |
| World Food Programme | WFP | Combats global hunger and responds to hunger emergencies.<br>The world's largest humanitarian agency fighting hunger. | http://www.wfp.org/ |
| World Health Organization | WHO | Produces health guidelines and standards, helps countries address public-health issues, and supports and promotes health research.<br>*Note:* The World Health Assembly (WHA) is WHO's decision-making body and sets WHO policies. | http://www.who.int/en/ |
| **Other UN Organizations with Potential Interest in Nutrition** | | | |
| CODEX Alimentarius | CODEX | Harmonizes international food standards to protect consumer health and promote fair practices in food trade.<br>Its science-based recommendations include standards for food hygiene, maximum limits for food additives and residues of pesticides and veterinary drugs, and maximum limits or codes for preventing chemical and microbiological contamination is part of the FAO. | http://www.fao.org/fao-who-codexalimentarius/codex-home/en |
| International Labor Organization | ILO | Brings together governments and employers to set labor standards and develop work policies and programs. | http://www.ilo.org/global/lang--en/index.htm |
| Joint United Nations Program on HIV/AIDS | UNAIDS | Serves as leading advocate for global action against HIV and AIDS.<br>Not a single UN agency but combines expertise and resources of multiple agencies. | http://www.unaids.org/ |
| United Nations Development Program | UNDP | Works to eradicate poverty and reduce inequalities and exclusion.<br>Helps countries develop policies, leadership skills, partnering abilities, institutional capabilities, and resilience to sustain development results. | http://www.undp.org/ |
| United Nations Educational, Scientific, and Cultural Organization | UNESCO | Known as the United Nations'"intellectual" agency. Builds networks among nations to mobilize for education, to build intercultural understanding, to pursue scientific cooperation, and to protect freedom of expression. | http://en.unesco.org/ |
| United Nations Environment Programme | UNEP | Sets global environmental agenda, promotes implementation of environmental dimension of sustainable development, and serves as an authoritative advocate for the global environment. | http://www.unep.org/ |

## TABLE 12.1 *(continued)*

| Organization | Abbreviation | Description | Website |
|---|---|---|---|
| United Nations High Commissioner for Human Rights | UNHCHR | Represents world's commitment to universal ideals of human dignity and promotes and protects all human rights. | http://www.ohchr.org/EN/Pages/Home.aspx |
| United Nations High Commissioner for Refugees | UNHCR | Protects and assists refugees around the world. | http://www.unhcr.org/en-us |
| United Nations Population Fund | UNFPA | Works to expand possibilities for women and young people to lead healthy, productive lives. | http://www.unfpa.org/ |
| United Nations Research Institute for Social Development | UNRSID | Undertakes multidisciplinary research and policy analysis on social dimensions of contemporary development issues to ensure that social equity, inclusion, and justice are central to development thinking, policies, and practices.<br>Acts as autonomous research institute within UN system. | http://www.unrisd.org/ |
| United Nations University | UNU | Contributes through collaborative research and education to efforts to resolve pressing global problems of human survival, development, and welfare.<br>Acts as global think tank and postgraduate teaching organization. | http://unu.edu/ |
| **Non-UN Organizations with Potential Interest in Nutrition** | | | |
| World Bank Group | | Group of five associated development institutions, including: (1) the International Bank for Reconstruction and Development (IBRD), which lends to governments of middle-income, creditworthy low-income countries; (2) the International Development Association (IDA), which provides interest-free loans and grants to governments of poor countries; (3) the International Finance Corporation (IFC), which is the largest global development institution focused exclusively on the private sector; (4) the Multilateral Investment Guarantee Agency (MIGA), which promotes foreign direct investment into lower-income countries to support economic growth, reduce poverty, and improve people's lives; and (5) International Centre for Settlement of Investment Disputes (ICSID), which provides international facilities for conciliation and arbitration of investment. | http://www.worldbank.org |
| Asian Development Bank | | Helps its more than 60 members and partners by providing loans, technical assistance, grants, equity investments to promote social and economic development. | http://www.adb.org/about/main |

One UN organization is highly active in the area of nutrition: the WHO and its policy body, the World Health Assembly. The WHA has established specific Global Nutrition Targets for 2025 (**FIGURE 12.8**) which are focused on improving maternal, infant, and young child nutrition. Unfortunately, older adults are not included in these targets.

UN member states have committed to monitoring progress on these nutrition targets. A range of other UN multilateral organizations may be engaged in international nutrition research and programs or have an interest in nutrition, including **CODEX Alimentarius**, which harmonizes international food standards (Table 12.1). Multilateral organizations that are not

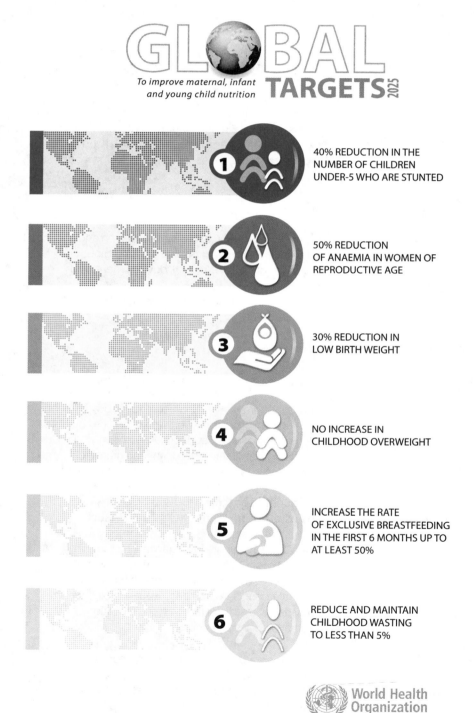

**FIGURE 12.8** 2025 World Health Organization global nutrition targets

part of the United Nations and may be related to international nutrition research include the World Bank Group and the Asian Development Bank (Table 12.1).

## Bilateral Organizations

**Bilateral organizations** are governmental agencies from a single country that provide aid to lower-income countries. History, politics, and geography—including a country's past territorial relationships—often play a role in a bilateral organization's funding decisions. One of the largest bilateral organizations is USAID. This organization and several others, including bilateral organizations from other industrialized countries that may be involved in international nutrition research, are described in **TABLE 12.2**.

**TABLE 12.2** Examples of bilateral organizations

| Organization | Abbreviation | Description | Website |
|---|---|---|---|
| **US Organizations** | | | |
| Biomarkers of Nutrition for Development Program | BOND | Harmonizes processes for making decisions about what biomarkers are best for supporting research, program development, evaluation, and generation of evidence-based policy. Partnership of US National Institute of Child Health and Human Development (NICHD) and others representing global food and nutrition enterprises. | https://www.nichd.nih.gov/global_nutrition/programs/bond/pages/index.aspx |
| International Micronutrient Malnutrition Prevention and Control Program | IMMPaCt | Works to eliminate vitamin, and mineral deficiencies among global vulnerable populations primarily by focusing on helping eliminate deficiencies in iron, vitamin A, iodine, folate, and zinc. Program of the Centers for Disease Control and Prevention (CDC). | http://www.cdc.gov/immpact/index.html |
| United States Agency for International Development | USAID | Seeks to empower and support other countries through collaborative partnerships to foster sustainable development. Often contracts its support for health and nutrition programs through international health agencies. | https://www.usaid.gov/ |
| **Other Nations' Organizations** | | | |
| Australian Agency for International Development | AUSAID | Works to promote prosperity, reduce poverty, enhance stability, make performance count, make environment performance driven. Focuses on Indo-Pacific region. | http://dfat.gov.au/aid/pages/australias-aid-program.aspx |
| Canadian International Development Agency | CIDA | Maintains significant bilateral aid programs focusing on increasing food security, stimulating sustainable economic growth, securing future of children and youth, and supporting governance. Focuses on countries based on need, capacity to benefit from development assistance, and alignment with Canadian foreign policy priorities. | http://www.international.gc.ca/development-developpement/index.aspx?lang=eng |

*(continues)*

**TABLE 12.2** (continued)

| Organization | Abbreviation | Description | Website |
|---|---|---|---|
| Department for International Development in the United Kingdom | DFID | Leads United Kingdom's work to end extreme poverty and build safer, healthier, and more prosperous world.<br>Works to end need for aid by creating jobs, unlocking potential of girls and women, and helping save lives during humanitarian emergencies. | https://www.gov.uk/government/organisations/department-for-international-development |
| European Union Aid | EUROPEAID | Focuses on reducing world poverty; ensuring sustainable economic, social, and environmental development; and promoting democracy, rule of law, good governance, and respect of human rights.<br>Implements programs and projects around the world wherever assistance is needed. | http://ec.europa.eu/europeaid/home_en |
| German Agency for Development Cooperation | GIZ | Develops sustainable and effective solutions in countries worldwide. | https://www.giz.de/en/html/worldwide.html |
| Japan International Cooperation Agency | JICA | Supports socioeconomic development, recovery, or economic stability of lower-income regions.<br>Advances activities around pillars of field-oriented approach, human security, enhanced effectiveness, efficiency, and speed. | http://www.jica.go.jp/english/ |
| Norwegian Agency for Development Cooperation | NORAD | Focuses on climate change, democracy, education, energy, global health, higher education, macroeconomics, and oil for development. | https://www.norad.no/en/front/ |
| Swedish International Development and Cooperation Agency | SIDA | Works to reduce world poverty.<br>Conducts reform with Eastern Europe nations.<br>Distributes humanitarian aid. | http://www.sida.se/English/ |
| Swiss Agency for Development and Cooperation | SDC | Supports countries in their efforts to overcome poverty and development-related problems.<br>Places special emphasis on fragile states and countries affected by conflict | https://www.eda.admin.ch/sdc |

# Nongovernmental Organizations

**Nongovernmental organizations (NGOs)**, also known as *private voluntary organizations*, are defined by the United Nations as not-for-profit voluntary citizen's groups that are organized on local, national, or international levels to address issues in support of the public good. NGOs are typically free from governmental control and can address a range of issues such as economic empowerment, humanitarian aid, emergency relief, environmental protection, and social justice. Traditionally, these groups have primarily humanitarian or cooperative rather than commercial objectives.

NGOs are a heterogeneous group that may be best understood by considering their orientation and level of operation. The Global Development Research Center categorizes the orientation of NGOs' scopes of work as charitable, service, or participatory.

- A *charitable orientation* may lead to direct provision and distribution of food, clothing, or medicine or to provision of housing, schools, or disaster relief. The involvement of beneficiaries in the development and delivery of the charitable programs can vary.
- A *service orientation* includes activities such as providing health, family planning, or education services. Programs are often designed by the NGO, and its beneficiaries participate not only in receiving the services but also in implementing them.
- A *participatory orientation* is characterized by self-help projects that beneficiaries help implement by contributing cash, tools, land, materials, or labor.

- An *empowering orientation* helps people develop a clearer understanding of the social, political, and economic factors affecting their lives, and it strengthens their awareness of their own potential power to control their lives. These groups may develop spontaneously or through the facilitation of an existing NGO.[28]

NGOs' levels of operations relate to their organizational interactions and can range from community-based to national or international. Additional NGO classifications include size of the organization, thematic scope, geographic scope, and funding levels. Although NGOs function independently from governments—without direct government oversight or representation—some NGOs may receive government funding. Other sources for NGO funding include foundations, citizens and volunteers, religious groups, businesses, and the private sector. Examples of NGOs that may be involved in international nutrition assessment and research are detailed in **TABLE 12.3**. Examples of several specific nutrition programs and projects of top-ranking NGOs are found in **TABLE 12.4**.

**TABLE 12.3** Examples of NGOs

| Organization | Abbreviation | Description | Website |
|---|---|---|---|
| Alliance for Global Food Security (US Food Aid and Security) | | Implements emergency development programs that build capacity of local communities, enterprises, institutions.<br>Comprises private voluntary organizations committed to eradicating hunger, malnutrition, and food insecurity and reducing poverty.<br>Operates in more than 100 lower-income countries. | http://foodaid.org/ |
| American Jewish World Service | AJWS | Combines power of grants to human rights advocates in lower-income countries with efforts to persuade US government to adopt laws and policies benefiting people in lower-income countries. | https://ajws.org/ |
| CARE | | Works around the globe to save lives, defeat poverty, achieve social justice. | http://www.care.org/ |
| Catholic Relief Services | CRS | Assists the poor and the vulnerable.<br>Works with Catholic institutions and structures as well as other organizations. | http://www.crs.org/ |

*(continues)*

**TABLE 12.3** (continued)

| Organization | Abbreviation | Description | Website |
|---|---|---|---|
| Concern Worldwide | | Global community of humanitarians, partners, community members, supporters, donors, and volunteers who share common vision of world where no one lives in poverty, fear, or oppression and all can exercise their rights to decent standard of living; and can access opportunities and choices essential to long, healthy, creative lives; and can be treated with dignity and respect. | http://www.concernusa.org/ |
| Food for the Hungry International | FHI | Seeks to end all forms of human poverty by actively partnering with churches, leaders, and families to build transformational relationships, usher in justice, and renew communities. | http://www.fh.org/ |
| Food Fortification Initiative | | Works to improve health by advocating for fortification in industrial grain mills. Specializes in wheat flour, maize flour, and rice. | http://www.ffinetwork.org/ |
| Bill & Melinda Gates Foundation | | Partners with organizations worldwide to address global development (hunger and poverty), global health (harnessing advances in science to save lives), and global policy and advocacy (build strategic partnerships to advance work). | http://www.gatesfoundation.org/ |
| Global Alliance for Improved Nutrition | GAIN | Acts as catalyst to building alliances between governments, businesses, and civil society and to finding and delivering solutions to complex problems of malnutrition. Focuses on children, girls, and women to help end cycle of malnutrition and poverty. | http://www.gainhealth.org/ |
| Global Child Nutrition Foundation | GCNF | Helps countries develop and operate successful, sustainable school-feeding programs. | http://gcnf.org/ |
| Helen Keller International | HKI | Works to save and improve the sight and lives of world's vulnerable by combatting causes and consequences of blindness, poor health, and malnutrition. | http://www.hki.org/ |
| International Committee of the Red Cross | | Takes action to ensure humanitarian protection and assistance for victims of armed conflict and other violent situations. | https://www.icrc.org/en |
| International Council for Control of Iodine Deficiency Disorders | ICCIDD | Advocates to governments, citizens, and development agencies a priority commitment to iodine nutrition through multidisciplinary approach that involves all relevant partners. | http://www.who.int/pmnch/about/members/database/iccidd/en/ |

## TABLE 12.3 (continued)

| Organization | Abbreviation | Description | Website |
|---|---|---|---|
| International Development Research Centre | IDRC | Funds research in lower-income countries to help find solutions to local problems and create lasting change. Contributes to Canada's foreign policy goals. | https://www.idrc.ca/ |
| International Food Policy Research Institute | IFPRI | Provides research-based policy solutions to sustainably reduce and end hunger and malnutrition in lower-income countries. | http://www.ifpri.org/ |
| International Federation of the Red Cross and Red Crescent Societies | IFRC | Acts before, during, and after disasters and health emergencies to meet needs and improve the lives of vulnerable people The world's largest humanitarian network. | http://www.ifrc.org/ |
| International Food Information Council | IFIC | Works to effectively communicate science-based information on health, nutrition, and food safety for the public good. | http://www.foodinsight.org/ |
| International Life Sciences Institute | ILSI | Provides science that improves human health and well-being and safeguards the environment. | http://ilsi.org/ |
| International Nutrition Foundation | | Builds capacity in lower-income country individuals/institutions in nutrition research, policy, programming so they can effectively address issues of food, nutrition/hunger in their countries | http://www.inffoundation.org/ |
| International Union of Nutritional Sciences | | Promotes advancement in nutrition science, research, and development through international cooperation. Encourages communication and collaboration among nutrition scientists to disseminate information in nutritional sciences through modern communication technology. | http://www.iuns.org/ |
| Islamic Relief USA | | Provides relief and development in working toward the goal of a world free of poverty. | http://irusa.org/ |
| Lutheran World Relief | LWR | Partners with other organizations around the world to end poverty, injustice, and human suffering. | https://lwr.org/ |
| Micronutrient Initiative | MI | Ensures world's most vulnerable—especially women and children—in lower-income countries get vitamins and minerals needed to survive and thrive. | http://www.micronutrient.org/ |

*(continues)*

| TABLE 12.3 (continued) | | | |
|---|---|---|---|
| **Organization** | **Abbreviation** | **Description** | **Website** |
| The Rockefeller Foundation | | Promotes well-being of humanity throughout the world.<br>Focuses on building greater resilience and advancing more inclusive economies. | https://www.rockefellerfoundation.org/ |
| Save the Children Fund | | Invests in childhood by giving children healthy starts and opportunities to learn while protecting them from harm. | http://www.savethechildren.org/site/c.8rKLIXMGIpl4E/b.6115947/k.B143/Official_USA_Site.htm |
| Scaling Up Nutrition | | Unites governments, civil societies, the United Nations, donors, businesses, and researchers in collective effort to improve nutrition.<br>Goal is a world without hunger or malnutrition. | http://scalingupnutrition.org/ |
| United Methodist Committee on Relief | UMCOR | Works to alleviate human suffering around the globe.<br>Programs include disaster response, health, sustainable agriculture, food security, and relief supplies. | http://www.umcor.org/ |
| World Council of Churches | WCC | Brings together churches, denominations, church fellowships in >110 countries and territories throughout the world.<br>Represents >500 million Christians.<br>Ecumenical Advocacy Alliance (EAA) focuses on common concerns for justice and human dignity; current issues include food security and sustainable agriculture. | https://www.oikoumene.org/en/what-we-do/eaa |
| World Vision | | Christian humanitarian organization<br>Works with children, families, and their communities worldwide to reach their full potential by tackling root causes of poverty and injustice. | http://www.worldvision.org/ |

## Partnership Organizations and Collaborations

Although many international nutrition-assessment and research efforts focus on the issue of malnutrition caused by lack of access to or knowledge about adequate, nutritious food, awareness is also growing about the issue of disease-associated malnutrition among international populations, particularly older adults. The European Society for Parenteral and Enteral Nutrition has published a consensus statement on the diagnostic criteria for malnutrition.[29] Many international organizations—typically partnerships with healthcare professional organizations, governmental groups, and the private sector—have been formed to help address disease-associated malnutrition. Other types of international collaborations include groups joined together to address frailty, chronic disease, or other health issues (**TABLE 12.5**).

**TABLE 12.4** Examples of nutrition programs among top-ranked NGOs*

| | |
|---|---|
| Bangladesh Rural Advancement Committee (BRAC): http://www.brac.net | This development organization is dedicated to alleviating poverty by empowering the poor in a dozen countries around the world. It is viewed as the largest nongovernmental development organization in the world when measured by numbers of employees and people it has helped. Its nutrition program works at the household and community levels to create malnutrition awareness. Shasthya shebika (health volunteers) and nutrition promoters visit families to provide counseling, coaching, and demonstrations. The program also distributes micronutrient powder sachets to prevent anemia and provides supplementary food to manage acute malnutrition in mothers and children. |
| Doctors Without Borders (Medecins Sans Frontieres): http://www.doctorswithoutborders.org | Helps people worldwide where the need is greatest, delivering emergency medical aid to people affected by conflict, epidemics, and disasters and those who are exclusion from health care. Malnutrition is one of more than 15 medical issues identified by the organization. Although its primary focus is on young children, it also identifies adolescents, pregnant and breastfeeding women, the elderly, and the chronically ill as vulnerable populations. Its feeding programs provide ready-to-use therapeutic food to treat malnutrition. |
| The Danish Refugee Council: https://drc.dk/ | Organization formed after World War II in response to the 1956 Soviet Invasion of Hungary, which led to a European refugee crisis. The humanitarian organization now serves more than 30 countries by providing aid during conflict. Provides emergency food and voucher programs, trains refugees in agriculture, and gives agricultural grants. |
| OXFAM International: https://www.oxfam.org/ | An international confederation of 18 organizations working together with partners and local communities to find practical, innovative ways for people to fight poverty. Offers substantial food aid in response to both natural disasters and those caused by human action, assists small-scale farmers in adopting sustainable practices and adapting to climate change, and works to reform the food system through its GROW campaign. |
| Mercy Corps: https://www.mercycorps.org/ | Originally founded as the Save the Refugees Fund. Now a leading global organization with a mission to alleviate suffering, poverty, and oppression through the development of secure, productive, and just communities. Works to streamline nutrition education on how to prevent malnutrition among the most vulnerable (children and pregnant and lactating women). Other nutrition education focuses on safe food-handling techniques and nutritional requirements, as well as addressing cultural food taboos. Also takes responsibility for diversifying food production, emphasizing nutrient-dense foods, introducing biofortification into traditional foods, and supporting small-scale farmers. |

*These NGOs were among the top 500 ranked by ngoadvisor.net. Ngoadvisor.net's 2015 rankings used public data to score NGOs on impact, innovation, and governance.

**TABLE 12.5** Examples of partnership organizations and collaborations

| Organization | Abbreviation | Description | Website |
|---|---|---|---|
| **Disease-Associated and Malnutrition-Related** | | | |
| Canadian Malnutrition Task Force | CMTF | Standing committee of the Canadian Nutrition Society, focuses on education, data aggregation, development of best practices, and influencing policy. | http://nutritioncareincanada.ca/ |
| The European Nutrition for Health Alliance | ENHA | Works with key stakeholders to improve nutritional care across Europe by actively promoting: the implementation of nutrition risk screening across Europe, public awareness, appropriate reimbursement policies, and medical education. Launched Optimal Nutritional Care for All campaign to facilitate greater screening for risk of disease-related malnutrition and undernutrition and implement nutritional care across Europe. Members include European nutrition, geriatric, healthcare, insurance, and industry groups. | http://www.european-nutrition.org |
| feedM.E. | | Works to increase global awareness, education, action on malnutrition Works with healthcare systems and communities to help bring global change to the local level. Members include Latin American nutrition professionals and industry. | https://nutritionmatters.com/ |
| The Malnutrition Task Force | | Addresses avoidable and preventable malnutrition in older adults. Works with partners in hospitals, care homes, local authorities, and private and voluntary organizations. Members include UK nutrition and industry groups. | http://www.malnutritiontaskforce.org.uk |
| **Frailty or Chronic-Disease Related** | | | |
| Canadian Frailty Network | CFN | Facilitates evidence-based research, knowledge sharing, and clinical practices that improve healthcare outcomes for frail elderly Canadians, their families, and caregivers. Members include funded investigators and others working with funded projects as well as the general public. | http://www.cfn-nce.ca/ |

**TABLE 12.5** *(continued)*

| Organization | Abbreviation | Description | Website |
|---|---|---|---|
| European Innovation Partnership on Active and Healthy Ageing | | Pursues a "triple win for Europe: (1) enabling European Union (EU) citizens to lead healthy, active, independent lives while aging; (2) improving sustainability and efficiency of social and healthcare systems boosting and improving competitiveness of markets for innovative products and services; and (3) responding to aging challenges at both the EU and global levels, thus creating new opportunities for businesses.<br>Overarching target: increase average healthy lifespan by two years by 2020.<br>Members include professional groups, public authorities, and industry. | http://ec.europa.eu /research/innovation -union/index _en.cfm?section=active -healthy-ageing |
| International Obesity Consortium | IOC | Conducts research to identify common and unique dietary, behavioral factors contributing to obesity and related diseases (including diabetes and cardiovascular disease) in different countries.<br>Uses information to develop country-specific interventions for effective, sustainable weight loss and improved health.<br>Formed by Jean Mayer, US Department of Agriculture Human Nutrition Center on Aging at Tufts University.<br>Members include United States and eight other countries. | http://hnrca.tufts.edu/ioc/ |
| Joint Programming Initiative | JPI | Provides holistic approach to develop and implement research agenda to understand interplay of factors known to directly affect diet-related diseases.<br>Works to discover new relevant mechanisms.<br>Contributes to development of actions, policies, innovative products and diets with aim of drastically reducing burden of diet-related diseases.<br>Members include 25 countries (primarily European). | http://www .healthydietforhealthylife .eu/index.php |

## Private-Sector Organizations

The private sector is engaged in nutrition assessment and research across the globe to help quantify nutrition problems and identify effective solutions. **Private-sector organizations** may support the nutrition research of NGOs and partner with organizations and even governments through corporate foundations. Private-sector organizations may also directly fund primary nutrition research to develop new commercial products. **TABLE 12.6** provides examples of several multinational corporations engaged in international nutrition research.

**Recap**  Five different types of organizations may be involved in international nutrition-related research: multilateral organizations, bilateral organizations, nongovernmental organizations, partnership organizations and collaborations, and private-sector organizations. How these organizations engage in an international nutrition-research project depends on their scope. Many internationally focused organizations have a strong interest in nutrition, and a successful collaboration across multiple types of organizations can help achieve meaningful nutrition and public-health outcomes.

**TABLE 12.6** Examples of private-sector organizations

| Organization | Description of Nutrition Research | Website |
|---|---|---|
| Abbott | Committed to increasing awareness of critical role nutrition plays in improving patient outcomes with research in emerging field of health economics and outcomes research and in developing and clinically validating new solutions to address greatest needs. | http://www.abbott.com/ |
| Danone | Strives to support food as key asset to reinforce healthy living globally. Scientific approach is rooted in food styles and local needs as tailored to each person's culture or local environment. | http://www.danone.com/ |
| Mars | Conducts fundamental research at cutting edge of plant science, human and pet health and nutrition, food science, materials science, and computational science. | http://www.mars.com/ |
| Mondelez | Invests in research to develop technology-based solutions to help improve nutritional profile of its products and better meet needs of consumers. | http://www.mondelezinternational.com/ |
| Nestle | Seeks to support public health by investing in both individual- and population-based scientific research to deliver better nutrition for current and future generations. | http://www.nestle.com/ |
| Unilever | Collaborates with research partners to understand how food affects health and what the motivators are for behavior change. Contributes to latest thinking on nutrition security and sustainable diets. | https://www.unilever.com |

# How is an International Nutrition-Research Problem Defined?

**Preview** Many UN and WHO global development goals are related to malnutrition, provide a framework for identifying specific nutrition disorders, and are supported by foundational research and global trend data that may be useful in helping define an international nutrition-research problem.

The global nutrition agenda can serve as an important framework for helping to define an investigator's international nutrition-research problem. Global nutrition problems reside within the scope of food availability and the capacity of the human body to use nutrients from the food that is available. One factor that cannot be overlooked is **food safety**; indeed, food safety is an essential component of dietary quality. Although food safety's importance is well understood when considering nutrition issues in lower- and middle-income countries, it may not be considered as fundamental for the dietary quality of higher-income countries. Yet food-borne illness is a serious problem that causes morbidity and mortality in countries worldwide.

International nutrition-research problems can be categorized into those relevant to general food insecurity and those associated with malnutrition—specifically, protein-energy undernutrition, disease-associated malnutrition, obesity, and micronutrient deficiencies. In international nutrition, the high prevalence of protein-energy malnutrition and micronutrient deficiencies results mainly from environmental factors, including poor sanitation and hygiene—increasing the risk of infections—and a lack of education on age-specific diets, which contributes to poor or inadequate food intake. This section addresses how the goals of global organizations such as the United Nations and WHO underscore international nutrition-research problems. An international nutrition-research problem can be seen in how the global goals of these organizations are related to specific nutritional disorders that can be characterized as tangible research problems and the types of resources that are available to help define an international nutrition research problem.

## Links Between an International Nutrition-Research Problem and the Global Nutrition Agenda

When evaluating ideas for an international nutrition-research study, it is important to consider that research tied to UN or WHO development goals will likely be the most viable in lower- and lower-middle income countries because they can garner increased resources when they positively affect development goals. Two critical areas are **protein-energy undernutrition (PEU)**—particularly in children—and obesity. As documented in the *Essential Nutrition Actions Improving Maternal, Newborn, Infant, and Young Child Health and Nutrition* report of 2013, globally close to 101 million children under five years of age were underweight and 165 million were stunted at the same time that some 43 million were overweight or obese.[6] This is the reality of malnutrition in lower- and lower-middle income countries today; the rising tide of obesity affects some sectors of their populations although a large portion that is undernourished and stunted remains. This duality needs to be taken into account when considering an international nutrition-research problem along with its complex causes. The assessment of the problem and its solutions will likely require actions across multiple sectors of society; accordingly, the assessment should be evidence based and pursued in the context of international policies and resources.

To help conceptualize the scope of an international nutrition-research problem and narrow its complexity, consider the two major global initiatives forging global health outcomes: the UN Millennium Development Goals for 2015 (Figure 12.2) and the subsequent UN Sustainable Development Goals and Targets for 2030 (Figure 12.4). These goals and targets focus on social development and incorporate multisector interventions. Furthermore, they establish responsibility targets through monitoring and accountability frameworks.

The UN Millennium Development Goals arose from ambitious social development targets—including education, health, nutrition, water, and sanitation—and were an effort to rally the world around global development. As summarized by researchers Chopra and Mason,[30] the UN Millennium Development Goals formed the basis for multilateral global health institutions to collaborate and address extreme poverty with time-bound and quantified targets to achieve by 2015. The eight goals ranged from eradicating extreme hunger and poverty (goal 1) to developing a global partnership for development (goal 8). In between were goals focused on reducing child mortality (goal 4) and improving maternal health (goal 5).

Reducing child mortality and improving maternal health are among the greatest successes of the UN Millennium Development Goals program.[30] A more recent **United Nations Children's Fund (UNICEF)** and WHO report documented that between 1990 and 2014 the prevalence of stunting declined from 39.6% to 23.8%.[31] To improve maternal health under UN Millennium Development goal 5, countries committed to reducing maternal mortality by three-fourths between 1990 and 2015. Since 1990, worldwide maternal deaths have dropped by 44% from approximately 532,000 in 1990 to an estimated 303,000 in 2015, with nearly all occurring in low-resource settings and most of which were preventable.[32] During this same time, the approximate global lifetime risk of a maternal death fell considerably from 1 in 73 to 1 in 180. These are significant accomplishments, but poverty and poor health remain critical global issues. A review of the literature by Fehling et al.[33] on articles related to UN Millennium Development Goals identified a range of important concerns about the global goals, including limitations in their formulation, structure, content, and implementation. If the next generation of global development goals can address such limitations, there could be an even greater positive impact on the health and well-being of people worldwide.

The UN established the UN Sustainable Development Goals (Figure 12.4) as its newest set of global goals and targets. These goals are categorized as five P's—people, planet, prosperity, peace, and partnership—and include 17 goals and 169 targets (eight times the number of UN Millennium Development Goals targets). The UN Sustainable Development Goals build on the UN Millennium Development Goals and focus on completing what those goals did not achieve. The new goals and targets became effective in 2016 and will be guiding international development decisions and research until 2030.

Like the UN Millennium Development Goals, the UN Sustainable Development Goals can be useful in identifying research problems of international nutrition relevance. For example, goal 2—end hunger, achieve food security and improved nutrition, and promote sustainable agriculture—is built around the possible factors affecting or facilitating adequate food resources and includes women, children, and older adults in its targets. Others such as goal 3—ensure healthy lives and promote well-being for all at all ages—have targets to reduce mortality by 2030. These include reducing the global maternal mortality ratio to less than 70 per 100,000 live births and ending preventable deaths of newborns and children under five years of age—with all countries aiming to reduce neonatal mortality to at least as low as 12 per 1,000 live births and under-five mortality to at least as low as 25 per 1,000 live births. Indeed, these two goals provide a range of targets for maternal, child, and older adult morbidity and mortality that are specifically related to malnutrition.

The Global Burden of Disease, Injuries, and Risk Factors Study (GBD) has been analyzed to determine the current status of 33 health-related UN Sustainable Development Goal indicators. The GBD may be a potential resource for international nutrition research by being an open, collaborative, and independent study that comprehensively measures epidemiological levels, trends of disease, and the worldwide risk factor burden with more than 1870 individual collaborators from 124 countries and three territories across the full range of development. Using the GBD results, researchers were able to identify countries with the largest improvements between 1990 and 2015 and provide a basis for monitoring the health-related indicators of the UN Sustainable Development Goals.[34]

Supporting the UN Sustainable Development Goals are the **WHO Global Nutrition Targets for 2025** (Figure 12.8) that are specific to maternal and child nutrition. The Global Nutrition Targets are important to consider when defining international nutrition-research problems because their targets represent priority areas for action, catalyze global change, and are regularly monitored by the WHO for progress. In addition, the targets establish absolute and quantitative thresholds, which is a shift in approach from the UN Millennium Development Goals' percentage-decline targets. This will result in a greater focus on evaluating inequalities across countries.[35]

## Identifying Specific Nutritional Problems Inherent in the Global Health and Nutrition Goals

A common denominator of the UN and WHO global health and nutrition goals is malnutrition, which makes identifying an international nutrition-research problem much more tangible. For example, one form of malnutrition—undernutrition—can occur as an acute or chronic condition, depending on duration and types of limitations in the diet. *Chronic* describes a dietary intake that is inadequate in essential nutrients, particularly micronutrients such as vitamins and minerals, over a protracted period of time. On the other hand, *acute* is a sudden reduction in food intake or diet quality and can occur along with pathological processes such as infections that occur secondary to disease. PEU develops when there are limitations in diet quality (energy sources and protein), which may lead to wasting or stunting. PEU can be sudden and total (starvation) or gradual. Severity ranges from subclinical deficiencies to obvious wasting (with edema, hair loss, and skin atrophy) to starvation. In lower-income countries, PEU affects children who do not consume enough calories or protein; in higher-income countries, PEU is more common among the institutionalized elderly (although often not suspected) and among patients with disorders that decrease appetite or impair nutrient digestion, absorption, or metabolism.

The diagnosis of PEU in international populations may include taking a clinical history to determine primary and secondary causes and possible associated factors. In most cases, PEU is caused by limited access to foods and their nutrients, although common causes in the elderly can be disability, chronic disease, and depression. PEU can also result from fasting or anorexia nervosa. Secondary causes may include gastrointestinal disorders as well as factors interfering with the food intake (e.g., poor infant-feeding practices), poor digestion (e.g., parasitic infection and pancreatic insufficiency), or poor absorption (e.g., viral or bacterial diarrhea, inflammatory bowel disease, and irritable bowel syndrome). The physical examination for a diagnosis of PEU may include measurements of height and weight, inspection of body fat distribution, anthropometric measurements of lean body mass, and nutrition-focused physical examinations of the body (as further discussed in previous chapters).

Internationally, the micronutrient deficiencies most commonly related to chronic malnutrition are vitamin A deficiency, iodine-deficiency disorders, and iron-deficiency anemia. Vitamin A deficiency has well-recognized clinical signs, including night blindness and corneal damage (known as *xerophthalmia*), but these are difficult to assess accurately by surveys. Increasingly, the incidence and prevalence of vitamin A deficiency have been assessed by other methods, of which "the only biochemical parameter validated and found practical for routine survey use is serum retinol concentration."[36] One agreed cutoff point is 20 µg/dL, and the criterion for establishing a public-health problem is greater than 15% prevalence. The term *subclinical* has generally been dropped, and now low serum retinol can be referred to as vitamin A deficiency, meaning the state of inadequate vitamin A nutrition. For clarity, the term used here is *low serum retinol* (<20 µg/dL, which is the same as <0.7 µmol/L).

Iodine-deficiency disorders include goiter, which is clinically recognized as an iodine deficiency, but low urinary iodine (<100 µg/L) has also been used. Iodine deficiency is associated with various morbidities, depending at which point in the life cycle it occurs. In pregnancy and early life, it causes mental retardation, stunted growth, and other developmental abnormalities, which are largely irreversible. In later life, it reduces intellectual capacity and productivity, which can be reversed with increased iodine intakes. The UNSCN's sixth report on world nutrition provides guidelines on how to use measures of the incidence of goiter surgery and low urinary iodine to establish regional trends in iodine deficiency.

Anemia is best assessed by measuring hemoglobin concentrations rather than clinical signs. Anemia in the general (nonpregnant) female population is assessed as hemoglobin <12g/dL; in pregnancy, it is determined to be hemoglobin <11 g/dL (taking into account the increased blood volume in pregnancy and resulting hemodilution). Anemia is often caused by iron deficiency, but a lack of other nutrients may also cause it, including folic acid, $B_{12}$, and vitamin A. In addition, anemia can result from disease, such as through malabsorption and iron losses from intestinal parasites or the destruction of red blood cells in malaria.[37]

## Resources Available to Help Define an International Nutrition-Research Problem

In developing a potential international nutrition-research problem, many WHO resources may be useful.

### WHO Resources

The first is WHO's **Nutrition Landscape Information System (NLiS)**. This web-based system dynamically brings together all existing WHO global nutrition databases and other existing food and nutrition-related data from partner agencies. It provides automated country profiles and user-defined downloadable data. Data presented in the country profiles are based on the UNICEF conceptual framework and are organized around child malnutrition. Data contain information about low birth weight, maternal malnutrition, vitamin and mineral deficiencies, health services, food security, caring practices, commitment, capacity, and meta-indicators describing general conditions and contextual factors that may affect nutrition actions.[38]

Another important area to consider when defining an international nutrition-research problem is the potential for the results to help drive specific nutrition actions. The WHO has developed its Landscape Analysis on Countries' Readiness to Accelerate Action in Nutrition to help assess where and how best to invest to accelerate action in nutrition. Specifically, the landscape analysis examines the readiness of stakeholders' commitment and capacity to scale up evidence-informed interventions. The landscape analysis focuses on countries with high levels of chronic undernutrition, including the 36 high-burden countries identified by *The Lancet* Nutrition Series, which are home to 90% of the world's stunted children, and additional countries that have undertaken in-depth country assessments.[10] The landscape analysis has three components:[39]

1. development of country typologies for "readiness,"
2. in-depth country assessments, and
3. the NLiS.

A third WHO tool that may be useful in helping define an international nutrition-research problem is the **Global Database on the Implementation of Nutrition Action (GINA)**. This database provides information on the implementation of many nutrition policies and interventions and invites users to directly submit their own data. Users can share information on how programs are implemented, including country adaptations and lessons learned.[40]

## Reports from Other Organizations

In addition to these WHO databases, reports from other groups can also be helpful resources for identifying potential international nutrition-research problems. In 2013, for example the Sackler Institute for Nutrition Science published *A Global Research Agenda for Nutrition Science*, which was the outcome of a collaborative process between academic and not-for-profit researchers and the WHO. The collaboration identified three topic areas as critical "focus areas" for concentrating future nutrition research:[41]

1. environmental and societal trends affecting food and nutrition among vulnerable groups;
2. unresolved issues of nutrition in the life cycle; and
3. delivery of intervention and operational gaps.

Many of the specific gaps defined under each focus area reflect the nutrition problems raised earlier in this chapter.

The *Global Nutrition Report* is an annual peer-reviewed publication produced by an independent expert group. In 2016, it had contributions from more than 100 people, including leading researchers and practitioners working across the world and the malnutrition spectrum.[42] The report regularly identifies and tracks global health and nutrition issues and is defined as the only independent and comprehensive annual review of the state of the world's nutrition. It provides examples of change and identifies opportunities for action.

The 2016 report focused on the global goal of ending malnutrition by 2030: "Few challenges facing the global community today match the scale of malnutrition, a condition that directly affects one in three people." "Malnutrition and diet are by far the biggest risk factors for the global burden of disease: every country is facing a serious public-health challenge from malnutrition."[42] The report included 10 measures, the six WHO Global Nutrition Targets for 2025 (Figure 12.8)—which have been previously discussed—and two of the WHO's targets in the Global Monitoring Framework for the Prevention and Control of Noncommunicable Diseases:

1. Experience no increase in obesity and diabetes (in adults and adolescents).
2. Achieve a 30% reduction in average population salt intake.

One key finding of the report important for nutrition researchers was that "Today's data and knowledge are not sufficient to maximize investments." The report identified a need for a "data revolution" for nutrition, stating that the "scarcity of data prevents us from identifying and learning from real progress at the global and national levels." One of the report's five calls for action was "Collect the right data to maximize investments," specifying that "data gaps are a significant roadblock to nutrition progress throughout the world" and that "every country has a different nutrition context and should gather the national and subnational data it needs to understand—and act on—its own unique situation." Further, the report identified that the "absence of data is a fundamental impediment to determining real progress at the global

and national levels, hiding inequalities within countries and making it more difficult to hold governments accountable."[42]

In discussing the *Global Nutrition Report*, the **World Food Programme (WFP)** states that "data aren't telling us the whole story" and "there is a major lack of data to tell us what is and isn't working, whom to target and how to reach them. This is hampering efforts to reduce global malnutrition. In many cases these data exist but aren't readily available."[43]

One report from the Bill & Melinda Gates Foundation stated, "Better data [are] needed to define the problem of malnutrition, diagnose its root causes, design interventions, and track progress." The foundation further reported that it is "developing new tools and platforms to enable timely collection of data and improve its analysis and use" and to "support global efforts to standardize the collection and monitoring of nutrition data and use evidence to develop effective policies and guidelines."[44]

Finally, in defining an international nutrition-research problem, it is also important to consider the geopolitical, economic, sociological, clinical, and public-health dimensions. As explained in a joint statement of the UN Platform on the Social Determinants of Health,

> It was long believed that, as countries developed, noncommunicable disease would replace communicable disease as the main source of ill health. However, there is now evidence that the poorest in lower-income countries face a triple burden of communicable disease, noncommunicable disease and socio-behavioral illness. In this context of the epidemiological transition, there is growing recognition that noncommunicable diseases are one of the major causes of mortality and morbidity globally. The causes and determinants of noncommunicable diseases are wide ranging and include exposure to environmental toxins, unhealthy diets and various forms of malnutrition, tobacco use, excess salt and alcohol consumption, and increasingly sedentary lifestyles. These proximal drivers are, in turn, linked to broader social conditions, such as low and insecure income, poor housing and working conditions, inadequate transportation systems, and misguided agricultural and education policies.[45]

USAID's **Strengthening Partnerships, Results, and Innovations in Nutrition Globally (SPRING)** has developed resources that promote **systems thinking** and specifically help integrate

## HIGHLIGHT

### Systems Thinking for Global Nutrition Action

*People don't live their lives in health sectors or education sectors or infrastructure sectors, arranged in tidy compartments. People live in families and villages and communities and countries, where all the issues of everyday life merge. We need to connect the dots.*

*– Robert Zoellick, former head of the World Bank (2010); USAID. Systems Thinking and Action for Nutrition. Spring Working Paper. March 2015.*

In the rapidly changing field of nutrition, professionals must remain dynamic and continually identify the changing needs of any given population. Providing nutrition care at the population level cannot simply be accomplished with one method alone. The traditional approach to thinking about or trying to solve one corner of a puzzle may not be enough to tackle complex issues. Therefore, focusing on the entire system rather than just one piece can improve problem-solving skills and create more effective solutions.

System thinking acknowledges that a system is an organized whole comprising interdependent parts. In theory, an impact within one part of the system will affect other parts. This approach works by expanding the view to consider the "bigger picture" rather than isolating smaller parts of the system. For example, building a grocery store within a desolate rural community would fail or only provide a short-term solution to the issue of malnutrition. Those community members would require jobs to afford grocery items, knowledge on what to buy, roads, transportation systems, and food cooking and storage methods, to name a few of many needs. When considering nutritional interventions and solutions, other parts of the system must be addressed or at least considered.

USAID's Strengthening Partnerships, Results, and Innovations in Nutrition Globally (SPRING) has identified several cross-cutting factors that "influence, interact and impact one another and nutrition outcomes" (**FIGURE A**). These include:

- policies and governance,
- infrastructure and markets,
- inputs and services,
- information and communication,
- financing,
- household resources, and
- the sociocultural environment.

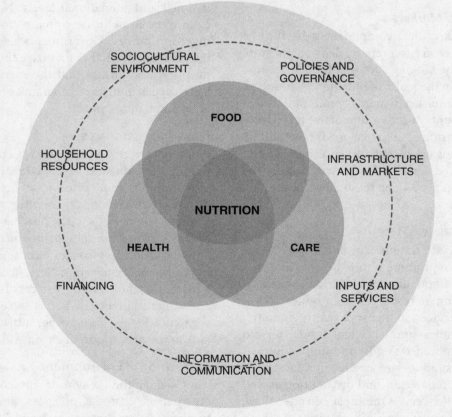

**FIGURE A** Systems thinking in action as applied to nutrition

societal dimensions—such as those identified previously—into international nutrition research (highlight 1). SPRING is "dedicated to strengthening global and country efforts to scale up high-impact nutrition practices and policies."[46]

### Policies and Governance

Policies and governance affect food, health, education, and the environment, although their impact varies according to adherence and enforcement. The World Health Organization published its *Global Nutrition Policy Review* (2013) to summarize the nutrition policy findings from 123 countries.

Overall, the report found that the existing nutrition policies did not adequately respond to the nutrition challenges that countries and regions are facing today. The review uncovered many flaws within current nutrition-focused policies. First, the majority of nutrition policies did not include evidence-informed interventions (e.g., complementary feeding, food fortification, folic acid and iron supplementation). Nutrition policies also did not have clear goals, targets, timelines, or deliverables; did not specify roles and responsibilities; did not include outcome evaluations with appropriate indicators; and did not have an adequate budget for the actual policy implementation.

### Infrastructure and Markets

A less obvious but critical component is having the infrastructure necessary to prepare, deliver, and store foodstuffs properly. Making sure that food is accessible is a battle within the realm of nutrition. A country's infrastructure and market dynamics profoundly affect nutrition. Each country needs a supportive infrastructure (e.g., roads, bridges, electrical grids) that allows communities to engage in nutritional programs and purchase healthy, diverse foods. Prices within the market system also need to be reasonable for the surrounding population.

### Inputs and Services

Despite an increased awareness of nutritional needs, "the workforce to promote those actions is often insufficient and unqualified." Nutrition programming requires human resources to produce foods, provide quality services, and ensure safety, yet nutrition policies do not assign sufficient funds to train people for the required tasks. In addition to human resources, many supplies are needed for food production, storage, preparation, and distribution as well as health-service delivery.[1] One must consider these finer details when developing an organizational plan and nutrition solution.

### Information and Communication

Changes in policy, financing, and accessibility, for example, will do little good without effective communication. Nutrition programs can only reach their full potential when knowledge is shared and populations are motivated and committed to achieve success. The transmission of information is invaluable for improved teamwork, support, and coordination.

Unfortunately, nearly 775 million adults worldwide are illiterate, which translates into one in five adults. Illiteracy in rural communities must be considered when trying to communicate a message. By using multiple modes of communication, organizations can reach more people (e.g., radio and television broadcasts, community meetings and presentations, email blasts, brochures, newspaper articles, social networking sites). However, to save time, an organization should assess the prevailing technologies within a community to decide which communication strategies will be most beneficial.

### Financing

In recent years, governments have begun to take seriously the issue of nutrition, although the necessary levels of aid and financing to deal with it still lag behind political ambition. For nutrition interventions to go into effect, financial support is required at both the national and subnational levels. New funding strategies must draw in new donors and maintain existing contributors. Governments need to boost their budgets for the sectors that have the strongest link to nutrition and ensure that the spending is appropriately used if nutrition programs are to have a long-term population impact.

### Household Resources

Household access to resources such as income, technology, and education are important basic drivers of nutrition.[1] As food prices rise, households may try to replace pricier groceries with cheaper sources of calories, which leads to the purchase of lower-quality foods. Lack of household income can also cause a household decrease in caloric consumption, contributing to eventual undernutrition. Access to technology allows households to have access to safe food, water, and sanitation services. Education equips households with knowledge about proper nutrition practices and aids in the prevention of chronic illnesses.

### Sociocultural Environment

The sociocultural environment consists of a society's beliefs, customs, practices, and behaviors. Cultural rules classify items as "edible" or "inedible" and become the basis for dietary choices. Social structures and norms mediate the interactions between all of the interrelated components previously described. Social roles, relationships, and policies in settings such as schools, neighborhoods, places of worship, and healthcare settings influence perceptions of resources and services as well as nutrition-related behaviors and decisions around what is produced, purchased, prepared, consumed, or thrown away.

> **Recap**  The UN and WHO health and development goals and related reports and databases are guideposts for identifying and quantifying international nutrition problems for investigation and research. More important is the true need for international nutrition research to delineate problems and potential solutions. The absence of nutrition data has been identified as a "fundamental impediment" to determining real progress at the global and national levels on topics such as malnutrition, hiding inequalities within countries, and making it more difficult to hold governments accountable.

## ▶ What is Different About the International Nutrition-Research Process?

> **Preview**  The process for international research can be different than the domestic research process, a point to consider when determining the time and resources needed to successfully plan and complete an international nutrition-research project.

The core elements of international nutrition research are aligned with those delineated in other chapters earlier in this book. However, there are many unique considerations, principles, and adaptations that will likely influence the international research process. Fortunately, a range of internationally related resources may be useful.

### Ethical, Legal, and Regulatory Considerations

Ethical, legal, and regulatory considerations are fundamental to good research design. Conducting research outside the United States does not eliminate the need to adhere to these standards; in some cases, international guidelines may be even more stringent than domestic

requirements. In general, when research is conducted outside the United States, investigators must comply with both US regulations and local policies and regulations governing the international research sites.

The **Nuremberg Code**, developed in 1947 after World War II, helped form the basis for today's ethical, legal, and regulatory framework for research on human subjects. The Nuremburg Code was developed as a result of the brutalities of Nazi medical researchers and reflects the belief that human beings must voluntarily consent before participating in research.[47] In 1962, the World Medical Association (WMA) developed and ratified the first version of the Declaration of Helsinki, which further delineated ethical principles for human subject researchers, particularly the ethical complexities of conducting such research in foreign countries. The WMA has continued to amend the declaration through the years.[48]

Several decades later in the United States, revelations about the Tuskegee experiment in which several hundred poor black Southern males were left untreated in a government-funded research project, led to enactment of the National Research Act in 1974.[49] The act created the National Commission for the Protection of Human Subjects of Biomedical and Behavioral Research. One of the commission's initial charges was to develop basic ethical principles and guidelines for biomedical and behavioral research on human subjects; these were subsequently published as the *Belmont Report* in 1979. The report emphasized three ethical principles:[50]

1. *Respect for persons*, which underlies the principle of informed consent where participants are given relevant information in a comprehensible format and voluntarily agree to participate
2. *Beneficence*, which means the researcher should work to minimize risks to participants and maximize benefits to participants and society and
3. *Justice*, which addresses the distribution of the burdens and benefits of research—for example, one group in society should not bear the costs of research while another group reaps the rewards

These three principles were later operationalized into the detailed rules and procedures of the **Common Rule**, which is more formally known as the US Federal Policy for the Protection of Human Subjects. The Common Rule outlines the basic provisions for institutional review boards (IRBs), informed consent, and assurances of compliance (an organization's guarantee it will follow required policies and procedures) and is applied to research funded by federal agencies and federally funded universities (even for their own self-funded research).[51] The **Office for Human Research Protections** of the Department of Health and Human Services (HHS) is the federal office that oversees the system protecting the rights, welfare, and well-being of research subjects and ensures that federal research meets the Common Rule standards. Their focus is education, compliance, regulation, and policy setting.[52]

## Other Guiding Principles

The Office for Human Research Protections has established the guideline that "human subjects outside of the United States who participate in research projects conducted or funded by HHS receive an equal level of protection as research participants inside the United States."[53] Thus, at a minimum, the framework established by the Common Rule applies to federally funded international research.

Many universities have their own offices on human subject research to help ensure Common Rule standards are followed and to govern their own IRBs. Susan Rose of the University of Southern California Office for the Protection of Research Subjects has outlined eight universal ethical principles for international research:[54]

1. Collaborative partnership
2. Social value
3. Scientific validity
4. Fair selection of participants
5. Favorable risk-benefit ratio
6. Peer review
7. Informed consent and
8. Respect for participants built in

Rose stressed that researchers should be prepared to justify why a foreign population is needed and identify the potential value and applicability of the investigation to other populations. She further reminded researchers of the need to practice cultural sensitivity and engage community leaders in identifying and addressing the effects of spiritual, moral, and legal values and to limit any potential concerns for coercion such as that related to socioeconomic status. Rose also cautioned against "helicopter" research in which investigators engage in data or sample collection and then leave the site with no follow-up. She reminded investigators to consider financial and injury protection options for their research teams and subjects because US laws and regulations may not apply.[54]

The lack of infrastructure in some developing countries can make obtaining approvals from governments and ethics organizations that are equivalent to IRBs difficult, but they are generally necessary, as is ongoing local government oversight.[54] Even if a local ethics committee review is not required, additional documentation may be needed to meet the requirements for the US institutions that are supporting the research or have study oversight. For example, the University of Pittsburgh's Research Protection Office requires documentation of these considerations.

For minimal risk studies in which international regulations do not require a local ethics review:

- A memo of cultural appropriateness authored by an "individual completely independent of your study who is highly familiar with the culture of the region where the research will be conducted" is required *and*
- Documentation that the local regulations do not require a local ethics review, with "direct references to the local regulations that state ethics review is not required; or an Acknowledgement of Unregulated Research Activities letter confirming that local ethics review is not required."

For minimal risk studies in which international regulations require a local ethics review, a letter of review from the local ethics review committee is required.

For greater than minimal risk studies, a formal ethics review within the country where the research will be conducted is required and may be addressed by the country's department of ministries or other relevant governmental entities if there is no ethics review committee.

The University of Pittsburgh's Research Protection Office also strongly encourages investigators to collaborate with individuals or organizations having expertise in the region to help in "identifying appropriate research sites, navigating the local regulations and policies, understanding culture, local infrastructure, overcoming language barriers [and] increasing community partnership." The office states that when enrolling non–English-speaking research subjects, "investigators must have a plan to manage communications with participants during *all phases* of study participation. Given that participants may have questions or concerns at any time, Investigators must be prepared to manage communication beyond the consent process and data collection."[55] Additional cultural considerations for international nutrition research are discussed in the Highlight Cultural Rules for International Nutrition Research.

## Adaptation of Nutrition-Assessment Methods, Tools, and Resources

Many nutrition-assessment methods, tools, and resources have been identified and described in detail in previous chapters of this book. Many of these may

## HIGHLIGHT

### Cultural Rules of the Road

When planning to conduct international nutrition assessment and research, investigating the social rules of the local culture is essential before international colleagues, organizations, and governments can be engaged. What may be a natural practice to the researcher might be viewed as disrespectful to others. An investigator who becomes familiar with cultural norms can raise his or her level of cultural competency.

Cultural competency is the ability of an individual to understand and respect values, attitudes, beliefs, and morals that differ across cultures and to consider and respond appropriately to these differences in planning, implementing, and evaluating health education and nutrition programs and clinical interventions. General considerations to take into account when working with individuals from different cultures include modesty and privacy, eye contact, communication, handshakes and touching, and beliefs about illnesses and medical conditions.

### Modesty and Privacy

Be aware that people in many cultures have different views of how to maintain their modesty. A researcher may need to consider both his or her own clothing as well as the dress for study participants (hospital gowns, etc.). For example, foreign women visiting or working in Saudi Arabia are required by law to wear abayas that fully cover their bodies. In some cultures, it may not be appropriate for medical or staff or investigators to perform physical exams or tests on members of the opposite sex.

### Eye Contact

Although eye contact is a respectful way of demonstrating attention in Western culture, Hispanic, Asian, and Middle Eastern cultures view eye contact as a sign of disrespect or as a sign of sexual interest when between members of the opposite sex. Thus, if members of these cultures do not make eye contact, it likely is not a lack of attentiveness or a sign of dishonesty as it might be interpreted in the American culture.

### Communication

When engaging in conversation, the researcher should be mindful of both verbal and nonverbal gestures. Consciously making an effort to maintain appropriate body language, gestures, and physical distance when speaking with someone can go a long way in helping gain their trust and support. Suggestions include the following.

- Keep a conversational tone. Loudness may be associated with aggression, so it may be best to maintain a soft, calm voice.
- Be aware that the meaning of speech can also be altered significantly by tone and character of voice.
- Remember silence can have a variety of meanings, including disagreement and approval, in addition to being a natural part of conversation.
- Be aware that head nods and smiles may not always mean comprehension.
- Try not to interrupt a speaker. This can ruin attempts to establish a relationship.
- Remember that rules about social distance vary with different groups of people. Learn to detect this by watching people's reactions.

### Handshakes and Touching

Keep in mind that handshake rules can vary across cultures, so before traveling to a new country, find out the cultural norms. Consider these guidelines.

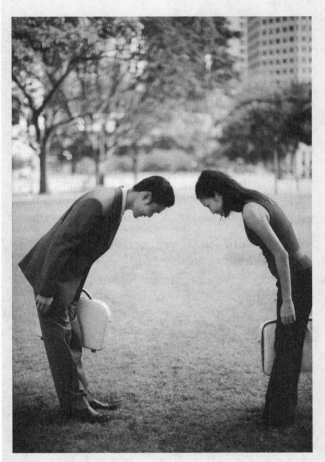

© Floresco Productions/Getty Images.

- Be mindful that some customs prohibit handshakes or any contact between different genders.
- Always shake hands with the right hand. In many cultures, the left is used for bodily hygiene.
- Consider that light touching in some cultures may be more appropriate during a handshake than a firm touch would be (e.g., Japan, South Korea, Taiwan).
- Remember that some cultures use gestures other than handshakes as a greeting (e.g., bowing in Japan).

### Beliefs About Illnesses and Medical Conditions

If planning to conduct disease-related nutritional research, take the time to investigate how the local culture perceives its own conditions. For example, individual or group counseling on carbohydrate counting to manage type 2 diabetes may not be successful approach if locals believe their diabetes was caused by supernatural forces rather than their dietary patterns. Other common cultural beliefs about causes of illness include the following.

- Illness is caused by a disharmony between the mind and body.
- Illness is the result of karma, so it is an inevitable consequence from this or a previous life.
- Health is controlled only though God.
- Illness is caused by witchery imposed by someone else.
- Illness can come from envy or wishing another individual were ill.
- Other reasons for illness include ghosts, breaking taboos, the evil eye, and possession by evil spirits.

Although much of the lower- and lower-middle-income countries are now incorporating more so-called Western medicine into their treatment strategies, keep in mind that "traditional" therapies and approaches to healing are still used broadly in the world. For example, in Africa, as much as 80% of the population uses traditional medicine for its primary health care.

http://www.nccccurricula.info/culturalcompetence.html. Modified from: National Center for Cultural Competence Georgetown University Center for Child and Human Development. Definitions of cultural competence. Curricula enhancement module series. https://nccc.georgetown.edu/curricula/culturalcompetence.html. Accessed December 1, 2016. http://www.who.int/mediacentre/factsheets/2003/fs134/en/. Modified from: World Health Organization. Traditional medicine. http://www.who.int/mediacentre/factsheets/2003/fs134/en/ 2003. Accessed December 1, 2016.

be appropriate for use in international nutrition-research settings. However, the investigator will need to consider the specific applicability of the methods and tools to a given study population, local infrastructure, and available resources.

## Standards for Desirable Nutrient Intake

Recommendations for nutrient intake can vary by population and country. The WHO's Department of Nutrition for Health and Development, in collaboration with the **Food and Agriculture Organization (FAO)**, continually "reviews new research and information from around the world on human nutrient requirements and recommended nutrient intakes" and makes specific recommendations and suggests nutrient requirements. These agencies identify this as a "vast and never-ending task, given the large number of essential human nutrients." WHO notes that the evidence is increasing on the importance of micronutrients for immune function, physical work capacity, and cognitive development, including learning capacity in children.[56]

Many countries adopt the WHO and FAO dietary recommendations and requirements, but other countries use the information as a base to develop their own standards for dietary patterns and desirable nutrient intakes. The scope of the WHO and FAO recommendations includes protein, energy, carbohydrates, fats and lipids, and many vitamins, minerals, and trace elements. Specific nutrient requirements and dietary recommendations are available online.[57]

### Measuring Nutrient Intake

Because of the global importance of addressing micronutrient deficiencies, the WHO has established a Vitamin and Mineral Nutrition Information System—formerly known as the Micronutrient Deficiency Information System—to strengthen surveillance worldwide. It is part of WHO's mandate to assess the micronutrient status of populations, monitor and evaluate strategies for the prevention and control of micronutrient malnutrition, and track related trends over time.[58]

### Food and Nutrition Surveys and Computerized Food and Nutrition Analysis Systems

Certainly, surveying dietary patterns and analyzing food intake on a global scale can be a challenge. An important resource is the FAO's **International Network of Food Data Systems (INFOODS)**. This worldwide network of food-composition experts aims to improve the quality, availability, reliability, and use of food-composition data. INFOODS is also a forum for international harmonization and support for food-composition activities. The network is organized into several regional data centers and provides guidelines, standards, compilation tools, databases, capacity-development tools, policy advice, advocacy tools, and technical assistance at the country level.[59]

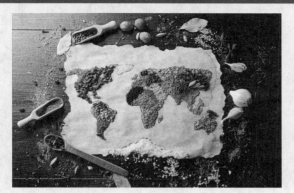

© Africa Studio/Shutterstock.

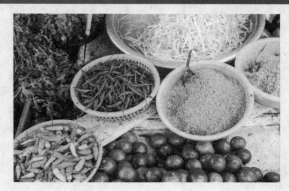

© Elena Ermakova/Shutterstock.

## Cultural Competency

*Randi S. Drasin, MS, RDN*

As our society continues to grow in the United States, there is more diversity when it comes to diet and food practices. Religion, culture, and ethnicity all play a part in our world, so our profession and perspective are ever changing. Health care providers must continue to learn and expand our knowledge to include cultural awareness and competency as nutrition professionals.

So what is cultural competence, you ask?

*Cultural competence is the ability to understand, appreciate, and interact with persons from cultures and/or belief systems other than one's own, based on various factors.[1]*

Registered Dietitian Nutritionists are well versed in the science of food and nutrition, but we also must be conscious of how culture plays a significant role in all people's choices about what they eat, when they eat, how they eat, and with whom they eat.

In our culture, multiple groups have their own sets of dietary practices. Although we cannot be expected to learn them all, it is the best practice to do some research before meeting with a specific client or group in order to provide the best possible care. With that being said, the centrality of food in our lives involves multiple sets of rules, rituals, restrictions, and traditions that revolve around festivities, weddings, birthdays, funerals, political holidays, festivals, fairs, and religious celebrations. To earn the trust and build relationships with our clients and patients, we must be able to offer nutrition guidance that fits their lifestyle.

It is fundamental for health and nutrition professionals to increase awareness of food traditions and the incredible variety of foods, herbs and spices, fruits and vegetables that have evolved over the years

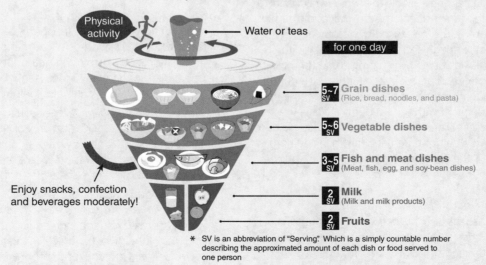

**Japanese food guide spinning top**

Do you have well-balanced diet?

Physical activity

Water or teas

for one day

**5~7 SV Grain dishes** (Rice, bread, noodles, and pasta)

**5~6 SV Vegetable dishes**

**3~5 SV Fish and meat dishes** (Meat, fish, egg, and soy-bean dishes)

**2 SV Milk** (Milk and milk products)

**2 SV Fruits**

Enjoy snacks, confection and beverages moderately!

\* SV is an abbreviation of "Serving". Which is a simply countable number describing the approximated amount of each dish or food served to one person

Reproduced from Food and Agriculture Organization of the United Nations. Food-based dietary guidelines. http://www.fao.org/nutrition/education/food-based-dietary-guidelines /regions/countries/japan/en/. Updated 2005. Accessed June 23, 2017.

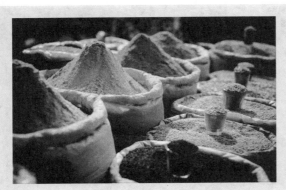

© Curioso/Shutterstock.

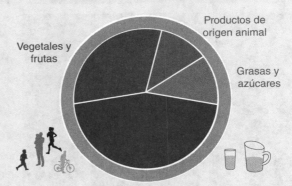

**Costa Rica**

**CÍRCULO DE LA ALIMENTACIÓN SALUDABLE**

Productos de origen animal

Vegetales y frutas

Grasas y azúcares

Cereales, leguminosas y verduras harinosas

Reproduced from Food and Agriculture Organization of the United Nations. Food-based dietary guidelines–Costa Rica. http://www.fao.org/nutrition/education/food-based-dietary-guidelines/regions/countries/costa-rica/en. Updated 2010. Accessed June 23, 2017.

and throughout the cultures. Countless ways of food preparation and food service have enriched our food horizons and expanded our view of what constitutes a healthy diet. Therefore, understanding the many aspects of other cultures is indispensable in any communication.

Although it would be a great professional perk, we cannot be expected to travel to every country or be a member of every culture, so to become culturally competent we need to read about the vast majority of cultural food practices and beliefs around the world. The Academy of Nutrition and Dietetics provides resources and research that can benefit any nutrition or health care provider and provide support in understanding how to provide the best treatment options when it comes to the diversity of regional foods and diets.[2] For instance, a practitioner working with a client from Japan and another from the Netherlands would make quite different diet recommendations based on geography, tradition, and culture, and the client would tend to view the nutrition advice in the context of his or her own unique culture. As practitioners, our goal would be to provide the best possible healthy diet recommendations within each cultural setting.

Many resources are available to anyone who wants to stay culturally relevant. Aside from studying food pyramids from other countries, be sure to look to resources from the Academy of Nutrition and Dietetics such as "Cultural Food Practices—Tip Sheets," which provides a summary of traditional foods and practices in countries all around the world. Academy members have developed these tip sheets in collaboration with the Academy affiliate, the American Overseas Dietetic Association. To find these tip sheets, go to www.eatrightinternational.org In addition, a great resource is the Food and Agriculture Organization of the United Nations at www.FAO.org.

### References

1. Segen, JC. *Segen's Medical Dictionary*. Huntington Valley, PA: Farlex; 2011. http://medical-dictionary. thefreedictionary.com/cultural+competence.

2. Fox M. Global food practices, cultural competency, and dietetics. *J Acad Nutr Diet*. 2015; 115(3):342-348. http://dx.doi.org/10.1016/j.jand.2014.12.019.

### Other Resources

Mahan KL, Escott-Stump S. Guidelines for dietary planning. In: Escott-Stump S, Earl R. eds. *Krause's Food and Nutrition Therapy*. 12th ed. St. Louis, MO: Saunders Elsevier; 2008; 337–362.

Conner SL. Think globally, practice locally: Culturally competent dietetics. *J Acad Nutr Diet*. 2015; 115 (5) (Suppl.):S5. http://dx.doi.org/10.1016/j.jand.2015.03.015.

Fox M. (2015). Global Food Practices, Cultural Competency, and Dietetics. *J Acad Nutr Diet*. 2015; 115 (3):342-348. http://dx.doi.org/10.1016/j.jand.2014.12.019.

Pelzel J. Championing cultural competence. Food Insight. 2014; February 25. http://www.foodinsight .org/Championing_Cultural_Competence.

Goody C, Drago L. Introduction: Cultural competence and nutrition counseling. In: Goody C. ed. *Cultural Food Practices*. Washington, DC: American Dietetic Association; 2009. http://www.eatrightstore.org/~ /media/eatrightstore%20documents/books%20 and%20publications/culturalguideintro.ashx.

Elnakib S. *Understanding the Diverse Culinary Traditions of Islam*. Washington, DC: Academy of Nutrition and Dietetics; 2016. http://www.eatrightpro.org /resource/news-center/in-practice/dietetics-in-action /understanding-the-diverse-culinary-traditions-of-islam.

California Department of Social Services. *Cultural Considerations in Nutrition and Food Preparation*. http:// www.cdss.ca.gov/agedblinddisabled/res/VPTC2/9%20 Food%20Nutrition%20and%20Preparation/Cultural _Consider_in_Nutrition_and_Food_Prep.pdf

### Anthropometry

According to the WHO,

> Anthropometry provides the single most portable, universally applicable, inexpensive and noninvasive technique for assessing the size, proportions and composition of the human body. It reflects both health and nutritional status and predicts performance, health and survival. As such, it is a valuable, but currently underused, tool for guiding public health policy and clinical decisions.[60]

Just as nutrient recommendations may vary across populations, so too can growth and anthropometric standards. Many countries again rely on the recommendations and standards of the WHO. The WHO child growth standards were developed using data collected in the WHO Multicentre Growth Reference Study. Its website documents how the physical growth curves and motor milestone windows of achievement were developed. The site also offers application tools to support implementation of the growth standards.[61]

The WHO also maintains a **global database on body mass index**, an interactive surveillance tool for monitoring the global epidemic of overweight and obesity or "globesity." Overweight and obesity are associated with many diet-related and chronic diseases, including diabetes mellitus, cardiovascular disease, stroke, hypertension, and certain cancers that paradoxically coexist with undernutrition in developing countries. The database provides both national and subnational adult overweight and obesity prevalence rates by country, year of survey, and gender. The information is presented interactively as maps, tables, graphs, and downloadable documents.[62]

### Biochemical Methods in Nutritional Assessment

Biomarkers are medical signs and symptoms that can be accurately observed and reproducibly measured. Many biomarkers have been well characterized and can be used to correctly predict relevant clinical outcomes across methods of treatment and study populations. In other cases, however, biomarkers may be assumed to be valid, but the measures may not be relevant to the intervention or the study population.

In the United States, the Eunice Kennedy Shriver National Institute of Child Health and Human Development has established the **Biomarkers of Nutrition for Development (BOND)** program to provide information and services that support the entire food and nutrition research and global health enterprise by developing consensus on accurate assessment methodologies. The methodologies have international application, can serve a variety of users,

and have the overall goal of improving the health of mothers and children. The tools for accurate nutrition assessment include those measuring exposure (i.e., what has been consumed, including bioavailability), status (i.e., where an individual or a subgroup falls relative to an accepted cutoff such as adequate, marginal, or deficient), function or role of a nutrient within the body, and effect or impact of an intervention on nutrient status and function. Over the past several years, BOND has convened panels for a many nutrients of public-health significance and has published descriptions of assessment tools for iron, iodine, folate, zinc, vitamin A, and vitamin $B_{12}$. The BOND website includes links to these documents and other tools that may be useful in designing international nutritional assessment and research.[63]

One BOND program, the Biomarkers Reflecting Inflammation and Nutritional Determinants of Anemia project, focuses on developing a database to inform global guidelines on the assessment of anemia and micronutrient status and to guide future research.[64] Iron is of particular interest because there are so many nutritional and non-nutritional causes of anemia.[65] One report profiles examples of integrating iron nutrition assessment and research with the implementation of iron-intervention programs.[66]

Another BOND program, the Inflammation and Nutritional Science for Programs/Policies and Interpretation of Research Evidence (INSPIRE) project, provides guidance for researchers on the interactions between nutrition, immune function, and the inflammatory response. The proceedings of the INSPIRE workshop provide a good start for exploring these issues and planning interventions.[67]

In international settings, the basic biochemical methods used in nutrition assessment may need to be adapted in some ways to fit the study population and meet ethical, cultural, resource, and other potential restrictions. The researcher is responsible for ensuring that the tests are standardized and calibrated against international measures and populations. For example, standardization programs exist for serum cholesterol determinations, blood glucose levels, and the 25-hydroxy vitamin D test. If a blood draw is needed, the WHO has published best-practice guidelines.[68]

One practical blood-collection and sampling method to consider is dried blood spot sampling, which has been used to screen newborn babies for congenital metabolic diseases for more than fifty years. For the analysis, a spot of blood (from a heel stick in infants) is placed on filter paper and allowed to air dry. Thus, the blood sample does not require cold storage. A circular punch (about 3 mm) of the spot is then removed, eluted with solvent, and analyzed. Protocols have been published for the analysis of many different analytes (the constituents being measured) in dried blood spots.[69]

In addition to requiring a minute amount of blood, dried blood spot sampling has the added advantage of easy collection, often by nonprofessionals. Both benefits can be important in an international setting. Dried blood spot sampling has been studied for many nutrients, including:

- Vitamin A[70]
- Iodine[71]
- Vitamin D[72] and
- Trans fatty acids[73]

Indeed, modern technology, combined with high sensitivity and specificity, means that many nutrient biomarkers (including metabolites, lipids, vitamins, minerals, and many types of peptides and proteins) can now be analyzed with tiny amounts of blood or tissue.

### Clinical Assessment of Nutritional Status

Internationally, the clinical assessment of nutritional status in institutions often employs similar tools to those used domestically. Watson et al.,[74] in a review of nutrition as a vital sign, profiled the use of malnutrition-assessment tools and determined that several countries, including the United Kingdom, Canada, New Zealand, and Australia, have "more advanced tools and policies to integrate malnutrition screening and intervention into routine medical care than does the [United States]."

Watson et al. recognized the following:

- The British Dietetic Association recommends embedding screening by using a validated tool like the Malnutrition Universal Screening Tool (MUST) that supports rapid intervention.[75]
- Canada has worked to develop and validate a tool known as Seniors in the Community: Risk Evaluation for Eating and Nutrition, Version II.[76]
- The Dietitians Association of Australia recommends a range of validated screening tools, including the MUST and Malnutrition Screening Tool.[77]
- A study of more than 21,000 patients in Europe and Israel found that malnutrition screening for hospitalized patients was most frequently done with instruments developed locally.[78]

As part of its Joint Programming Initiative (JPI), the European Union has launched its own knowledge hub on **Malnutrition in the Elderly (MaNuEL)**. The hub brings together 22 research groups from seven countries to build better research capacity across Europe on malnutrition in the elderly. It will contribute to a common and shared understanding on the definition of malnutrition, the etiology and prevalence of malnutrition in older persons, preferred screening tools, and effective interventions in different healthcare settings.[79]

### Assessment of Functional Status and Health-Related Quality of Life

In addition to evaluating the usual signs and symptoms of nutritional and diet-related problems, it is also important to consider functional status assessment. There are many different and relatively straightforward methods for doing this. The Instrumental Activities of Daily Living screen identifies difficulties in carrying out various cognitive activities that are necessary in most societies for individuals to remain independent. The Activities of Daily Living screen focuses on physical functions such as the ability to ambulate and toilet oneself without assistance. Other assessments such as the Mini Mental State Examination focus on mental state. There are also specialized functional status indicators that may be helpful if dealing with a special population such as individuals suffering from arthritis. If possible, use forms of the screens or assessments that have been specifically validated for the country or population being studied.

Another useful dimension of health to consider is the individual's health-related quality of life. This can be assessed by short self-administered tools. One well-regarded questionnaire is the 36-item Short Form Survey.[80] Two even shorter self-administered versions that are culturally appropriate in many settings are the physical component score and the mental component score.

### Health Promotion and Disease Prevention and Treatment

A tool that may be useful for international nutrition research related to health promotion, disease prevention, and treatment is the WHO **e-Library of Evidence for Nutrition Actions (eLENA)**, which is an online library of evidence-informed guidance for nutrition interventions. It is available in all six official languages of the WHO—Arabic, Chinese, English, French, Russian, and Spanish—and serves as a single point of reference for the latest nutrition guidelines, recommendations, and related information such as:[81]

- Available scientific evidence supporting the guidelines
- Biological, behavioral, and contextual rationale statements and
- Commentaries from invited experts

## International Research Standards and Resources

International research regulations and procedures are highly variable. Most foreign regulations however are based on the foundational ethical guidelines and principles of the International Conference of Harmonization (ICH)[82] and the **Council for International Organizations of Medical Sciences (CIOMS)**.[83]

The ICH is focused on pharmaceutical products. The CIOMS serves a much broader role, facilitating international biomedical research—especially when coordination is needed between multiple international associations and national institutions—and collaborating with the United Nations and its agencies. Information on research standards is also available through the Association of Clinical Research Organizations, which helps advocate for safe and ethical clinical trials and provides information and support for clinical research organizations that conduct thousands of clinical trials in more than 140 countries globally.[84]

The HHS Office for Human Research Protections has an international program[52] that offers resources for international research, including:

- The **International Compilation of Human Research Standards**, a listing of more than 1000 laws, regulations, and guidelines on human subjects protections in more than 100 countries and from several international organizations;[85]
- **clinical trials registries**, a listing of 24 clinical trials registries from around the world;[86]
- Ethical Codes and Research Standards, which links to the codes and standards previously discussed in this chapter; and[87]
- Equivalent Protections, which links to reports related to how international research standards may or may not provide protection similar to those established in the United States.[88]

Other international research resources include those from the **Fogarty International Center** of the US National Institutes of Health. The center supports and facilitates global health research conducted by US and international investigators, builds partnerships between health research institutions in the United States and abroad, and helps train the next generation of scientists to address global health needs. The center's listing of e-resources for global health researchers identifies many no- or low-cost training courses, massive open online courses (MOOCs), course materials (presentations, videos, reading lists, visual aids, articles), resource centers, and resource networks.[89]

## Political Considerations

The international context for nutritional research is also unique. The researcher must deal with two different societies: his or her own native society and the place in which the research is being carried out. The level of scientific knowledge, scientific customs, mores, and ways of doing business and conducting research may be radically different from that in the researcher's country of origin. Thus, an approach that may be scientifically correct may be culturally, economically, or politically unacceptable. When others are arrayed against the research project, science may not win the day.

Cultural sensitivity and competence are important but are only part of the labyrinth of international research that must be solved to navigate these unfamiliar shores successfully. Legislative, executive, and judicial agencies of a country's government may differ widely in their power and the degree to which they will choose to intervene in research efforts. Bias and suspicion of foreigners, doubt about the need to put tried and true traditional practices to the test, and many other factors must also be addressed. For all of these reasons, it is important to identify country nationals who are willing and able to help and partner in the research effort. They are also needed to serve as trustworthy, honest, and knowledgeable guides to their local systems. Such collaboration can help the investigator successfully make his or her way through these unfamiliar structures and challenges.

**Recap** Researchers should be prepared to justify why a foreign population is needed for their research and to identify the potential value and applicability of the investigation to other populations. Cultural and political concerns are important in planning international research. Additional considerations are possible adaptations that may be needed in nutrition-assessment methods and tools to fit the study population and any potential resource constraints. A variety of resources are available to help address these issues.

## ▶ What Solutions have been Developed to Address International Nutrition Problems?

**Preview** Scientific evidence and in-country politics play important roles in international nutrition research, and nutrition assessment is fundamental for helping determine the effectiveness of nutrition solutions on health outcomes.

The FAO has advised that nutrition assessment is the best way to determine "whether or not people's nutritional needs are effectively being met, once food is available and easily accessible. Nutrition assessment provides timely, high-quality and evidence-based information for setting targets, planning, monitoring and evaluating [programs] aiming at eradicating hunger and reducing the burden of malnutrition."[90] Thus, nutrition assessment can be effective in helping determine whether specific international nutrition interventions and solutions have been successful.

In-country, at the national level, it is particularly important that rational research practices are followed in assessing nutrition problems and developing science-based nutrition solutions. This process involves three major steps: (1) assessment of nutritional risk, (2) planning and development of national **food and nutrition policy**, and (3) implementation of nutrition interventions through a **food and nutrition action plan** with follow-up monitoring and evaluation. Ideally, a country's health officials who develop and implement food and nutrition policies and programs already have a framework of procedures and thus ask and answer in a logical manner the types of questions described in the following section.

## Nutrition Assessment at the National Level

Assessing nutritional risk explores the relationship between a population's consumption (i.e., dietary exposure) of a nutrient, food constituent, food, or group of foods; identified risk factors (e.g., elevated weight, blood pressure, serum cholesterol); and specified health outcomes (dietary deficiency disease, chronic disease, or death). The state of the art today is to rely on an evidence-based risk assessment rather than on the opinions or guesses of those in authority as was often the case in years past. These advances in risk assessment depend on high-quality evidence, such as research involving a nutrition assessment, being made available to policy makers so subsequent decisions can be made.

Key questions to ask in designing the nutrition assessment include the following:

1. **What is the nutrition-related problem and how severe is it?** Consider whether the nutrition-related problem can be easily quantified and evaluated with standard nutrition-assessment tools and measures and how results of the nutrition assessment compare to similar populations and global standards.

2. **Who is afflicted or at risk?** The group at risk of nutrition problems may have similarities that involve biological characteristics, socioeconomic status, occupation, or place of residence. From the biological standpoint, some groups such as infants, children, teenagers, pregnant, and lactating women; those who are ill and frail; and older adults have high nutritional requirements and may be especially vulnerable to undernutrition and malnutrition. One method used to identify these persons on the national level is to carry out a population-based survey with a representative sample of the population; this is done in countries such as the United States, Korea, and the Philippines, among others. A second method is to use a "list-based survey" of institutional populations (such as those in jails, nursing homes, and others), of groups known to be at high risk of malnutrition (patients with HIV or AIDs, cancer patients) or of persons in an area afflicted with a particular problem (natural disaster, war, etc.). Individuals in these settings are then examined to determine their nutrition problems.

In the United States, Canada, New Zealand, the European Union, and many other higher-income countries, formal processes are already in place for regularly assessing nutrient intakes, developing food and nutrition policies, and implementing food and nutrition action plans and programs. Similar systems are coming into use in other countries as well. Publications reviewing the evidence for nutrient requirements and for assessing and planning intakes are available from the US National Academy of Sciences' Food and Nutrition Board and relevant government agencies in other countries.

3. **Where is the problem?** Geographic distribution may be important. An area hit by a hurricane or famine is likely to have many individuals with similar nutritional problems.

4. **When does the problem occur?** Some nutrition problems occur only at certain times, such as during the rainy season, when other seasonal variations affect the food supply, or at the end of the month when the elderly poor run out of money from their pensions.

5. **Why does the problem occur?** Diet-related diseases may be the result of too little food, lack of a single nutrient (e.g., iodine, vitamin D, iron, or folic acid), excessive nutrient intakes (e.g., excess calories, sodium, saturated fat, sugars, or alcohol), toxicities (e.g., excessive alcohol intake, contaminants, or intake of food-borne pathogens causing illness), and chronic diseases (such as type 2 diabetes) or conditions that affect the ability to use the food.

## Planning and Development of National Food and Nutrition Policies

Once specific nutritional problems have been identified and assessed, attention turns to what can be done about them. The next steps involve a logical process of developing a strategy for managing the identified nutrition risks or problems. Ideally, the processes of risk assessment should be separated from risk management because the skills required differ. Risk assessors describe and quantify the risk. Risk management involves deciding what should be done about the potential risk and what the policy options are for doing it. Separation of the two processes lessens the tendency of either or both groups to over- or underestimate risk or for risk assessors to insist on a certain set of solutions without considering larger societal issues. The scientific evidence from the risk assessment, along with economic and political dimensions of the problem are considered by public-health officials and other decision makers, who frequently are part of a national **Food and Nutrition Council** or similar body with responsibility for **food control**, **food policy**, food and nutrition policy, and food-security regulation.

The political process is important for local governments to take action. Local governments need to consider how much potential interventions will cost, whether specific solutions are worthwhile, who benefits, how interventions will be implemented, and how solutions will be monitored, assessed, and ultimately valued. Thus, the decision about what can be done about a nutrition problem includes a realistic assessment of capabilities and resources for managing it. For some problems, nutritional solutions alone will suffice; for the many more complex nutrition problems— such as poverty-related malnutrition—interventions may not be easy or obvious because nutrition may be only a small part of the overall systemic solution.

Asking whose problem is being solved and for what purpose is important. Technical knowledge and skills are indispensable for problem solving, but effective interventions are ultimately only as good as the processes that define the problems and solutions. Open and inclusive (often referred to as "transparent") processes produce policies that are more likely to be acceptable to the majority of citizens. Closed (or nontransparent) decision-making processes often give preference to the interests of the few and may be regarded as unfair. Other decisions to be made are who should implement the policy and cover the costs. The human capital and other resources needed and expenses entailed must be calculated and paid. These costs must be weighed against competing uses of the same resources for other nutrition and health policies and programs, such as those targeting food safety or **food sustainability**.

## Implementation of Food and Nutrition Action Plans, Monitoring, and Evaluation

Translating food and nutrition policies into national action plans and programs follows. It is often helpful to scale up by starting small with a pilot program and then expanding. Opinions can vary on the best approach to take for implementing nutrition action plans and interventions, because individual policy makers can interpret the same scientific evidence differently. Cultural factors also come into play and can affect decisions on how and when to proceed.

Ultimately, whatever the nutrition action plan may be, it is important to have a system in place for monitoring the results of the solution. A system for regular monitoring and evaluation should be implemented right along with the intervention, not as an afterthought. Do not assume that the nutrition intervention will work simply "because it is the right thing to do" and that the nutrition action plan will be carried out exactly as developed. There is little evidence that things usually work out this way. Monitoring and evaluation must be put into place before implementation to assess what is actually occurring. It will be difficult, if not impossible, to determine what has gone on "after the fact" if the original implementation plan lacked built-in monitoring.

Evaluation reveals whether the policy and action plan need to be refined and reintroduced or abandoned and what parts of an intervention may need to be retrofitted or changed to help the program advance. The reality is, there is no perfect international nutrition solution, and modifications must often be made. Most nutrition programs are not flawless as initially implemented, and successful programs make the changes needed to move forward. In addition, in-the-field research rarely follows along exactly with the rational, step-by-step process described previously, but having such a model as an ideal may be helpful in anticipating potential pitfalls and bottlenecks that could ultimately derail an international nutrition-research project.

## Classification of International Nutrition Solutions Using the Social Ecological Model

There are seemingly as many types of international nutrition interventions and solutions as there are organizations that help develop and support them.

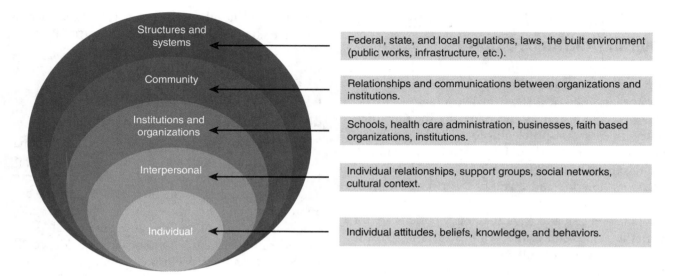

**FIGURE 12.9** Social ecological model

One way to classify types of international nutrition solutions is with the Centers for Disease Control and Prevention's **social ecological model** (**FIGURE 12.9**). This model describes five levels of influence on health behavior: (1) individual, (2) interpersonal, (3) institutional and organizational, (4) community, and (5) structural and system.

When considering the effectiveness of international nutrition interventions and solutions, several of the WHO resources identified earlier in this chapter may be useful. One is GINA, which has information on the implementation of numerous nutrition policies and interventions and also provides an opportunity for users to directly submit their own data.[40]

Examples of different international nutrition interventions and solutions—particularly those listed as top actions in the GINA database—are described in the following sections and classified based on the social ecological model.

## Individual Level: Breastfeeding and Complementary Feeding

Educating mothers and families to encourage breastfeeding and appropriate complementary feeding is an important individual-level nutrition intervention that has been part of UNICEF's work for decades. UNICEF has developed a set of generic tools for community-based infant and young child feeding counseling. The tools guide local adaptation, design, planning, and implementation using an interactive

and experiential adult learning approach. In addition, the tools are regularly updated to include lessons learned from their use, such as how to offer guidance on home fortification of complementary foods.[91] Promoting sound feeding practices is also important for the WHO, which has led the development of policies and recommendations and maintains an active **Global Data Bank on Infant and Young Child Feeding**.[92]

## Interpersonal Level: Growth Monitoring and Promotion

Growth monitoring and promotion programs measure and chart children's weights and use this information to counsel parents and motivate them to take actions that help improve growth. Growth-monitoring and growth-promotion programs have been in place for many years, and UNICEF has been one of the lead agencies involved in this effort.

Unlike other types of interventions that are more technical in nature—such as food fortification—the success of growth-monitoringand growth-promotion programs depends on both the technical interventions and the programs' acceptance and use by parents and other caretakers. Debate has continued about the effectiveness and feasibility of these programs to prevent malnutrition and, more specifically, the added value of growth monitoring to growth promotion. In a 1990 report for USAID titled *Growth Monitoring and Promotion: The Behavioral Issues*, Ann Brownlee commented, "Due to the necessity for active involvement of mothers, health workers and the community in growth monitoring and promotion activities, this child survival strategy has been one of the most difficult to implement."[93]

Nearly 30 years later, this challenge remains. Bilal et al.[94] reported that several studies have shown discrepancies between the purpose and the practice of growth-monitoring and growth-promotion programs. Based on their own research, they concluded that these programs are unlikely to succeed if mothers lack awareness of proper child-feeding practices or are not supported by their husbands.

## Institutional and Organizational Level: School Feeding and Food Distribution

The WFP is the largest humanitarian provider of school meals worldwide, providing school meals to more than 20 million children every year. As the WFP explains, nearly every country has a school meals program and governments recognize school meals are an essential tool for the development and growth of children, communities, and society in general (**FIGURE 12.10**).[95]

The WFP is the UN's frontline agency in fighting world hunger. Its programs respond to emergencies, help prevent future hunger, and use food to build assets and help communities become more food secure. The WFP brings food assistance to more than 80 million people in 80 countries. WFP expertise includes food-security analysis, food procurement, and logistics. Increasingly, the WFP is also focusing on nutrition. In addition to designing programs that directly treat and prevent malnutrition, WFP works to develop long-term solutions and influence the broader policy dialogue on food and nutrition security. They are integrating nutrition considerations into other areas of work—even those that previously did not have improved nutrition as an explicit goal—to address the underlying causes of malnutrition.[96]

## Community Level: Food Fortification and Micronutrient Supplementation

Food fortification is a frequent community-level nutrition solution. In the United States, food fortification has been a common practice and a requirement for some foods for so long that many Americans may not give it much thought. However, globally, the decision to fortify food products is often made by individual food manufacturers because food fortification is voluntary in many countries. Approximately 50 countries, including the United States, require mandatory fortification of certain food staples with specific nutrients to improve public health (for example, fortification of enriched flour with folic acid to reduce the risk of neural tube birth defects). The United States and some other countries also have restrictions on which foods may be fortified and at what levels.[97]

The Food Fortification Initiative is a public, private, and civic partnership to help country leaders plan, implement, and monitor fortification programs. The focus is on industrially milled wheat flour, maize flour, and rice. The initiative's website has an interactive map that includes country-specific information on grain production, legislation, nutrients added, milling-industry information, and nutrient-deficiency indicators.[98]

Vitamin A, iron, and folic acid supplementation are the most common nutrient-related actions listed in the GINA database. According to the Micronutrient Initiative, more than 2 billion people suffer from micronutrient deficiencies and cannot lead healthy, productive lives. Iron deficiency impairs the mental development of more than 40% of the developing world's infants. The Micronutrient Initiative works to improve the lives of some 500 million people in more than 70 countries and provides more than 75% of the global need for vitamin A.[99]

## Structural and System Level: Dietary Goals and Food-Based Dietary Guidelines

Dietary goals and food-based dietary guidelines are policy-level nutrition solutions. WHO's GINA database identifies dietary goals and food-based dietary guidelines as one of the top 10 global nutrition actions countries have implemented. The FAO reports that more than 100 countries have developed food-based dietary guidelines that are adapted to their nutrition situation, food availability, culinary cultures, and eating habits. The FAO helps member countries develop, revise, and implement food-based dietary guidelines and food guides based on current scientific evidence. It also reviews the progress on development and use of dietary guidelines. The FAO website offers detailed, interactive information on dietary guidelines from all member countries, including the official name, publication year, review process, stakeholders,

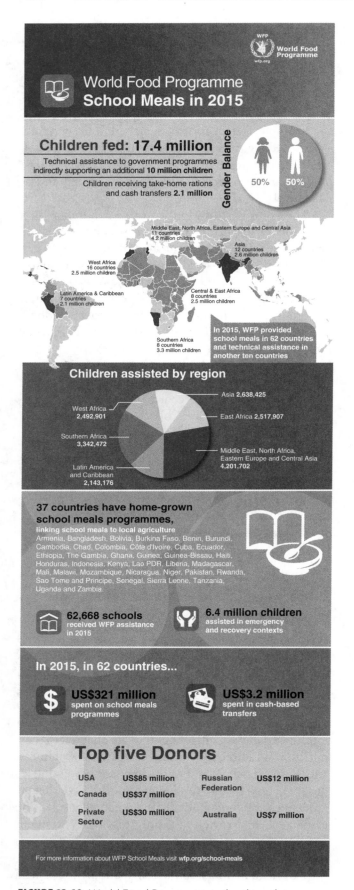

**FIGURE 12.10** World Food Programme school meals program

intended audience, food guide model, messages, and resources in the native language.[100] The United Nations offers a healthy diet fact sheet that warns an "unhealthy diet and lack of physical activity are leading global risks to health.[101]

**Recap** Nutrition assessment provides important baseline and follow-up data for helping design international nutrition research to identify important nutrition problems and determine the effectiveness of international nutrition solutions. The framework for many international nutrition interventions has been in place for many years and includes nutrition assessment as an important element.

## ▶ Chapter Summary

Nutrition assessment lays the foundation of the scientific evidence base for determining an international nutrition program's impact on growth and health outcomes. The nutritional threats to the world's population are shifting; although undernutrition remains a significant problem, obesity and other diet-related diseases as well as an increasingly older population are also affecting the health, survival, and developmental capacities of countries around the globe.

Defining international nutrition-assessment and research problems presents many challenges. Success demands an analysis of how the problem and its solutions will likely require actions across and from multiple sectors of society, including economic development, water sanitation and hygiene, and education. The assessment itself should be evidence based and pursued in the context of international policies and resources. Also, it involves being able to relate the problem to an individual country's interests, which are most often linked to global goals that affect the health, survival, and developmental capacity of populations. At the core of these problems is malnutrition in all its forms. Malnutrition is a major issue that can affect the citizens of a global region, a country, or an area within a country, and it ultimately impairs their ability to contribute to achieving their country's full economic development potential. For this reason, reducing malnutrition is a common target of the global goals. However, malnutrition has multiple causes, and its assessment emphasizes the application of food and nutrition knowledge, policy, and research to improve the health of populations.

Global organizations such as the United Nations and the WHO recognize this and have helped develop specific goals and targets as seen in the UN Millennium Development Goals and UN Sustainable Development Goals that are implemented at the household, community, national, and international levels to reduce malnutrition and improve nutritional status. The need for a focus on malnutrition is critical because the majority of people in most lower-income countries remain food insecure and nutritionally deprived with respect to both macronutrients (notably protein and fat) and essential micronutrients. At the same time, many of these countries are experiencing a "nutrition transition," with ever-increasing rates of overweight and obesity and a graying populace, as overall the population of the world is growing older. The United Nations and its agencies have not really developed or promoted nutrition programs focused on older adults, even though nutrition and older adults are included in the UN Sustainable Development Goal targets. This provides an opportunity for nutrition assessment and international research and specific program development.

Global goals provide a framework that gives a sense of the relevance of malnutrition and those at higher nutritional risks, and global goals also provide coherence in the use of available resources. Global goals are not necessarily top-down; instead, they help identify those targets that meet the criteria of clarity, conciseness, and measurability to improve the lives of the world's growing population. In doing so, they help delineate opportunities for international nutrition-assessment and research problems.

The world has just entered the UN-declared **Decade of Action on Nutrition**. International nutrition assessment and research can play a pivotal role in affecting these actions by providing the scientific evidence base for identifying nutrition problems and targeted solutions. This chapter has explored the different types of organizations that may be involved in international nutrition-related research. It has discussed the resources for nutrition-intervention approaches to be implemented at the household, community, national, and international levels to improve nutritional status. Finally, it has emphasized that the process for international nutrition assessment and research differs in several unique ways, and it has outlined principles and adaptations that are probable determinants of success.

 **CASE STUDY**

### Cross-Cultural Study of Iron Deficiencies

You have an opportunity to participate in Boston University's study-abroad program in Zanzibar, Tanzania. One of your projects for your research-methods course is to design a population health study that would compare biomarkers and prevalence of iron-deficiency anemia among teenage girls living in Zanzibar and teenage girls living in Massachusetts.

#### Questions:

1. Identify four possible organizations that may be interested in funding this type of research.
2. Define biomarkers that could potentially discriminate against iron-deficiency anemia.
3. Discuss the difference(s) between iron-deficiency anemia and anemias from other nutrient deficiencies.
4. Describe methods you could use to rule out parasitic disease, hemoglobinopathy, and other pathologies that can lead to iron-deficiency anemia.
5. Identify international and domestic databases that could be used to gather preliminary information on anemia rates and existing intervention programs for teenage girls in Zanzibar and in Massachusetts.
6. Use this information to outline your proposed research methods.

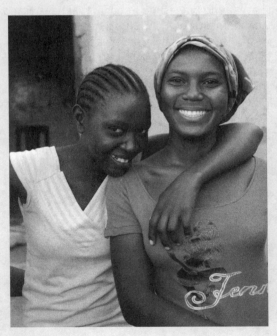

© Jake Lyell / Alamy Stock Photo.

## CASE STUDY

### Stunting in Bangladesh

Globally, the prevalence of growth stunting in children under 5 years of age has decreased, yet it remains a significant problem for many lower-income countries.

You have been awarded a $100,000 grant from the Bill & Melinda Gates Foundation for a project to reduce stunting in Bangladeshi children under 5 years of age. As you move through this chapter, consider how your research project may benefit Bangladesh, because it links to the global health agenda.

#### Questions:

1. What specific biomarkers will you measure?
2. What nutrition-assessment methods do you plan to use?
3. Are there any specific genetic conditions or environmental issues that could be a concern?
4. What domestic and in-country levels of approval will you need to secure?
5. How will you present your research plan to the appropriate authorities within the Bangladeshi government?
6. What are your plans for evaluation and follow-up?

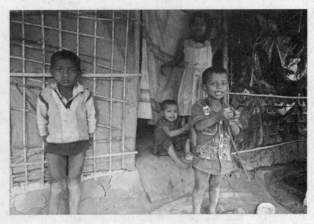

© Wadi Alias/Shutterstock.

## CASE STUDY

### Studying Nutrition in the Elderly

You have found interesting research that has tracked cohabitating families in Indonesia over time and suggests that cohabitation has a *negative* impact on parental survival rate. You wonder if there are potential negative impacts on nutrition and other health outcomes, too. In reviewing the material in this chapter, consider how you would conduct a research study in Indonesia to compare the nutritional and functional status of elderlies (ages 85 years and older) who live independently versus those living with their children.

#### Questions:

1. What organizations would potentially be interested in funding this type of study?
2. What biomarkers for nutrition would you evaluate and use?
3. What validated tools to measure functional status would you evaluate and use?

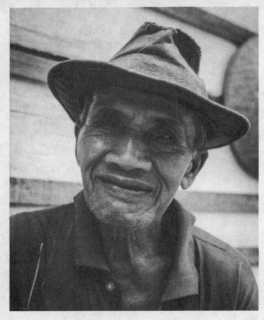

© Gilang Pandu Akbar / EyeEm/Getty Images.

# Learning Portfolio

## Key Terms

*Belmont Report*
Bilateral organizations
Biomarkers of Nutrition for Development (BOND)
Clinical trials registries
CODEX Alimentarius
Common Rule
Council for International Organizations of Medical Sciences (CIOMS)
Decade of Action on Nutrition
e-Library of Evidence for Nutrition Actions (eLENA)
First 1000 Days
Fogarty International Center
Food and Agriculture Organization (FAO)
Food and nutrition action plan
Food and Nutrition Council
Food and nutrition policy
Food control
Food policy
Food safety
Food sustainability
Global Database on the Implementation of Nutrition Action (GINA)
Global Data Bank on Infant and Young Child Feeding
Global database on body mass index
*Global Nutrition Report*
International Network of Food Data Systems (INFOODS)
International Compilation of Human Research Standards
Malnutrition in the Elderly (MaNuEL)
Multilateral organizations
Nongovernmental organizations (NGOs)
Nutrition Landscape Information System (NLiS)
Nuremberg Code
Office for Human Research Protections
Partnership organizations and collaborations
Protein-energy undernutrition (PEU)
Private-sector organizations
*Rome Declaration on Nutrition*
Social ecological model
Strengthening Partnerships, Results, and Innovations in Nutrition Globally (SPRING)
Stunted growth
Scaling Up Nutrition (SUN)
Systems thinking
UN Decade of Action on Nutrition
United Nations Children's Fund (UNICEF)
UN Millennium Development Goals
UN Standing Committee on Nutrition (UNSCN)
UN Sustainable Development Goals
US Agency for International Development (USAID)
WHO Global Nutrition Targets for 2025
World Food Programme (WFP)
World Health Assembly (WHA)
World Health Organization (WHO)

## Study Questions

1. Stunted growth among children is defined by which anthropometric index?
   a. Weight for height
   b. Height for age
   c. Weight for age
   d. Body mass index

2. Stunted growth among children younger than age five is associated with which one of the following?
   a. Decreased risk of early exposure to adverse conditions
   b. Decreased infection rates
   c. Increased mortality risk
   d. Reversible damage to a child's brain development

3. The first 1000 days is the period of time from:
   a. the child's second through fifth birthday.
   b. the child's first through fifth birthday.
   c. the beginning of pregnancy until the child's second birthday.
   d. birth until the child's second birthday.

4. When considering the issue of obesity, which of the following is true?
   a. Most of the world's population now lives in countries where overweight and obesity kill more people than underweight.
   b. The world is on track to meet the WHO global target of no increase in obesity or diabetes beyond the levels of 2010.

c. Approximately 90% of the world's health budgets are spent on obesity and associated diseases.

d. Worldwide obesity has remained constant since 1980.

5. Which one of the following is true for the UN Decade of Action on Nutrition?

a. It concluded in 2015 with the implementation of the UN Sustainable Development Goals.

b. It is focused solely on ending hunger worldwide.

c. It set overall global targets, and member countries cannot vary from these global targets.

d. It specifically calls on governments to set national nutrition targets and milestones for 2025 based on internationally agreed-on indicators.

6. Which two organizations will lead implementation of the Decade of Action on Nutrition (2016–2025)?

a. The World Health Organizations and the Food and Agricultural Organization

b. The World Health Assembly and Food for the Hungry International

c. The Global Alliance for Improved Nutrition and the Bill & Melinda Gates Foundation

d. The International Committee of the Red Cross and the Rockefeller Foundation

7. The population of the world is aging. Which one of the following statements is true?

a. By 2020, 150 countries will be "superaged," with more than 20% of their populations older than 65.

b. The graying population shift is occurring much more quickly in higher-income countries.

c. Older adults are not a nutritionally high-risk population.

d. To date, UN agencies have developed few if any international nutrition programs that specifically target older adults and their unique nutritional needs.

8. Which type of organization may be involved in international nutrition-related research?

a. Nongovernmental organizations

b. Vertical organizations

c. Trilateral organizations

d. Traditional organizations

9. Which one of the following descriptions of a UN agency is correct?

a. The Food and Agriculture Organization works with governments to resolve food insecurity and social reform.

b. The World Food Programme is the world's largest humanitarian agency fighting hunger.

c. The United Nations Children's Fund serves as leading advocate for global action against HIV and AIDS.

d. CODEX Alimentarius works to promote safe, secure, and peaceful use of nuclear technologies.

10. Which one of the following statements about bilateral organizations is true?

a. They never consider a country's past history, politics, and geography when making funding decisions.

b. They are governmental agencies from multiple countries that provide aid to lower-income countries.

c. They are governmental agencies from a single country that provide aid to lower-income countries.

d. They include the Asian Development Bank and UNICEF.

11. Which one of the following statements about nongovernmental organizations is true?

a. They are often known as public voluntary organizations.

b. They are typically free of governmental control but may receive government funding.

c. They are a homogeneous and similar group of organizations addressing humanitarian aid needs.

d. They are groups that have primarily commercial rather than humanitarian or cooperative objectives.

12. Which one of the following is one of the greatest successes of the UN Millennium Development Goals?

a. Reduced food-borne illnesses

b. Reduced child mortality

c. Reduced obesity

d. Decreased poverty rates

13. Which one of the following statements is true about the UN Millennium Development Goals?

a. They were derived from the US Millennium Declaration of 2000.

b. They have been replaced by the UN's 17 Sustainable Development Goals for 2030.

c. They includes 12 goals.

d. They are not useful for identifying research problems of international nutritional relevance.

14. Internationally, which micronutrient deficiency is most commonly related to chronic malnutrition?
    a. Potassium deficiency
    b. Vitamin K deficiency
    c. Calcium deficiency
    d. Vitamin A deficiency

15. Which resource may be helpful in defining an international nutrition-research problem?
    a. The US Department of Defense's satellite tracking system
    b. WHO's Nutrition Landscape Information System
    c. The national vulnerability database
    d. The national register information system

16. The Nuremberg Code:
    a. was developed in 1918 after World War I.
    b. was developed as a result of the Tuskegee trials.
    c. helped form the basis for today's ethical, legal, and regulatory framework for research using human subjects.
    d. states that the voluntary consent of a human subject is not necessary.

17. Which principle is emphasized by the *Belmont Report*:
    a. Transparency
    b. Beneficence
    c. Participation
    d. Independence

18. Which one of the following statements about the Common Rule is true?
    a. It is a UN federal policy for the protection of human subjects.
    b. It outlines the basic provisions for an institutional review board.
    c. It is regulated by the UN's Department of Economic and Social Affairs.
    d. It does not apply to federally funded research.

19. Which federal office "oversees the system protecting the rights, welfare, and well-being of research subjects and ensures federal research meets the Common Rule standards"?
    a. The HHS Office for Human Research Protections
    b. The HHS Office for International Research
    c. The World Agency Office for Human Rights
    d. The FAO Office for Research Justice

20. "helicopter research" is when?
    a. Investigators hover outside of people's homes in hopes of enrolling them in a research study

b. Investigators collect their data and then leave the site without any follow-ups

c. Investigators bribe potential research subjects with gifts to join a study

d. Investigators stay in a research site longer than they are allowed to by the country's officials

21. When planning to conduct international research, investigators should understand the social rules of that local culture. Which one of the following is a good cultural practice?
    a. Always shake hands with the left hand because the right is assumed in many cultures to be used for bodily hygiene.
    b. Lack of eye contact shows inattentiveness, therefore an investigator should ask colleagues and study participants to look him or her in the eye when speaking.
    c. Try to interrupt the speaker to establish dominance and gain respect.
    d. Keep a conversational tone. Loudness may be associated with aggression, so it may be best to maintain a soft, calm voice.

22. In international settings, the basic methods used to collect information for nutrition assessment may need to be adapted in some ways. What is an example of an adaptation cited in this chapter?
    a. Triceps skinfold thickness measurements
    b. Midarm-circumference measurements
    c. Body mass calculations
    d. Dried blood spot sampling

23. Functional status measures include which one of the following?
    a. The Acute Emotional Inventory
    b. The Instrumental Activities of Daily Living Screen
    c. The Cognitive Ability Exam
    d. The Cognitive Function Test

24. Which one of the following has been identified as a validated malnutrition screening tool?
    a. Individual nutrition-assessment tool
    b. Malnutrition Universal Screening Tool
    c. Nutrition Indicator Checklist
    d. Subjective Nutrition Risk Index

25. Key questions recommended to ask in designing a nutrition assessment include which one of the following?
    a. What is the nutrition-related problem and how severe is it?
    b. What nutrition problems have been routinely solved before?

c. What nutrition policies need to be implemented to solve the nutrition-related problem?

d. What nutrition-related interventions have failed in this region?

26. True or false? Open and inclusive (often referred to as "transparent") processes produce policies that are more likely to be acceptable to the majority of citizens.
    a. True
    b. False

27. When should a system for regular monitoring and evaluation be implemented?
    a. At the start of the nutrition intervention
    b. Halfway through the nutrition intervention to assess progress
    c. At the conclusion of the nutrition intervention
    d. Interventions and research studies do not require systems for monitoring and evaluation.

28. In the social ecological model, how many levels of influence are there on health behavior?
    a. 3
    b. 4
    c. 5
    d. 6

29. School-feeding and food-distribution programs fall into which level on the social ecological model?
    a. Individual level
    b. Interpersonal level
    c. Institutional and organizational level
    d. Community level

30. In considering food fortification and micronutrient supplementation, which one of the following statements is true?
    a. All countries require mandatory fortification of certain food staples.
    b. Vitamin D and iodine supplementation are the most common nutrient-related actions listed in the GINA database.
    c. The Food Fortification Initiative is a public, private, and civic partnership to help country leaders plan, implement, and monitor fortification programs.
    d. The Micronutrient Initiative provides more than 75% of the global need for vitamin C.

## Discussion Questions

1. Consider how Guatemala could design and implement a specific nutrition project related to the UN Decade of Action on Nutrition. Describe the project and how nutrition-assessment research could help establish a baseline. Discuss what specific nutrition-assessment methods would be used.

2. Using question 1, consider how Guatemala could design and implement a specific nutrition project related to the UN Decade of Action on Nutrition.

3. Describe the project and discuss potential roles and involvement from civil society, the private sector, and academia in actively supporting the government's engagement in the project.

4. Compare and contrast the UN's Millennium Development Goals and UN Sustainable Development Goals. Discuss their pros and cons, value and importance, opportunities and limitations, and suggest potential changes and reasons for the changes.

5. What are specific examples of biomarkers that could be used to measure both dietary intake and nutritional status of vitamin D for older adults (65 years and older) living in rural China?

6. If you could choose only one food or food ingredient to fortify in Zambia, what would it be? What would be the five most important nutrients you would choose to fortify the food or food ingredient with and why? What specific nutrient-deficiency indicators would you evaluate and in what populations to determine the potential effectiveness of the food or food ingredient fortification?

## Activities

### Individual Activities

1. Compare and contrast at least two nutrition-assessment methods for their:
   a. validity,
   b. feasibility, and
   c. potential cost
      to study the impact of a vitamin A supplementation program on pregnant women, infants, and preschool-aged children living in Sudan.

2. Use the WHO Global Database on Body Mass Index to profile adult underweight, overweight, and obesity prevalence rates for a selected country in Asia.
   i. Plot two graphs (one for each gender) of the prevalence rates over the past decade for the three weight categories.
   ii. Identify the data sources used for the body weight information in the selected country.
   iii. Describe how you would use the database information to support a nutrition-assessment component of a research project studying the potential impact of the country's dietary guidelines on adult body weight trends over the past decade.
   Source: http://www.who.int/nutrition /databases/bmi/en/

## Group Activity

1. NGOs Focusing on the First 1000 Days
   a. Identify five nongovernmental organizations that include a focus on the first 1000 days.
   b. Assign each member of the group a different NGO to investigate and identify the following:
      i. Organization profile, including history, orientation, size, thematic scope, mission, geographic scope, funding levels and sources, and collaboration with other organizations; and

      ii. 1000 days program overview, including description, budget, strategic fit with NGO's thematic scope, countries included, and program reviews and evaluations.
   c. Come back together as a group and compare the five NGOs' similarities and differences and potential for impact in various regions of the world. Discuss how working with each NGO to implement a nutrition-assessment research project in a country it supports could help benefit the NGO and the individual country.
2. Organizations involved in international nutrition related research
   a. Identify and differentiate the five different types of organizations involved in international nutrition related research.
   b. Assign each member of the group a different research organization to investigate and identify the following:
      i. organization profile, including history, orientation, size, thematic scope, mission, geographic scope, funding levels and sources, and collaboration with other organizations.
      ii. What drives each type of organization's research agenda?
   c. Come back together as a group and discuss your findings.

## Online Resources

### UN Sustainable Development Goals

This United Nations Sustainable Development knowledge platform shows all 17 of the global UN Sustainable Development Goals that UN member countries have committed to meet by 2030. Click on each goal for details about the individual targets and more information about the goal:

http://www.un.org/sustainabledevelopment/sustainable -development-goals/.

### Scaling Up Nutrition

This SUN website provides details about the movement. SUN is based on the principle that everyone has a right to food and good nutrition. The program is unique in bringing together different groups of people—governments, civil society, the United Nations, donors, businesses, and scientists—in a collective action to improve nutrition:

http://scalingupnutrition.org/

### United Nations Division for Social Policy and Development Ageing

Every second, two people in the world turn 60 years old. The UN Division for Social Policy and Development Ageing website provides resources and information about UN programs on aging. What is most striking about this site is its limited focus on nutrition when compared to the UN's maternal and child programs: https://www.un.org/development/desa/ageing/

### National Institute of Child Health and Human Development (NICHD) Biomarkers of Nutrition for Development (BOND) Program

Biomarkers are the foundation of nutrition assessment. The BOND website provides information about how they are creating a unified approach to examine the scientific basis for choosing appropriate biomarkers for:

- assessing the function and effect of diet and nutrition on health and disease in individuals and populations and

■ supporting the development and evaluation of evidence-based programs and policies to improve diet and nutrition as a way to improve health.

https://www.nichd.nih.gov/global_nutrition/programs/bond/Pages/index.aspx

### FAO

Includes links to assessment tools, information to help develop countries' capacities to collect data, and country-specific nutrition information based on food consumption:
http://www.fao.org/nutrition/assessment/en/.

### UNICEF

Provides an overview of UNICEF's nutrition programs: http://www.unicef.org/nutrition/.

### US Agency for International Development (USAID)

Provides an overview of USAID nutrition projects (https://www.usaid.gov/what-we-do/global-health/nutrition/projects) and provides an overview of one of these projects, the US global hunger and food-security initiative:
https://www.feedthefuture.gov/

### WFP

Provides an overview of WFP's nutrition programs: https://www.wfp.org/nutrition.

### WHO

Provides an overview of WHO's nutrition programs: http://www.who.int/nutrition/en/.

### FAO

Video on current global nutrition challenges—for adults and children—and the need for global nutrition policies (in preparation for the Second International Conference on Nutrition):

http://www.fao.org/news/audio-video/detail-video/en/?uid=10571.

### UNICEF

Video on stunting:
http://www.unicef.org/nutrition/index_68726.html

### UN Sustainable Development Goals

Educational video for children explaining the sustainable development goals:
http://worldslargestlesson.globalgoals.org/d

### WFP

Eight "must-see" videos on world hunger (https://www.wfp.org/stories/8-must-see-videos-hunger-

and-nutrition) and a video on "nutrition in 2 minutes" (http://www.wfp.org/videos/nutrition-2-minutes-0)

### WHO

What is the double burden? Introductory video for the Second International Conference on Nutrition: http://www.who.int/nutrition/topics/WHO_FAO_ICN2_videos_doubleburden/en/.

### edX

Massive Open Online Course (MOOC) providing free university courses including food security and sustainability, health and wellness, nutrition and health, and the ethics of eating:
https://www.edx.org/.

### FAO

E-learning center for agriculture and food-security professionals (http://www.fao.org/elearning/#/elc/en/courses/NUTR), including a food-composition data course
(http://www.fao.org/elearning/#/elc/en/course/FCD).

### Fogarty International Center, US National Institutes of Health

E-learning resources for global health researchers, including training courses, MOOCs, course materials, resource centers, and resource networks:
https://www.fic.nih.gov/Global/Pages/training-resources.aspx.

### UNICEF

E-learning training course with Cornell University to enhance the competencies and build the capacity of UNICEF staff and counterparts involved in Infant and Young Child Feeding (IYCF) programs in lower income countries (https://www.nutritionworks.cornell.edu/UNICEF/about/) and an e-learning course on nutrition in emergencies (http://www.unicef.org/nutrition/training/).

### SuperCourse (SC)

Online repository of lectures, research methods, materials on global health; includes network of about 2 million scientists in 174 countries sharing a free library of more than 198,000 lectures in 33 languages: http://www.pitt.edu/~super1/.

### USDA and Food and Nutrition Technical Assistance (FANTA)

E-learning course on nutrition, including common nutritional deficiencies, the magnitude of malnutrition in different populations, groups most vulnerable to malnutrition, causes of undernutrition, and key indicators.

The site also includes major population-based interventions to improve nutritional status: https://www.globalhealthlearning.org/course/nutrition -introduction.

**WFP**

E-learning toolkit and resources on food-security analysis: http://learning.vam.wfp.org/.

**Food and Agriculture Organization (FAO)**

Infographic on why food and nutrition education is needed (http://www.fao.org/3/a-c0064e.pdf) and an interactive map on the constitutional right to adequate food (http://www.fao.org/right-to-food-around-the -globe/en/).

**National Academies Press**

Workshop summaries and publications include Exploring Shared Value in Global Health and Safety—Workshop Summary (https://www.nap.edu/read/23501 /chapter/1), Investing in Global Health Systems—Sustaining Gains, Transforming Lives (https://www.nap .edu/read/18940/chapter/1), including Health in Global Frameworks for Development, Wealth, and Climate Change—Workshop Summary (https://www.nap.edu /catalog/18554/including-health-in-global-frameworks -for-development-wealth-and-climate-change).

**Scaling Up Nutrition**

The SUN "Why Nutrition" page provides infographics on the cycle of good nutrition and the scale of malnutrition: http://scalingupnutrition.org/nutrition/the-importance -of-good-nutrition/.

**United Nations Children's Fund**

UNICEF's child nutrition interactive dashboard 2015: http://data.unicef.org/resources/child-nutrition -interactive-dashboard-2015-edition.html#.

**World Food Programme**

Nine WFP infographics about hunger: https://www .wfp.org/students-and-teachers/teachers/blog/nine -infographics-will-help-you-teach-hunger.

**World Health Organization**

WHO infographic on the double burden of malnutrition: http://www.who.int/nutrition/double-burden -malnutrition/infographic_print.pdf?ua=1.

**WHO**

Tracking tool for the 2025 Global Nutrition Targets to Improve Maternal, Infant, and Young Child Nutrition: https://extranet.who.int/sree/Reports?op=    vs&path = %2FWHO_HQ_Reports/G16/PROD/EXT/Targets _Menu&VSPARAM_varLanguage=E&VSPARAM _varISOCODE=ALB.

**WHO and National Institutes on Aging**

Global Health and Aging Report with graphic on increasing burden of chronic noncommunicable disease in low-income countries: http://www.who.int/ageing/publications/global _health.pdf.

# References

1. United Nations (UN) System's Forum on Nutrition. SCN's 26th Session: Making History. July 1999. http://www.unscn .org/layout/modules/resources/files/scnnews18.pdf. Accessed September 24, 2016.
2. First Report on the World Nutrition Situation. http://agris .fao.org/agris-search/search.do?recordID=XF19880106879. Accessed September 24, 2016.
3. UN System Subcommittee on Nutrition. UNSCN Publications. https://www.unscn.org/en/resource-center/UNSCN-Publications. Accessed September 24, 2016.
4. United Nations Children's Fund (UNICEF). Undernutrition contributes to nearly half of all deaths in children under 5 and is widespread in Asia and Africa. 2017. UNICEF Data: Monitoring the Situation of Children and Women. http://data.unicef.org /nutrition/malnutrition.html.
5. United States Agency for International Development (USAID). Multi-Sectoral Nutrition Strategy 2014–2025. https://www .usaid.gov/sites/default/files/documents/1864/1000-days -brief-508.pdf. Accessed September 24, 2016.
6. World Health Organization (WHO). Essential Nutrition Actions. 2013:146. http://www.who.int/nutrition/publications/infantfeeding /essential_nutrition_actions/en/. Accessed September 24, 2016.
7. UN System Subcommittee on Nutrition. Scaling Up Nutrition Movement. http://www.unscn.org/en/sun-scaling-up/. Accessed September 24, 2106.
8. US Department of Health and Human Services (HHS). Global Statistics. Global HIVAIDS Epidemic. https://www.aids .gov/hiv-aids-basics/hiv-aids-101/global-statistics/. Accessed September 24, 2016.
9. US Agency for International Development (USAID). The Essential Role of Nutrition in the HIV and AIDS Response. https://www.usaid.gov/what-we-do/global-health/hiv-and -aids/technical-areas/essential-role-nutrition-hiv-and-aids -response. Accessed September 24, 2016.
10. The Lancet. 2008 Maternal and Child Undernutrition Series. http://www.thelancet.com/series/maternal-and-child -undernutrition. Accessed September 24, 2016.
11. The Lancet. 2013 Maternal and Child Nutrition Series. http:// www.thelancet.com/series/maternal-and-child-nutrition. Accessed September 24, 2016.
12. WHO. Globalization, Diets and Noncommunicable Diseases. 2002; 185. http://apps.who.int/iris/bitstream /10665 /42609/1/9241590416.pdf. Accessed September 24, 2016.

13. WHO. Global Strategy on Diet, Physical Activity and Health. 2004:21. http://www.who.int/dietphysicalactivity/strategy /eb11344/strategy_english_web.pdf. Accessed September 24, 2016.

14. UN General Assembly. Political Declaration of the High-Level Meeting of the General Assembly on the Prevention and Control of Non-Communicable Diseases. 2012. http:// www.who.int/nmh/events/un_ncd_summit2011/political _declaration_en.pdf. Accessed September 24, 2016.

15. WHO. Global Action Plan for the Prevention and Control of Noncommunicable Diseases 2013–2020. 2013; 55. http://apps .who.int/iris/bitstream/10665/94384/1/9789241506236_eng .pdf?ua=1. Accessed September 24, 2016.

16. UN. United Nations Global Nutrition Agenda. 2014; 48. http://unscn.org/files/Activities/SUN/UN_Global_Nutrition _Agenda_final.pdf. Accessed September 24, 2016.

17. WHO, Food and Agriculture Organization (FAO) of the United Nations. United Nations Decade of Action on Nutrition. 2016. http://www.who.int/nutrition/decade-of-action/info_flyer .pdf?ua=1. Accessed September 24, 2016.

18. FAO, WHO. Conference Outcome Document: Rome Declaration on Nutrition. Rome, Italy; 2014: 6. http://www .fao.org/3/a-ml542e.pdf. Accessed September 24, 2016.

19. FAO, WHO. Conference Outcome Document: Framework for Action. 2014: 8. http://www.fao.org/3/a-mm215e.pdf. Accessed September 24, 2016.

20. WHO. Obesity and Overweight. 2016. http://www.who.int /mediacentre/factsheets/fs311/en/. Accessed September 24, 2016.

21. WHO. Noncommunicable diseases and mental health. 9 Voluntary Global Targets. http://www.who.int/nmh/ncd -tools/definition-targets/en/. Accessed September 24, 2016.

22. Petroff A. World getting "super-aged" at scary speed. CNN. 2014. http://money.cnn.com/2014/08/21/news/economy/aging -countries-moodys/. Accessed September 24, 2016.

23. Jackson R, Macaranas R, Peters T. *US Development Policy in an Aging World.* 2013:34. https://csis-prod.s3.amazonaws.com /s3fs-public/legacy_files/files/publication/130517_Jackson _USDevelPol_web.pdf. Accessed September 25, 2016.

24. WHO, National Institute on Aging, National Institutes of Health, HHS. *Global Health and Aging.* 2011: 32. http://www .who.int/ageing/publications/global_health.pdf.

25. UN. *Vienna International Plan of Action on Aging.* 1983: 50. http://www.un.org/es/globalissues/ageing/docs/vipaa.pdf. Accessed September 24, 2016.

26. WHO. *Multisectoral Action for a Life Course Approach to Healthy Ageing: Draft Global Strategy and Plan of Action on Ageing and Health.* 2016: 37. http://apps.who.int/gb/ebwha /pdf_files/WHA69/A69_17-en.pdf.

27. UN. Sustainable Development Goal 2. https://sustain abledevelopment.un.org/sdg2. Accessed September 24, 2016.

28. The Global Development Research Center. Types of NGOs. http://www.gdrc.org/ngo/ngo-types.html.

29. Cederholm T, Bosaeus I, Barazzoni J, et al. Diagnostic Criteria for Malnutrition—An ESPEN Consensus Statement. *Clin Nutr.* 2015; 34(3):335-340. doi:10.1016/j.clnu.2015.03.001.

30. Chopra M, Mason E. Millennium development goals: Background. *Arch Dis Child.* 2015; 100(Suppl 1):S2-S4. doi:10.1136/archdischild-2013-305437.

31. UNICEF, WHO, World Bank Group. Levels and Trends in Child Malnutrition UNICEF-WHO-World Bank Group Joint Child Malnutrition Estimates Key Findings of the 2014 Edition. 2015: 6. http://www.unicef.org/media/files/JME _2015_edition_Sept_2015.pdf. Accessed September 24, 2016.

32. WHO. Maternal mortality. 2015. http://www.who.int /mediacentre/factsheets/fs348/en/.

33. Fehling M, Nelson B, Venkatapuram S. Limitations of the millennium development goals: A literature review. *Glob Public Health.* 2013; 8(10):1109-1122. doi:10.1080/17441692. 2013.845676.

34. GBD 2015 SDG Collaborators. Measuring the health-related Sustainable Development Goals in 188 countries: A baseline analysis from the Global Burden of Disease Study 2015. *Lancet.* 2016. doi:http://dx.doi.org/10.1016/S0140-6736(16)31467-2.

35. Murray CJ. Shifting to sustainable development goals— Implications for global health. *N Engl J Med.* 2015; 373:1390-1393. doi:10.1056/NEJMp1510082.

36. Sommer A, Davidson F. Assessment and control of vitamin A deficiency: The Annecy accords. *J Nutr.* 2002; 132:S2845-2850.

37. Burger S, Pierre-Louis J. *How to Assess Iron Deficiency Anemia and Use the Hemocue.* New York, NY: Helen Keller International; 2002: 97. http://pdf.usaid.gov/pdf_docs /Pnacw824.pdf.

38. WHO. Nutrition Landscape Information System (NLiS). http:// www.who.int/nutrition/nlis/en/. Accessed September 24, 2016.

39. WHO. Landscape Analysis on Countries' Readiness to Accelerate Action in Nutrition. http://www.who.int/nutrition /landscape_analysis/en/. Accessed September 24, 2016.

40. WHO. Global Database on the Implementation of Nutrition Action (GINA). http://www.who.int/nutrition/gina/en/.

41. Arabi M, Hsieh A, McLean M. *A Global Research Agenda for Nutrition Science.* 2013: 28. http://www .nutritionresearchagenda.org/pdf/Sackler-Agenda-121313 -WEB.pdf. Accessed September 24, 2016.

42. *Global Nutrition Report: From Promise to Impact Ending Malnutrition by 2030.* 2016: 157. http://ebrary.ifpri.org/utils /getfile/collection/p15738coll2/id/130354/filename /130565.pdf.

43. World Food Programme. *5 Takeaways from the Global Nutrition Report.* http://www.wfp.org/stories/5-takeaways -global-nutrition-report.

44. Bill & Melinda Gates Foundation. *Nutrition Strategy Overview.* http://www.gatesfoundation.org/What-We-Do/Global -Development/Nutrition. Accessed September 24, 2016.

45. UN. *Health in the Post-2015 Development Agenda: Need for a Social Determinants of Health Approach.* 2016: 18. http:// www.who.int/social_determinants/advocacy/UN_Platform _FINAL.pdf?ua=1. Accessed September 24, 2016.

46. USAID. SPRING Strengthening Partnerships, Results, and Innovations in Nutrition Globally. https://www.spring-nutrition .org/. Accessed September 24, 2016.

47. *Br Med J.* 1996; 313(7070):1448.

48. World Medical Association. *WMA Declaration of Helsinki: Ethical Principles for Medical Research Involving Human Subjects.* http://www.wma.net/en/30publications/10policies/b3/. Accessed September 24, 2016.

49. Centers for Disease Control and Prevention. The Tuskegee Timeline. http://www.cdc.gov/tuskegee/timeline.htm. Accessed September 24, 2016.

50. HHS. *The Belmont Report.* 1979. http://www.hhs.gov/ohrp /regulations-and-policy/belmont-report/. Accessed September 24, 2016.

51. *Code of Federal Regulations.* Title 45 Public Welfare Department of Health and Human Services Part 46 Protection of Human Subjects. Vol 45 CFR 46. 1991. http://www.hhs.gov /ohrp/regulations-and-policy/regulations/45-cfr-46/index .html. Accessed September 24, 2016.

52. HHS. Office for Human Research Protections. http://www.hhs.gov/ohrp/. Accessed September 24, 2016.

53. HHS. International. http://www.hhs.gov/ohrp/international. Accessed September 24, 2016.

54. Rose S. Considerations for International Research. https://oprs.usc.edu/files/2017/04/International-Research_2012.pdf. Accessed September 24, 2016.

55. University of Pittsburgh Human Research Protection Office. International Research. http://www.irb.pitt.edu/node/297. Accessed September 24, 2016.

56. WHO. Dietary Recommendations/Nutritional Requirements. http://www.who.int/nutrition/topics/nutrecomm/en/. Accessed September 24, 2016.

57. WHO. Nutrient Requirements and Dietary Guidelines. http://www.who.int/nutrition/publications/nutrient/en/. Accessed September 24, 2016.

58. WHO. Vitamin and Mineral Nutrition Information System (VMMNIS). http://www.who.int/vmnis/en/. Accessed September 24, 2016.

59. FAO. About INFOODS. http://www.fao.org/infoods/infoods/en/. Accessed September 24, 2016.

60. WHO. Physical Status: The Use and Interpretation of Anthropometry. http://www.who.int/childgrowth/publications/physical_status/en/. Accessed September 24, 2016.

61. WHO. The WHO Child Growth Standards. http://www.who.int/childgrowth/en/. Accessed September 24, 2016.

62. WHO. Global Database on Body Mass Index (BMI). http://www.who.int/nutrition/databases/bmi/en/. Accessed September 24, 2016.

63. National Institutes of Health. Biomarkers of Nutrition for Development (BOND) Program. https://www.nichd.nih.gov/global_nutrition/programs/bond/Pages/index.aspx. Accessed September 24, 2016.

64. Suchdev PS, Namaste SML, Aaron GJ, et al. Overview of the Biomarkers Reflecting Inflammation and Nutritional Determinants of Anemia (BRINDA) project. *Adv Nutr.* 2016; 7(2):349-356. doi:10.3945/an.115.010215.

65. Raiten DJ. Iron: Current landscape and efforts to address a complex issue in a complex world. *J Pediatr.* 2015; 167(4):S3-S7. doi:10.1016/j.jpeds.2015.07.013.

66. Raiten DJ, Neufeld LM, De-Regil L-M, et al. Integration to implementation and the micronutrient forum: A coordinated approach for global nutrition. Case study application: Safety and effectiveness of iron interventions. *Adv Nutr.* 2016; 7(1):135-148. doi:10.3945/an.115.008581.

67. Raiten DJ, Sakr Ashour FA, Ross AC, et al. Inflammation and Nutritional Science for Programs/Policies and Interpretation of Research Evidence (INSPIRE). *J Nutr.* 2015; 145(5):1039S-1108S. doi:10.3945/jn.114.194571.

68. WHO. *WHO Guidelines on Drawing Blood: Best Practices in Phlebotomy.* 2010. http://apps.who.int/iris/bitstream/10665/44294/1/9789241599221 _eng.pdf.

69. McDade T, Williams S, Snodgrass J. What a drop can do: dried blood spots as a minimally invasive method for integrating biomarkers into population-based research. *Demography.* 2007; 44(4):899-925.

70. Fallah E, Peighambardoust S. Validation of the use of dried blood spot (DBS) method to assess Vitamin A status. *Health Promot Perspect.* 2012; 2(2):180-189. doi:10.5681/hpp.2012.021.

71. Zimmermann M, de Benoist B, Corigliano S, et al. Assessment of iodine status using dried blood spot thyroglobulin: Development of reference material and establishment of an international reference range in iodine-sufficient children. *J Clin Endocrinol Metab.* 2006; 91(12):4881-4887. doi:10.1210/jc.2006-1370.

72. Hoeller U, Baur M, Roos FF, et al. Application of dried blood spots to determine vitamin D status in a large nutritional study with unsupervised sampling: The Food4Me project. *Br J Nutr.* 2016; 115(2):202-211. doi:10.1017/S0007114515004298.

73. Gupta R, Abraham RA, Dhatwalia S, Ramakrishnan L, Prabhakaran D, Reddy KS. Use of dried blood for measurement of trans fatty acids. *Nutr J.* 2009; 8:35. doi:10.1186/1475-2891-8-35.

74. Marie Farrell KW. Nutrition as a vital sign: Progress since the 1990 multidisciplinary nutrition screening initiative and opportunities for nursing. *J Nurs Care.* 2015; 4(1). doi:10.4172/2167-1168.1000224.

75. BDA. Nutritional Screening, Assessment, and Treatment. https://www.bda.uk.com/improvinghealth/healthprofessionals/nutritional_screening. Accessed September 24, 2016.

76. Keller HH. Promoting food intake in older adults living in the community: A review. *Appl Physiol Nutr Metab Physiol Appliquée Nutr Métabolisme.* 2007; 32(6):991-1000. doi:10.1139/H07-067.

77. Evidence based practice guidelines for the nutritional management of malnutrition in adult patients across the continuum of care. *Nutr Diet.* 2009;66:S1-S34. doi:10.1111/j.1747-0080.2009.01383.x.

78. Schindler K, Pernicka E, Laviano A, et al. How nutritional risk is assessed and managed in European hospitals: A survey of 21,007 patients findings from the 2007-2008 cross-sectional nutrition day survey. *Clin Nutr Edinb Scotl.* 2010; 29(5): 552-559. doi:10.1016/j.clnu.2010.04.001.

79. JPI. MaNuEL, the Knowledge Hub on Malnutrition in the Elderly. http://www.healthydietforhealthylife.eu/index.php/news/232-manuel-the-knowledge-hub-on-malnutrition-in-the-elderly. Accessed September 24, 2016.

80. RAND Health. 36-Item Short Form Survey (SF-36). Santa, Monica, CA: RAND Corporation. http://www.rand.org/health/surveys_tools/mos/36-item-short-form.html. Accessed September 24, 2016.

81. WHO. About eLENA. 2017. http://www.who.int/elena/about/en/. Accessed September 24, 2016.

82. ICH. Efficacy Guidelines. http://www.ich.org/products/guidelines/efficacy/article/efficacy-guidelines.html. Accessed September 24, 2016.

83. Council for International Organizations of Medical Sciences. *International Ethical Guidelines for Biomedical Research Involving Human Subjects.* 2017; 113. http://www.cioms.ch/publications/layout_guide2002.pdf. Accessed September 24, 2016.

84. ACRO. Home page. ACRO. http://acrohealth.org/. Accessed September 24, 2016.

85. HHS. http://www.hhs.gov/ohrp/international/compilation-human-research-standards/index.html. 2010; October 15. Accessed September 24, 2016.

86. HHS. Listing of Clinical Trial Registries. http://www.hhs.gov/ohrp/international/clinical-trial-registries/index.html. 2016; March 4. Accessed September 24, 2016.

87. HHS. Ethical Codes & Research Standards. http://www.hhs.gov/ohrp/international/ethical-codes-and-research-standards/index.html. 2016; February 19. Accessed September 24, 2016.

88. HHS. Equivalent Protections. http://www.hhs.gov/ohrp/international/equivalent-protections/index.html. 2016; March 4. Accessed September 24, 2016.

89. National Institutes of Health. E-learning Resources for Global Health Researchers. https://www.fic.nih.gov/Global/Pages/training-resources.aspx. Accessed September 24, 2016.

90. FAO. Nutrition Assessment. http://www.fao.org/nutrition/assessment/en/. Accessed September 24, 2016.

91. UNICEF. Community Based Infant and Young Child Feeding. http://www.unicef.org/nutrition/index_58362.html. Accessed September 24, 2016.

92. WHO. WHO Global Data Bank on Infant and Young Child Feeding. 2017. http://www.who.int/nutrition/databases/infantfeeding/en/. Accessed September 24, 2016.

93. Brownlee A. *Growth Monitoring and Promotion: The Behavioral Issues.* 1990: 110. http://pdf.usaid.gov/pdf_docs/PNABG752.pdf.

94. Bilal SM, Moser A, Blanco R, Spigt M, Dinant GJ. Practices and challenges of growth monitoring and promotion in Ethiopia: A qualitative study. *J Health Popul Nutr.* 2014; 32(3):441-451.

95. UN World Food Programme. School Meals. 2017. https://www.wfp.org/school-meals. Accessed September 24, 2016.

96. UN World Food Programme. Our Work. 2017. http://www.wfp.org/our-work. Accessed September 24, 2016.

97. International Food Information Council Foundation. Food Fortification in Today's World. http://www.foodinsight.org/Newsletter/Detail.aspx%3Ftopic%3DFood_Fortification_in_Today_s_World. Accessed September 24, 2016.

98. Food Fortification Initiative. http://www.ffinetwork.org/country_profiles/index.php. Accessed September 24, 2016.

99. Nutrition International. http://www.micronutrient.org/. Accessed September 24, 2016.

100. FAO. *Food Based Dietary Guidelines.* http://www.fao.org/nutrition/education/food-dietary-guidelines/home/en/. Accessed September 24, 2016.

101. WHO. Healthy Diet. September 2015. http://www.who.int/elena/healthy_diet_fact_sheet_394.pdf?ua=1.

# Appendix A

## CONSORT 2010 Checklist of Information to Include When Reporting a Randomised Trial*

| Section/Topic | Item no. | Checklist item | Reported on page no. |
|---|---|---|---|
| **Title and abstract** | | | |
| | 1a | Identification as a randomized trial in the title | |
| | 1b | Structured summary of trial design, methods, results, and conclusions (for specific guidance see CONSORT for abstracts) | |
| **Introduction** | | | |
| Background and objectives | 2a | Scientific background and explanation of rationale | |
| | 2b | Specific objectives or hypotheses | |
| **Methods** | | | |
| Trial design | 3a | Description of trial design (such as parallel, factorial) including allocation ratio | |
| | 3b | Important changes to methods after trial commencement (such as eligibility criteria), with reasons | |
| Participants | 4a | Eligibility criteria for participants | |
| | 4b | Settings and locations where the data were collected | |
| Interventions | 5 | The interventions for each group with sufficient details to allow replication, including how and when they were actually administered | |
| Outcomes | 6a | Completely defined prespecified primary and secondary outcome measures, including how and when they were assessed | |
| | 6b | Any changes to trial outcomes after the trial commenced, with reasons | |
| Sample Size | 7a | How sample size was determined | |
| | 7b | When applicable, explanation of any interim analyses and stopping guidelines | |
| **Randomization** | | | |
| Sequence generation | 8a | Method used to generate the random allocation sequence | |
| | 8b | Type of randomization; details of any restriction (such as blocking and block size) | |
| Allocation concealment mechanism | 9 | Mechanism used to implement the random allocation sequence (such as sequentially numbered containers), describing any steps taken to conceal the sequence until interventions were assigned | |
| Implementation | 10 | Who generated the random allocation sequence, who enrolled participants, and who assigned participants to interventions | |

| Section/Topic | Item no. | Checklist item | Reported on page no. |
|---|---|---|---|
| **Randomization** | | | |
| Blinding | 11a | If done, who was blinded after assignment to interventions (for example, participants, care providers, those assessing outcomes) and how | |
| | 11b | If relevant, description of the similarity of interventions | |
| Statistical methods | 12a | Statistical methods used to compare groups for primary and secondary outcomes | |
| | 12b | Methods for additional analyses, such as subgroup analyses and adjusted analyses | |
| **Results** | | | |
| Participant flow (a diagram is strongly recommended) | 13a | For each group, the numbers of participants who were randomly assigned, received intended treatment, and were analyzed for the primary outcome | |
| | 13b | For each group, losses and exclusions after randomization, together with reasons | |
| Recruitment | 14a | Dates defining the periods of recruitment and follow-up | |
| | 14b | Why the trial ended or was stopped | |
| Baseline data | 15 | A table showing baseline demographic and clinical characteristics for each group | |
| Numbers analyzed | 16 | For each group, number of participants (denominator) included in each analysis and whether the analysis was by original assigned groups | |
| Outcomes and estimation | 17a | For each primary and secondary outcome, results for each group, and the estimated effect size and its precision (such as 95% confidence interval) | |
| | 17b | For binary outcomes, presentation of both absolute and relative effect sizes is recommended | |
| Ancillary analyses | 18 | Results of any other analyses performed, including subgroup analyses and adjusted analyses, distinguishing prespecified from exploratory | |
| Harms | 19 | All important harms or unintended effects in each group (for specific guidance see CONSORT for harms) | |
| **Discussion** | | | |
| Limitations | 20 | Trial limitations, addressing sources of potential bias, imprecision, and, if relevant, multiplicity of analyses | |
| Generalizability | 21 | Generalizability (external validity, applicability) of the trial findings | |
| Interpretation | 22 | Interpretation consistent with results, balancing benefits and harms, and considering other relevant evidence | |
| **Other Informationg** | | | |
| Registration | 23 | Registration number and name of trial registry | |
| Protocol | 24 | Where the full trial protocol can be accessed, if available | |
| Funding | 25 | Sources of funding and other support (such as supply of drugs), role of funders | |

*We strongly recommend reading this statement in conjunction with the CONSORT 2010 Explanation and Elaboration for important clarifications on all the items. If relevant, we also recommend reading CONSORT extensions for cluster randomized trials, noninferiority and equivalence trials, nonpharmacological treatments, herbal interventions, and pragmatic trials. Additional extensions are forthcoming: for those and for up-to-date references relevant to this checklist, see www.consort-statement.org.

# Appendix B

## STROBE Statement—Checklist of Items that Should be Included in Reports of Observational Studies

| | Item No | Recommendation |
|---|---|---|
| **Title and abstract** | 1 | (a) Indicate the study's design with a commonly used term in the title or the abstract<br>(b) Provide in the abstract an informative and balanced summary of what was done and what was found |
| **Introduction** | | |
| Background/rationale | 2 | Explain the scientific background and rationale for the investigation being reported |
| Objectives | 3 | State specific objectives, including any prespecified hypotheses |
| **Methods** | | |
| Study design | 4 | Present key elements of study design early in the paper |
| Setting | 5 | Describe the setting, locations, and relevant dates, including periods of recruitment, exposure, follow-up, and data collection |
| Participants | 6 | (a) *Cohort study*—Give the eligibility criteria, and the sources and methods of selection of participants. Describe methods of follow-up<br>*Case-control study*—Give the eligibility criteria, and the sources and methods of case ascertainment and control selection. Give the rationale for the choice of cases and controls<br>*Cross-sectional study*—Give the eligibility criteria, and the sources and methods of selection of participants<br>(b) *Cohort study*—For matched studies, give matching criteria and number of exposed and unexposed<br>*Case-control study*—For matched studies, give matching criteria and the number of controls per case |
| Variables | 7 | Clearly define all outcomes, exposures, predictors, potential confounders, and effect modifiers. Give diagnostic criteria, if applicable |

| | Item No | Recommendation |
|---|---|---|
| Data sources/measurement | 8* | For each variable of interest, give sources of data and details of methods of assessment (measurement). Describe comparability of assessment methods if there is more than one group |
| Bias | 9 | Describe any efforts to address potential sources of bias |
| Study size | 10 | Explain how the study size was arrived at |
| Quantitative variables | 11 | Explain how quantitative variables were handled in the analyses. If applicable, describe which groupings were chosen and why |
| Statistical methods | 12 | (a) Describe all statistical methods, including those used to control for confounding<br>(b) Describe any methods used to examine subgroups and interactions<br>(c) Explain how missing data were addressed<br>(d) *Cohort study*—If applicable, explain how loss to follow-up was addressed<br>*Case-control study*—If applicable, explain how matching of cases and controls was addressed<br>*Cross-sectional study*—If applicable, describe analytical methods taking account of sampling strategy<br>(e) Describe any sensitivity analyses |
| **Results** | | |
| Participants | 13* | (a) Report numbers of individuals at each stage of study—eg numbers potentially eligible, examined for eligibility, confirmed eligible, included in the study, completing follow-up, and analysed<br>(b) Give reasons for non-participation at each stage<br>(c) Consider use of a flow diagram |
| Descriptive data | 14* | (a) Give characteristics of study participants (eg demographic, clinical, social) and information on exposures and potential confounders<br>(b) Indicate number of participants with missing data for each variable of interest<br>(c) *Cohort study*—Summarise follow-up time (eg, average and total amount) |
| Outcome data | 15* | *Cohort study*—Report numbers of outcome events or summary measures over time<br>*Case-control study*—Report numbers in each exposure category, or summary measures of exposure<br>*Cross-sectional study*—Report numbers of outcome events or summary measures |
| Main results | 16 | (a) Give unadjusted estimates and, if applicable, confounder-adjusted estimates and their precision (eg, 95% confidence interval). Make clear which confounders were adjusted for and why they were included<br>(b) Report category boundaries when continuous variables were categorized<br>(c) If relevant, consider translating estimates of relative risk into absolute risk for a meaningful time period |

| | Item No | Recommendation |
|---|---|---|
| Other analyses | 17 | Report other analyses done—eg analyses of subgroups and interactions, and sensitivity analyses |
| **Discussion** | | |
| Key results | 18 | Summarise key results with reference to study objectives |
| Limitations | 19 | Discuss limitations of the study, taking into account sources of potential bias or imprecision.<br>Discuss both direction and magnitude of any potential bias |
| Interpretation | 20 | Give a cautious overall interpretation of results considering objectives, limitations, multiplicity of analyses, results from similar studies, and other relevant evidence |
| Generalisability | 21 | Discuss the generalisability (external validity) of the study results |
| **Other information** | | |
| Funding | 22 | Give the source of funding and the role of the funders for the present study and, if applicable, for the original study on which the present article is based |

*Give information separately for cases and controls in case-control studies and, if applicable, for exposed and unexposed groups in cohort and cross-sectional studies.

**Note:** An Explanation and Elaboration article discusses each checklist item and gives methodological background and published examples of transparent reporting. The STROBE checklist is best used in conjunction with this article (freely available on the Web sites of PLoS Medicine at http://www.plosmedicine.org/, Annals of Internal Medicine at http://www.annals.org/, and Epidemiology at http://www.epidem.com/). Information on the STROBE Initiative is available at www.strobe-statement.org.

# Appendix C

## PRISMA 2009 Checklist

| Section/Topic | | Checklist item | Reported on page # |
|---|---|---|---|
| **Title** | | | |
| Title | 1 | Identify the report as a systematic review, meta-analysis, or both. | |
| **Abstract** | | | |
| Structured summary | 2 | Provide a structured summary including, as applicable: background; objectives; data sources; study eligibility criteria, participants, and interventions; study appraisal and synthesis methods; results; limitations; conclusions and implications of key findings; systematic review registration number. | |
| **Introduction** | | | |
| Rationale | 3 | Describe the rationale for the review in the context of what is already known. | |
| Objectives | 4 | Provide an explicit statement of questions being addressed with reference to participants, interventions, comparisons, outcomes, and study design (PICOS). | |
| **Methods** | | | |
| Protocol and registration | 5 | Indicate if a review protocol exists, if and where it can be accessed (e.g., Web address), and, if available, provide registration information including registration number. | |
| Eligibility criteria | 6 | Specify study characteristics (e.g., PICOS, length of follow-up) and report characteristics (e.g., years considered, language, publication status) used as criteria for eligibility, giving rationale. | |
| Information sources | 7 | Describe all information sources (e.g., databases with dates of coverage, contact with study authors to identify additional studies) in the search and date last searched. | |
| Search | 8 | Present full electronic search strategy for at least one database, including any limits used, such that it could be repeated. | |
| Study selection | 9 | State the process for selecting studies (i.e., screening, eligibility, included in systematic review, and, if applicable, included in the meta-analysis). | |
| Data collection process | 10 | Describe method of data extraction from reports (e.g., piloted forms, independently, in duplicate) and any processes for obtaining and confirming data from investigators. | |
| Data items | 11 | List and define all variables for which data were sought (e.g., PICOS, funding sources) and any assumptions and simplifications made. | |
| Risk of bias in individual studies | 12 | Describe methods used for assessing risk of bias of individual studies (including specification of whether this was done at the study or outcome level), and how this information is to be used in any data synthesis. | |
| Summary measures | 13 | State the principal summary measures (e.g., risk ratio, difference in means). | |

| Section/Topic | | Checklist item | Reported on page # |
|---|---|---|---|
| Synthesis of results | 14 | Describe the methods of handling data and combining results of studies, if done, including measures of consistency (e.g., I2) for each meta-analysis. | |
| Risk of bias across studies | 15 | Specify any assessment of risk of bias that may affect the cumulative evidence (e.g., publication bias, selective reporting within studies). | |
| Additional analyses | 16 | Describe methods of additional analyses (e.g., sensitivity or subgroup analyses, meta-regression), if done, indicating which were specified. | |
| **Results** | | | |
| Study selection | 17 | Give numbers of studies screened, assessed for eligibility, and included in the review, with reasons for exclusions at each stage, ideally with a flow diagram. | |
| Study characteristics | 18 | For each study, present characteristics for which data were extracted (e.g., study size, PICOS, follow-up period) and provide the citations. | |
| Risk of bias within studies | 19 | Present data on risk of bias of each study and, if available, any outcome level assessment (see item 12). | |
| Results of individual studies | 20 | For all outcomes considered (benefits or harms), present, for each study: (a) simple summary data for each intervention group (b) effect estimates and confidence intervals, ideally with a forest plot. | |
| Synthesis of results | 21 | Present results of each meta-analysis done, including confidence intervals and measures of consistency. | |
| Risk of bias across studies | 22 | Present results of any assessment of risk of bias across studies (see Item 15). | |
| Additional analysis | 23 | Give results of additional analyses, if done (e.g., sensitivity or subgroup analyses, meta-regression [see Item 16]). | |
| **Discussion** | | | |
| Summary of evidence | 24 | Summarize the main findings including the strength of evidence for each main outcome; consider their relevance to key groups (e.g., healthcare providers, users, and policy makers). | |
| Limitations | 25 | Discuss limitations at study and outcome level (e.g., risk of bias), and at review-level (e.g., incomplete retrieval of identified research, reporting bias). | |
| Conclusions | 26 | Provide a general interpretation of the results in the context of other evidence, and implications for future research. | |
| **Funding** | | | |
| Funding | 27 | Describe sources of funding for the systematic review and other support (e.g., supply of data); role of funders for the systematic review. | |

# Glossary

## 0-9

**24-hour recall** Structured interview that asks participants to recall all foods and beverages consumed in the preceding 24 hours.

## A

**Acceptable macronutrient distribution range (AMDR)** Range of intakes for a particular energy source that are associated with reduced risk of chronic disease while providing adequate intakes of essential nutrients.

**Adequate intake (AI)** The nutrient intake that appears to sustain a defined nutritional state or some other indicator of health (e.g., growth rate or normal circulating nutrient values) in a specific population or subgroup. AI is used when there is insufficient scientific evidence to establish an EAR.

**Adiposity** Part of the body composition known as body fat mass or tissue, including two predominant compartments, visceral and subcutaneous fat; also known as *adipose tissue*.

**Advocacy research** Attempts to influence the formal and informal policies established by policy makers and other stakeholders.

**Alternate hypothesis** A hypothesis that states the nature of the relationship should one be present and that there will be a difference between the two variables in the population being studied.

**Android** Apple-shaped body type in which weight is primarily in the upper part of the body, such as the abdomen; more common in males and associated with increased health risk.

**Anorexia nervosa (AN)** Restriction of energy intake relative to requirements; leads to a significantly low body weight in the context of age, sex, developmental trajectory, and physical health. Condition includes an intense fear of gaining weight or of becoming fat and persistent behavior that interferes with weight gain even at significantly low weights. Disturbance in the way someone perceives her or his body weight or shape with a persistent lack of recognition of the seriousness of the current low body weight.

**Anthropometry** Measurements taken of various parts of the human body; used for population comparisons for determining body composition and nutritional status.

**Applied research** Inquiry using the application of scientific methodology with the purpose of generating empirical observations to solve critical problems in society.

**Atherosclerosis** Type of "hardening of the arteries" in which cholesterol and other substances in the blood build up in arterial walls. As the process continues, the arteries to the heart can narrow, cutting down the flow of oxygen-rich blood and nutrients to the heart.

## B

**Basal Energy Expenditure (BEE)** The basal metabolic rate (BMR) extrapolated to 24 hours. Often used interchangeably with REE.

**Basic research** Research that follows the scientific method and focuses on exploring unknown information. Also known as *fundamental* or *pure* science.

**Behavioral Risk Factor Surveillance System (BRFSS)** National health survey administered by telephone and conducted by individual state health departments to look at behavioral risk factors such as smoking, alcohol use, physical inactivity, and diet.

**Behavior theories** Psychological theories that attempt to explain how people behave by identifying and modeling constructs or variables that temporally and statistically predict behavior.

**Belmont Report of 1979** Report published in 1979 by the National Commission for Protection of Human Subjects of Biomedical and Behavioral Research that set forth the basic ethical principles and guidelines for the conduct of research of human sublets.

**Beneficence** The ethical principle that focuses on maximizing good results while minimizing harms.

**Bias** Any tendency that prevents unprejudiced consideration of a research question.

**Bilateral organizations** Governmental agencies from a single country that provide aid to developing countries; one of the largest is the United States Agency for International Development (USAID).

**Binge-eating disorder (BED)** Recurring episodes of eating significantly more food in a short period of time than most people would eat under similar circumstances, with episodes marked by feelings of lack of control. Someone with binge eating disorder may eat too quickly, even when he or she is not hungry. The person may have feelings of guilt, embarrassment, or disgust and may binge eat alone to hide the behavior. This disorder is associated with marked distress and occurs, on average, at least once a week over three months.

**Bioelectric impedance analysis (BIA)** Single-frequency or multifrequency system for measuring body composition using measurements of resistance and reactance or the impedance of electrical conductivity of the body to determine total body water, body fat percentage, and fat-free mass.

**Biomarker or Biological marker** Biological measures, such as urine, feces, and blood, used to perform a clinical/nutritional assessment.

**Biomarkers of Nutrition for Development (BOND)** Partnership program of the US National Institute of Child Health and Human Development (NICHD) and other organizations representing global food and nutrition enterprises; harmonizes processes for making decisions about what biomarkers are best for use in support of research, program development, evaluation, and the generation of evidence-based policies.

**Body cell mass (BCM)** Way to assess body composition that evaluates the cellular functions of the components of the body (muscle, viscera, blood, and brain).

**Body composition (BC)** Distribution of protein, fat, water, and minerals that make up the human body.

**Body mass index (BMI)** Measure of body fat that is the ratio of the weight of the body in kilograms to the square of its height in meters.

**Bulimia nervosa (BN)** Is a serious, potentially life-threatening eating disorder characterized by a cycle of bingeing and compensatory behaviors such as self-induced vomiting designed to undo or compensate for the effects of binge eating.

**Bureau of Labor Statistics** Federal agency that keeps track of all data related to US employment.

# C

**Cachexia** A complex metabolic syndrome associated with underlying illness and characterized by loss of muscle with or without loss of fat mass. The prominent clinical feature of cachexia is weight loss in adults (corrected for fluid retention) or growth failure in children (excluding endocrine disorders).

**Cardiovascular disease (CVD)** Any abnormal condition characterized by dysfunction of the heart and blood vessels. CVDs include atherosclerosis (especially coronary heart disease, which can lead to heart attacks), cerebrovascular disease (e.g., stroke), and hypertension (high blood pressure).

**Carryover effects** When the effect of a previous treatment carries over to influence the response to the next treatment.

**Case-control studies** Studies that compare two groups of people—those with the disease or condition under study (cases) and similar group of people who do not have the disease or condition (controls).

**Client-centered** An approach to counseling that initiates and monitors changes based on the client's needs rather than counselor-identified needs.

**Client history** This section of nutritional assessment data gathering includes personal history; medical, health, and family histories; treatments and complementary alternative medicine use; and social history.

**Clinical trials registries** Listing of 24 clinical trials registries from around the world; maintained by the Human Research Protections International Program of the US Department of Health and Human Services.

**Coaching** An approach to counseling that is a partnership to promote wellness.

**CODEX Alimentarius** Part of the UN Food and Agriculture Organization; harmonizes international food standards to protect consumer health and promote fair practices in food trade.

**Cognitive Behavior Therapy (CBT)** Psychotherapeutic approach to helping clients improve their perceptions of self, situations, and environment as a way to change their behavior.

**Cognitive interviewing** Formative work completed to be sure the questions and answers in a questionnaire or interview script are understood by the target interviewee population.

**Cohort studies** Studies in which exposures of interest are assessed at baseline in a group (cohort) of people; health outcomes occurring over time are then related to baseline exposures.

**Common Rule** Detailed federal rules and procedures that set US policy for the protection of human subjects.

**Complete counterbalancing** When all possible orders of presentation are included in an experiment.

**Computer-based diet-assessment application** Software loaded onto a single or only a few computer hard drives or onto a network system. Users are limited to the location and availability of the computer with the software.

**Computerized tomography (CT)** Scanning method involving an x-ray tube and a receiver to produce an image that is used as a diagnostic test to detect the presence of tumors, vascular diseases, pulmonary emboli, or aortic aneurysms.

**Conditionally indispensable amino acids** Amino acids that can be made by the body under many circumstances; under some other circumstances, they cannot be made in a sufficiently reliable way to meet the body's needs.

**Conflict of interest** A set of circumstances that creates a risk that professional judgment or actions regarding a primary interest will be unduly influenced by a secondary interest.

**Construct validity** The underlying constructs that can be inferred from observed behaviors.

**Consumer expenditure survey data** Information on US food supply and Americans' purchasing habits.

**Content validity** Indicates whether the instrument items reflect various part of the content domain.

**Control condition** The effect that exists in the absence of an experimental treatment.

**Controls** Technique used to prevent additional variables from influencing the outcome of an experiment.

**Council for International Organizations of Medical Sciences (CIOMS)** Organization that facilitates international biomedical research and coordination between multiple international associations and national institutions.

**Counterbalancing** When a series of sequences is administered in such a way that it balances out order effects.

**Creatinine clearance** Test that measures the rate at which a waste produced called *creatinine* is "cleared" from the blood by the kidneys.

**Creatinine height index (CHI)** Measurement of a 24-hour urinary excretion collection of creatinine that is generally related to the individual's muscle mass and an indicator of malnutrition, particularly in young males.

**Criterion validity** The extent to which an instrument correlates with an external reference.

**Cross-sectional studies** Studies that include measurements on a group of individuals at a single interval in time so that the exposure of interest and the outcome of interest are measured at the same time.

**Crossover design** A clinical trial in which groups of human subjects receive two or more interventions in a particular order.

**Cultural competence** Understanding the importance of social and cultural influences on the beliefs and behaviors of individuals.

**Cutoff point** Anthropometric indicator below which either individuals or populations will require an intervention or therapy.

# D

**Decade of Action on Nutrition** UN-declared period of international nutrition assessment and research that can affect global nutrition by providing the scientific evidence base for identifying nutrition problems and helping to offer targeted solutions.

**Declaration of Helsinki of 1964** Declaration developed by the World Medical Association (WMA) with the purpose of elaborating on the ethical principles for medical research with human subjects that were previously presented in the Nuremberg Code.

**Densitometry** Method for evaluating body volume and density to estimate percentage of body fat and fat-free mass

such as underwater weighing and air-displacement plethysmography.

**Dependent variable** The variable or *outcome variable* that is measured in research that is assumed to be influenced by the independent variable. The variable that captures the outcome of an intervention.

**Descriptive study** Study in which information is collected without changing the environment (no manipulation occurs).

**Diabetes mellitus (DM)** Chronic disease in which uptake of blood glucose by body cells is impaired, resulting in high glucose levels in the blood and urine. Type 1 is caused by decreased pancreatic release of insulin. In type 2, target cells (e.g., fat and muscle cells) lose the ability to respond normally to insulin.

*Dietary Guidelines for Americans* A set of national guidelines released by the federal government every five years that provides evidence-based recommendations for diet and physical activity to all healthy Americans two years of age and older.

**Dietary history** Questionnaire that uses open-ended and closed-ended questions and is conducted by a trained interviewer to collect dietary information through a 24-hour recall, a three-day food diary, and a checklist of commonly eaten foods.

**Dietary recall (24-hour)** Open-ended questionnaire administered by a trained interviewer to collect information on food-preparation methods and food consumption throughout a subject's typical day.

**Dietary Reference Intake (DRI)** A framework of dietary standards that includes Estimated Average Requirement (EAR), Recommended Dietary Allowance (RDA), Adequate Intake (AI), and Tolerable Upper Intake Level (UL).

**Dispensable amino acids (AA)** Amino acids that our bodies are able to make under virtually all circumstances.

**Double-blind study** An experiment designed to test the effect of a treatment or substance by using groups of experimental and control subjects; neither the subjects nor the investigators know which treatment is being administered to which group.

**Dual-energy x-ray absorptiometry (DXA)** Three-compartment method using low dose x-rays to assess body composition, both regional and whole body, in adults and children.

**Dynamometer** Tool used to assess grip strength by measuring static force in kilograms or pounds; can be measured by isokinetic, electrical, digital, or electronic means.

# E

**e-Library of Evidence for Nutrition Actions (eLENA)** Library that provides evidence-informed guidance for nutrition interventions; available in six languages.

**eButton** Button with a built-in camera and sensors worn on the chest to capture images of eating occasions and other health-related behaviors.

**Energy density** The amount of energy a food or beverage provides per weight of the food or beverage (kcals/gm).

**Energy expenditure** Energy needed to complete physical functions such as breathing, digesting food, and physical movement.

**Epidemiology** The branch of medicine that deals with the incidence, distribution, and possible control of diseases and other factors relating to health.

**Erythropoiesis** Production of red blood cells.

**Essential fat** Adipose tissue that surrounds and protects organs, bones, and the nervous system; needed to maintain health.

**Estimated Average Requirement (EAR)** The intake value that meets the estimated nutrient needs of 50 percent of individuals in a specific life-stage and gender group.

**Estimated Energy Requirement (EER)** Dietary energy intake that is predicted to maintain energy balance in a healthy adult of a defined age, gender, weight, height, and level of physical activity consistent with good health.

**Estimated glomerular filtration rate (eGFR)** Stands for *estimated glomerular filtration rate*; a number based on blood test for creatinine, a blood waste product, as a measure of kidney function.

**Evidence-based nutrition practice** According to the Academy of Nutrition and Dietetics, it is the "use of systematically reviewed scientific evidence in making food and nutrition practice decisions by integrating the best available evidence with professional expertise and client values to improve outcomes."

**Exempt research** Risk-free research. Review by an IRB is not required in such cases.

**Experimental research design** A design in which all factors are held constant except those that are manipulated by the researcher to help determine the results and cause and effect of a process or procedure on the experimental group.

**Experiment** A test under controlled conditions that is run to demonstrate a known truth, to examine the validity of a hypothesis, or to determine the efficacy of something that has not been tried before.

# F

**Face validity** The extent to which an instrument is assumed to measure a characteristic based on the participants' judgment.

**Factorial design** A design that investigates the independent and interactive effect that two or more independent variables have on the dependent variable.

**Factors** A categorical variable with two or more values that are commonly referred to as *levels*.

**Familiarization** Becoming well acquainted with something. In research, subjects repeated exposure to certain tests or procedures can lead to familiarization.

**Fat-free mass (FFM)** Part of body composition representing lean body tissue.

**First 1000 Days** Period of time from the beginning of pregnancy through a child's second birthday that has been identified as a critical window of opportunity to break the intergenerational cycle of malnutrition.

**Five A's** Style of counseling based on *assess* (ask) about the problem or issue, *advise* on possible solutions, *agree* with client on client-centered goals, *assist* the client in determining solutions to barriers, and *arrange* for follow-up.

**Flesch-Kincaid grade reading level** Reading grade evaluation of written material based on the number of words in a sentence, the number of syllables in the words, and the total sentences.

**Fogarty International Center** Office of the US National Institutes of Health that supports and facilitates global health research conducted by US and international investigators; maintains an online listing of e-resources for global health researchers.

**Food- and nutrition-related history** This section of nutritional assessment data gathering includes food and nutrient intake, food and nutrient administration, medication/herbal supplement use, knowledge/beliefs, food and supplies availability, physical activity, nutrition quality of life.

**Food-consumption record** Method of data collection in which a trained surveyor observes a subject's in-home food preparation and consumption habits.

**Food-frequency questionnaire (FFQ)** Questionnaire in the form of a checklist that asks respondents how often and how much food they consumed over a specific time period.

**Food and Agriculture Organization (FAO)** UN agency that works with governments to achieve food security and ensure people have regular access to enough high-quality food to lead active, healthy lives.

**Food and nutrition action plan** Structured set of steps showing how to develop and implement a food and nutrition policy.

**Food and Nutrition Council** National group or mechanism that oversees the development, implementation, and evaluation of national action plans through an intersectoral approach.

**Food and nutrition policy** Umbrella term for a course or principle of action that incorporates public-health concerns into food-related concerns in order to lead to more concerted, intersectoral actions (defined as actions affecting health outcomes undertaken by groups outside the health and nutrition sectors).

**Food control** Mandatory regulatory activity and enforcement by local or national authorities with the goals of providing consumer protection to ensure that all foods (from production, handling, storage, processing, and distribution) are safe, wholesome, and fit for human consumption; conform to quality and safety requirements; and are honestly and accurately labeled as prescribed by law.

**Food fortification** Addition of certain essential vitamins and minerals to staple foods to improve their nutritional composition and reduce dietary deficiencies within a population.

**Food policy** Course or principle of action related to food that is proposed or adopted by a government or organization, and the policy does not necessarily or explicitly include public-health concerns.

**Food record** Record of all foods and beverages consumed over a designated period of time.

**Food safety** Assurance that food will not cause harm to the consumer when it is prepared or eaten according to its intended use.

**Food security** Exists when all people always have physical and economic access to sufficient, safe, and nutritious food to meet their dietary needs and food preferences for an active and healthy life.

**Food sustainability** Ways and means by which food is produced and distributed that respect Earth's natural processes and enhance a community's environmental, economic, and social well-being.

**Four-components model** Model used for evaluating body composition; includes body fat mass, fat-free mass, bone, and total body water.

**Frontal-occipital circumference** Same as head circumference; measured until age three to assess brain development.

# G

**Global Data Bank on Infant and Young Child Feeding** Online resource developed by the UN World Health Organization that pools information from national and regional surveys and studies on the prevalence and duration of breastfeeding and complementary feeding.

**Global database on body mass index** The World Health Organization's interactive surveillance tool for monitoring the global epidemic of overweight and obesity; provides both national and subnational adult underweight, overweight, and obesity prevalence rates by country, year of survey, and gender.

**Global Database on the Implementation of Nutrition Action (GINA)** Database that provides information on the implementation of numerous nutrition policies and interventions and includes opportunities for users to directly submit their data.

*Global Nutrition Report* Annual peer-reviewed, independent publication that identifies and tracks global health and nutrition issues; is defined as the only independent and comprehensive annual review of the state of the world's nutrition.

**Greater than minimal risk** Type of research that may involve physical or psychological stress. In this type of case, a thorough review needs to be conducted by an IRB.

**Gynoid** Pear-shaped body type characterized by smaller fat cells in the hips and thighs; more common in females; presents a low health risk.

# H

**Handgrip strength (HGS)** Quick quantitative index for assessing upper-body strength and a good predictor of health changes, morbidity, and mortality for adults and children.

**Health Belief Model (HBM)** Behavioral theory comprising perceptions of susceptibility to a disease or condition, severity of the disease or condition, barriers to achieving a behavior, benefits to the behavior, and self-efficacy for accomplishing the behavior. May also include cues to action.

**Health disparity** Health outcome that is seen to a greater or lesser extent between different populations.

**Health literacy** The degree to which individuals have the capacity to obtain, process, and understand basic health information and services needed to make appropriate health decisions.

**Healthy Eating Index (HEI)** Measure of diet quality assessing adherence to the *Dietary Guidelines for Americans* used to monitor diet quality in the United States and examine the relationship between dietary quality and health-related outcomes, the quality of food-assistance packages, menus, and the US food supply.

**Healthy eating patterns** Styles of eating and drinking that are routine and follow key principles of the *Dietary Guidelines for Americans*.

**Healthy People 2020 (HP 2020)** A set of goals and objectives with 10-year targets designed to guide national health promotion and disease prevention efforts to improve the health of all people in the United States.

**Height velocity** Measurement for detecting growth abnormalities early in the course of all types of chronic illness.

**Hemochromatosis** When iron collects in the parenchymal cells of several organs, predominantly the liver, followed by the heart and pancreas. Disorder can cause organ dysfunction and result in death.

**Hemolysis** Rupture or destruction of red blood cells.

**Human Immunodeficiency virus (HIV)** Is a virus that affects the immune system, gradually damaging it until it can no longer fight off infection and disease. The HIV infects the cells of the immune system. However, for reasons that scientists don't fully understand, HIV remains resistant to the immune system's efforts to eliminate it.

**Hypercholesterolemia** The presence of greater than normal amounts of cholesterol in the blood.

**Hypervitaminosis** A condition of abnormally high storage levels of vitamins that can lead to toxic symptoms.

**Hypoparathyroidism** State of decreased secretion or activity of parathyroid hormone (PTH). This leads to decreased blood levels of calcium (hypocalcemia) and increased levels of blood phosphorus (hyperphosphatemia).

**Hypothesis** Statement of prediction that can be evaluated, measured, or analyzed.

**Hyptertension** Long-term high blood pressure; when resting blood pressure consistently exceeds 140 mm Hg systolic or 90 mm Hg diastolic.

# I

**Image-assisted dietary assessment (IADA)** Capturing images of eating occasions to objectively observe and record dietary intake. It may support traditional methods of obtaining intake data or serve as a primary food record.

**Independent variable** The variable that is assumed to affect the dependent variable or outcome. In experimental research, it is the intervention or treatment that is varied by the research to affect the dependent variable.

**Indirect calorimetry** Metabolic carts are used to measure the amount of heat produced by a subject by determination of the amount of oxygen consumed and the amount of carbon dioxide eliminated. The overall resting energy expenditure or resting metabolic rate (RMR) is determined through an equation. Indirect calorimetry is considered the gold standard for predicting calorie needs at rest, however, due to cost of equipment, staff time and patients that are not able to participate in the test, it is not routinely used in healthcare settings.

**Indispensable amino acids** Amino acid that cannot be synthesized by the organism and thus must be supplied in its diet.

**Inflammatory response** A response of the body to an injurious agent, characterized by signs such as: tumor or swelling; pain; heat; loss of function; or erythema (redness of the skin or mucous membranes).

**Informed consent** A document that shows respect for a subject's' self-determination and ability to make an informed, rational, and voluntary decision to participate in a research study.

**Institutional review board (IRB)** Institutional group that has been formally assigned to review and monitor biomedical research with human subjects.

**Internal motivation** Motivation that derives from a person's own thoughts or feelings.

**International Compilation of Human Research Standards** Listing of more than 1000 laws, regulations, and guidelines on human subjects protections in more than 100 countries; maintained by the Human Research Protections International Program of the US Department of Health and Human Services.

**International Network of Food Data Systems (INFOODS)** Worldwide network of food composition experts run by the the UN's Food and Agriculture Organization that also serves as a forum for international harmonization and support for food-composition activities.

**Internet-based diet-assessment application** Assessing dietary intake from anywhere and anytime when an Internet connection is available.

**Interprofessional** The coordinated care of patients by a collaborative team of healthcare providers

# J

**Justice** When all subjects are provided equitable and fair treatment by researchers; each person can then access the benefits of science.

# K

**Kwashiorkor** Is a nutritional disorder most often seen in regions experiencing famine. It is a form of malnutrition caused by a lack of protein in the diet. People suffering from kwashiorkor typically have an extremely emaciated appearance in all body parts except their ankles, feet, and belly, which swell with fluid.

**Kyphoscoliosis** Deformity of the spine characterized by abnormal curvature of the vertebral column in the coronal and sagittal planes. Term is a combination of *kyphosis* and *scoliosis*.

# L

**Latin square** Counterbalancing technique used to control for order effects without having all possible orders. Its $n \times n$ array is filled with $n$ different symbols, each occurring exactly once in each row and exactly once in each column. This ensures that all possible orders are received by different subjects

**Learner-centered approach** Similar to a client-centered approach but in an educational setting. The learning determines what the client would prefer to learn as opposed to the teacher.

**Lipodystrophy** A disorder of adipose tissue characterized by a selective loss of body fat. Patients with lipodystrophy have a tendency to develop insulin resistance, diabetes, a high triglyceride level (hypertriglyceridemia), and fatty liver.

**Literature review** Reading, analyzing, and synthesizing existing published research to summarize what is and is not known in a specific topic area.

**Longitudinal study** An observational research method in which data are repeatedly gathered for the same subjects over a period of time.

# M

**Magnetic resonance imaging (MRI)** Closed system using strong magnetic field to obtain a view of the chemical composition of body tissue and visual images of organs, structures, and tissues.

**Malnutrition** An acute, subacute, or chronic state of nutrition in which a combination of varying degrees of overnutrition or undernutrition with or without inflammatory activity have led to a change in body composition and diminished function.

**Malnutrition in the Elderly (MaNuEL)** Knowledge hub launched by the Joint Programming Initiative of the European Union; brings together 22 research groups from seven countries to build better research capacity on malnutrition in the elderly.

**Malnutrition Universal Screening Tool (MUST)** Is a five-step screening tool to identify adults, who are malnourished, at risk of malnutrition (undernutrition), or obese. It also includes management guidelines which can be used to develop a care plan.

**Medical nutrition therapy (MNT)** Nutritional diagnostic, therapeutic, and counseling for the purpose of disease management; furnished by a registered dietitian or nutrition professional.

**Meta-analysis** The process of using statistical integration of the results of several studies to reach an independent conclusion.

**Minimal-risk research** Research in which the risk of harm is no greater than the risk encountered in daily life or routine examinations.

**Mini Nutrition Assessment (MNA)** Is a validated nutrition screening and assessment tool that can identify older adult patients age 65 and above who are malnourished or at risk of malnutrition.

**Monitoring** Collection and analysis of quantitatively accurate measures from representative samples of a population in order to observe diet and health trends with precision.

**Morbidity rate** Frequency with which diseases appear in a population.

**Mortality rate** Number of deaths in a population per unit of time.

**Motivational interviewing (MI)** Client-centered approach in which the counselor or coach guides the conversation with the client to explore ambivalence.

**Multilateral organizations** Organizations funded by multiple governments that provide support to many different countries; examples include the UN's World Health Organization (WHO), Food and Agriculture Organization (FAO), and World Food Programme (WFP).

**Multilevel randomized design** Experimental design that has more than two levels of the independent variable, with *level* referring to the number of variations of the independent variable.

# N

**National Commission for the Protection of Human Subjects of Biomedical and Behavioral Research** Commission of experts generally recognized as the first national bioethics commission; developed the Belmont Report.

**National Health and Nutrition Examination Survey (NHANES)** Series of cross-sectional, nationally representative surveys conducted in mobile examination units to assess the health and nutrition status of adults and children. The surveys combine interviews and physical examinations and monitor changes over time by gathering information on dietary intake, biochemical tests, physical measurements, and clinical assessments.

**National Health Examination Survey (NHES)**

**National Institutes of Health Revitalization Act of 1993** Legislation that directs the National Institutes of Health to establish guidelines for the inclusion of women and minorities in clinical research.

**National Nutrition Monitoring System (NNMS)** Comprehensive, coordinated program for nutrition monitoring and related research in the United States.

**National Research Act of 1974** Legislation signed into law that created the National Commission for Protection of Human Subjects of Biomedical and Behavioral Research.

**Nitrogen balance** Measure of nitrogen input minus nitrogen output.

**Nongovernmental organizations (NGOs)** Not-for-profit or voluntary citizen's groups organized on various levels—local, national, and international—to address issues in support of the greater public good; examples include CARE, the Food Fortification Initiative, and the Bill & Melinda Gates Foundation.

**Nonprotein calories** Simply the calories in the diet coming from carbohydrates and fats only.

**Nonquantitative food frequency questionnaire** Simple FFQ that asks participants how many times a year, month, week, or day they eat a particular food or nutrient in question.

**Null hypothesis** Experimental hypothesis used when formally testing a hypothesis for statistical significance; holds that there will be no difference between the two variables in the population being studied.

**Nuremberg Code** Code developed in 1947 after trials of convicted Nazi war criminals; helped form the basis for today's ethical, legal, and regulatory framework of research using human subjects.

**Nutrient density** A description of the healthfulness of foods. Foods high in nutrient density are those that provide substantial amounts of vitamins and minerals and relatively few calories; foods low in nutrient density are those that supply calories but relatively small amounts of vitamins and minerals (or none at all).

**Nutrition-focused physical exam (NFPE)** A systematic way of evaluating an individual from head to toe, paying attention to his or her physical appearance and function to discover signs and symptoms related to malnutrition, nutrient deficiency, and toxicity.

**Nutrition-focused physical examination (NFPE)** Is a systematic head-to-toe examination of a patient's physical appearance and function to help determine nutritional status by uncovering any signs of malnutrition, nutrient deficiencies, or nutrient toxicities.

**Nutritional assessment** Is a structured way to establish nutritional status and energy-requirements by objective measurements and whereby, completed with objective parameters and in relation to specific disease-indications, an adequate (nutritional-) treatment can be developed for the patient.

**Nutritional biomarker** Any organic test that can be used as an indicator of nutritional status as it relates to intake or metabolism of dietary components.

**Nutritional epidemiology** An area of epidemiology that involves research to examine the role of nutrition in the etiology of disease, monitor the nutritional status of populations, and develop and evaluate interventions to achieve and maintain healthful eating patterns among populations.

**Nutritional status** The state of an individual's overall health and body as influenced by levels of nutrients and diet.

**Nutrition assessment** A method of identifying and evaluating data needed to make decisions about a nutrition–related problem or diagnosis.

**Nutrition Care Process (NCP)** Systematic approach to providing high-quality nutrition care. This standardized model is intended to guide registered dietitian nutritionists in delivering nutrition therapy.

**Nutrition Care Process and Model (NCPM)** A pictorial conception that shows the steps of the Nutrition Care Process as well as internal and external factors that influence the NCP's application.

**Nutrition Care Process Terminology (NCPT)** A controlled vocabulary used to depict the distinctive activities of nutrition and dietetics in completing nutrition assessments, nutrition diagnoses, nutrition interventions, and nutrition monitoring and evaluation.

**Nutrition diagnosis** Used to identify and define a particular nutrition problem that can be solved or symptoms that

can be managed through nutrition interventions by a nutrition and food professional.

**Nutrition intervention** The action taken by the nutrition and dietetics professional to correct or manage a nutrition problem.

**Nutrition Landscape Information System (NLiS)** Web-based system that dynamically brings together all existing WHO global nutrition databases and other existing food and nutrition-related data from partner agencies.

**Nutrition literacy** Reflection or evaluation of the client's understanding of nutrition information.

**Nutrition screening** The first-line process of identifying patients who are already malnourished or at risk of becoming so; nutritional assessment is a detailed investigation to identify and quantify specific nutritional problems.

# O

**Obesity** A body mass index at or above 30 kg/m².

**Observational studies** Type of study in which individuals are observed and variables of interest are measured. No attempt is made to affect the outcome.

**Office for Human Research Protections** Office in the US Department of Health and Human Services that oversees the system and protects the rights, welfare, and well-being of research subjects and ensures that federal research meets the standards set forth in the Common Rule.

**Opportunistic infection** Is an infection caused by pathogens (bacteria, viruses, fungi, or protozoa) that take advantage of an opportunity not normally available, such as a host with a weakened immune system, an altered microbiota (such as a disrupted gut flora), or breached integumentary barriers.

**Outcome expectancies** What a person expects will occur following a particular action or behavior.

# P

**Partnership organizations and collaborations** Groups formed in partnership with healthcare professional organizations, governmental groups, and the private sector; examples include the European Nutrition for Health Alliance and the International Obesity Consortium.

**Patient-generated subjective global assessment (PG-SGA)** A nutrition assessment tool adapted from the Subjective Global Assessment which includes seven components for assessment: weight, food intake, nutrition impact symptoms, activities and function, medical condition, metabolic stress, and physical examination. The questions regarding short-term weight loss and nutrition impact symptoms increase the Scored PG-SGA's sensitivity to changes in nutrition status over a short period of time. A scored PG-SGA has also been developed.

**Pediatric Nutrition Surveillance System (PedNSS)** National public-health surveillance system in coordination with the Centers for Disease Control and Prevention that monitored the growth, anemia, and breastfeeding status of low-income US children who participated in federally funded maternal and child health nutritional programs. Discontinued in 2012.

**Percentile** Position of an individual on a given reference distribution comprising 100 points.

**PES statement** Statement that address three elements: a problem (P), its etiology (E), and its signs and symptoms (S).

**Phototransduction** Process by which light is converted into electrical signals in the rod, cone, and photosensitive ganglion cells of the retina of the eye. The rod cells and the cone cells are retinal specialized photoreceptors.

**Physical activity** Any body movement that works muscles and requires more energy than resting; generally refers to movement that enhances health.

**Placebo effect** Way of describing, quantifying, and understanding everything that surrounds a placebo treatment.

**Placebo** Sugar or cellulose pill that has little or no physiological effect in and of itself.

**Predictive equations for estimating energy needs** Equations that have been developed and validated which estimate resting metabolic rate and used in place of conducting indirect calorimetry.

**Pregnancy Nutrition Surveillance System** National public-health surveillance system in coordination with the Centers for Disease Control and Prevention that monitored risk factors associated with infant mortality and poor birth outcomes among low-income pregnant women in federally funded maternal and child health programs. Discontinued in 2012.

**Private-sector organizations** Businesses and industries that may support the nutrition research of nongovernmental organizations (NGOs) and others through corporate foundations; they may also directly fund primary nutrition research to develop new commercial products.

**Prospective study** Study that assesses exposures of interest for a group of individuals at baseline, follows them over time, and compares them for a particular outcome.

**Protein-energy undernutrition (PEU)** Form of malnutrition that occurs when there are limitations in diet quality (energy sources and protein) that may lead to wasting or stunting.

# Q

**Qualitative data** Data that are derived from interviews, discussions, or focus groups.

**Qualitative research** Primarily exploratory research used to gain an understanding of underlying reasons, opinions, and motivations. Provides insights into the problem or helps develop ideas or hypotheses for potential quantitative research.

**Qualitative research** Type of research that focuses on behavior in natural settings or studies small groups in a particular setting. Data gathered in qualitative research are nonnumerical and presented in language and or pictures.

**Quantitative** Data that are derived from surveys, biochemical, dietary, or anthropometrics that are recorded or scored numerically.

**Quantitative food frequency questionnaire** See FFQ.

**Quantitative research** Type of research that focuses on gathering numerical data and generalizing it across groups of people to explain a particular phenomenon.

# R

**Randomized assignment** Random placement of subjects into control and experimental groups.

**Reactivity bias** Occurs when a subject changes behavior as result of participation in a study. An example is changing dietary behavior as a result of being asked to keep a food record.

**Recall bias** Occurs when a subject remembers past events differently than how they truly occurred.

**Recommended Dietary Allowance (RDA)** The nutrient intake levels that meet the nutrient needs of almost all (97 percent to 98 percent) individuals in a life-stage and gender group.

**Registered dietitian nutritionist (RDN)** Registered dietitian (RD) who wants to emphasize the nutrition aspect of his or her credential to the public and other health practitioners. Both RDs and RDNs are accredited by the Commission on Dietetics Registration of the Academy of Nutrition and Dietetics.

**Relative risk (RR)** The extent of an association between an exposure and the likelihood of developing the outcome of interest in the exposed group relative to the unexposed group.

**Relative validity** Compares a new measurement method with one or more established methods believed to have greater degree of demonstrated face validity.

**Reliability** the ability of a method to produce the same results on several occasions.

**Research** Systematic process of collecting, analyzing, and interpreting information or data to answer questions to extend knowledge.

**Research proposal** Proposal to conduct research that is submitted to a funding agency.

**Research question** Question that needs to be answered through systematic testing, evaluation, and analysis.

**Respect for persons** Treatment of persons that includes two moral requirements—the requirement to acknowledge autonomy and the requirement to protect those with diminished autonomy.

**Resting Energy Expenditure (REE)** The minimum energy needed to maintain basic physiological functions (e.g., heartbeat, muscle function, respiration). The resting metabolic rate (RMR) extrapolated to 24 hours. Often used interchangeably with BEE.

**Resting metabolic rate (RMR)** Is the major component of total energy expenditure which is the amount of energy the body requires for vital functioning.

*Rome Declaration on Nutrition* Declaration resulting from the Second International Conference on Nutrition (ICN2) held in 2012. The declaration commits countries to eradicate hunger and prevent all forms of malnutrition worldwide, particularly undernutrition in children and anemia in women and children (among other micronutrient deficiencies), as well as reverse the trend in obesity.

# S

**Sarcopenia** Is a condition characterized by loss of skeletal muscle mass and function. Sarcopenia is a syndrome characterized by progressive and generalized loss of skeletal muscle mass and strength and it is directly correlated with declines in physical function, physical disability, and decreased quality of life, and death.

**Sarcopenic obesity** A condition in which excess energy intake, physical inactivity, low-grade inflammation, insulin resistance and changes in hormonal milieu leads to obesity and changes in muscle composition and quality.

**Saturation** Point in qualitative work where no additional themes or concepts emerge from interviews.

**Scaling Up Nutrition (SUN)** Global push for action and investment to improve maternal and child nutrition.

**Screeners** Shorter version of a food-frequency questionnaire that focuses on specific components of a diet such as fruit and vegetable intake or calcium intake.

**Scurvy** A deficiency disease caused by inadequate amounts of vitamin C in the diet. Symptoms of scurvy include bleeding gums, corkscrew hair, and petechial hemorrhage.

**Self-efficacy** Belief that one is capable of achieving a goal or mastering a skill.

**Semiquantitative food frequency questionnaire** FFQ in which participants are given an example of a portion size.

**SenseCam** Small camera-based recording device worn around the neck that captures a subject's eating episodes and other health behaviors.

**Skinfold thickness** Early technique of measuring subcutaneous fat by specially designed calipers; used with formulas that include a person's age and gender to estimate the percent of body fat.

**SMART goals** Goals that are Specific, Measurable, Achievable, Reasonable, and Timely.

**Social-approval bias** Occurs when subjects respond in a manner consistent with social norms or expectations, although it does not represent true behavior. For example, a subject reports consuming four to five cups of fruits and vegetables per day because he or she believes that is what the interviewer wants to hear.

**Social Cognitive Theory (SCT)** Behavioral theory that focuses on four areas: (1) competencies and skills, (2) expectancies and beliefs, (3) evaluative standards, and (4) personal goals.

**Social ecological model** Model that describes five levels of influence on health behavior (1) individual, (2) interpersonal, (3) institutional and organizational, (4) community, and (5) structural and system.

**Stages of change** Behavioral theory that evaluates a person's readiness to change, including the stages of precontemplation, contemplation, preparation, action, maintenance, and termination.

**Strengthening Partnerships, Results, and Innovations in Nutrition Globally (SPRING)** Project of the United States Agency for International Development (USAID) that is dedicated to strengthening global and country efforts to scale up high-impact nutrition practices and policies.

**Stunted growth** Condition reflecting the failure to reach linear growth potential as a result of suboptimal health or nutritional conditions or both.

**Subcutaneous adipose tissue (SAT)** Approximately 10% of total body fat; found between muscles and subcutaneous tissue.

**Subjective global assessment (SGA)** A validated nutritional assessment tool that measures nutritional status based on the features of a patient history (weight change, dietary intake change, gastrointestinal symptoms that have persisted for greater than two weeks, and functional capacity) and physical examination (loss of subcutaneous fat, muscle wasting, ankle or sacral edema and ascites).

**Subjective global assessment (SGA)** Is a validate nutritional assessment tool that measures nutritional status based on the features of a history (weight change, dietary intake change, gastrointestinal symptoms that have persisted for greater than 2 weeks, and functional capacity) and physical examination (loss of subcutaneous fat, muscle wasting, ankle/sacral edema and ascites).

**Surveillance** System of data collection of superficial and rapid measures used to determine if a population-based intervention is indicated.

**System thinking** Approach that acknowledges a system is an organized whole composed of interdependent parts; takes into account the "bigger picture" rather than isolating smaller parts of a system.

# T

**T-score** Index for assessing risk or documented osteoporosis; calculated based on bone density of a healthy 30-year-old person to determine bone mineral density and strength.

**Telehealth** Health promotion and disease management using telecommunications.

**Theory of Reasoned Action** Behavioral theory that determines to predict behavior through assessment of attitudes and beliefs, subjective norms, perceived behavioral control, and intention to perform the behavior.

**Thermic effect of activity (TEA)** The amount of energy required to meet the energy demands of any physical activity.

**Thermic effect of food (TEF)** The energy used to digest, absorb, and metabolize energy-yielding foodstuffs. It constitutes some 10 percent of total energy expenditure but is influenced by various factors.

**Three-components model** Model used to evaluate body composition; includes body fat mass, fat-free mass, and bone.

**Tolerable upper intake level (UL)** The maximum levels of daily nutrient intakes that are unlikely to pose health risks to almost all of the individuals in the group for whom they are designed.

**Total body potassium (TBK)** Component or method used to assess nutritional status and body composition.

**Total body water** Sum of extracellular and intracellular water that correlates with fat-free mass as compared to intracellular water; nutritional index that correlates with body cell mass.

**Translational science** Field of investigation that focuses on understanding the scientific and operational principles underlying each step of the translational process.

**Two-components model** Model for evaluating only body fat mass and the body's fat-free mass.

# U

**Ultrasound** Scanning method for isolating and distinguishing body fat and lean tissue based on reflected ultrasound waves and differences in the acoustic impendence between tissues.

**UN Decade of Action on Nutrition (2016–2025)** Era declared by the United Nations in 2016 to trigger intensified action that will end hunger and eradicate malnutrition worldwide while ensuring universal access to healthier and more sustainable diets.

**United Nations Standing Committee on Nutrition (UNSCN)** The United Nations' food and nutrition policy harmonization forum.

**United Nation's Children's Fund (UNICEF)** UN organization that works to bring attention to and mobilize resources to address challenges facing children.

**UN Millennium Development Goals** Goals adopted by the United Nations in 2000 that are interdependent and influence health; UN member states agreed to try to achieve these goals by 2015.

**UN Sustainable Development Goals** Goals adopted by the United Nations in 2015 that focus on ending poverty, protecting the planet, and ensuring prosperity for all as part of a new sustainable development agenda; each of the 17 goals has specific targets to be achieved by 2030.

**US Agency for International Development (USAID)** Federal agency that seeks to empower and support other countries through collaborative partnerships that foster sustainable development.

# V

**Validity** The ability of an instrument to measure what it is intended to measure.

**Visceral adipose tissue (VAT)** Hormonally active component of total body fat that possesses unique biochemical characteristics that influence several normal and pathological processes in the human body. An abnormally high deposition of visceral adipose tissue is known as *visceral obesity*.

**Vitamin and Mineral Nutrition Information System (VMNIS)** The World Health Organization's system for assessing the micronutrient status of populations, monitoring and evaluating the effect of strategies for preventing and controlling micronutrient malnutrition, and tracking related trends over time.

**Vulnerable population** A group of people who are relatively (or absolutely) incapable of protecting their own interests and may be exposed to social, economic, legal, psychological, or physical harm.

# W

**Weight to length** Ratio measure used in calculating body mass index.

**WHO fracture-risk assessment tool (FRAX)** Computerized screening tool that incorporates *T*-score along with risk factors (smoking, family history, and lifestyle) to estimate a person's risk for such bone diseases as osteoporosis.

**WHO Global Nutrition Targets for 2025** Specific global nutrition goals established by the World Health Organization through its World Health Assembly (WHA); targets include improving maternal, infant, and young child nutrition. UN member states have committed to monitoring progress on these targets through 2025.

**World Food Programme (WFP)** UN program with a mission to combat global hunger and respond to hunger emergencies; the world's largest humanitarian agency fighting hunger.

**World Health Assembly (WHA)** The World Health Organization's decision-making body and policy-setting organization.

**World Health Organization (WHO)** Organization that produces health guidelines and standards, helps countries address public-health issues, and supports and promotes health research worldwide.

# Y

**Youth Risk Behavior Surveillance System (YRBSS)** Surveillance system used to examine health risk behaviors that significantly contribute to the leading causes of death, disability, and social problems among the nation's youth and young adults.

# Z

**Z-scores** Standardized measures that are comparable across ages, sexes, and measures.

# Index